ASTRA

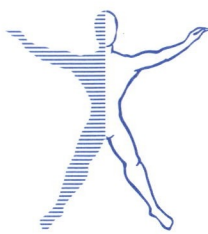

ADVANCING ANAESTHESIA

Provided as a service to medicine
by Astra Pharmaceuticals Ltd

To: ST. JOHNS HOSPITAL
ANAESTHETIC DEPT.

Date: 29/10/98

Representative: DAWN PARYNO

Laser Applications in Oral and Maxillofacial Surgery

Laser Applications in Oral and Maxillofacial Surgery

Guy A. Catone, DMD

Associate Professor, Allegheny University of the Health Sciences,
MCP • Hahnemann School of Medicine, Allegheny Campus
Assistant Professor, Department of Oral and Maxillofacial Surgery
University of Pittsburgh Medical Center
Private Practice
Pittsburgh, Pennsylvania

Charles C. Alling III, DDS, MS

Adjunct Professor
University of Iowa School of Dentistry
Private Practice
Oral and Maxillofacial Surgery
Birmingham, Alabama

W.B. SAUNDERS COMPANY
A Division of Harcourt Brace & Company
Philadelphia • London • Toronto • Montreal • Sydney • Tokyo

W.B. SAUNDERS COMPANY
A Division of Harcourt Brace & Company

The Curtis Center
Independence Square West
Philadelphia, Pennsylvania 19106

Library of Congress Cataloging-in-Publication Data

Laser applications in oral and maxillofacial surgery / [edited by] Guy A. Catone, Charles C. Alling, III.—1st ed.

p.   cm.

ISBN 0–7216–5020–1

1. Mouth—Laser surgery.   2. Jaws—Laser surgery.   3. Face—Laser surgery.   I. Catone, Guy A.   II. Alling, Charles C.
[DNLM: 1. Surgery, Oral—methods.   2. Laser Surgery.
WU 600 L343 1996]

RK530.5.L37 1997   617.5′ 2059—dc20

DNLM/DLC   95–45035

LASER APPLICATIONS IN ORAL AND MAXILLOFACIAL SURGERY   ISBN 0–7216–5020–1

Printed in the United States of America.

Last digit is the print number: 9   8   7   6   5   4   3   2   1

To Winston, Anna, and Donna for their many years
of patience, understanding, and support of my academic pursuits.
G.A.C.

The purpose of his learning: patients.
The target of his teaching: patients.
The priority of his practice: patients.
The beneficiaries of his professionalism: patients.
My contributions for this book are dedicated to him:
Dr. Guy A. Catone
C.C.A.

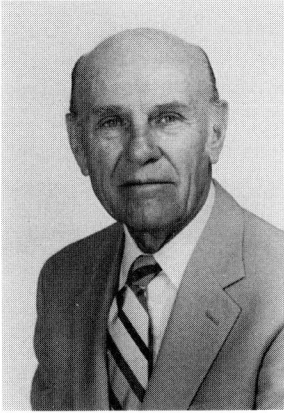

Dedication

This book on the rapidly evolving application of the technology of the laser to surgical problems in oral and maxillofacial surgery is dedicated to the memory of Dr. Fred A. Henny, an internationally renowned oral and maxillofacial surgeon who was a mentor to a generation of promising young surgeons in an equally expanding field of surgical endeavor. His life and work served as a paradigm for the modern oral and maxillofacial surgeon; his self-imposed role was to serve as a guide for an entire surgical specialty because his wisdom advocated the changes that were to have profound influences on the role of the oral and maxillofacial surgeon in the spectrum of head and neck maladies.

Dr. Henny graduated from the University of Michigan School of Dentistry in 1935, and following surgical training, he became Chief of the Oral and Maxillofacial Surgery Department at Henry Ford Hospital until 1970. He then became Associate Chairman of the Department of Oral and Maxillofacial Surgery at Sinai Hospital of Detroit, a post he held until 1977.

He served as President of the Michigan Dental Association and Editor of the *Michigan Dental Association Journal.* He was President of the American Association of Oral and Maxillofacial Surgeons, an association that he was instrumental in reorganizing, and served as Editor of the *Journal of Oral and Maxillofacial Surgery* for 13 years.

Dr. Henny was the founding President of the International Association of Oral and Maxillofacial Surgeons and received citations of honor from the surgical societies of Canada, Australia-New Zealand, Cuba, Guatamala, Greece, and Great Britain. Dr. Henny received the initial Distinguished Service Award from the American Association of Oral and Maxillofacial Surgeons in 1970, and was one of the first Americans in any discipline to be inducted as a Fellow of the Royal College of Surgeons of England. His surgical colleagues in the global community were legion and represented the most distinguished and accomplished in their native countries. His prescience was to encourage the cross-fertilization of knowledge, clinical skills, and technology across the illusory barriers of the surgical specialties and to develop lasting bonds with medicine and its specialties.

Dr. Henny remained a loyal alumnus of the University of Michigan throughout his career, and received the Sesquicentennial Alumnus Award from that institution in 1977. Years earlier, he was president of the Chalmers J. Lyons Academy, an organization of specialists in oral and maxillofacial surgery formed in honor of Dr. Lyons, a distinguished surgeon long associated with the University of Michigan. He was pivotal in the establishment of the Chalmers J. Lyons Memorial Lecture in Oral and Maxillofacial Surgery in 1952, which is presented annually during the yearly meeting of the Association. Dr. Henny received the William J. Gies Foundation Award in 1977, a coveted honor in his specialty.

The 1984 annual scientific sessions of the American Association of Oral and Maxillofacial Surgeons were dedicated to Dr. Henny for his pioneering achievements in the specialty. During that same meeting, the Education and Research Foundation initiated the Fred A. Henny Fellowship that provides an individual with the opportunity to conduct clinical and basic research studies in oral and maxillofacial surgery on a postgraduate level at an accredited institution in the United States or abroad. He received the Education and Research Foundation's first Torch Award in 1984, an award that recognizes individuals who have provided exemplary services or made significant contributions in fostering the mission of the Foundation.

Dr. Henny's life was one of long days and consistent achievement, but a significantly important part was dedicated to the intimate art of resident education. He achieved this by his obvious surgical skills, his humane approach to the protection of his patients, and by a subtle, if not gentle, inculcation of these attributes to his housestaff. For those of us who were his wards, we still feel his guiding hand in the surgical theater.

Guy A. Catone
Charles C. Alling

Contributors

Charles C. Alling III, DDS, MS
Adjunct Professor, University of Iowa School of Dentistry; Private Practice, Oral and Maxillofacial Surgery, Birmingham, Alabama
Complications and Side Effects of Laser Surgery

Timothy J. Atkinson, DDS
Clinical Assistant Professor, West Virginia University, Morgantown, West Virginia; Adjunct Associate Clinical Professor, Hahnemann University, Philadelphia, Pennsylvania; Associate in Oral and Maxillofacial Surgery, Geisinger Medical Center, Danville, Pennsylvania
Fundamentals of the Carbon Dioxide Laser

Guy A. Catone, DMD
Associate Professor, Allegheny University of the Health Sciences, MCP • Hahnemann School of Medicine, Allegheny Campus; Assistant Professor, Department of Oral and Maxillofacial Surgery, University of Pittsburgh Medical Center; Private Practice, Pittsburgh, Pennsylvania
Qualitative Laser Physics in Maxillofacial Surgery; Photobiology of Lasers in Oral and Maxillofacial Surgery; Laser Management of Intraoral Surface Lesions; Lasers in Periodontal Surgery; Laser Surgery of the Temporomandibular Joint; Cutaneous Facial Laser Resurfacing

Terry A. Fuller, MS, PhD
Adjunct Assistant Professor, Department of Urology, Jefferson Medical College, Philadelphia, Pennsylvania; Adjunct Associate Professor, Biomedical Engineering, Northwestern University, Chicago, Illinois; President and CEO, Fuller Corporation, Vernon Hill, Pennsylvania; Executive Vice President

and CEO, Surgical Laser Technologies, Montgomeryville, Pennsylvania
Wavelength Conversion Effect–Contact and Free-Beam Laser Surgery

Edward Halusic Jr, DMD
Associate Professor, Division of Oral and Maxillofacial Surgery, Department of Surgery, Medical College of Pennsylvania and Hahnemann Medical School, Allegheny University, West Campus, Pittsburgh, Pennsylvania; Chairman, Subdivision of Oral and Maxillofacial Surgery and Dentistry, Department of Surgery, Frick Hospital and Community Health Center, Mount Pleasant, Pennsylvania
Photobiology of Lasers in Oral and Maxillofacial Surgery; Cutaneous Facial Laser Resurfacing

Michael G. Koslin, DMD
Private Practice, Oral and Maxillofacial Surgery; Active Staff, Brookwood Medical Center, Health South Medical Center, Birmingham, Alabama
Laser Surgery of the Temporomandibular Joint

Jeffrey Moses, DDS
Adjunct Assistant Professor, Department of Oral and Maxillofacial Surgery, University of California, Los Angeles, California; President and Director, Pacific Clinical Research Foundation; Private Practice, Encinitas, California
Lasers for Use in Cosmetic Maxillofacial Surgery

Frank L. Nelson, DDS, JD
Oral Surgeon; Forensic Examiner; Attorney at Law, Birmingham, Alabama
Medical-Legal Considerations in Laser Surgery

M. Anthony Pogrel, MB, ChB, BDS, FRCS

Professor and Chairman, and Department of Oral and Maxillofacial Surgery, University of California, San Francisco, California
Laser Management of Malignant Lesions of the Head and Neck

James H. Quinn, DDS

Professor, Oral and Maxillofacial Surgery, Louisiana State University, New Orleans, Louisiana; Private Practice, Oral and Maxillofacial Surgery, Metairie, Louisiana
Laser Surgery of the Temporomandibular Joint

John Sexton, DMD, MSD

Instructor, Oral and Maxillofacial Surgery, Harvard University School of Dental Medicine, Boston, Massachusetts; Chief, Oral and Maxillofacial Surgery, Director, Maxillofacial Trauma Service, Beth Israel Hospital, Boston, Massachusetts
Laser Management of Vascular and Pigmented Lesions

Robert A. Strauss, DDS

Associate Professor, Director, Residency Training Program, Department of Oral and Maxillofacial Surgery, Medical College of Virginia, Richmond, Virginia
Laser Management of Discrete Lesions; Laser-Assisted Uvulopalatoplasty

Edward Teeple, MD

Associate Professor, Anesthesiology, Allegheny Hospital, Pittsburgh, Pennsylvania
Laser Safety in Anesthesia and Oral and Maxillofacial Surgery

Preface

A scientific discovery heralded by the prescience of no less a mind than that of Einstein, lasers within the first half of the twentieth century have been associated with other laboratory curiosities as a technology searching for an application. Despite the inertia of being a dramatic, often fanciful technology with initial limited pragmatic uses, the physical concept of the generation of radiant energy by stimulated emission and the explosion in the manufacturing of a multitude of laser devices—each possessing unique characteristics related to photobiology and power—have more than vindicated lasers as mere scientific oddities to be featured at laseriums and laser shows.

Lasers are not unique to this kind of development and eventual scientific acceptance. Indeed, the gift of general anesthesia given to humanity by the dental profession was associated early on with popular experimentation (ether and nitrous oxide "frolics"). Popular expositions using laser devices for purely decorative purposes may have enhanced their mystery and general acceptance so much so that patients often inquire if the most mundane operative procedure can be performed with a laser.

With the host of clinical applications of laser energy growing each day and the number of available laser products growing with advances in overall technology, such as the parallel development of novel software and new methodologies of creating laser energy, the surgeon is hard pressed to keep informed much less acquire new skills in all laser devices. Observations concerning the early history of lasers, their rapid recent development, their association with other enabling modern technology, and their unique properties when compared with traditional surgical armamentarium (sharp scalpel, diathermy, cryosurgery) compelled the editors to offer a text that would speak specifically to the unique problems faced by the oral and maxillofacial surgeon. To that end, the editors assembled a group of competent contributors willing to address their colleagues on the use of various laser devices in solving surgical problems in a wide spectrum of conditions from orofacial lesions to facial cosmetic applications involving endoscopy and facial skin resurfacing.

Recognizing the constant flux of this field and the format chosen, individual chapters were composed to be read as chapters and also to be useful as sources of reference data. This structure has resulted in a modicum of redundancy. Therefore, qualitative laser physics, use of power settings and wavelength, for example, may be encountered in several sites in the overall text. Fortunately, some repetition may be helpful when learning what may be a new field for some and also for tracking down specific data to be used in a given clinical setting.

As a result of the outline and substance of the text, the surgeon should gain both fundamental information on basic laser physics (how lasers work); the effects of laser energy of various types, wavelengths, and power on skin, mucosa, and contiguous tissues; laser safety; legal ramifications; and common lasers used in the specialty. There are a number of chapters devoted to specific uses and anatomic sites. Thus, despite the rapid sophistication of laser radiant energy use and evolving devices in all surgical specialties, the reader is offered a foundation on which to place yet another useful device into those most precious surgical instruments—one's hands.

Contents

Color Plates

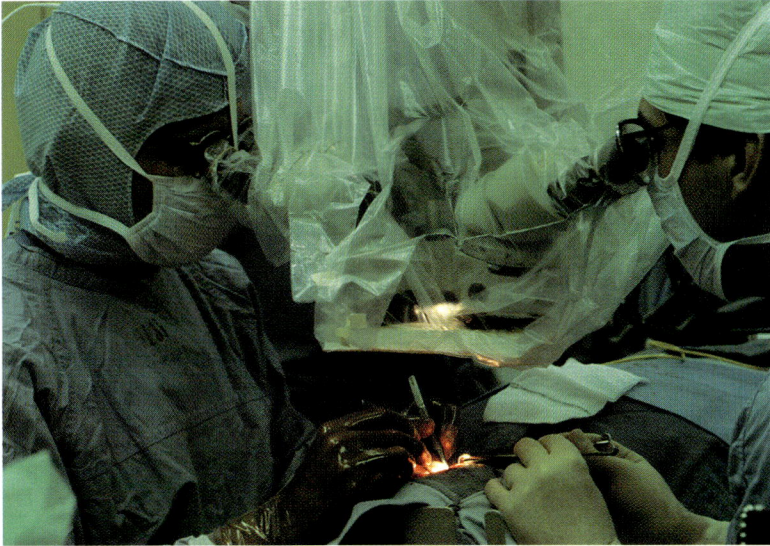

COLOR PLATE 1. The use of the microscope with a built-in laser and coaxial soft target laser beam. In this instance, the surgeon and the assistant can see the operative field without distortion of the image for the assistant, thus enabling the assistant to be much more effective. Once again, as in the single-operator microscopes with coupled carbon dioxide lasers, the beam is controlled with the index finger of the operator while the arc of the beam and its direction and sweep are controlled with the thumb and index finger. (Courtesy of Dr. Edward Halusic, Mount Pleasant, Pennsylvania.)

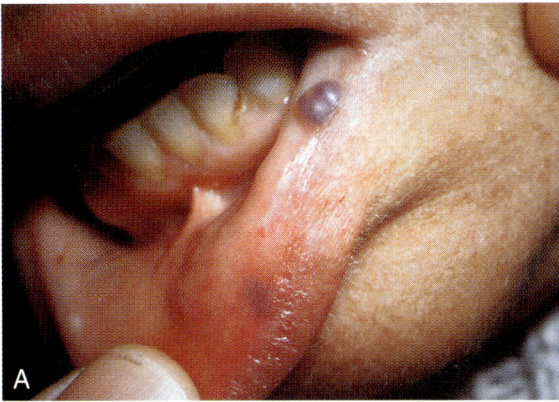

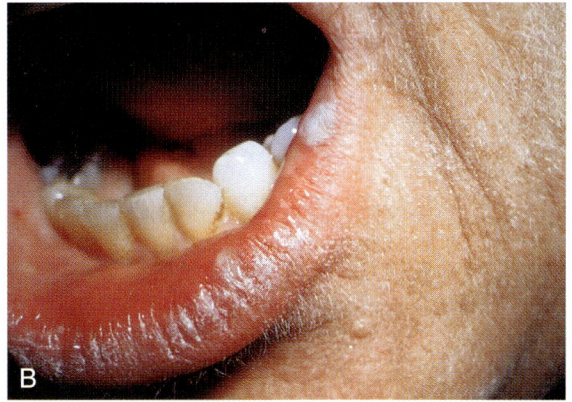

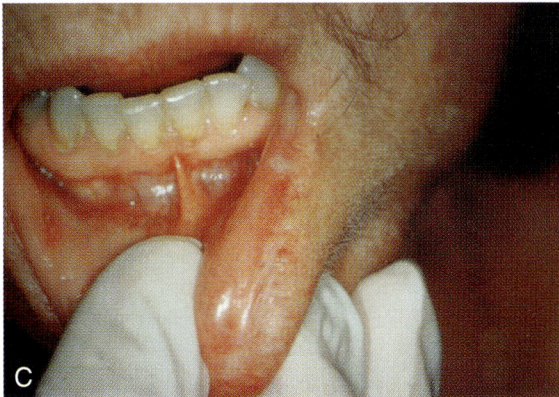

COLOR PLATE 2. *A*, Sixty-one-year old woman with two venous lakes involving the left lower lip. *B*, Immediately after treatment. *C*, Three weeks after treatment.

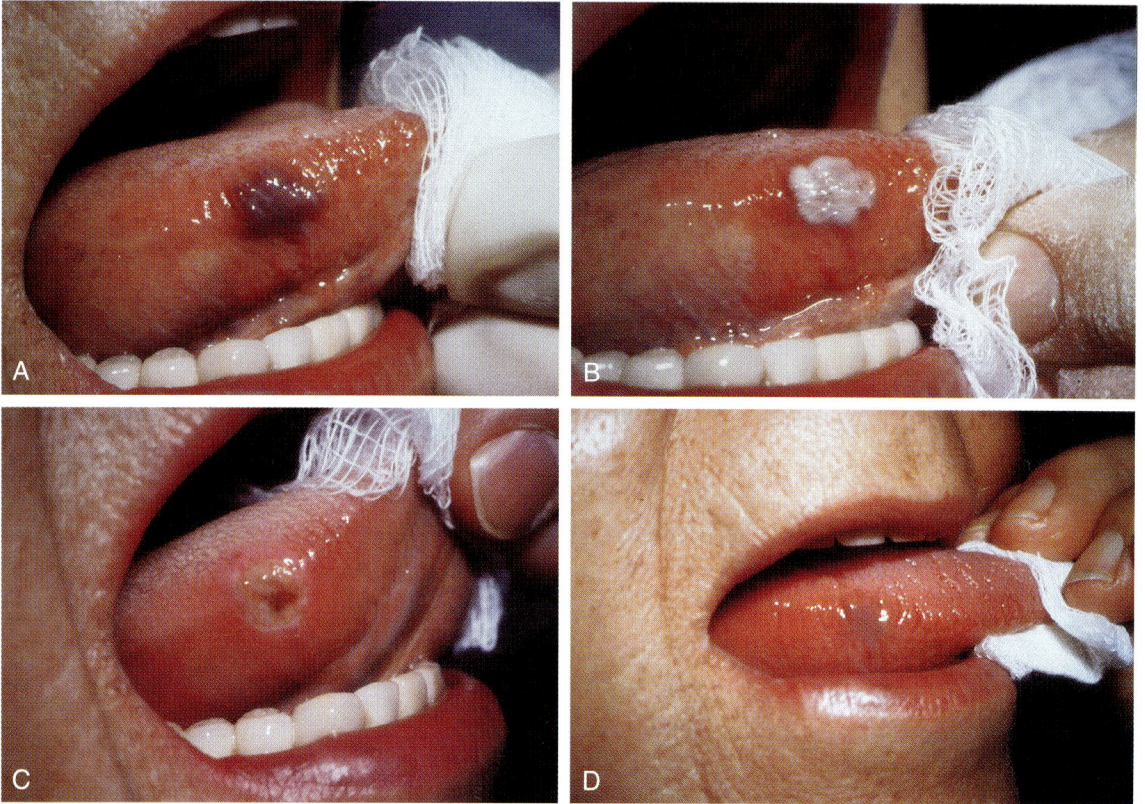

COLOR PLATE 3. *A*, Seventy-two-year-old female with a hemangioma involving the right posterolateral border of the tongue. *B*, Immediately after treatment. *C*, One week after treatment. D, After treatment.

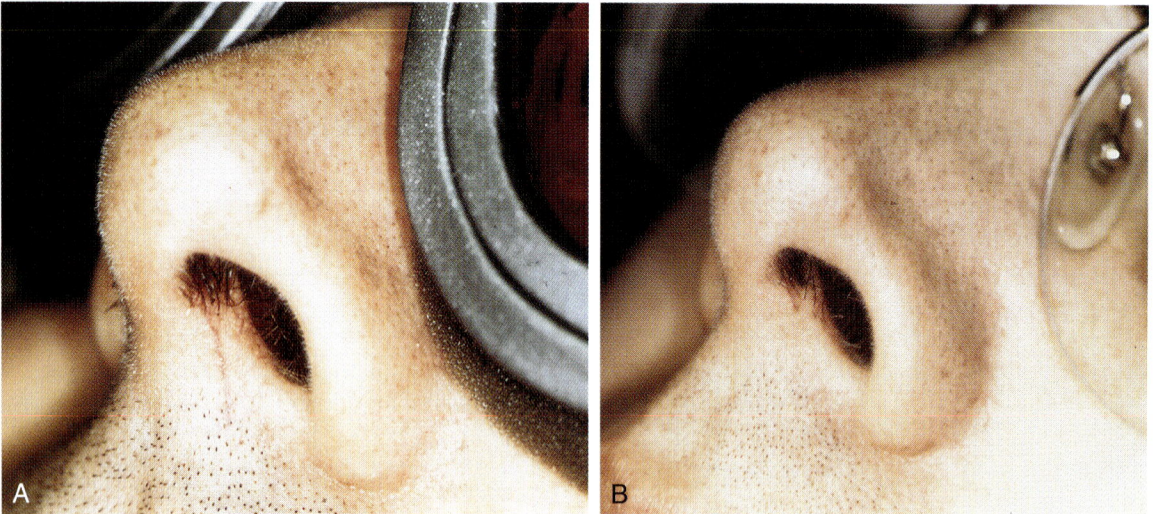

COLOR PLATE 4. Pulsed-dye laser. Telangiectasia. *A*, Preoperative appearance. *B*, Postoperative appearance.

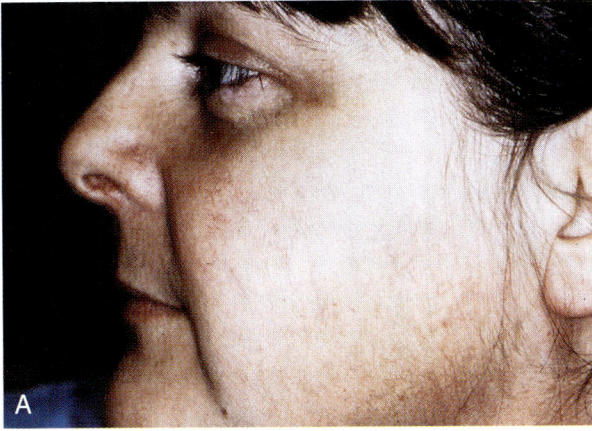

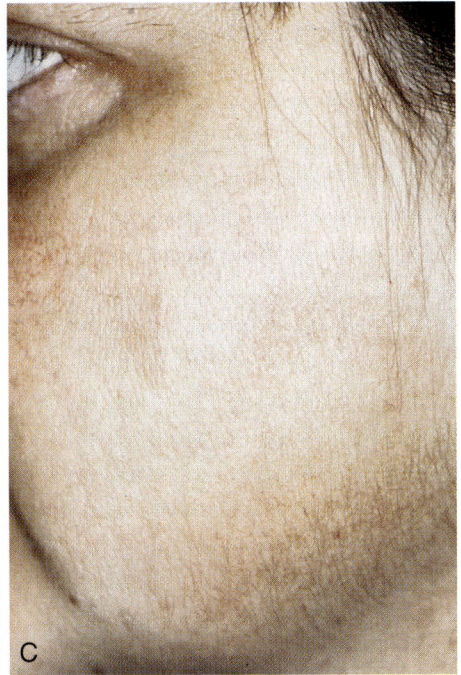

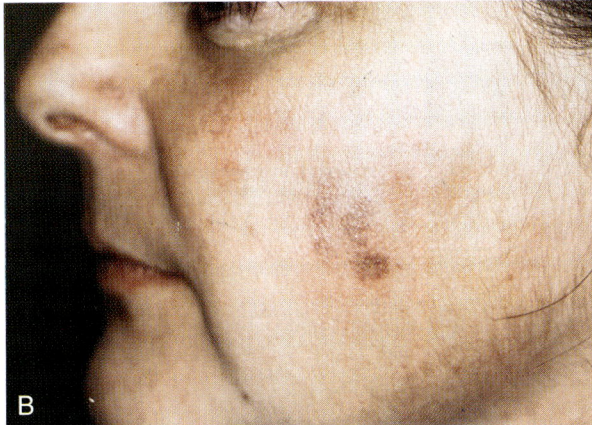

COLOR PLATE 5. Pulsed-dye laser. Small vessel ectasias of the face. *A*, Preoperative appearance. *B*, Postoperative appearance (1 to 2 weeks). *C*, Postoperative clearing.

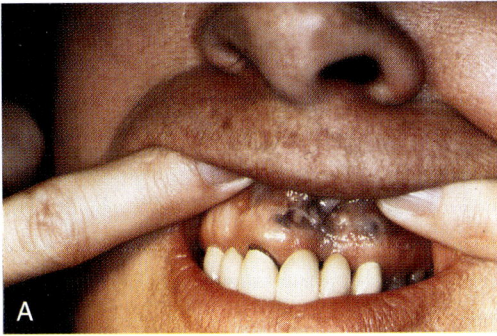

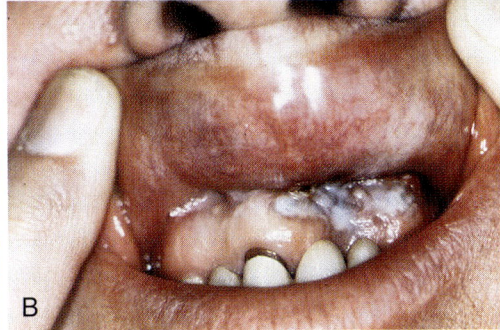

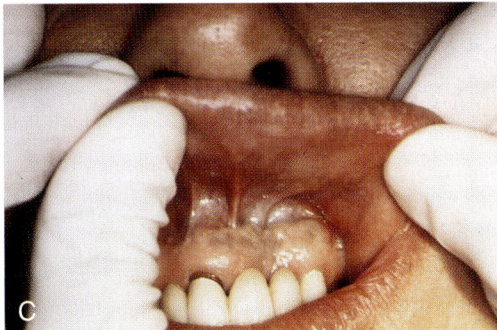

COLOR PLATE 6. Q-switched YAG. Amalgam tattoo. *A*, Preoperative appearance. *B*, Immediately after surgery. *C*, Postoperative appearance.

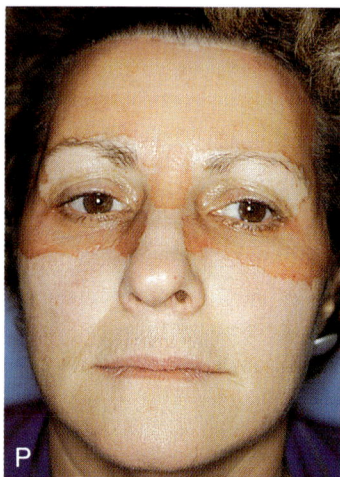

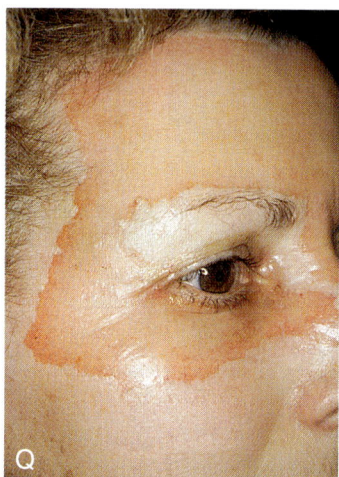

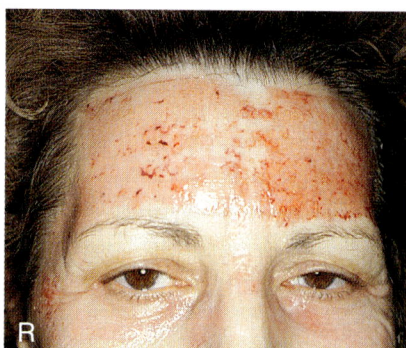

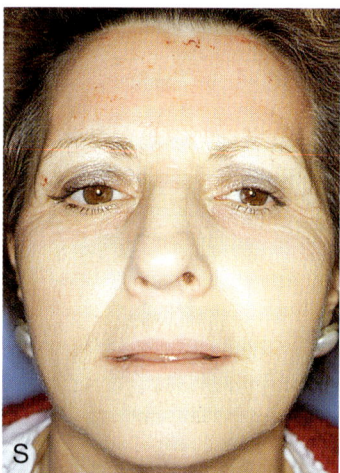

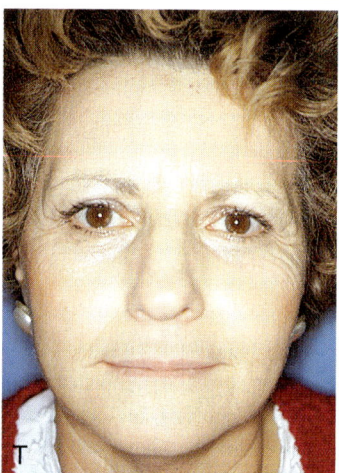

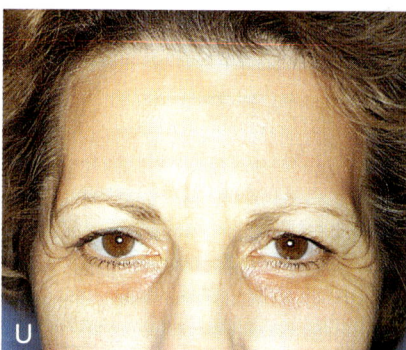

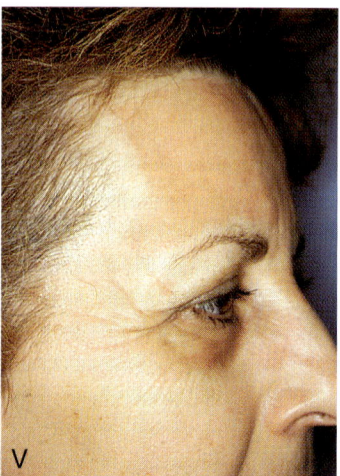

COLOR PLATE 7. *P* and *Q*, One day after laser resurfacing *R*, One week after laser resurfacing. *S*, Ten days after laser resurfacing. *T*, Ten days after laser resurfacing with make up. *U* and *V*, Twenty-four days after laser resurfacing.

Laser Applications in Oral and Maxillofacial Surgery: Introduction

GUY A. CATONE, DMD
CHARLES C. ALLING III, DDS, MS

The term *laser* is an acronym for *l*ight *a*mplification by the *s*timulated *e*mission of *r*adiation, which serves to explain most but not all the critical physical interactions that occur within a laser generating cavity. Surgeons do not necessarily have to be fully tutored on the complex physics required to create the various forms of laser radiant energy. However, it is pragmatic to have a general knowledge of stimulated emission so that one can evaluate newer laser technologies and understand how lasers affect biologic tissues. This book is dedicated to the oral and maxillofacial applications of the laser and provides the reader with a modicum of fundamental information about lasers, their basic physics, and photobiologic effects; free-beam versus contact types; safety precautions; and terminology. The core chapters describe the use of lasers to solve oral and maxillofacial problems. These chapters on laser applications demonstrate the evolution of laser radiation within the specialty of oral and maxillofacial surgery and provide practical information on the use of laser radiant energy in such areas as control of oral leukoplakia, discrete oral mucosal lesions, angiodysplasias, and oral malignancy, as well as semi-elective or elective procedures, including pre-prosthetic and periodontal surgery, temporomandibular arthroscopy, including open joint procedures, uvulopalatostomy (LAUP), and cosmetic surgery using the emerging technology of endoscopy and laser facial resurfacing.

Lasers have evolved as optional surgical instruments for over 30 years from a concept expounded by Albert Einstein as early as 1917. From these early beginnings as laboratory curiosities, lasers have been embraced by all surgical specialties. The initial skepticism, while appropriate and still a part of any novel applications of the laser, was directed to the question of whether the use of lasers possessed significant advantages over the use of conventional surgical instrumentation. This skepticism received a dramatic rebuttal by the early successes of the helium-neon laser in the management of retinal detachment and the expanding uses of lasers in ophthalmology. Lasers by no means supplant traditional surgical armamentaria but can be used in combination with conventional techniques and have found extraordinary success in laser-assisted laparoscopy and in neurosurgical and skull base procedures.

As with all technologies, there are significant advantages and disadvantages in their applications. The advantages of laser surgery are numerous and involve the actual properties of the laser and its applications. The disadvantages of the laser arise from the extraordinary power of its radiant energy and the complexities in the generation of the beam. The significant advantages of the laser in surgery are its ability to coagulate, vaporize, or incise tissue based on its power and the time of application on tissue. Certain lasers are more effective in coagulating bleeding vessels and thereby assist in providing a relatively dry surgical field. There is a reduction in the thermal damage to contiguous nontarget tissue and an apparent reduction in postoperative tissue edema presumably arising from reduced mechanical tissue trauma. The surgeon is able to use precision in the application of laser energy to affect only the diseased tissue with marginal injury to vital organs, especially when the laser is transmitted through a coaxial system within a microscope, which permits enhanced visual and physical access to target tissue. Further access to target tissue is provided by phototransmission through flexible quartz fibers or waveguides, or both. The latter provides tactile sense to the hand of the surgeon when contact tips or waveguides are used. The laser beam or its energy characteristics can be modified to produce selective tissue ablation and to provide selective tissue effects by the use of specific tissue photosensitizing agents. One can change lasers or laser wavelengths to enhance selective tissue absorption. Investigators have reported a decreased incidence of postoperative pain, presumably owing to the interdiction of neural afferent pathways by the laser, as well as a decrease in wound contraction owing to the reduction in stimulation of tissue myoepithelial and fibroblastic cellular elements, thus leading to less scarring. More recently, lasers have been used in the welding of arteries and neural repair. Finally, lasers have been constantly used in new applications, such as facial resurfacing and endoscopic facial cosmetic surgery.

As with any technology, there are significant disadvantages. Of primary consideration are radiant energy hazards to the patient, surgeon, and operative team from inadvertent exposure, resulting in laser skin burns, eye damage, and even blindness. There have been disastrous reports of injury or death of the patient from the ignition of endotracheal tubes by errant laser energy, which was further fueled by anesthetic gases used during surgery. There have been reports of electrocution from the laser device due to the high voltages necessary to generate laser energy, and thermal injuries and or fires have been caused by heat produced by such high voltages or leakage of thermal energy from the physical reaction within the laser cavity. Other disadvantages include the great expense of laser equipment and service fees, the need for additional training of the surgeon and operating team, special wiring and plumbing requirements, and continuing maintenance and upgrading of an evolving technology. The earlier lack of portability of the laser machines has become a relative disadvantage with the advent of portable devices possessing significant power and versatility. Enterprising companies now lease equipment for use in the surgical office.

Historical Considerations

The 1917 seminal publication by Einstein of "Zür Quanten Theorie der Stralung"[1] contained the elements of the conceptual basis for stimulated emission of radiant energy that was to form the foundation of modern laser physics. When combined with the principles of quantum mechanics promulgated by Nails Bohr and the fabrication of optical resonators[2] known in the nineteenth century, Gordon and others, much later in 1955 were the first to demonstrate the stimulated emission of microwaves within the electromagnetic spectrum. In 1958, Schawlow and Townes[3] revealed that it was possible to stimulate emission of radiant energy in the form of photons in the infrared and visible or optical portions of the spectrum, which rapidly led to the development of the laser. The first working laser was constructed by Maiman[4] in 1960 by exciting a ruby rod with intense pulses of light from a flash lamp. The so-called ruby laser emanated pulses of light radiation of 0.69 microns of one-millisecond duration or less within the visible portion of the electromagnetic spectrum. The first actual continuously generating laser was attributed to Javan and colleagues[5] in 1961 who used a mixture of helium and neon. The "HeNe" laser was of low power, but it advanced the concept of laser energy practicability by its continuous mode and continues to be used as a coaxial spotter for the laser beams of more powerful lasers.

In 1961, several major advances in laser technology led to the development of lasers with increasing power output such as the neodymium-in-glass laser invented by Snitzer,[6] which also could be operated in a pulsed mode and far outpowered the ruby laser and possessed a wavelength of 1.06 microns. Later, Johnson and Nassau[7] developed the first solid-state neodymium laser which used the neodymium ion as a dopant in calcium tungstate ($CaWO_4$). In this same year, Johnson invented a laser device that was the forerunner of the Nd:YAG laser by using a neodymium ion–doped yttrium-aluminum-garnet (YAG) rod. Both the helium:neon and the YAG lasers were characterized by a limited absorption of their wavelengths in nonpigmented biologic tissue. Physicists soon appreciated that there was a differential absorption of laser radiation by biologic tissue, and a continuing search was begun to develop lasers with specific tissue absorptive characteristics based on known tissue chromophores (melanin and hemoglobin).

One of the most practical lasers used in oral and maxillofacial surgery was developed by Patel[8] in 1964. This was the first continuous-wave carbon dioxide (molecular) gas laser emitting light radiation in the infrared zone of the electromagnetic spectrum. The importance of this laser arose from its high-power continuous output and an infrared wavelength of 10.6 microns, which was found to be completely absorbed by most biologic tissue. By the appropriate application of lenses, the beam of the carbon dioxide laser could be narrowly focused to a small spot size, thus permitting the laser beam to ablate a specific volume of tissue by thermal effects and vaporization. This laser was the first laser to enable the surgeon to create a well-controlled, precise tissue effect that resulted in an ability to produce an incision similar to a scalpel as well as a debulking or ablative ability for use in tumor surgery. The properties of the carbon dioxide laser were extended by Polanyi and coworkers[9] in 1970, who enhanced the laser as an experimental tool for surgical research and later invented and designed hand-held instruments that could be used with the laser on biologic tissues.

The early YAG and carbon dioxide lasers were known as free-beam lasers because the laser handpiece did not come into contact with the tissue to be lased. The physical nature of the beam or wavelength of the carbon dioxide laser was too large to be propagated through flexible quartz fibers, whereas the smaller wavelength of the neodymium:YAG laser enabled an increased versatility so that at first this laser could be used through endoscopes via fiberoptic technology to control gastrointestinal hemorrhage. Later advances in the Nd:YAG laser focused the beam at the tip of sapphire contact probes mounted on the distal end of the quartz fiber, further enabling the surgeon to have greater control of power and application. Also, the tactile sense that was lost in the use of the free beam laser was restored to the surgeon. In 1985, DiaKuzono and Joffe[10] developed synthetic contact probes that have been further refined by scientists at Surgical Laser Technologies (Oaks, Pennsylvania). Contact probes for oral and maxillofacial surgery are mounted on a handpiece, usually with a convenient finger trigger to provide precision of mucosal and skin incisions with the added benefit of superb hemostasis and to avoid the relatively uncontrolled wide and deep thermal damage of the free-beam laser. To attempt to mimic these significant advantages of the contact-probe YAG laser while keeping the advantages of the carbon dioxide laser, various laser companies have developed impressive waveguides that come very close to the properties of the contact tips yet possess the power and wave characteristics coveted by surgeons in the carbon dioxide devices. These devices have superb tissue handling abilities and can be used in office settings with power outputs of 20 watts. Such versatile carbon dioxide lasers can be used for the full gamut of oral and maxillofacial procedures from simple biopsies to uvulopalatostomy.

Other laser devices such as the argon and the holmium:YAG systems are of importance to the specialist in oral and maxillofacial surgery. Bridges[11] of the Hughes Research Laboratories developed the argon laser in 1964. Radiant energy generated by the argon laser is produced by the infusion of a current of high electrical energy into the laser cavity containing argon gas as the laser medium. Indeed, the argon laser is an ion laser in which the active medium is an ionized rare gas. The argon radiant energy has at least two emission lines in the blue-green (0.488 and 0.514 microns) and weaker lines in the ultraviolet and near-infrared portions of the electromagnetic spectrum.

Early use of the argon laser focused on the treatment and management of angiodysplasias, especially those occurring in the head and neck region. Newer laser devices have encroached on the clinical successes of the argon laser, however, many surgeons still find it the device of choice in vascular anomalies. It was the first laser to be used in the management of port wine stains and continues to have a role in the treatment of these congenital lesions. Such congenital lesions in the orbitofacial region can occur as isolated entities or as part of a multiform syndrome such as Sturge-Weber disease. The argon laser has its advantages in the ability of its beam to be absorbed by tissue chromophores such as hemoglobin and melanin. Historically, the argon laser pointed the way for the development of ever-increasingly specific lasers possessing wavelengths that could be more selectively absorbed by target tissues, thus sparing contiguous and subjacent healthy tissues. More recently, the pulsed dye laser, tunable wavelength lasers, Q-switched ruby lasers, and copper-vapor lasers have exhibited superior results in selected lesions. Although there has been continuing improvement in selectivity of laser wavelengths for given susceptible tissues, in the absence of more sophisticated devices, the argon laser has significant usefulness for lesions such as deep purple, nodular vascular facial lesions in adults and other vascular entities, including telangiectasias, venous lakes, angiofibromas, and angiomas.

The last two decades have witnessed the development of increasingly powerful and wavelength enhancements in the semiconductor lasers including a new generation of tunable solid-state lasers. An example of the newer solid-state laser with oral and maxillofacial applications is the holmium:YAG laser, which, like all such lasers is based on rare earth ions (holmium), which can be stimulated to emit near 2.1 microns. The holmium is doped onto the YAG crystal along with erbium and thulium, the latter two dopants acting as sensitizers that absorb the pump light and transfer this energy to the holmium ions in the lattice of the crystal. At this juncture, the holmium laser has applications in arthroscopy of the temporomandibular joint because of the ability of this wavelength to be transmitted effectively through a water medium.

The future promise of laser radiant energy directed at solving problems of oral and maxillofacial surgery can only be realized by a relentless scholasticism and academic integrity combined with healthy skepticism. In the end, the yield of this promise will derive from painstaking controlled clinical trials by objective scientists and clinicians.

REFERENCES

1. Einstein A: Zür Quanten Theorie der Stralung. Phys Zeit 18:121, 1917.
2. Gordon JP, Zeigler HJ, Townes CH: The Maser—new type of amplifier, frequency standard and spectrometer. Physiol Rev 99:1264, 1955.
3. Schawlow AL, Townes CH: Infrared and optical red maser. Physiol Rev 112:1940, 1958.
4. Maiman TH: Stimulated optical radiation in ruby. Nature 187:493, 1960.
5. Javan A, Bennet WR, Herrott DR: Population inversion and continuous optical Maser oscillation in a gas discharge containing a HeNe mixture. Physiol Rev Letter 6:106, 1961.
6. Snitzer E: Optical Maser action on Nd3 + Ba crown glass. Physiol Rev Letter 7:444, 1961.
7. Johnson LF, Nassau K: Proceedings of the Institute of Radio Engineers. 49:1704, 1961.
8. Patel CKN: Interpretation of CO_2 optical laser experiments. Physiol Rev Letter 12:588, 1964.
9. Polanyi TG, Bredemeier HC, Davis TW: A CO_2 laser for surgical research. Med Biol Eng Comput 8:541, 1970.
10. DiaKuzono N, Joffe SN: Artificial sapphire probe for contact photocoagulation and tissue vaporization with the Nd:YAG laser. Med Instr 19:July–August, 1985.
11. Bridges WB: Laser oscillation in singly ionized argon in the visible spectrum. Applied Physics Letters 4:128, 1964.

SECTION One

CHAPTER 1

Qualitative Laser Physics in Maxillofacial Surgery

GUY A. CATONE, DMD

Since their introduction to medicine and surgery over 30 years ago, lasers have found increasing application in the majority of surgical disciplines including oral and maxillofacial surgery. Coincident with the general broadening and innovative evolution of the specialty of oral and maxillofacial surgery, newer laser designs have found a special niche in the discipline. In contrast to conventional instrumentation and other adjunctive equipment used to enhance surgery, it is important that the surgeon should possess at least a fundamental understanding of qualitative laser physics and essential operation of those lasers most useful in clinical practice. No less important to the surgeon is the photobiology of specific types of lasers and the manner in which lasers are selected for specific surgical tasks. (See Chapter 2.) Each laser device has a different effect on biologic tissues. Therefore, knowledge of the properties of radiant energy generated by various laser systems is essential in the choice of a laser to solve various surgical problems. It is the purpose of this chapter to present fundamental physics common to most laser systems.

HISTORICAL PERSPECTIVES

The hypothetical origins and conceptual basis of a laser or *l*ight *a*mplification by the *s*timulated *e*mission of *r*adiation were enunciated by Einstein.[1] The basic physical principles on which laser radiation is formed were known as early as the 1930s.[2] In the 1960s, a series of lasers were produced that were capable of operating in a pulsed manner, the first being a ruby laser invented by Maiman.[3] The carbon dioxide laser, which operated in the infrared

portion of the electromagnetic spectrum, was fabricated by Patel and colleagues in 1964.[4] Following this discovery, there was rapid development of multiple laser systems and the production of continuously operating carbon dioxide lasers with higher power.[5] Parallel to these developments was the design by Johnson in 1961 of a laser with a wavelength of 1.06 microns using a neodymium (Nd)-doped yttrium-aluminum-garnet (YAG) rod.[6] These early carbon dioxide and YAG lasers were free-beam lasers in the sense that the laser instrument did not contact the target tissue.

More recently, in the early 1980s, the contact laser concept was developed by collaboration between Dikuzono and Joffe, who experimented with synthetic sapphire tips, with the laser energy conducted via optical fibers. The tips were designed for various surgical tasks, and thus, the tips had a number of shapes and sizes. The neodymium YAG laser energy was transmitted via an optical quartz fiber with the operator holding a handpiece directing the tip against the target tissue. Used in this manner, via fiberoptic technology, hemostasis was enhanced and the laser provided a tactile sensation to the operator while not possessing the deep penetration or thermal injury characteristic of the free-beam YAG laser systems.[7]

The first argon laser was developed by Bridges in 1964. The argon laser is an ion laser in which the active lasant is an ionized rare gas. The importance of argon radiation is its wavelength in the blue-green and weaker lines in the ultraviolet and near-infrared portions of the electromagnetic (EM) spectrum and its role in the treatment of cutaneous and mucosal vascular angiodysplasias.[8–11]

For many years the CO_2, the Nd:YAG, and the

argon were the major lasers used in the surgical specialties. During the 1980s, the pulsed-dye laser, Q-switched ruby, copper vapor, and holmium lasers have exhibited superior results in selected surgical cases. The pulsed-dye laser and the copper vapor laser have been very successful in the treatment of angiodysplasias.[11–14] The newer solid-state lasers such as the holmium:YAG laser have found application in arthroscopic surgery of the temporomandibular joint. These holmium lasers are based on rare earth ions similar to neodymium. The holmium laser emits near 2.1 microns and, its energy, therefore, can be transmitted via optical fibers.[15–19] The development of laser technology with increasing variation in wavelength and power that could be predictably controlled led to enhancements that were necessary for surgical applications.

LASER RADIANT ENERGY

Electromagnetic (EM) Spectrum

Generally, lasers function within the so-called optical spectrum. This is that portion of the electromagnetic spectrum (Fig. 1–1) that includes the far or longer wavelength radiation through the visible portion seen by the human eye and including the ultraviolet segment just before the microwave part of the EM spectrum. The portion of the optical

spectrum occupied by visible light detected by the human eye is less than 0.1%. Physicists and engineers consider light as consisting of not only that which is appreciated by the human eye, but beyond that narrow definition to include the portions next to the visible spectrum including the infrared and ultraviolet regions. Admittedly, optical radiation and light cannot specifically be used synonymously with laser radiation and laser light but the generation of laser radiation is by and large bounded by that portion of the EM spectrum with gamma radiations or high-frequency radiation in the extreme ultraviolet and microwave radiation at the long wavelength boundary of the infrared region. Thus, lasers are torches of radiation from within the EM spectrum emitting beams of energy that parenthetically possess special properties that enable their use for surgical applications.

GENERATION OF LASER ENERGY

The word laser is an acronym that actually names the device as well as the process by which laser radiation is generated. Laser, or *Light Amplification by Stimulated Emission of Radiation*, is a mnemonic term that describes the process in which a certain laser medium or lasant within a resonator space is energized by internal or external energy sources to produce an excited population of atoms, molecules,

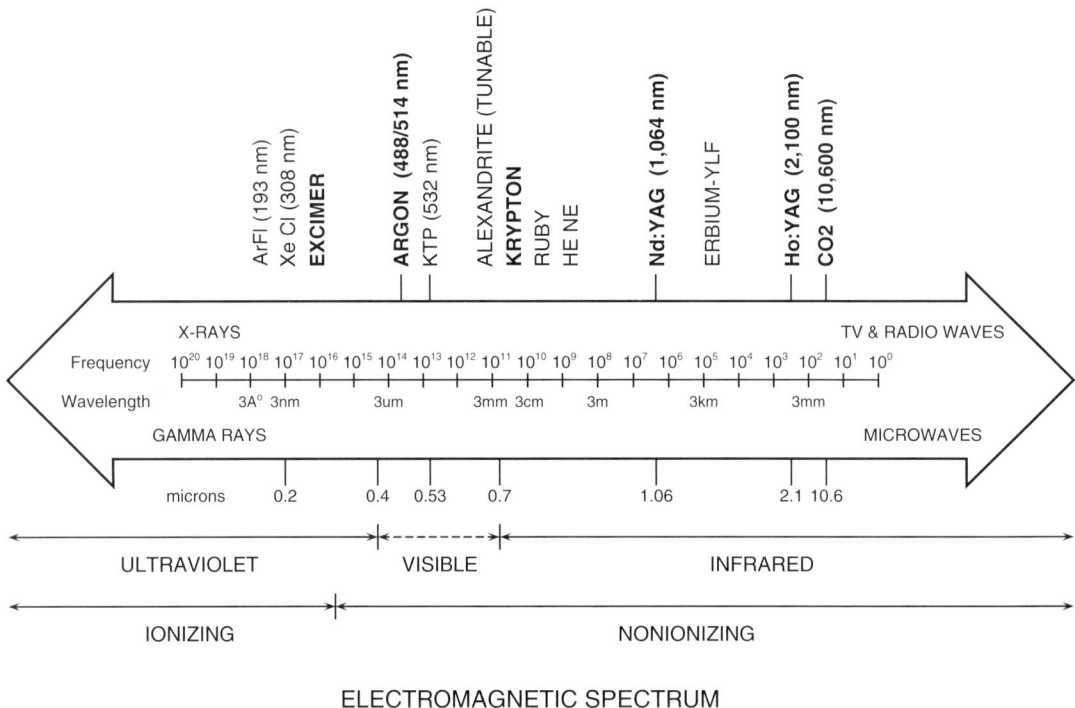

FIGURE 1–1. The accepted electromagnetic (EM) spectrum. All lasers are represented on the EM spectrum depending on their specific wavelength.

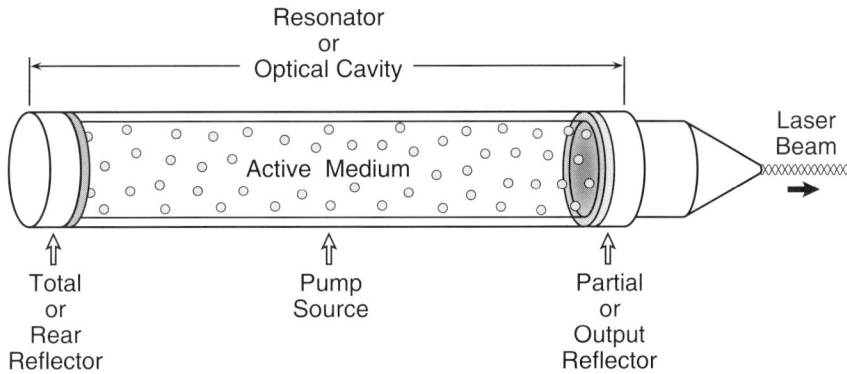

FIGURE 1–2. The fundamental components of a laser. The lasant is composed of a laser medium consisting of a species that is the name of that laser. The species can consist of ions, atoms, and molecules.

and rare gas (species). The energy within a resonator space reaches a population inversion in which the greatest cohort of species is in an excited state and in which photons are emitted and amplified within a laser cavity. The radiant energy is released as a laser beam.

To understand the generation of laser radiation, it is probably expeditious to consider the fundamental design of the laser cavity, the system that houses the actual physical reaction that eventually results in the production of the laser beam. The fundamental components of a laser system include a resonant cavity housing an active medium that has the ability to produce a population inversion, which is discussed later, and energy input, either external or internal (Fig. 1–2). The active medium is housed by a cavity and bounded by two mirrors. These mirrors are designed to reflect photons completely on one end and partially on the other end of the cavity. Consequently, one end is completely reflective, and the other is semireflective and semitransparent to allow the radiant energy to exit the resonant cavity. Within the design of the laser device may be apertures to actually shape the beam and shutters designed to control the power or magnitude of the energy and its periodicity. With the combination of two mirrors that are essentially parallel (which is a state that is very difficult to achieve physically and is not practical in commercial surgical lasers but is useful to the present discussion), the mirrors are placed at either end of the laser cavity consisting of, for simplicity, a cylinder.

The mirrors are separated by a fixed distance (d), forming a Fabry-Perot interferometer (Fig. 1–3),

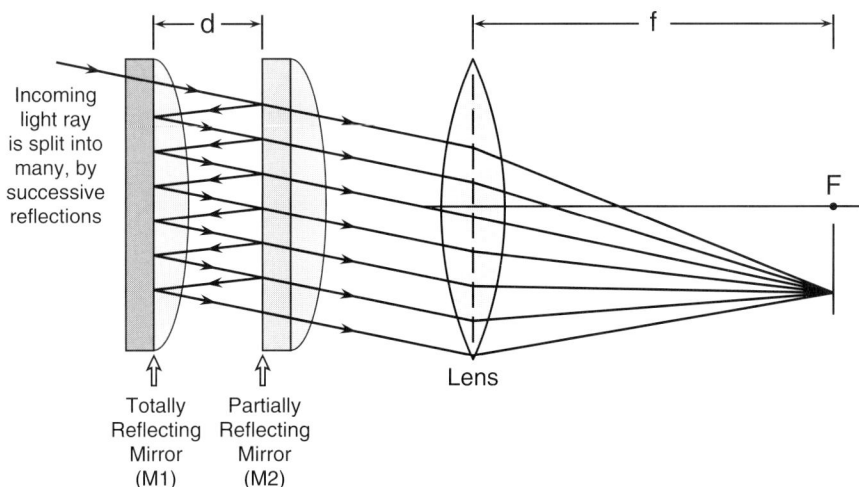

FIGURE 1–3. The Fabry-Perot interferometer is made up of two mirrors M1 and M2, which are separated by a distance, d. Light of a given wavelength (gamma) after entering the interferometer will experience multiple reflections. Because mirror M2 is partially reflective, some light will pass out of the device. These light waves are then focused by the lens to a specific locus in the focal plane F, at which point interference takes place.

which uses the physical principle of interference. Interference occurs when two or more waves simultaneously penetrate some material, forming a combined wave. The result is a larger wave having a higher amplitude and thus deeper troughs. If these waves are in phase, they are said to be constructively interfering or exhibit constructive interference. Such light produced by constructive interference is brighter. The opposite can also occur, that is, destructive interference, in which the waves are not in phase. In such a case, the wave is of reduced amplitude and thus has less brightness. Indeed, if the two waves are of the same amplitude, the process of destructive interference means that the waves cancel and result in darkness. Light formed by laser action within the cavity from the active medium (to be discussed) has a certain wavelength (λ). The more the process of constructive interference occurs, the more consistent a wavelength is produced by the laser cavity. Photons of light travel a distance of 2d over each previous ray, which means that the distance is only 2d if the rays are perpendicular to the mirrors. Then constructive interference occurs if 2d is equal to mλ, where m is an integer. Constructive interferences occur between all rays if the wavelength is equal to 2d/m (λ = 2d/m). In this system, only certain wavelengths are consistent and result in constructive interference and thus a bright output. This critical factor means that a laser of a given length can emit light only of certain wavelengths that will fit within the resonant cavity formed by its mirrors. The concept of constructive/destructive interference is also paramount in the design and fabrication of the dielectric mirrors that are used in most laser systems (Fig. 1–4).

The generation of laser radiant energy is singularly dependent on designing and forcing the light within the laser cavity to travel between the mirrors and be reflected theoretically infinitely through a process termed optical feedback (Fig. 1–5). One could conceive of the mirror system within the laser cavity as a completely silvered mirror opposed by a parallel partly silvered mirror that allows some light to leave the resonant cavity and to be emitted as a collimated beam of laser energy. The laser cavity is designed so that enough light reflects back into the laser cavity to continue the laser action within the laser medium. The process, however, is much more complex, as are the dielectric mirrors, not only in their composition but also in their shape. It is not surprising that the mirrors forming the ends of the laser cavity are not the same kinds of mirrors that one would find in everyday use. Indeed, it is very difficult to maintain parallelism if one designs a laser based on parallel flat plane or so-called planar mirrors. Theoretically, one would have to continually adjust the mirrors for parallelism. Otherwise, a resonation of the beam to and fro would not occur and, indeed, amplification would be difficult (see later).

In lasers such as the argon laser, the mirrors are made of glass but do not have reflective surfaces as such. These mirrors are the dielectric mirrors (discussed above), which rely on a constructive interference phenomenon to produce significant reflectivity. Within the dielectric system, there are alternative layers of high refractive index materials, such as titanium oxide, and low refractive index materials, such as silicon oxide (see Fig. 1–4). Remarkably, these materials are deposited on a glass

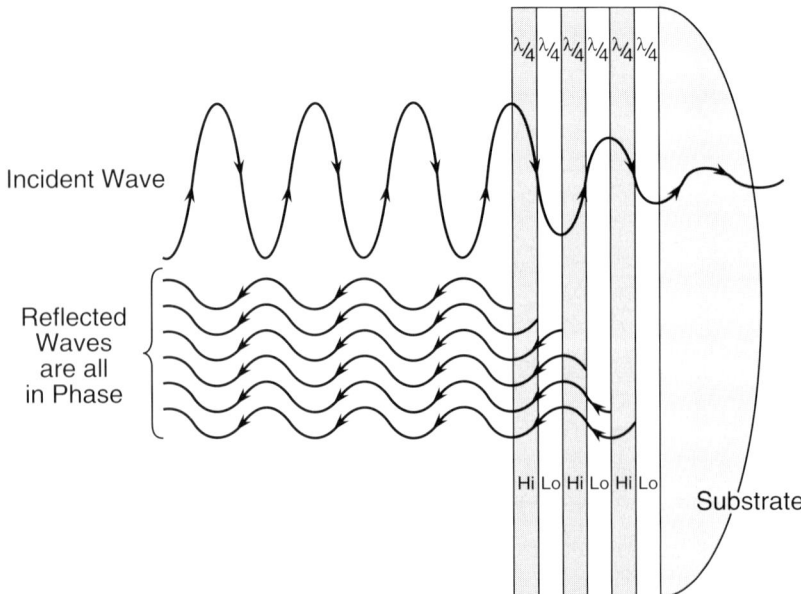

FIGURE 1–4. This is a magnification of a section of the laser dielectric mirror. This shows an alternation of glasses of high (Hi) and low (Lo) refraction indices. By alternating the glasses as indicated, all reflections are forced to be in phase, resulting in a constructive interference and controlled reflectance.

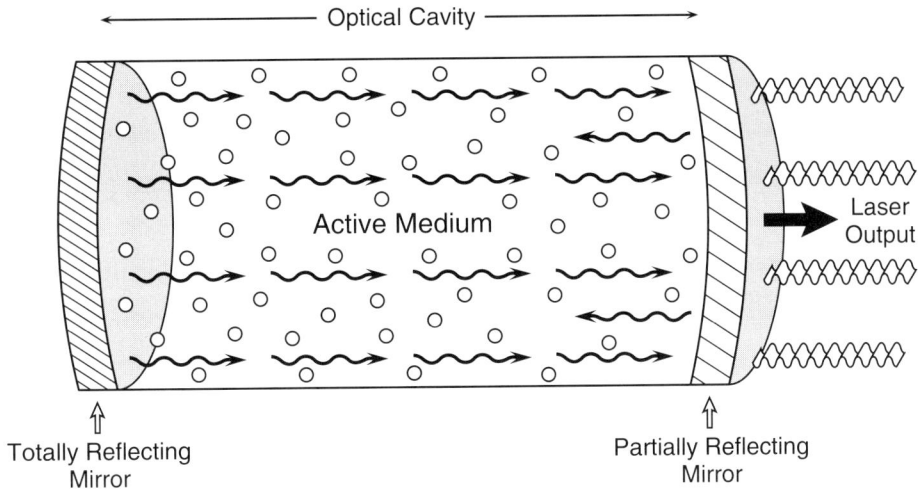

FIGURE 1–5. A schematic of optical feedback in the laser chamber. One mirror is highly reflective, and the other permits a small amount of incident light to be released as useful output.

substrate and each layer is designed to be one quarter of a wavelength thick. By alternating the pattern of high and low refractive index materials, the light waves are reflected from successive surfaces and undergo a phase change equivalent to one half wavelength or 180 degrees on reflection from high-index materials. No phase change occurs on reflection from low-index materials; thus, the result is that all reflected rays are interfered with constructively, and light of this particular wavelength is kept inside the laser cavity, causing stimulated emission only at a specific controlled wavelength. The resulting waves that do not constructively interfere leak out of the system, and therefore, stimulated emission does not occur at those wavelengths. This alternating pattern results in all reflections that are in phase, causing constructive interference and a controlled reflectance from the mirror. Depending on the number of layers within the mirror, a direct linear relationship is observed with a number of layers. Consequently, as the number of layers increases up to 20 or more, the reflectance will approach 100% for at least one particular wavelength, as in a gas laser. One mirror is nearly a perfect reflector, and the other is 99% reflective, resulting in 1% of light at the desired wavelength emerging as the incident laser beam.

In summary, most medical and surgical lasers are not designed to operate with the plane parallel mirror system. These systems of planar mirror cavities are prone to small malalignment and also they will produce a poorly controlled beam shape. In the planar system, there is no specific axis that most photons would be forced to resonate upon so that, theoretically, the laser beam could resonate along several disparate axes, causing output that is spotty and randomly changing in time. It is much more

efficient to produce a curved mirror cavity, such as the curved planar configuration or the confocal resonator (Fig. 1–6).

The actual optical cavity itself can be of many different shapes and materials. The simplest design is set up with one of the mirrors (M_1) having a reflectivity of 100%, and the other (M_2) having a reflectivity of less than 1% to 10%, which are called the total reflector and the output coupler, respectively. One can imagine an optical cavity with a cylindric or rectangular shape. There are also elliptic optical cavities or pumping chambers with a rod and lamp at the ellipse foci. Circular chambers also are made with the lamp and rod parallel to one another. The pumping chamber or optical cavity sometimes is constructed of a reflecting or scattering material, for example, ceramic or a polished metal. It is certainly not always circular. Weaker light that is not optically pumped to threshold is constantly leaking through the output coupler M_2. However, if optical pumping or excitation of the species within the cavity or active medium has reached a so-called population inversion, then the light wave will experience gain to offset this small loss. The beam will gradually get weaker until the gain just balances the loss.

If, for example, the total reflector and the output coupler equal 100% and 1%, respectively, then the light wave would have to increase by 1% in passing through the laser cavity or rod twice to just balance the 1% loss through the output coupler and out of the cavity. As alluded to earlier, the gain just equal to the loss is called the laser threshold. If the excitation increases or optical pumping of the active medium is enhanced above the threshold, this gives rise to a rapid increase in the beam power. In any laser cavity, only specific wavelengths will be

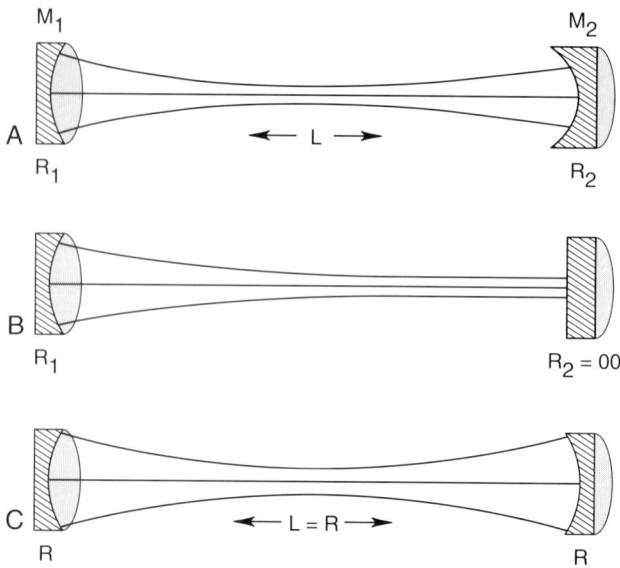

FIGURE 1–6. Examples of curved mirror cavities: *A*, general form; *B* curved/plane shape; and *C*, confocal resonator. (L, Length of the laser cavity; M_1, totally reflecting mirror; M_2, partially reflecting mirror; R_1 and R_2, differing radii of curvature of the mirrors of M_1 and M_2. These radii determine the shape and dimensions of the laser beam. As one can see from the diagram, changes in the radius of curvature offers different beam patterns. In *C*, the length of the laser cavity is equal to the radius of curvature or equal to the diameter of a circle represented by the radius of R; in this case, R = R.)

capable of resonation as they reflect back and forth between the mirrors. A prerequisite to ensure resonance, and therefore, constructive interference and thus amplification, is that the length of the cavity should be a whole number of half wavelengths. That is to say, because $L = n \times$ the fraction $\lambda/2$ (where L is the length of the laser cavity and n is an integer), one can then use the equation that the frequency times the wavelength ($f\lambda$) is equal to the speed of light and reformatting $f = \lambda c/2L$. The frequencies within the laser cavity thus established are known as the cavity modes or, more clearly, the axial modes of the cavity. The cavity is extraordinarily long with regard to the actual wavelength of the emitted light from the active medium. The quantity n is thus an extraordinarily large number approximately 10^6, with a frequency difference between adjacent modes (known as the mode spacing) that is relatively small within the value of the order of several hundred megahertz (MHz).

PROPERTIES OF LASER LIGHT

There are several important properties of laser light that distinguish it from white light. These singular properties of laser light that make it useful for surgery are monochromaticity, directionality, coherence, and brightness. For over two centuries, there has been controversy surrounding the precise physical character of light or EM radiation. Light can be viewed both as a particle and as a wave, and behaves as both in certain physical instances. A light wave can be thought of as a stone dropped into a pool of water. The wave that radiates away from the impact point has an amplitude, frequency, and wavelength. The peak of the wave or its vertical height is called the amplitude, and this is related analogously to the intensity of a light wave. The number of wave peaks per second passing a specific static measuring point is the frequency of the wave expressed in light as hertz. Measuring the distance from one peak to the trough is called the wavelength. In light radiation, the wavelength and frequency determine the actual energy level of light and how it is distinguished or positioned within the EM spectrum. Longer wavelengths in the EM spectrum, such as infrared, produce lower energy, and they include not only infrared but microwaves, television waves, and radio waves. Shorter wavelengths have higher energy and include ultraviolet, x-ray, and gamma radiation.

Laser radiation is an intense beam of light that generates energy in the wavelengths that range from the near-ultraviolet to the near-infrared frequencies. The energy thus generated by a laser beam and its position within the EM spectrum are determined by the wavelength and frequency of the light wave. Whether or not the laser light is visible or invisible to the human eye depends on the medium used to generate laser light, the lasant. The carbon dioxide, Nd:YAG, helium-neon (HeNe), argon, and holmium:YAG lasers are of current interest and value to the oral and maxillofacial surgeon. The method by which radiation is generated from these systems is of clinical importance to the surgeon and will be discussed further.

The notion that light is composed of packets of independent energy units was advanced by Sir Isaac Newton. Much later in the 20th century, the concept of quanta was used by Neils Bohr and Einstein to reconcile the concept that light was composed of packets of energy. Later, Einstein proposed the concept that light emanates in currents of massless particles referred to as photons, each photon carrying a specific quantum of energy and associated with a specific wavelength. This is the accepted theory and terminology used in laser physics. However, neither the wave concept nor the particulate concept fully explains all of the properties and observations of radiant light and other forms of EM radiation.

Monochromaticity

Lasers emit light that is monochromatic or specifically a single wavelength. This contrasts greatly with a typical incandescent light bulb, which emits colors of the entire spectrum, usually wavelengths from ultraviolet through the entire visible and then into the infrared range of 500 nm or more. An example of monochromaticity is the ability of a laser to selectively destroy tumor cells that have absorbed a particular dye such as hematoporphyrin derivative (HPD) or other tissue photosensitizer while not injuring contiguous or overlying cells. Lasers of varying types emit an individual wavelength or specified wavelengths, and indeed, some can be tuned to different wavelengths based on the desires of the operator. Importantly, each type of target tissue absorbs a given wavelength far better than others. This factor is based on the specific consistency of the tissue, its thickness, and significant tissue chromophores such as melanin and hemoglobin.

Directionality

There is little divergence of the laser as it exits the laser device, and the beam can travel a considerable distance with very little movement away from parallelism. Most gas or solid-state lasers emit laser beams with a divergence angle of approximately a milliradian. In other words, they will spread out to one meter in diameter after traveling a kilometer.

This also explains why laser light is extraordinarily hazardous. By not diverging over distance, laser light maintains brightness. For example, after traversing 10 meters across a large room, the beam could still be within a range of 10 mm across, still concentrated enough to be dangerous.

Coherence

Coherence is a property of laser light that occurs when there is some fixed-phase relationship between two waves of laser light. There are two types of coherence of laser light, longitudinal and transverse. The longitudinal type of coherence represents a time or temporal coherence along the longitudinal beam axis, whereas transverse or spatial coherence refers to coherence across the beam. Thus, each wave is in phase with the other (Fig. 1–7). Both longitudinal and transverse coherence are produced by the process of stimulated emission and by resonation or optical feedback. Coherence thus causes the collimation of a laser beam over extremely large distances and allows the beam to accept extremely fine focusing. Any given laser beam can be focused only to a diameter equal to the wavelength of the specific laser. There is, of course, a finite coherent length or that distance over which the light produced is in actual phase; however, for conventional light sources, that distance is, for practical purposes, 0.

Brightness

Another property of laser light that distinguishes it from conventional light sources, is that of brightness. This property arises from the parallelism or collimation of the laser light as it moves through space maintaining its concentration and, thus, the characteristic brightness. This high-brightness factor translates to high concentrations of energy when the laser is focused on a small spot. Conventional

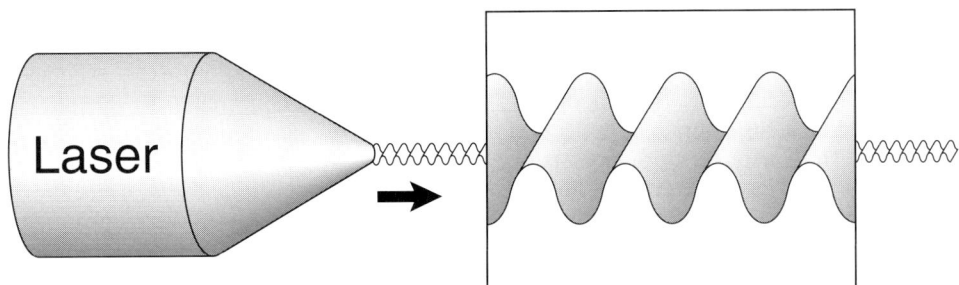

FIGURE 1–7. A radiant light source from a laser is characterized by transverse coherence if the wavelength is constant, that is, not changing in time and possessing spatial coherence if the waves are in step across the beam.

light sources can be focused, but the ultimate image is much larger than the microscopic focal spot of the laser beam. This focusing of the brightness of the laser beam is what the surgeon depends on to elevate the temperature of tissues or to cut or vaporize. Although there is dependence on defraction limitations, that is the focal spot can only equal the length of the specific laser wavelengths, there are instances in which the laser light can be concentrated microscopically to extremely high levels, resulting in atoms within the target zone becoming ionized as a result of the EM field energy's ability to strip electrons from the outer atomic shells and directly ionize the tissue. This forms a disruptive pattern referred to as an optical plasma, and this pattern can be used to cut tissues and is useful in ophthalmology.

QUANTUM ELECTRONICS

To understand how a laser produces radiant energy in the form that it does, it is important to understand the basic principles of quantum electronics, which is a term for laser physics that is usually associated with academic research but nonetheless, describes the physical principles that will result in a useful laser beam for surgical purposes. The basic requirements for laser activity are the active medium or lasant, a population inversion through quantum electronics, and some form of optical feedback or optical resonation (see Fig. 1–2). The understanding of quantum electronics and laser action necessarily may present some repetition. This is because the principles of laser physics tend to be organic such that one particular physical action affects another and another, producing a cascade effect, ultimately resulting in the laser beam.

Active Medium

Most lasers are named with regard to the substance that is used to create the actual laser light. This is referred to as the active medium or the lasant. The active lasant may be in the form of a gas, atoms, or ions, all of which are referred to by the laser physicist as the species. This is a convention, even though the mechanisms by which they produce laser light at an atomic, ionic, or molecular level are different. Thus, neon gas produces laser light in the helium:neon laser, argon ions in the argon laser, gas molecules in the carbon dioxide laser, ionic impurities in a solid-state crystalline Nd:YAG laser (Nd ions are responsible for laser action), and chromium ions in the ruby laser. Finally, holmium is the ion that is responsible for the laser action in the holmium:YAG laser. Although

these characteristic elements or molecules are the main source of laser light, there may be other ingredients within the resonator cavity that assist in the alteration of the quantum state of the species, thus resulting in radiant energy. An example is the carbon dioxide laser, in which helium and nitrogen atoms assist in the processes of activation and deactivation.

Energy Level

The singular concept of laser physics that directly relates to the use of surgical lasers is the concept of energy level. This applies to the energy or excitation level of a laser medium. The energy that the laser medium possesses at any given time is related directly to the application of external or internal energy from a source that is specific for the laser system. For example, in order to excite a species of a lasant, one may need an electrical discharge, as in a gas medium, for example, the carbon dioxide laser or the helium:neon, or krypton, laser. It may be a chemical reaction or an external high-powered radiant source, such as a xenon or krypton flash lamp. In the latter instance, the solid-state crystalline laser medium such as the Nd:YAG or ruby laser is excited by a flash lamp energy source. This causes a process called optical pumping, in which energy is driven into the resonant chamber or cavity. This energy is used to change the energy level or quantum state of the lasant species, atoms, molecules, and ions, which results in one or more quantum reactions.

The energy level is the quantum state of an atom or molecule and species, which ranges from a base or ground level of 0, or the lowest possible energy level, to a higher level in which this species is driven to a state of excitation. In this state of excitation, a quantum process called stimulated emission can occur. Species can exist in only certain thermodynamically allowed discrete energy states. The energy status is very much like the rungs of a ladder in which an electron can exist on any rung but not able to occupy areas between rungs. Electrons or parts of every ion or species are permitted to have certain energies that correspond to orbits of certain sizes. These orbits do not exist at equal distances, but nonetheless, conceptually it is useful to consider this status in three dimensions. When there is a shift of a species from one energy level to another, this is called transition. The movement or transition of an electron to a lower energy level results in the emission of radiant energy. This radiant energy is emitted as a discrete packet of energy termed a photon, whose energy is equal to that given up by the electron. To equate this particular photon's energy to the electromagnetic radiation or wave produced, this energy is proportionate to the frequency of the emitted light wave.

Similarly, if the species absorbs a photon of an appropriate energy, this may cause an electron within the species to move to a higher energy level, thus producing excitation. When there is a shift of the species from one energy level to another, this is called, as mentioned earlier, a transition or, in the case of a large population of species, a population inversion. There is a specific required absorption of energy level equal to the difference in energy between the two levels to make this excitation change transition possible. The ability of an active medium or lasant to be optically pumped or excited to a higher energy level in which a greater quantity or cohort above the population of the species is at a higher energy level is a major property that enables the active medium to act as the source of laser radiant energy. Similarly, a reduction from a higher energy level to one of lesser energy is called decay or de-excitation, which is characterized by the release of the energy of transition.

Pursuant to understanding laser action, consider the diagram that represents energy levels from ground level or minimum energy to the highest energy level attainable by a species: atom, ion, or molecule. E_0 represents the ground state at thermal equilibrium. Most of the energy of an atom or ion in isobaric conditions exists at this minimal energy level. Transitions to various energy levels, such as E_1, E_2, E_3, E_4, and E_n (Fig. 1–8), can occur through several quantum accepted mechanisms. These mechanisms have been explained by Einstein as three types of radiative transitions within atoms or processes in which an electron either absorbs or emits light. These mechanisms are referred to as stimulated absorption, spontaneous emission, and stimulated emission. During laser action, all three processes occur simultaneously. Stimulated emission produces the monochromatic, coherent, direc-

tional radiation output. The important concept in physics is that each atom or molecule has a particular emission spectrum; that is, the particular wavelength of light that is emitted is characteristic of that particular element. Moreover, individual atoms or molecules at isobaric conditions have a specific absorption spectrum, that is, a set of particular wavelengths that can be absorbed that is uniquely characteristic of that atom or molecule, and it is the same set of wavelengths that characterizes the elements or species emission spectrum.

In quantum mechanisms, atoms or species can exist only in discrete energy states. As alluded to earlier, the electrons that are within the orbitals of an atom have quantum acceptable energy levels that correspond to the orbits of the electrons. These orbitals are not necessarily equal in spacing, and the distance between orbitals corresponds to the kinetic and electrostatic potential between the states, which is usually expressed in electron volts (eV). When an electron moves to a lower energy state or orbital, a photon of light is emitted. The energy of the photon is equal to that given up by the electron. In EM wave terms, the energy produced by the photon is proportional to the frequency of the associated light wave. On the other hand, absorption of an energy packet in the form of a photon of the right kind of energy causes an electron of a certain orbital to move to a higher orbital or energy level, causing excitation of the atom.

In summary, the energies and distances between orbitals with the quantum acceptable energy states are specific for each chemical element, and thus, the absorption and emission spectrums are characteristic, or a fingerprint, for each element. The nature of radiant light produced can be quantified or measured in three ways: (1) as the wavelength of a light wave, (2) as a frequency of oscillation of a wave, and (3) as the energy within a photon of radiation. Usually, the wavelengths are measured in micrometers when lasers are employed for medical and surgical reasons. The mathematical relationship between the photon produced and the frequency or wavelength (λ) is $E = h\nu$.

E is the energy of the photon, h is Planck's constant $6.63 + 10^{-34}$ J, or $4.14 + 10^{-14}$ eV. J is Joules and eV is electron volts, both of which represent energy. Typically, the energy, however, is measured in electron volts. One electron volt is the energy required to move an electron through the potential of one volt. The frequency is measured in Hertz (Hz), or the number of oscillations per second.

There are at least three basic energy levels seen in laser physics. These are electronic, vibrational, and rotational levels. Electronic levels can be understood when the diagram of an atom is considered; these levels involve the actual electron configura-

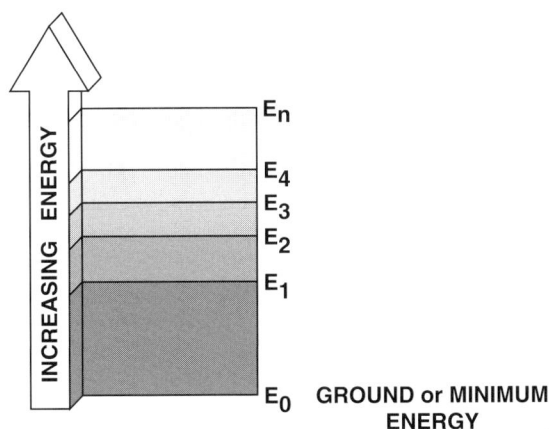

FIGURE 1–8. A typical energy diagram.

tion or orbitals in a species. The consideration of energy levels is more easily understood when the atomic model is used and optical pumping is the methodology that causes excitation of the atoms. In the case of a hydrogen atom, electrons are elevated to existing electron orbitals as they move away from the nucleus, eventually attaining a large enough amount of energy to escape from the nucleus. Energy transitions that occur in laser physics involve those electrons in the outer orbitals, and the orders of magnitude of the energies consist of an electron volt or more corresponding to the wavelengths in the near infrared, the visible, and the ultraviolet. Moving closer to the nucleus, transitions involve higher energies corresponding to the far-ultraviolet or gamma emissions and are less favorable for laser action. Energy transitions through vibrational levels involve the vibration of atoms within a molecule when molecules shift from one vibrational state to another, producing distortions of the molecule. These distortions result in transitions that have specific energies of a fraction of an electron volt and correspond to infrared wavelengths. Moreover, rotational levels involving the quantitized rotation of molecules entail energies clinically 0.001 to 0.1 eV and correspond to the far-infrared or submillimeter wavelengths. These latter vibrational and rotational energy transitions are typical of the carbon dioxide laser system (see Chapter 5).

The atomic model fits the description of the generation of laser energy and the description of stimulated emission much easier from a didactic standpoint. In considering our model of the hydrogen atom, as earlier, the visible portion of the hydrogen emission spectrum consists of several wavelengths specific for the element from a deep red color to a blue-green color, ranging from 656 nm to 486 nm, respectively. The diagram of the energy levels of the hydrogen atom has specific allowable energies based on quantum mechanics (Fig. 1–9). In viewing the energy diagram, one plots the energy as increasing upward, as a ladder. However, the spacing between each rung of the ladder is not uniform. Thus, the amount of energy required to transfer from one rung to the next is different. The ground state of the hydrogen atom is -13.6 eV. Others above this state are considered to be excited states, thus having excess energy. In the excited state, the normal process of gaining stability is to move from the state of excitation, for example, from the second stage to the first stage, moving from -1.51 to -3.40 eV. For the electron to do this, it must give up energy in the form of a photon, which has an energy of 1.89 eV or 3.40 to 1.51 eV. This first stage of release of photon energy has a wavelength of 656 nm, which corresponds to the first kind of light, that is, deep red that is produced by the

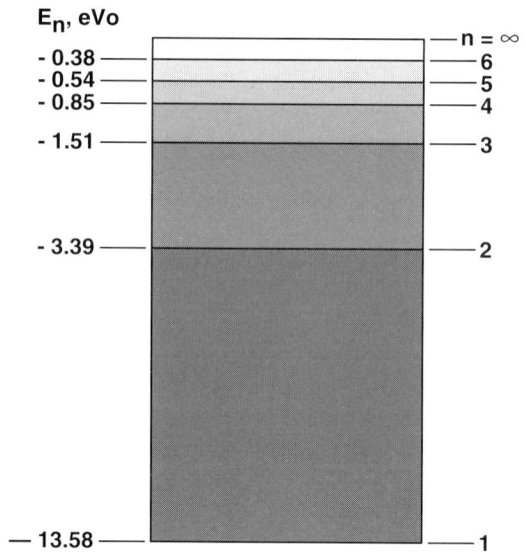

FIGURE 1–9. The energy level diagram specific for hydrogen. Note quantum mechanic acceptable energy levels. The energy is plotted as increasing vertically—the ground state at the lowest level, and the excited states above. Kinetic and electrostatic potential energy of the electron of hydrogen corresponding to each energy level is noted in electron volts. (E_n, increasing energy levels perhaps to infinity; eVo, electron volts.)

hydrogen emission spectrum. If hydrogen is in an excited state by the application of external energy or perhaps by the excitation process internally from another hydrogen atom, the electron in the orbital absorbs this photonic energy and then moves to a second excited state. So the electron would move from -3.40 to -1.15 eV, absorbing 1.89 eV of energy. In quantum mechanics, this can occur only if the absorbed photon has exactly the amount of photonic energy -1.89 because according to the laws of quantum mechanics, there does not exist a state between 3.40 and 1.51 eV. Thus, the loss or emission of a photon occurs for a transition from higher to lower energy states, and absorption of a photon produces a transition from a lower to a higher state (see the sections entitled Spontaneous Emission and Spontaneous Absorption).

Once we consider the energy diagram for an atomic system, external light in the form of a pump light or flash lamp raises the atom from 0, or ground level, to an energy level called E_n (Fig. 1–10). Photons possessing energies equaling the difference between E_n minus 0, or ground state, can accomplish this. The two laser levels U and L correspond to upper and lower levels of energy, respectively. The electrons remain in level U in excitation for longer periods than in the higher energy level B or the lower level L. Electrons rapidly decay from L to 0. In the transition from U to L, the wavelength of laser light is produced. The Y axis corresponds to the small increments of energy input into the

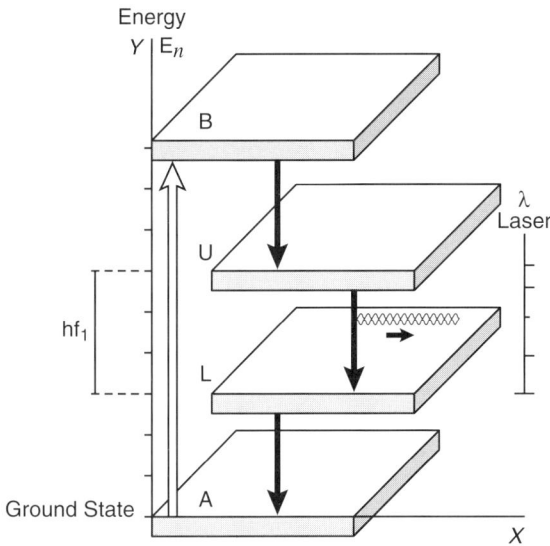

FIGURE 1–10. Energy level diagram representing an atom in a lasant. The ground state is represented by A. An external or internal energy state will pump the atom to level B. It is known that only those photons possessing energies corresponding to the difference between A and B can raise the atomic energy level. The levels relating to the production of laser radiant energy are represented by planes U and L, upper and lower, respectively. Excited species will remain in level U for longer periods than in L or B. E_n, energy level; Planck's constant × frequency = energy of the wavelength.

to hf. (h = Planck's constant, c = speed of light, λ = wavelength)

$$E_\lambda \text{ (photon energy)} = hc/\lambda$$

In the energy diagram for an atom given earlier (see Fig. 1–9), a laser operating at a specific wavelength produces a specific beam that has discrete packets of photon energy that are equivalent; this is in contrast to the broad band of incoherent light from an ordinary light bulb containing many wavelengths and energies, and photonic energies that are not equivalent. If a laser is operating at a wavelength, for example, 1.064 microns, the individual photonic energy remains constant. The surgeon or scientist changes the total energy delivered simply by increasing or decreasing the quantity of photons. In the figure mentioned earlier, the absorption and emission of photonic energy are indicated by vertical arrows, the length of which corresponds to the energies of the photons involved. The optical pumping consists of energizing the active medium with a light source or energy source in the case of optical pumping, a flash lamp or continuous arc lamp with many photons consisting of as large a cohort of photons possessing energies consistent with the energy equal to the ability to pump an atom from the ground level 0 on the X axis to an energy level represented by E_n. The absorption of the population of atoms at ground level making the transition to E_n is then rendered to an excited state.

The potential energy caused by transition from the 0 or ground state to a higher energy level gradually decays to lower energy levels apparently from one quantum level to another, emitting photons each time. The atom resides in a specific quantum level for a given period of time before emitting a photon and then moving to another level. It is important to remain at the upper state of quantum energy for a longer period than either the highest level or the level just before reaching ground level because it enables the laser to be pumped at ever greater levels in a population consisting of the upper, or U, level in the diagram. This particular population of atoms consists of the population that is responsible for the laser beam. Each laser material or active medium is different relative to the amount of time spent on each level. This explains the so-called rise time, or the time it takes for a specific laser medium to be brought up to an energy state such that the number of atoms in an excited state for lasing is much greater than that that exists at lower levels or ground level. Ideally, the atoms should remain at the highest level for a short time and then at the lasing level (U in the diagram); they would remain for a longer period of time there, while at level L, there is a rapid decay or short

system that are quantum allowable energy states for a specific atom or molecule. Quantum mechanics, then, allows only these discrete levels of energy and are not allowed to have energies between these incremental levels. Importantly, in a typical situation under isobaric and isothermal conditions, the atoms within a lasant exist as a large population with the 0 level along the X axis. A transition from the 0 X axis level up the vertical Y coordinate represents an increase in the energy stored within the atomic system. The transition from the X axis ground level to the B level requires photons having precise energies corresponding to the difference between B −0 (ground state). Lasing, or the formation of a laser beam, occurs between levels U and L; photons remain in level U longer than level B or, in fact, L.

As mentioned earlier, it is important to understand that a light beam is regarded alternatively as a stream of discrete particles or photons and that there is a direct relationship between the wavelength of the light and the energy of a photon. This is expressed mathematically as photon energy equals hc/λ, which is equal to the energy of the wavelength. In wave motion, the frequency (f) of the wave is related to its wavelength and velocity by $f = c/\lambda$. This could be expressed as E_λ is equal period to ground level. The objective is to create a large population existing within the U level and lower populations at the E_n, B, and L levels. Ideally, for lasing action to occur, the status of the population in the U level must be greater than that in the L or lower level. When this occurs, it is termed a population inversion.

The physics of quantum mechanics govern all the transitions between various energy states or levels. In the excited states, populations of atoms decay to lower energy levels by making one or a series of quantum mechanically governed or allowed/determined transitions. Thus, there are certain transitions that are probable because atomic transitions are governed by laws of probability, while others are thousands to a million times less likely or so-called forbidden transitions. There are, thus, lifetimes of atoms existing in a particular transition level or the average time an atom exists in the initial state before emitting a photon and, thus, removing itself to a lower state. It may be that in allowable or statistically probable transitions, this would range from 10 to 100 nsec, while for the so-called forbidden transition, the lifetime would be a millisecond to a second, thus a million times longer.

Metastable states, which are states in the upper end of such forbidden transitions, may be important in many lasers because they will hold a species or atom in our example in an excited state for a longer period of time for practical applications. The various states of a species such as atoms and ions at electronic states and molecules by vibrational and rotational determinants are independent. However, they can change simultaneously in a single transition. In the case of atoms or ions in electronic transitions, these occur independently because these particles do not have vibrational and rotational states as in molecular species. In the molecular species, however, changes in vibrational states are accompanied by similar changes in rotational states. There are important differences between transitions involving shifts in only one kind of energy level and those involving simultaneous shifts between two or more types. In atoms or ions, such transitions between electronic energy levels are defined definitively at a specific wavelength. There is practical importance in this distinction because if a series of shifts occurs simultaneously as in molecular species, the transitional rate occurs over a range of wavelengths, and this is exemplified in the carbon dioxide and dye lasers, which produce a series of discrete lines in the EM spectrum, appearing as such in the carbon dioxide laser or as a continuum in the dye laser.

Spontaneous Absorption, Spontaneous Emission, and Stimulated Emission

Einstein demonstrated three related physical phenomena in 1917, which after a long period, found practical application in laser research and technology. These processes were defined as spontaneous emission, spontaneous absorption, and stimulated emission (Fig. 1–11). Excited species can release their excess energy to nonradiative processes such as collisions with other atoms or molecules in which such excess energy may be released in the form of heat, or by the emission of photons.

Spontaneous Emission

Consider the atomic system energy diagram in which an atom in level U emits at random a photon of energy hf in any direction and then drops to the lower energy state. Then there is a rapid decay to ground level. Therefore, spontaneous emission can occur when a species without the application of external energy falls from a higher energy level or higher state of excitation to a lower state and energy is spontaneously transmitted as EM radiation. This kind of emission occurs after a natural decay time, usually within nsec, and the frequency of such spontaneously emitted radiation, thus, its energy, is directly proportional to the difference between the higher U level and the lower L energy levels.

Spontaneous Absorption

Spontaneous absorption, on the other hand, occurs if an atom in level L absorbs a photon of energy hf or an incoming photon. In this case, the energy level of the atomic system is elevated from the L level to the U level. Thus, the incident energy is absorbed because the frequency of incoming radiation in the form of photons is proportional to the difference between the ground state and the excited state. Thus, in stimulated absorption, the atomic system is in the lower energy state absorbing a photon whose energy is exactly equal to the differential between U level and L level, thus raising the atom to a higher energy state.

In spontaneous emission, thermodynamic principles dictate the essential conditions in which species tend to remain at or drop to the lowest available energy level. At isobaric and isothermal equilibrium, a species is in the ground state, as earlier. The ground state population is then governed by increases in its energy. At equilibrium, the large cohort of the population of a species in the upper energy states is much smaller than that in the lowest energy state. At equilibrium then, the large numeric cohort of species possessing the lowest energy state results in a condition in which the stimulation of emission from the prevailing low level to higher levels could occur. It is, thus, more probable that any emitted photon would be absorbed by a lower energy level species than that it would result in

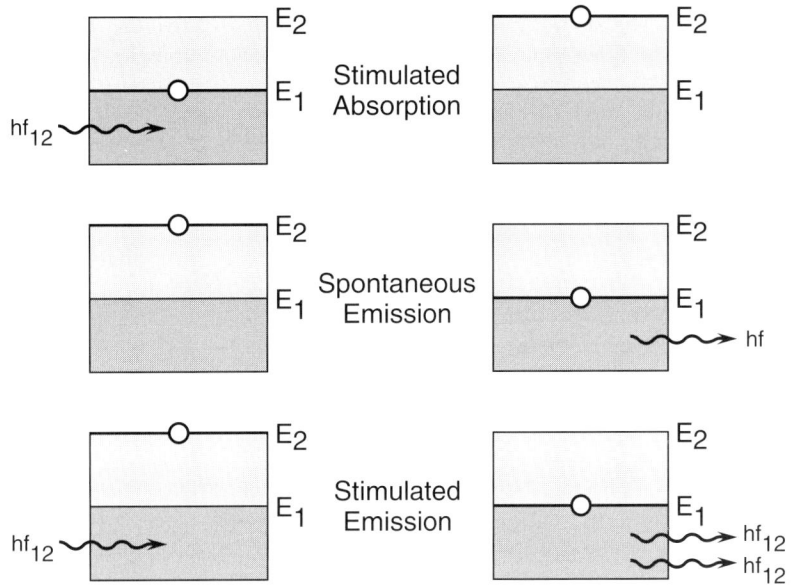

FIGURE 1–11. Processes of atomic transitions: Stimulated absorption, absorption of a photon of light of precisely the appropriate energy, raises the electron from lower energy state E_1 to an excited state E_2; spontaneous emission, an atom releases a photon without provocation as the electron falls from the higher to a lower energy state; stimulated emission, a photon of the identical radiant energy strikes an excited atom causing the emanation of a second identical photon in phase with the first photon and traveling in an identical direction. (hf, Planck's constant $\times$ frequency = energy of wavelength; hf_{12}, relative power of wavelength.)

stimulated emission from a species in a higher energy state.

Stimulated Emission and Population Inversion

A prerequisite for the origin of laser radiation is Einstein's concept of stimulated emission. Stimulated emission can occur if a species can be induced to possess a population existing in the higher energy levels, quantitatively considerably larger than those of the lower levels. This is considered to be a population inversion in a laser medium and is a fundamental prerequisite for laser action involving any species. Such excitation or population inversion occurs by several maneuvers and involves the input of energy into the active medium usually contained within the confined space of a resonator or laser cavity. The phenomenon of laser medium excitation involves the absorption of photons from an external or internal energy source. Collisions between electrons, ions, or other species within the laser medium and recombination of free electrons with ionized atoms and other mechanisms involving chemical reactions produce these excited species and also recombination of common carriers in a semiconductor and acceleration of electrons. All these processes lead to a population inversion. An incoming photon of energy hf can stimulate an atom in an excited state U to emit an extra photon, also at hf, then drop to the state L. The emitted photon travels directionally the same as the incoming photon and is in phase or in step with it in space and time. Assuredly, if the population of atoms within the L level are greater than those of the U level, then

under ordinary conditions, absorption prevails and the incoming light photons are absorbed. However, in contradistinction, if the population of the U level is greater than that of the L level, a state of excitation or population inversion and then stimulated emission prevails and the light waves will grow in intensity or brightness, experiencing gain rather than loss; thus a laser beam is formed.

Any species has an ability to absorb energy by the mechanism described earlier and indicated by measurements of what is known as absorption cross-section. These excitation probabilities or cross-sections involve such factors as the wavelength of the illuminating light, speed of incident electrons, or coincidences in the energy level structure of the species. Excitation is often a multiphasic phenomenon. One can point to carbon dioxide commonly used as a gas within the resonator cavity, but the elements nitrogen and helium also are essential for the lasing action to occur. Similarly, in the case of the helium:neon laser, electrons are passed through the active medium and transfer energy to the helium atoms, which, in turn, transfer the absorbed energy into less abundant neon atoms, which then emit the laser light.

To sum up, population inversion is critically dependent on radiative transitions within atoms, the processes in which an atom either absorbs or emits light—the three processes described by Einstein as stimulated absorption, spontaneous emission, and stimulated emission. In a laser medium in an active process, all three phenomena occur simultaneously, but it is stimulated emission that is critical for the lasing process. To understand population inversion, it is important to distinguish between these three phenomena. The simple line figure (see Fig. 1–11) shows that in the simplest energy state the ideal atom possesses two energy levels described as E_1 and E_2. In the case of stimulated absorption, the atom is initially in a lower state of energy and will absorb a photon whose energy is exactly equal to the difference between E_2 and E_1, and this will raise the atom to a higher energy state by means of this stimulated absorption. In spontaneous emission, the atom exists in a higher energy state and will, by a transition lifetime specific for that element, gradually drop to a lower energy level and emit a photon in the process. This photon is equal to the energy between E_1 and E_2, thus describing spontaneous emission.

Finally, if an atom exists in an already stimulated state or excited state during its time of transition to spontaneously drop to a lower energy level, a photon may come along of the energy exactly equivalent to that which the atom is waiting to emit. It is thought that a kind of resonance occurs between this external photon and the stimulated atom in which the atom emits a photon before it would have normally done so and, thus, is stimulated by the passing photon to emit its own photon of light earlier. The important thing to realize is that the emitted photon and the passing photon are absolutely identical in phase temporally and spatially, having the same wavelength, direction, and polarization. It could be stated that the statistical probability of an impact of an excited species by a photon possessing identical energy precisely equivalent to the transitional energy of that given species moving into a lower energy level is marginal at best, especially in the extraordinarily limited time observed as an excited species spontaneously resumes its lower energy level. However, useful laser media possess a population of such energy equivalent photons by the process of spontaneous emission, and this cohort of photons could initiate stimulated emission of other photons, thus resulting in an ever-increasing proliferation of stimulated emissions. Stimulated emission is essential for the lasing phenomenon and results in two photons of identical energy as earlier, emanating from the species of the lasing medium, traveling along the laser axis cavity, where they stimulate nearby already excited atoms that emit identical photons traveling in the same direction within the active medium.

CASCADE PROCESS OCCURS

In this process, photons travel parallel to the axis of the cylinder, and these have a far greater statistical probability of encountering other excited atoms and stimulating them to emit their energy leading to the ability of the photons to travel down the cylinder. This cascade process leads to amplification of light, which is characteristic of lasing action. A cascade of light that is parallel with the long axis of the laser cavity forms a collimated beam of intense radiant energy that is monochromatic, being emitted from the end of the laser cavity. The laser light is emitted from the cylinder in a beam that is in phase, both in space and time, and that is highly disciplined and, thus, coherent, which means that the wave forms are synchronized or in phase.

Thus, the singular requirement for laser activity and the production of radiant energy via a laser device, is the phenomenon of population inversion. In a population inversion, there are more atoms in a given excited state than in the next lower state. Power must be input by an artificial means to produce such a phenomenon in the active medium, because such a state is a paranormal condition. The principles of spontaneous absorption, spontaneous emission, and stimulated emission compete as existing phenomena in a laser cavity. Stimulated absorption and spontaneous emission depend on the number of atoms in the upper energy levels while stimulated emission depends on the number of atoms in the lower energy levels. Physics has shown us that under isobaric, isothermal conditions, the quantity of atoms in the lower energy state far outnumbers those in the upper energy states. For a population inversion to exist, at least two conditions must be overcome. Stimulated emission must predominate over stimulated absorption, producing more atoms in a laser medium in an excited state than in the state at lower energy levels. If the quantity is not high enough, then those photons that are emitted will be absorbed by atoms in lower energy levels. Qualitatively to produce lasing action, a prerequisite is to have more emission occurring than absorption. The process of stimulated emission must also counteract or predominate over spontaneous emission. To achieve this kind of result, the higher order lasing transition must be in a metastable state, as discussed earlier. In a metastable state, an excited atom will not quickly emit its photon as a spontaneous emission. This means that a stimulated photon, prior to the transition spontaneously from the higher state of an atom existing within the so-called metastable state, causes the metastable atom to emit another photon by stimulated emission because the metastable atom is able to remain in the excited state long enough to ensure such a proper photon of the correct wavelength to interact with it. A laser beam, thus, is produced of a coherency, directionality, and all the properties discussed concerning the attributes of such a radiant beam of energy.

A host of lasant materials are chosen consisting of species that sustain inverted energy populations, that is, energy states greater than ground state, and possess metastable states at the high end of the lasing transition. Examples of these are chromium, Nd, argon, neon, and ruby media, in which a population of species possessing higher energy levels than ground state will predominate the cohort of species of the ground state levels, inducing a population inversion of that specific lasant. A result of the inversion is that a photon of the energy of transition would be more probable to stimulate emission from the state of excitation than to be absorbed by the lower energy state. The result often is referred to by physicists as laser gain or amplification, that is, the difference between stimulated emission and absorption at that specific wavelength. Gain is a term that is a quantification of the percentage increase passed through the laser medium, per centimeter of distance through the medium, or indeed, the number of added photons generated per centimeter of laser medium. Laser gain is directly proportional to the difference between the probability of stimulated emission and the probability of absorption. Population inversions cease to exist if the lower levels of energy are not depopulated while the higher level is constantly quantitatively populated.

INDUCING POPULATION INVERSION BY PUMPING

The term pumping as used in laser technology means providing adequate energy to the species within a lasing medium in a form that induces them to proceed to a higher energy level or excited state, thus inverting the population of atoms from ground level to an excitation level. There are numerous methodologies of pumping laser media, such as optical, electrical discharge, radio frequency, chemical excitation, electron beam, using one laser to excite or pump another, and other more exotic methodologies such as alternating magnetic fields used in the free-electron laser and nuclear reactions

employed by x-ray lasers. As mentioned earlier, optical pumping seems to be better understood and is the prototype that a number of important lasers are based on. Using a flash lamp or intense incoherent radiation energy the ruby, the Nd:YAG laser, and electrical lasers of importance in maxillofacial surgery are the argon, carbon dioxide, and helium neon lasers. Other gas lasers including the helium:neon and carbon dioxide can be excited by manipulation of radio frequency. Diode lasers are often used to pump solid-state lasers, such as the Nd:YAG laser.

Although optical pumping using an external flash lamp is easy to describe, the physical mechanisms involved are complex. To begin, optical pumping is the application of external power in the form of radiant energy and involves the exposure of the active medium to this energy. The pumping mechanism that is achieved occurs in multiple stages or tiers. In the case of the Nd:YAG laser, some of the radiant light from the flash lamp is absorbed by the Nd ions in the YAG crystal. The Nd ions then are excited from their ground state to a state of excitation. In most cases, ions are pumped to the highest excitation tier and very quickly or spontaneously decay to the next lower state, all the time emitting photons at random. The important result is that the ions de-excite to a metastable state, and as mentioned earlier, they can remain so until an ion spontaneously emits a photon along the long axis of the crystal rod. This is the beginning of the process whereby the cascade phenomenon can produce stimulated emission via a photon being stimulated along the long axis of the rod, producing two identical photons that also continue along the axis of the rod and onward until two become four, four become eight, and the process continues, a process similar to that which occurs within a resonant cavity (Fig. 1–12). It is important to note that the ions that are stimulated or excited will be pumped to that excited state that is on a level higher than most other excited states of that ion. If they remain in the

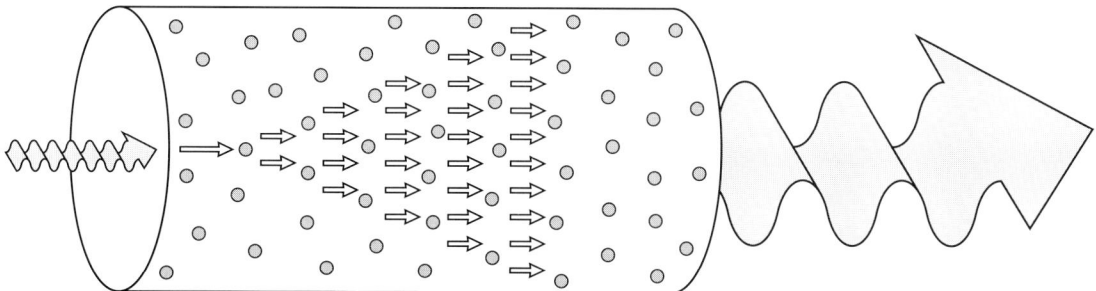

FIGURE 1–12. Stimulated emission in which radiant photons move longitudinally along the axis of the laser chamber and stimulate other proximal excited atoms to also emit additional identical photons that will travel with the same directionality as the other stimulated photons within the laser chamber. This is the cascade phenomenon, which is the sine qua non of laser radiation.

higher excited state for a long time, there is a probability of their being caused to emit by stimulated emission and dropping down to the actual ground state. It has been observed that during the end of the energy produced by the flash lamp, rather than ions moving to a high energy level, those in the higher level could actually be stimulated to de-excite. A population inversion is not achieved in this way.

Optical pumping, or most other physical pumping for that matter, is always to an unstable or metastable state. This metastable state is the next highest energy level, or tier, indicated. In this way, as mentioned earlier, the ions rest in this transitional state until being stimulated to emit by stimulated emission via a photon of the correct wavelength. The importance of the very unstable upper tier energy level and the second phase or metastable state in the active medium is that nearly every ion that is excited by pumping will end up in the second state or metastable state transition, which enables them to be available for stimulated emission. Each of the active laser media that is optically stimulated or pumped has its own unique number of tiers on which excited ions or atoms are stimulated to await higher excitation or decay to lower excitation levels or ground level. Therefore, if other states of the energy exist below the metastable state, then the energy required for optical pumping or the ease with which atoms can be pumped to metastable state may be easier in those instances in which the active medium has a tier or energy level below the metastable state that is not ground level. To pump from the ground level up to the metastable or the higher excitation levels is simply harder from the standpoint of energy input in time versus a level just below the metastable state in which the atoms or ions can be pumped very rapidly to the metastable state. This is a characteristic of the Nd:YAG laser, in which there are at least four known levels: higher energy, metastable, intermediate, and ground. There is a higher energy level prior to the metastable level in which fast decay occurs to the metastable level, then a transition that occurs from the metastable to an intermediate level. This intermediate level enables the Nd:YAG laser to be excited from the intermediate level above the ground state more rapidly, and therefore, the population inversion is achieved with greater ease.

Amplification

Amplification or oscillation is what is critical in the process called optical feedback. Amplification produced by stimulated emission is enhanced if the laser apparatus can reflect the photons along the longitudinal axis of the active medium within the cavity so they can produce even more stimulated emissions. As described earlier, this optical feedback is produced by causing the photons to bounce between mirrors placed on either side of the optical cavity. Within the optical or laser cavity, there is initially no EM radiation. This occurs only if the medium is pumped to the population inversion, where the atoms then emit spontaneously producing photons. These photons are multidirectional, and a great deal of the photons emanate away from the cavity and are thermally lost. The smaller number of photons mentioned earlier produced by spontaneous emission will travel perpendicular to the bounding mirrors remaining within the cavity, thus providing a constant source of continuing stimulated emission. As the light continues to reflect back and forth making round trips within the laser cavity (as many as 50 trips before being emitted through one of the partially reflective mirrors), the light is coherently amplified by this process. This constant stimulation by rebounding photons enabling stimulation of other species to emit other photons is the amplification part of the word laser. The actual beam of laser radiation that is generated within the laser cavity occurs because a fraction of the spontaneous emissions travel perpendicular to the mirrors and remain within the cavity; this fraction of spontaneous emission is the source of stimulated emission. The parallel mirror at the ends of the resonator chamber consist of a planar output mirror and a concave mirror. The mirrors focus the beam to a point outside the chamber. The planar mirror allows a portion of this light to escape the laser cavity through a number of design characteristics. The mirrors then provide a positive feedback mechanism by continual reflections, which is theoretically an infinite amplification system. This is practically impossible owing to losses from the cavity that restrict feedback and the degree of amplification by mirrors, thus coherently amplifying these perpendicular photons at the speed of light (3×10^8 meters per second) and enabling the laser to be pumped within nanoseconds.

Modes

When the nonplanar mirror is used, such a curved mirror creates wave fronts within the laser cavity that have finite radii of curvature that can produce noncircular beam profiles. These cross-sectional beam profiles are called transverse EM modes, or TEMs. The lower the mode pattern or TEM, and the smaller the spot size and the focal point of any given lens, then the longer the depth of focus for the particular spot size. The TEM mode or cross-sectional views of the beam affect the minimum spot size and the selectivity of the power density or irradiance that is available or chosen. Because the TEM_{00} mode is a smaller focused spot size, it is a desirable mode for surgical applications. Transverse EM modes describe the distribution of radiant energy across the beam profile or diameter and determine the distribution of the laser light within the beam and the nature of the beam focus. The TEM distribution determines whether or not the laser focus will occur at a precise circular pattern or form several patches of radiance distributed over a large area (Fig. 1–13). The TEM_{00} mode, or fundamental mode, has a gaussian distribution within the beam profile (Fig. 1–14). This means that this particular mode can be focused to the smallest possible spot of any of the transverse modes. The focus of the laser depends on the divergence of the beam and the angle by which the laser can deviate from true parallelism; collimation is defined by the equation $\Theta = 4 \times \lambda/\pi \ D_m$, where D_m is equal to the minimum beam diameter. The gaussian beam and its spot size can be calculated by the equation:

$$D = 4f\lambda/\pi D_m = F\Theta, \text{ where}$$

$$F = \text{lens focal length,}$$
$$D_m = \text{beam diameter at waist,}$$
$$\lambda = \text{laser wavelength}$$

The beam parameters can be elucidated in Figure 1–15, where one can see a beam parameter diagram showing the lens, the depth of focus, the focused spot size and focal length, and divergence of the beam. Although it is important to have a single-mode laser focused to the theoretically smallest spot size for that given wavelength, single-mode operation is not always feasible and the beam profile may be irregular in its shape. The irregular profile is referred to as multimode and may provide

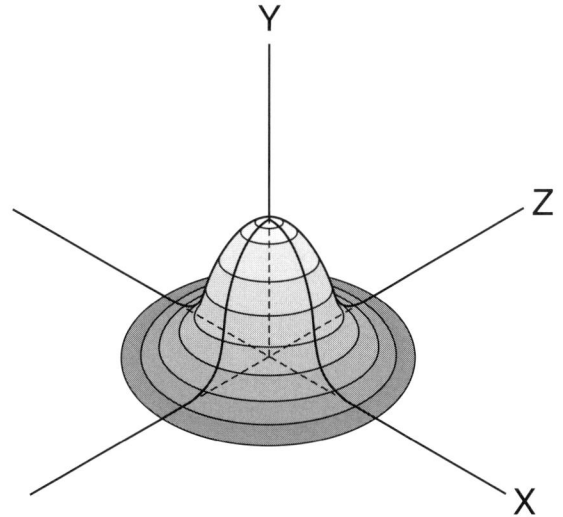

FIGURE 1–14. Three-dimensional representation of the gaussian beam profile produced by the fundamental mode. Shading of diagram shows a decrease in tissue effect as distance from the center increases.

higher energy levels that are required for operations other than tissue incision but may be more effective for debulking large tumors. In the design of the laser apparatus, it is not appropriate to consider the actual focal spot of a laser beam produced by a lens as that spot size that will be measurable on the tissue surface. Photobiology dictates that the actual spot size one observes on the substance of tissue is, in the main, larger than the spot size produced by the optics of the laser system. This larger spot produced on tissue is due to thermal conductivity from the impact site in a concentric manner. The spot size that is operationally effective is really the area of vaporization or photothermally affected tissue zone, which is dependent on the application and the specific mode of operation of the laser device.

In summary, the quality of a laser beam is characterized by at least two distinct types of modes, either transverse or longitudinal. Transverse modes define the nature of the cross-sectional profile of the beam or its pattern of intensity. Longitudinal modes are studied and are important in unusual applications in spectroscopy and communications but have little use in surgical applications. The TEM cross-sectional profiles directly affect the minimum spot size of the beam and thus the power density or irradiance produced by a laser. The reader is referred to the work of Fox and Li,[20] in which transverse modes are classified according to the number of nulls or the lack of presence of a laser beam that appear across the beam in two directions. The lowest order, or fundamental mode, TEM_{00}, describes a gaussian distribution in which

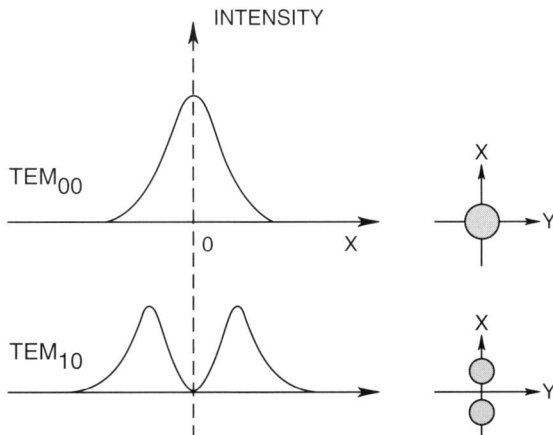

FIGURE 1–13. Schematics of transverse electromagnetic modes. Plotted diagrams on left are representative of laser focal spots produced at right.

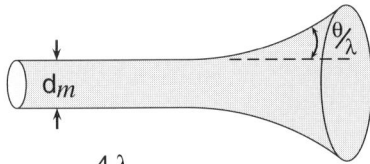

$$\theta = \frac{4\lambda}{\pi d_m}$$

λ = laser wavelength

d_m = beam diameter

BEAM DIVERGENCE SCHEMATIC

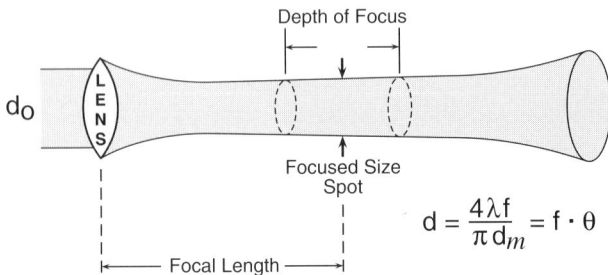

Depth of Focus

Focused Size
Spot

$$d = \frac{4\lambda f}{\pi d_m} = f \cdot \theta$$

Focal Length

BEAM DIAMETER SCHEMATIC

FIGURE 1–15. Beam divergence and beam diameter schematic (see text). (Redrawn after Fuller TA: Physics of surgical lasers. Lasers Surg Med 1:5–14, 1980. Copyright © 1980, John Wiley & Sons, Inc. Reprinted by permission of John Wiley & Sons, Inc.)

the intensity is greatest at the center and corresponds to the smallest focus spot size, and therefore is the mode that has significant application in maxillofacial surgery.

APPLICATION OF LASER POWER IN SURGERY

Continuous-Wave/Pulsed Lasers

Lasers are generally named by using the name of the active medium or lasant. It has been mentioned that the applied lasers in oral and maxillofacial surgery include the carbon dioxide, the Nd:YAG, the argon, and the holmium:YAG. In view of the disparate nature of these lasers, they can be operated in several different ways. In addition to the nature of the lasant, lasers are classified by their power output and wavelength. Laser radiant energy can be generated from a laser device in a continuous form or continuous wave (CW), or by discreet or single pulses or multiple timed pulses, termed pulsed modes. Most of the continuous-wave lasers can be operated in a so-called gated manner, thus permitting the inherently low power of the continuous-wave laser to be transmitted to tissue in bursts of radiant energy. The specific operation of a continuous-wave laser and its energy properties used in a pulsed mode are different than those of a specifically designed pulsed laser. In the pulsed laser, the energy that is incident on tissue is greater, and

each pulse is of shorter duration, typically under a millisecond compared with a continuous-wave laser.

For example, carbon dioxide lasers can be designed to be automatically set on so-called chopped pulse or chopped mode to deliver radiant energy to tissue in increments, thus avoiding thermal damage or conduction through nontarget tissue and allowing time for tissue cooling between energy bursts or pulses. The superpulse mode was developed to decrease thermal injury enhanced by cooling, providing higher peak powers within shorter duty cycles, that is, the ratio of time the laser beam has tissue contact versus the total time of the event. Within the industry, every new design of carbon dioxide laser has been developed or designed to decrease collateral thermal tissue damage and produce a char-free result. An example is UltraPulse, developed by Coherent Laser of Palo Alto, California. This mode is capable of delivering up to 250 to 300 millijoules of energy per pulse during a pulse of only a fraction of a millisecond. The quality of UltraPulse will allow true single-pulse tissue ablation, and the higher pulse energy results in the coldest, most char-free tissue response with the least amount of collateral thermal damage, indeed, as little as 50 microns, of those lasers in this category employing the chopped mode and superpulse. The reader is referred to a case report by Nazhat and Hazhat in which the UltraPulse was used in the treatment of endometriosis and laparoscopic-assisted vaginal hysterectomy.[21]

Both the continuous-wave and pulsed lasers can

be operated under a variant of pulse mode termed Q-switching. The Q-switching mode usually is permitted by using a fast shutter between the lasant and one of the mirrors. By closing the shutter of the resonant cavity, the energy within will tend to increase to magnitudes much higher than the threshold levels usually achieved with the shutter open. By this methodology, the energy within the resonant cavity can be increased in nanoseconds. Radiant energy can be released in a very short time upon opening the aperture of the shutter. This methodology has permitted energy several orders of magnitude higher than occurs without Q-switching, and the resulting laser beam is referred to as a giant pulse.[22]

Power Density

Power density is the most important factor in determining the effectiveness of any laser device. Power density coupled with power/time characteristics and the wavelength governs the ultimate effectiveness of the laser in surgical applications. As mentioned earlier, the quality of the laser beam, its transverse EM mode, is also critical in producing an appropriate configuration of the laser spot. To enhance the effectiveness of the laser beam diameter and to provide an increase in power, a coaxial focusing lens can reduce the diameter of the spot to produce greater power densities, thus enhancing tissue effects of the laser. It is easy to recognize that the power density will ultimately determine the ability of the laser to vaporize, excise, and coagulate biologic tissue.

To calculate power density expressed in watts per square centimeter, it can be shown that the power density (PD) is directly proportional to the wattage employed and inversely proportional to the area of the spot. Therefore

$$PD = \frac{Watts \times 100}{\pi R^2}$$

In the practical application of lasers, the PD is really a function of the spot size of the incident laser beam on the target tissue and the applied laser power in watts. This power in watts is determined by the surgeon, and the spot size is determined by the focal length of the coaxial lens selected by the surgeon either on the handpiece system or using the focal length of the lens system of a laser that is coaxial with a microscope. Moreover, the PD also depends on the TEM of the beam and characteristic wavelength of the laser. One can observe a direct proportional relationship between the focal length of the lens and the spot size of the beam, so that smaller focal sizes result in more intense power

density. An example of this is a carbon dioxide laser used with a microscope with a 400-mm focal length lens. The spot size is 0.8 mm as contrasted with a 50-mm lens, which will produce a spot size of 2.0 mm.

The characteristic wavelength of the laser and the actual absorption spectrum of biologic tissue that is its target will influence the percentage of the incident beam that actually is absorbed and causes biologic change. It is obvious that the higher the absorption of the tissue and the presence of tissue chromophores, compounds such as hemoglobin and melanin, as well as other biologic factors, for example, circulation or blood flow through a given tissue, the more effective the laser will be in producing surgical results. It has been mentioned that the size of the spot of the incident beam depends on the wavelength characteristic of the radiant energy produced by a given laser, so that focusing is directly related to the wavelength that is characteristic for that laser.

It can be demonstrated that shorter wavelengths result in smaller spot sizes if one keeps all other variables equal. Notably, the kind of laser one selects for a given procedure depends on the desired effects on the nature of the tissue disorder and its delivery system as opposed to its spot size only. An example of this is that the surgeon can obtain a much smaller spot size with an argon laser, again related to its smaller spot size as opposed to the larger spot size obtained with the carbon dioxide laser associated with its much larger wavelength. The two lasers are each selected to solve different surgical problems. Generally, the carbon dioxide laser is used to incise, excise, and vaporize certain lesions, whereas the argon laser is selected to have a specific tissue effect; that is, fibrosis of angiodysplasias that are deep to the epithelial surface of the skin. Most of the time, the transverse EM mode selected is the most fundamental, so that the most power is at the center of the beam (gaussian), thus producing very fine spots. Manipulation of the laser beam by the surgeon changes the diameter of the spot size and thus its effect on tissue. The surgeon also can change the time spent on tissue by the laser beam by simple modalities such as wiggling the beam, crosshatching, focusing, and defocusing.

ENERGY DENSITY

Energy density defines the power/time characteristics that determine the extent of tissue vaporization or coagulation. Not only are photobiologic effects determined by the impact of total power in watts of a given laser, but such tissue effects are also dependent on the power density and time of application. When using pulsed laser systems, power/time functions are extremely important. The surgeon can manipulate them directly on the console of the laser unit. The laser radiant exposure is measured in joules per square centimeter, which is calculated by multiplying power density and watts per square centimeter times the exposure time in seconds. The surgeon thus controls the total exposure of the target tissue to laser radiant energy, varying the power density and total radiant energy in joules by a factor of time.

To sum up, the oral and maxillofacial surgeon can control the amount of impact of the laser beam on target tissue by varying the power output of the laser in watts, the cross-sectional area of the spot, and the exposure time. The qualitative nature of the spot can also be controlled by use of an appropriate transverse electromagnetic mode. In most systems, as an example the carbon dioxide device, the output of power from the laser can be varied from milliwattages up to one hundred watts. The laser beam or area of the spot is controlled by changing the focal length of the lens, as mentioned in carbon dioxide systems, from 50 to 400 mm, with spot sizes of 2.0 to 0.8 mm, respectively. Spot sizes can also be varied by uncoupling or placing an appropriate lens system on a carbon dioxide handpiece. Selection of a smaller spot size for any wattage of power enhances the power density. The surgeon also can vary the cross-sectional area of the beam by working in and out of focus using focused or defocused modes. Moreover, in carbon dioxide devices, the incident beam first converges to its focal point on the tissue, governed by the lens, and then diverges. The surgeon can thus enlarge the spot size, thus lowering the power density for a given wattage.

An important concept in reducing thermal damage to collateral healthy tissue is to select the optimal power density as the highest value that can be safely controlled by the surgeon. It is useful to consider that contiguous tissue damage is directly proportional to the time of application of the beam and not specifically to the total wattage employed. This concept applies only where the power density is greater than 100 watts per square centimeter, because less than 100 watts per square centimeter is considered ineffectual. The longer the application of the beam, the greater the amount of total energy delivered to the tissue. The consequences of total energy are perceived either at the time of application or after surgery. Therefore, using the highest power density manageable with the shortest duration of application, the least collateral damage is observed. The time of exposure can be varied by using the continuous wave in single pulses or by using repetitive pulsed modes with pulse duration of one twentieth to one half of a second. Considering the use of continuous-pulsed lasers, the im-portant specification is usually expressed in terms of average power in watts, pulse repetition rate (PPS), and single pulse duration in seconds. From these data, the duty cycle can be derived.

Irradiance, Radiant Exposure, and Fluence

The power density that is expressed as the incident power per unit of area is also termed irradiance and is expressed also in watts per square centimeter. Radiant exposure or exposure dose is the total radiant energy incident on area target tissue per unit of tissue, and this is expressed in joules per square centimeter. The term fluence is used when a tissue surface is radiated by scattered laser energy as in photochemotherapy. Exposure dose or radiant energy often is referred to as fluence, whose units are expressed as joules per square centimeter. The power density or dose rate also is expressed as the fluence rate, which also uses the unit of watts per square centimeter. Fluence and fluence rate are in practical terms impossible to quantitate. The terms fluence and fluence rate are thought to be less accurate than the terms radiant exposure and irradiance. Apparently fluence has been used interchangeably with the more accurate term radiant exposure. The carbon dioxide laser, a device used in many types of oral maxillofacial surgery, is absorbed by a few cell layers; however, deeply penetrating laser energy is greatly scattered, and the concept of fluence then becomes more appropriate.

REFERENCES

1. Einstein A: Zur Quanten Theorie der Stralung. Phys Zeit 18:121, 1917.
2. Bertolotti M: Masers and Lasers. Bristol, Adam Hilger, 1983.
3. Maiman TH: Stimulated optical radiation in ruby. Nature 187:493–494, 1960.
4. Patel CKN, Faust WL, McFarlane RA: CW Laser action on rotational transitions of the Σu^+-Σg^+ vibrational band of CO_2. Bull Am Phys Soc 9:500, 1964.
5. Patel CKN, Tien PK, McFee JH: CW high power CO_2-N_2-H_3 laser. Appl Phys Lett 7:290–292, 1965.
6. Johnson LF: Optical maser characteristics of rare-earth ions in crystal. J Appl Physiol 34:897–909, 1961.
7. Dikuzono N, Joffe SN: Artificial sapphire probe for contact photocoagulation and tissue vaporization with the Nd:YAG laser. Med Instr 19:173–178, 1985.
8. Bridges WB: Laser oscillation in singly ionized argon in the visible spectrum. Appl Phys Lett 4:124–130, 1964.
9. Bridges WB: Ionized gas lasers. *In* Weber MJ (ed): CRC Handbook of Laser Science and Technology, Vol 2, Gas Lasers. Boca Raton, Florida, CRC Press, 1982, pp 171–269.
10. Arndt D, Noe JM: Lasers in dermatology. Arch Dermatol 118:293–295, 1982.
11. Dixon JA, Huether S, Rotering R: Hypertrophic scarring in argon laser treatment of port wine stains. Plast Reconstr Surg 73:771–779, 1984.

12. Shelnitz L, Garden JM: Applications of lasers for skin disorders. Comprehen Therap 18(9):28–31, 1982.
13. Gladstone GJ, Beckman H: Argon laser treatment of an eyelid margin capillary hemangioma. Ophthalmic Surg 14:944, 1983.
14. Tan OT, Carney M, Margolis R, et al: Histologic Response of Port-Wine Stains Treated by Argon, Carbon Dioxide, and Tunable Dye Lasers. Arch Dermatol 121:1016–1022, 1986.
15. Meller MM: Introduction to lasers. *In* Sherk HH (ed): Lasers in Orthopaedics. Philadelphia, J. B. Lippincott, 1990.
16. Trauner K, Nichioka N, Patel D: Pulsed Holmium: Yttrium-Aluminum-Garnet (Ho:YAG) Laser Ablation of Fibrocartilage and Articular Cartilage. Am J Sports Med 18:316, 1990.
17. Hendler BH, Gateno J, Mooar P, Sherk HH: Holmium YAG laser arthroscopy of the temporomandibular joint. J Oral Maxillofac Surg 50:931–934, 1992.
18. Fuller TA: The physics of surgical lasers. Laser Surg Med 1:514, 1980.
19. Carruth J, McKenzie AL: Medical Lasers, Science and Clinical Practice. Bristol and London, Adam Hilgar, Ltd., 1988.
20. Fox AG, Li T: Resonant modes in a laser interferometer. Bell System Tech J 40:453, 1961.
21. Nazhat C, Hazhat F: Treatment of endometriosis and laparoscopic assisted hysterectomy with the ultrapulse surgical laser: A case report. Update in GYN Laser Surgery. 1:140.5, 1991.
22. Dixon JA: Surgical Application of Lasers, 2nd ed. Chicago, IL, Year Book Medical Publishers, Inc, 1987.

CHAPTER 2

Photobiology of Lasers in Oral and Maxillofacial Surgery

GUY A. CATONE, DMD
EDWARD HALUSIC JR, DMD

A salient property of light and laser radiant energy (photons possessing high energy) is the results of its interaction with biologic tissues. The field of study involving the interactions of nonionizing electromagnetic radiation with biomolecules, and the resulting biologic reactions, is known as *photobiology*. The reaction of radiant energy with organic tissues depends on the nature of the light or that portion of the electromagnetic spectrum that has impacted the tissues, and on the character of the tissues so exposed. All photobiologic effects are both wavelength and dose dependent. The major reactions of laser radiant energy with living tissues involve photocoagulation, photovaporization, photochemical, and photophysical phenomena (Fig. 2–1). Claims reported in the literature assert comparatively low-energy lasers have a salubrious effect on wound healing.

The consequences of the incident laser radiant energy on biologic tissues, including skin, mucosa, odontogenic structures, and bone, is the result of a photobiologic tissue reaction and a photophysical reaction. The outcome of the photophysical event can be apparent in a microsecond; however, the final long-term reaction of laser-radiated tissue may be apparent only after some months. Tissue responses to laser radiation can be considered to be thermal or nonthermal processes. Thermal laser effects are known as *photocoagulation* and *photovaporization*. Nonthermal laser effects are related to a photomechanical response or to a photochemical phenomenon. What is observed as tissue laser ef-

fects are the result of the deposition of radiant energy and the manner in which such energy is manipulated, including the volume of tissue affected. Each category of laser exhibits different biologic effects; therefore, different ones are employed for different applications. Lasers are responsible for common tissue responses that the oral and maxillofacial surgeon must understand when laser radiation is incident on tissue.

When the surgeon chooses to lase skin or mucosa, these structures become the site for laser-induced photobiologic reactions; the optical properties of skin and mucous membrane must affect the response or outcome. The light energy must necessarily transfer through the stratum corneum before affecting involved tissues (Fig. 2–2). Thus, the variable thickness of the stratum corneum, its changes in a host of keratotic lesions, and its composition and morphology govern the deeper effects of the laser energy. When the stratum corneum is penetrated, lesional tissue is encountered, and the path of the light energy undergoes several alterations. It is absorbed, scattered, transmitted, or reflected by the anatomy of the tissues and existing chromophores such as melanin, oxygenated and reduced hemoglobin, and bilirubin, which are known to vary dynamically and among individuals (see Fig. 5–15). In the final analysis, qualitative understanding of the interaction and transfer of light radiation in skin and mucosa of photobiologic reactions induced by thermal light energy or photochemically mediated reactions enables the laser sur-

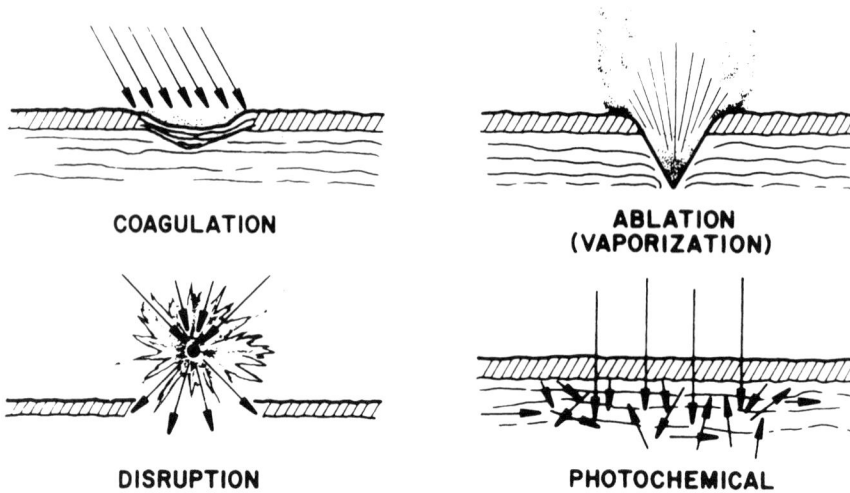

COAGULATION

ABLATION (VAPORIZATION)

DISRUPTION

PHOTOCHEMICAL

FIGURE 2–1. The photobiologic effects observed when radiant energy is incident on tissue is dependent on the physical parameters of the laser beam itself, that is, the lasant, wavelength, power density (watts), energy density (joules), pulsing characteristics (continuous wave, Q-switched, pulses per second, superpulse, UltraPulse [Coherent Laser, Palo Alto, Calif.]); the nature of the biologic tissue undergoing lasing (skin, mucosa); and whether the latter tissues have substantive changes that would alter the laser effects on them (e.g., hyperkeratosis, parakeratosis, presence of dense or vascular neoplastic cells). Photocoagulation is directly related to a temperature increase. When tissues are exposed to increasing radiant energies, rapid tissue heating occurs, resulting in photovaporization or ablation. Using the ultraviolet portion of the electromagnetic spectrum, photochemical interactions occur that change the biochemistry of the tissues (see the section entitled Biophysical Observations in the text). With increasing energy of irradiance, photochemical ablation of tissue is caused by photochemical disruption of intramolecular tissue bonds. During photophysical or disruption of tissues, extremely high irradiances cause a plasma effect and a shock wave in an extremely small volume of tissue. (From Sliney DH, Trokel SL: Medical Lasers and Their Safe Use. New York, Springer-Verlag, 1993, p 38.)

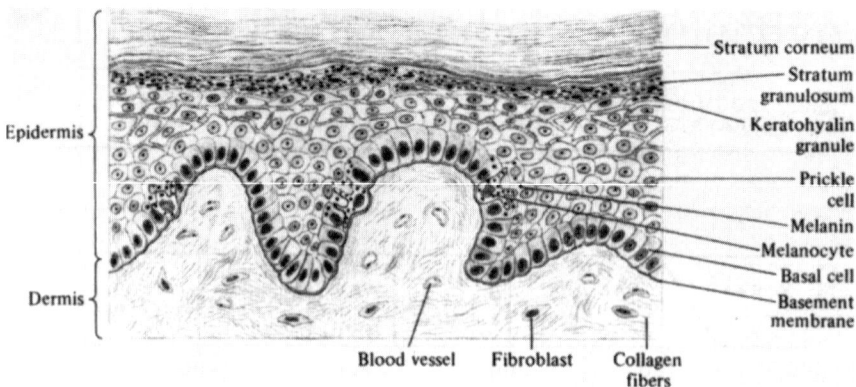

FIGURE 2–2. A representation of human skin. To affect the various cellular layers, the laser must be selected that is active within a given layer. For example, in the management of surface lesions, the surgeon need only deal with the more superficial skin strata; therefore, a laser that has a superficial penetrating property is used (carbon dioxide). When deeper epidermal layers or the papillary dermis must be lased, a laser with deeper penetration must be selected (argon, pulsed dye, or Nd:YAG). (From Parrish JA: Laser photomedicine: Selective laser-tissue interaction. *In* Dixon JA [ed]: Surgical Application of Lasers, 2nd ed. Chicago, Year Book Medical Publishers, 1987, p 36.)

geon to select an appropriate laser and provide individual or lesion-specific laser wavelength and energy parameters to manage lesions of the facial skin and oral mucosa more successfully (Fig. 2–3).

BIOPHYSICAL OBSERVATIONS

Commonplace experiences of incoherent light energy or light of lower energy yield (UVB or UVC) can cause a range of physical changes in skin, including significant erythema (sunburn), hyperpigmentation (effects on melanocytes), photokeratitis, and even malignancy (basal cell or squamous cell carcinoma, melanoma). Longer ultraviolet (UV) wavelengths in the UVA range (314 to 400 nm) of the electromagnetic spectrum can produce cataracts. The reaction of the epidermis to ultraviolet radiation is mainly a biochemical reaction, rather than a physical or thermal effect. An example of the former type of reaction is the formation of vitamin D by UV radiation.

The photons beyond 380 nm to 700 nm, the visible portion of the electromagnetic spectrum, are responsible for absorption by the pigmented elements in the pigmented epithelium and choroid of the eye, which results in stimulation of the photoreceptors (rods and cones) of the retina to allow for vision. Light from the UV and the visible spectrum affects the entire integumentary system and at higher intensity can result in heat-induced cell trauma.

The response of the skin to sunlight is an excellent paradigm for the changes in skin and mucosa induced by a laser and emphasizes that the process is not as straightforward as a thermal burn. Biochemical and histopathologic changes are observed in skin epidermis exposed to light energy of a wavelength greater than about 290 nm, which appears capable of penetrating the epidermis and causing degeneration of the prickle cell layer (a central microscopic feature in sunburned skin). The fact that a small amount of erythema-producing radiant energy can penetrate the epidermis, and the long latent period (several hours) between exposure and the manifestation of erythema, has led to the accepted notion that, as a result of the photochemical reaction, a substance is generated in the epidermis that diffuses to the microscopic vessels in the papillary layer of the dermis, causing vasodilatation. In vivo studies have demonstrated that minimal radiant energy that produces cutaneous erythema causes lysosomal membrane damage and release of hydrolytic enzymes. The fever associated with massive sun-induced skin damage could be due to diffusion of the hydrolytic enzymes into the dermis; moreover, human keratinocytes exposed to UVB release the cytokines interleukin-1 alpha and beta, which are also known as *endogenous pyrogens*.[1, 2]

It had also been found that there is a significant increase in prostaglandin E in the epidermis and dermis after UV radiation; therefore, it is speculated that this vasodilating substance is responsible for the erythema.[3] It has been shown that early UVB erythema is associated with significant elevations in prostaglandins E_2 (PgE$_2$) and I (prostacyclin) and 12-hydroxyeicosatetraenoic acid (12-HETE).[4, 5]

It is now known that a host of cytokines are responsible for the erythematous stigmata of overexposure to UV radiation (especially UVB). Some of these compounds have been identified as increases of PgE$_2$, PgI, PgF$_2$ alpha, and 12-HETE in basal cells, PgD$_2$ in mast cells, and PgI$_2$ in endothelial cells of the circulatory system of the subjacent dermis.[6] The importance of these studies involving the effects on skin of comparatively low-level light

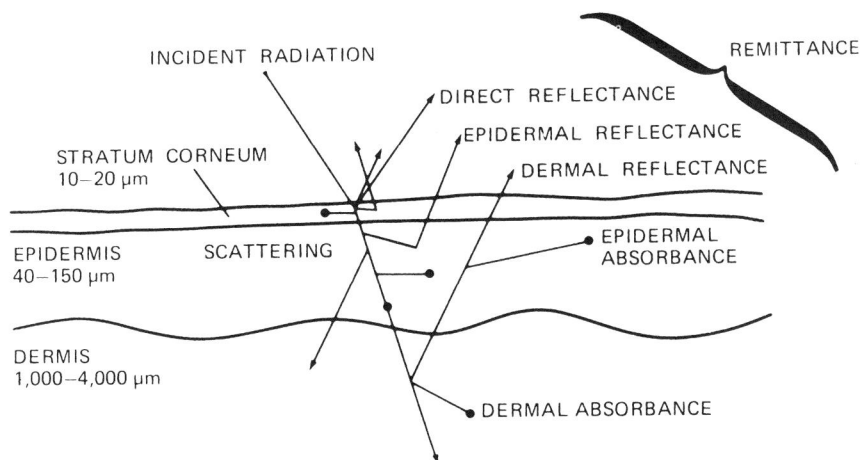

FIGURE 2–3. The multiple effects of radiant energy on skin and associated wavelengths. (From Parrish, JA: Laser photomedicine: Selective laser-tissue interaction. *In* Dixon JA [ed]: Surgical Application of Lasers, 2nd ed. Chicago, Year Book Medical Publishers, 1987, p 38.)

radiation is that such investigations serve as models for other studies involving laser effects on epidermis (epithelium) and dermis (lamina propria) and point the way to measures that can be taken to reduce collateral laser tissue damage.

Beyond the thermal effects of light on tissue, other effects have been suggested, such as red light on the phagocytotic index, wound healing, and hair growth.[7-9]

High-intensity light can give rise to heat damage in susceptible tissues. Indeed, a result of excessive laser radiation used inadvertently or therapeutically can be photocoagulation (discussed below). Besides the intensity of light radiation (power density, irradiance, time of tissue contact with incident beam, wavelength), the tissues can affect resultant laser effects, including (1) the absorption and scattering coefficients at a given wavelength, (2) power density and total irradiance of the beam on tissue, (3) total tissue impact time, (4) size of the irradiated tissue area, and (5) cooling properties of the tissue, such as blood flow[10] (Fig. 2–4).

PHOTOCOAGULATION

Laser radiant energy interacts with all tissues in several quantifiable ways: reflection, transmission, scattering, and absorption. It may appear obvious that, for, to exert its effect upon a given tissue, it must first be absorbed. Reflection from or transmission through tissue results in no observable laser-tissue interaction. Scattered laser energy is absorbed over a broader area or volume of tissue, thus diffusing the effects of the energy. If a laser incident to tissue with a normal body temperature of 37°C heats the tissues to 60°C for a limited time there is

no alteration in the *appearance* of the tissue structure; however, biologic tissues heated to temperatures over 60°C undergo coagulation. This coagulation phenomenon is the basis of most of the surgical applications of lasers. As a result of photocoagulation, proteins, enzymes, cytokines, and other bioactive molecules are heated to temperatures over 60°C, the result being instant denaturation.

The phenomenon of photocoagulation is critically dependent on the rate of energy transfer and is termed a thermochemical rate process. If radiant energy is delivered at a high intensity per unit of time (high irradiance), the result is high temperatures. Higher irradiances produce a more rapid increase in temperature and faster tissue coagulation, eventually exceeding 100°C. When this temperature is exceeded, the phenomenon of photovaporization is observed.

By inspection, photocoagulation appears as a whitening of the tissue surface. This surface change is the result of an alteration in the molecular structure of the tissue constituents, mainly collagen. Collagen has long been known to be a trihelical structure made up of long polypeptide protein chains linked in groups. When temperatures greater than 60°C are reached, the helical polymer is disrupted and the coils become randomized. The result is that the collagen fibers undergo significant shrinkage following photocoagulation. This physical event affecting collagen has a practical value during laser surgery: the lased tissues constrict against the proximal vasculature and the vessels shrink as a result of the collagen composition of their walls, which results in the enhanced hemostasis associated with the use of the laser. Laser damage to erythrocytes attracts a population of platelets, which encourage intraluminal thrombosis, further decreasing blood

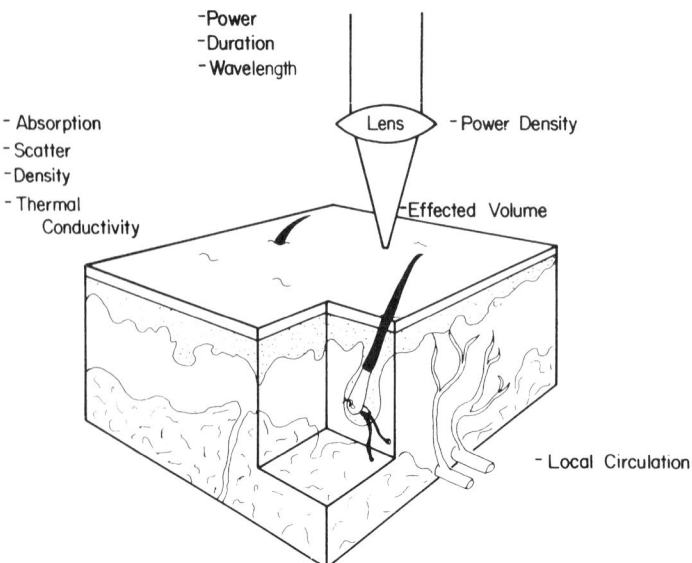

FIGURE 2–4. Laser and tissue parameters that determine photobiologic effects of radiant energy on tissue. (From Fuller TA: Fundamentals of lasers in surgery and medicine. *In* Dixon JA [ed]: Surgical Application of Lasers, 2nd ed. Chicago, Year Book Medical Publishers, 1987, p 23.)

loss. This latter mechanism may be less important than thermal contraction, which appears to be the primary hemostatic phenomenon; thrombosis is a secondary effect. Photocoagulation is said to be ideal after the radiant energy generates temperatures within the range of 50° to 100°C. At temperatures of 45° to 50°C, actual photocoagulation is seen after several seconds; in contrast, at temperatures near or greater than 100°C the phenomenon of photocoagulation occurs within fractions of a second.

The beam's irradiance (the amount of energy deposited in the tissue) is a product of the power of the laser and the duration the beam is in contact with the tissue. The irradiance is thus a critical variable in control of both expected and unwanted effects on target and collateral tissue. The surgeon seeks to control laser beam irradiance and duration of exposure to the target tissue and to limit exposure to contiguous tissue. By following this technique, the maximum temperature of 100°C is not exceeded by the surgeon manipulating exposure time using manual maneuvers and/or setting the parameters of the laser devise. The surgeon can choose a laser wavelength that produces larger or deeper tissue coagulation volumes. One can obtain deeper coagulation tracks within target tissue by using a laser with a wavelength that produces deeper penetration, such as the free-beam Nd:YAG laser (wavelength 1064 microns). When deep, larger volume photocoagulation energies are being used, the surgeon must be aware that undesirable and deeper coagulative alterations may not be evident on the surface of the target tissue. Surgeons can also choose a laser wavelength to cause selective coagulation of a tissue containing a so-called target chromophore, such as water, melanin, and reduced and oxygenated hemoglobin. Examples of lasers that are effective in a water medium are the erbium:YAG, and the holmium (2.1 microns). The carbon dioxide laser's energy is absorbed avidly by biologic tissue containing water; it is relatively ineffective through a water medium, as in a synovial joint. Thus, with the exception of the carbon dioxide laser, the latter lasers can transfer their energy through the water medium to affect target tissue because their wavelengths are marginally absorbed by water.[12]

The carbon dioxide laser is very useful in oral and maxillofacial surgery, and through its photobiologic effects on tissue, it can be used effectively in such exacting areas as laser facial resurfacing. This is because the carbon dioxide laser provides photocoagulation in deeper tissues through heat conduction because the absorption coefficient of its 10.6-micron wavelength is very high and it is, therefore, absorbed in the first 20 microns of tissue. Its energy is 90% absorbed within a depth of 100 microns, which is equivalent to a few cell diameters. The lateral necrosis of tissue observed with this laser is 41 to 85 microns.[13] It has been demonstrated in mammalian tissues that the peak temperature achieved by the carbon dioxide laser is 145°C, the heat of which is mostly lost in cell vaporization. There was an observed decrease in temperature to 45°C at 0.5 mm lateral to the laser beam, which may account for the comparative lack of extensive lateral thermal trauma.[14]

The surgeon must thus consider that only a portion of a laser beam incident on biologic tissues is effective or useful. A fraction is reflected from the tissue and lost to air and by transmission through a tissue such as the vitreous humor of the eye. The working laser radiant beam is thus that portion that is neither reflected nor transmitted. This fraction of the beam renders its radiant energy, usually in the form of heat, to the target tissue. Penetration of the beam, regardless of the nature of the laser device and the depth achieved versus photoheating effects, is ultimately associated with the probabilities of absorption and scattering. Scattering effects are observed to be statistically more probable in the optical and near infrared (IRA) portion of the electromagnetic spectrum, with very much less absorption in tissue. During the scattering phenomenon, photons of the laser beam are thrown off their course, resulting in loss of their original collimated direction. Lateral spread of the beam incident to the tissue is measured to be the same as the depth of penetration. The original concentrated power of a narrow beam is "diluted" over a greater volume of tissue. The argon, helium-neon, and Nd:YAG laser beams exhibit these properties (Table 2–1). Wavelengths greater than 1400 nm (IRB, IRC) demonstrate a higher probability of absorption, and maximum absorption is evident in an extremely thin layer on the tissue surface, with minimal lateral spread. An example of these latter properties is

TABLE 2–1. Relationships of Wavelength, Reflection, and Tissue Penetration

Lasing Medium	Spectrum	Wavelength (nm)	Power (W)	Tissue Reflect (%)	Penetration (mm)	PD 1 (W/mm²)
Nd:YAG	IRA	1064	100	90	1.5	0.02
HeNe	Red	633	0.001	90	1.5	0.02
Carbon dioxide	IRC	10,600	30	5	0.05	20

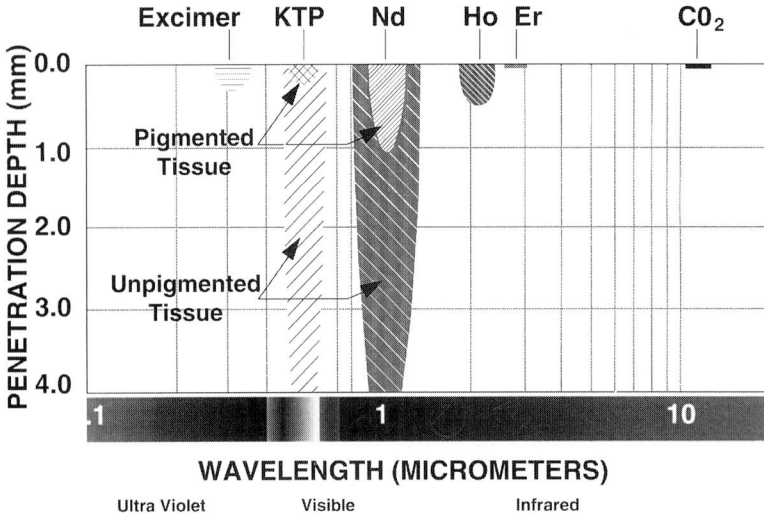

FIGURE 2–5. A comparison of the carbon dioxide laser with other popular surgical lasers, relating depth of penetration with wavelength. (Courtesy of Coherent Laser, Palo Alto, California.)

apparent in the carbon dioxide laser. For the surgeon, the phenomena of reflection, scattering, and absorption have practical value. The carbon dioxide laser thus exhibits intense absorption, which results in a high concentration of power in a thin layer of surface tissue with a dose of moderate power density. The intense absorption of carbon dioxide laser radiation can be explained by its wavelength.[15] A fundamental law of laser-tissue interactions is strong absorption means small penetration (Fig. 2–5 and see Fig. 5–17). The depth of penetration is plotted against the wavelength in microns. Laser penetration is also related to the presence of tissue chromophores, including water, where the absorption coefficient is plotted against the wavelength in microns in Figure 2–6. Since biologic tissue is

composed mainly of water, absorption of carbon dioxide radiant energy is maximal in the superficial layers of the skin and mucous membrane.

Exposure to a carbon dioxide laser beam produces a characteristic energy distribution in biologic tissue. Energy absorbed and dissipated in the superficial layers of the epithelium causes a vacant space, owing to the evaporation of tissue fluids and vaporization or burning of organic cellular matter. In the carbon dioxide system, only a fraction of the radiant energy, from absorption and thermal conduction, can penetrate deep and produce a zone of necrotic cells. Roodenburg[16] demonstrated that the zone of necrotic tissue in the depth of the laser crater is small. There is a layer of carbonized matter on the bottom of the crater, the depth of which is directly

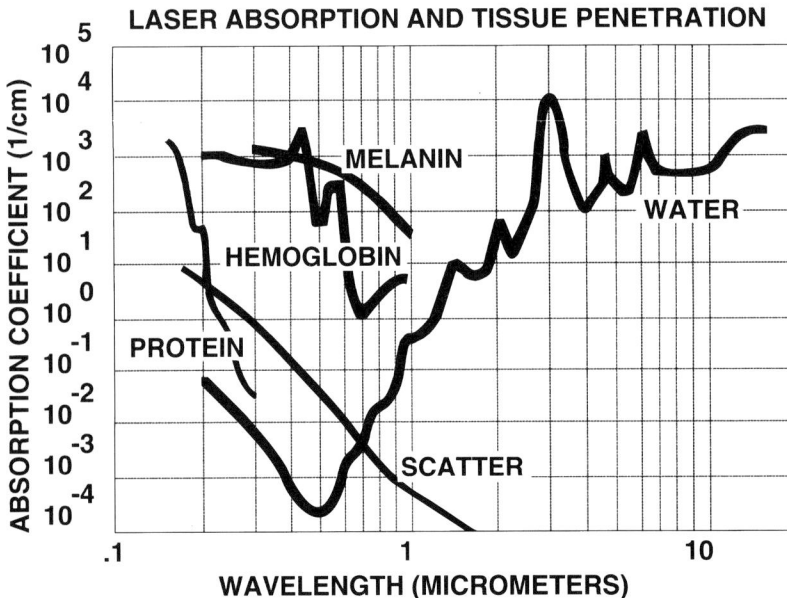

FIGURE 2–6. Laser penetration is also related to the presence of tissue chromophores. The absorption coefficient is plotted against the wavelength in micrometers. (Courtesy of Coherent Laser, Palo Alto, California.)

proportional to the energy density. The necrotic zone in the bottom of the crater increases as the power density increases. Histologically, the laser wound initiates healing by proliferation of epithelial cells from the borders of the wound and the ingrowth of fibrous tissue within the fibrin coagulum covering the wound site. There is a moderate inflammatory reaction with minimal edema. The wound epithelializes in 7 to 21 days, depending on its area. The healed laser wound epithelial layer initially is thin, with few identifying rete pegs. Within 60 days, there is the restoration of characteristic rete pegs. Also initially, there is the development of thick submucosal fibrous tissue, which shortly after lasing, decreases but is never entirely eliminated. Therefore, if one compares normal oral mucosa with lased mucosa, there is a 50% decrease in elasticity as compared with conventionally treated (with a sharp scalpel) mucosa, the latter demonstrating a 200% decrease in elasticity compared with normal mucous membrane. Because the carbon dioxide laser is well-absorbed by water, its penetration in blood is significantly limited, and when blood or blood vessels are struck by the carbon dioxide laser energy, a superficial and fragile layer of coagulated blood and blood elements is formed. Therefore, the carbon dioxide laser does not have hemostatic characteristics except for vessels 0.5 to 1.0 mm in diameter. Aranoff indicated that the carbon dioxide laser sealed lymph vessels, which would make it valuable in decreasing lymphatic spread of malignancies.[17] Aranoff's findings were supported by Oosterhuis in an investigation with experimental melanomas.[18] It is recommended by the majority of oncologic surgeons using lasers that the usual normal margins should be taken when using the carbon dioxide laser to manage malignant neoplasms.

An essential factor in the equation for the practical application of radiant energy in the form of power density (energy density) is the maneuver of the surgeon to limit the highest laser energy to the target tissues, or, in ablation, to the desired volume of pathologic tissue within limited times, thus sparing nontarget tissue by manipulating the laser beam with its power parameters to control the photophysical reactions on the target tissue. The extraordinarily rapid cell vaporization, with the loss of intracellular chemical mediators (cytokines), is posited to result in a markedly less intense local inflammatory response and consequently, less local pain, edema, and cicatrix formation.[19, 20] The final objective in laser surgery is to confine high photodensity and absorbance in tissue, permitting useful laser effects in desired pathologic tissue volumes (Fig. 2–7).

As noted, the carbon dioxide laser beam is highly absorbed within a distance of about 100 microns, causing rapid heating of the target tissue to 100°C. The extra energy provides the latent heat to cause cellular water to turn to steam. The nature of cellular destruction with the carbon dioxide laser enables

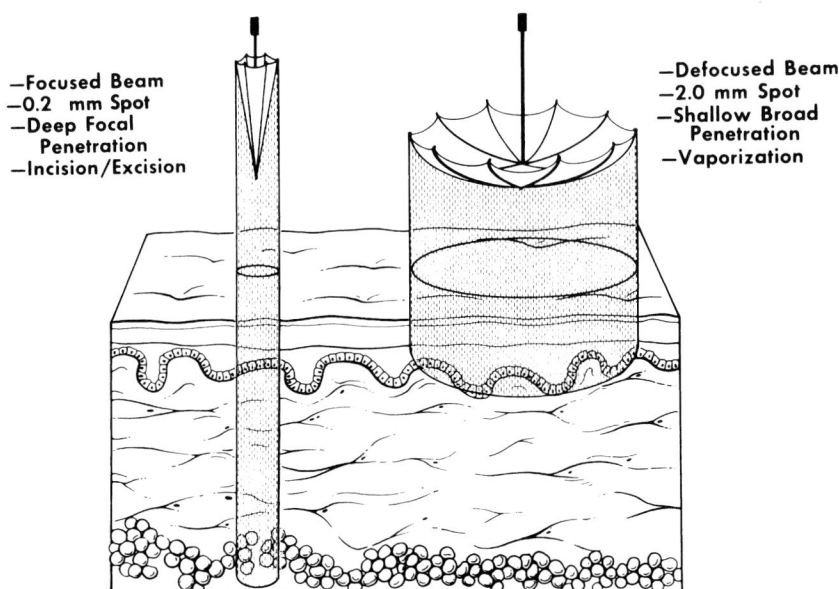

—Focused Beam
—0.2 mm Spot
—Deep Focal Penetration
—Incision/Excision

—Defocused Beam
—2.0 mm Spot
—Shallow Broad Penetration
—Vaporization

FIGURE 2–7. The effects of varying the power density and using focused versus defocused modes; in this case, the carbon dioxide laser is presented. Using the smaller focal spot or a focused mode permits a narrow laser impact trench and thus a deeper penetration or incisional character. (From Balin PL, Ratz JL: Use of the carbon dioxide laser in dermatologic surgery. *In* Ratz JL [ed]: Lasers in Cutaneous Medicine and Surgery. Chicago, Year Book Medical Publishers, 1986.)

the surgeon to see exactly what is occurring at the incident area of the beam-tissue interface. Each layer of cells in turn is vaporized and ablated: each cell is exploded in the path of the focal spot and cellular debris is evacuated as smoke or heated to incandescence in the path of the beam. The cellular residua remain as carbonized matter on the sides of the beam trench. For example, a 20-W beam with a uniform focal spot 2 mm in diameter penetrates 2.5 mm of tissue in 1 second. The high tissue absorption at 10,600 nm virtually eliminates lateral beam scatter, so contiguous tissue is not affected by any potential scatter. This property of the carbon dioxide laser is responsible for its use as a so-called light scalpel; additional advantages, for example, variable pulsing actions, are available, such as is provided by the UltraPulse modes (Coherent Laser, Palo Alto, Calif.).

PHOTOVAPORIZATION (PHOTOTHERMAL ABLATION)

Intense, highly focused laser radiation produces surface temperatures exceeding 100°C, which cause tissue vaporization. An instantaneous effect of a power density of approximately 20 W/mm^2 (which is generated by an incident carbon dioxide laser beam of 1 W/mm^2) is vaporization of the water in the cells and other tissue within a surface of about 0.05 mm thickness within one-eighth second. This must be compared with the average power of clinical lasers, which are up to 100 times as intense.[21] There is a thousandfold expansion of cells as cellular water is converted to steam and temperatures over 100°C destroy cellular protein. The volume of steam generated causes the cells literally to explode, releasing the confined steam. The production and explosive release of steam causes ablation of biologic tissue, which takes the form of a laser plume that consists of superheated steam and microscopic

particles. Debris or particles in the plume that lie randomly within the path of the laser beam are further heated, resulting in partial or complete combustion accompanied by smoke production and flashes of incandescence. With the carbon dioxide laser, the ablative process continues through each newly exposed tissue layer and is under the control of the laser surgeon. Photothermal or photovaporization is used for incision and removal of pathologic tissue. The instantaneous tissue volume expansion adjacent to the focused laser beam results in physical separation with reversible injury. With proper focusing and control a surgical incision can be produced (Fig. 2–8).[22]

The microscopic debris within the laser plume may be a source of hazard, as it has been shown variably to be completely vaporized or heated to incandescence. These particles are usually evacuated from the lased tissue site owing to the potential biohazards of airborne contaminants and possible pathogens (intact proteins and DNA fragments and possibly viable viruses).[23] Target tissue heated to temperatures above the heat of vaporization of free tissue water is carbonized and, therefore, further ablated, which provides another mechanism for tissue removal. The latter is possible because total desiccation of the tissue has occurred and with continued application of radiant energy increases the temperature of the tissue residua until temperatures between 300° and 400°C are measured. The result is tissue carbonization associated with outgassing and smoke. If temperatures exceed 500°C at isobaric conditions, tissues burn and evaporate. These effects—and which specific effect will be more or less prominent—depend on the type of laser used.[12]

During use of the carbon dioxide laser, vaporization of water prevents temperatures in the most superficial unlased cellular layer from exceeding 100°C; however, thermal energy conducted to deeper tissue planes produces a zone of permanent

Laser Incision of Tissue

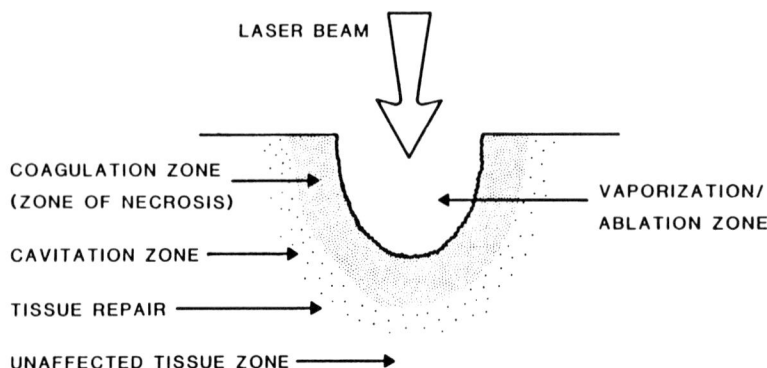

FIGURE 2–8. In laser incisional techniques, several tissue effects occur. There is a vaporization and ablation zone, as well as a zone of coagulation or tissue necrosis adjacent to the ablated zone. Pulsing the laser beam produces cavitation defects or the production of vacuoles by a thermomechanical wave. The sizes of the various zones are determined by the thermal conduction of the tissue, acoustic wave, and ultimately, the peak power and energy and optical penetration depth. (From Sliney DH, Trokel SL: Medical Lasers and Their Safe Use. New York, Springer-Verlag, 1993, p 44.)

heat damage evidenced by protein denaturation. This unseen zone of thermal damage is important during carbon dioxide laser surgery. The volume or thickness of the zone is directly proportional to the power density of the laser at the superficial lased tissue interface as well as on the duration of laser energy exposure. It can be understood by considering the observation that high power densities cause equally high removal of tissue. The heat from the most superficial lased cell layer, which could cause deeper tissue damage, simply cannot be conducted rapidly enough owing to the more rapid vaporization of the surface cells. Therefore, deeper penetration is avoided by the protective effect of rapid vaporization of more superficial cell layers. On the other hand, at lower power densities with equally small volumes of tissue, removal permits penetration of thermal energy to deeper tissue planes, resulting in a larger zone of injury. Similarly, when the laser is applied for longer periods, the deeper tissue damage is greater. If power density (in watts per millimeter) is plotted against the duration of laser application (in seconds), there is a graphic representation of the approximate dependence of the thickness of the zone of tissue injury on the power density and pulse duration (Fig. 2–7).

The power density varies for a single ablation crater or incision. Power density also varies across the diameter of the laser beam; the walls of the incision or laser trench are radiated only obliquely. In a deep narrow incision, the injury at the deepest penetration of the beam can be marginal, about 0.1 mm; however, lateral injury to tissue may extend to 1 mm. This observation has implications in using the laser to create an incision (light scalpel), avoiding unwanted injury to contiguous tissues. The surgeon should select a higher power density (i.e., greater than 5 W/mm². For photoablation or vaporization of larger masses of tissue it is necessary to use a larger focal spot size, which will result in a lower power density across the area of the beam. This ultimately causes deeper thermal tissue necrosis and should be factored in by the surgeon in planning the photovaporization procedure. After photovaporizing the more superficial cellular layers with the larger spot size it is recommended that the deeper layer be ablated using a higher power density, especially if important anatomic structures lie in the subjacent tissue.

The laser can be used in an incisive mode with high power density and small spot size while employing special pulsed-periodicity energy to impact the target tissue (UltraPulse, Coherent Laser, Palo Alto, Calif.). Incisions replicating that of a sharp scalpel are thus possible, and pedunculated lesions or neoplasms can be resected at their base with little bleeding. When the lesion is inaccessible to conventional instrumentation or incisive laser sur-

gery, the surgeon can use a photovaporization technique that employs a continuous-wave mode and can sweep the beam over the target tissue while defocusing it to achieve a larger spot size (3 to 4 mm) and enhance the control of the rate of penetration characteristic of the irradiance produced by defocused beams. Moreover, if the laser can operate at a high-order mode (i.e., greater than TEM_{oo} (Transverse Electromagnetic Mode), which is characterized by a gaussian spot pattern whose highest laser energy intensity is at the center (see Fig. 1–14), and the mode TEMo1 is used, an intensity spot pattern is produced with the greatest energy concentrated around the peripheral circumference of the focal spot; this will result in uniform penetration at the target area. The use of the defocused beam is associated with lower irradiance values (watts expressed in square centimeter per unit time), so that equilibrium damage (spread to nontarget tissue) may be greater than desired. It may, therefore, be appropriate to increase the power or wattage of the laser when using it in a defocused manner, to ensure maintenance of higher levels of irradiance.

The literature on laser surgery contains well-described classic findings in skin and mucous membranes related to the application of laser energy. The effects of the carbon dioxide laser on these tissues have been studied especially well. In all instances, these observations of the biologic effects of laser energy are directly dependent on the kind of laser used and all the important power-time and other beam parameters discussed earlier. Most investigations of the effects of laser energy on mucous membranes with comparison to other conventional surgical instrumentations such as sharp scalpel, diathermy, and cryosurgery have revealed histologic differences in the wounds and wound healing created by these modalities. Fisher and colleagues found in the canine model that scalpel wounds contracted significantly and displayed rolled margins that gradually flattened with time but were still detectable 42 days after wounding. In contrast, laser wounds caused by the carbon dioxide laser initially had a buff-colored base with adherent carbonized tissue fragments. Later, contraction occurred at the peripheral margins, the edge of the wound site being level with the adjacent tissue early in the postprocedure period. The laser wound, in contrast to the scalpel incision, was difficult to see at 28 days.[24] In later studies, Fisher and Frame confirmed the observations that mucosal wound healing after laser surgery contrasts with the accepted classic healing by secondary intention and the authors attributed the differences to the manner of tissue destruction by the laser beam. This was discussed earlier. A laser wound is not a burn in the commonly accepted sense of the word but rather is the result of almost instantaneous vaporization of intracellular fluid with immediate disintegration of the cell structure. Frame and Fisher said of the pattern of cell destruction that it occurs without the usual release of cytokines characteristic of acute inflammation. They also describe how the thin layer of denatured collagen on the surface of lased tissue acts as a relatively impermeable membrane immediately after lasing, thus reducing the amount of tissue irritation from the intraoral environment. Further, they attributed the comparatively low degree of wound contracture as being directly related to the small population of myofibroblasts seen in laser wounds. Myofibroblasts are now acknowledged to play a significant role in wound contracture.[25, 26]

Electron microscopic investigations in human skin and mucosal laser wounds have demonstrated the zone of photovaporization, which appears dark and structureless with no visible cellular morphology.[27] Swelling of the endothelial cells was a feature observed in the subepithelial connective tissue subjacent to the zone of laser wounding. Cellular organelles exposed to the laser appeared to be disrupted, whereas the desmosomes and hemidesmosomes and the nuclear membranes are comparatively well preserved in the surrounding lased tissue.[27, 28] Luomanen and Meurman used the electron microscope to elucidate more specifically alterations in soft tissues that could not be identified by light microscope alone.[29] They suggested that the laser-affected wound margins were not demarcated as definitively because of their observations that numerous ultrastructural changes in the lased areas did not show alterations with light microscopy. Further, Luomanen and Meurman speculated that this finding may explain the observation that the lased area appeared to be wider in the healing phase than after the initial lasing.

Thus, the photobiologic manner in which a laser causes tissue alterations consists of an instantaneous vaporization of intracellular fluid, organelles, and membranes, along with the extracellular fluid and denaturation of intracellular substance and proteins, especially collagen. In this manner, according to most investigators, there is limited release of intact chemical mediators of inflammation and, thus, less vigorous inflammatory response in adjacent tissues with a resultant decrease in edema.[25] Inflammation is further attenuated by the lack of irritation from physical or biochemical agents in the oral cavity as a result of the denaturation of surface collagen after lasing, which may function as an impermeable dressing. There is also delayed re-epithelialization and generally delayed healing of lased tissue. Delayed healing can be another manifestation of the decreased population of myofibroblasts characteristic of laser-induced wounds. In this setting, the comparative lack of myofibroblasts would tend to promote a larger area of the wound surface over which re-epithelialization would have to occur.[30] Delayed epithelialization may also be due to the inherent nature of epithelial turnover in humans as compared with most animal models studied.[31, 32] Wound contracture is dependent, in part, on myoepithelial cells; therefore, the relative paucity and disorientation in a laser wound results in an increased area to achieve epithelial coverage; however, there is some controversy about this mechanism.[33] Basu and colleagues made several observations that contradicted the earlier observations on myofibroblasts and sealed nerve endings in laser wounds. In healing glossectomy wounds of rats Basu's group demonstrated a significant population of myofibroblasts and few sealed nerve endings, despite the fact that the latter finding has been used to explain the relative lack of pain after laser surgery.[34]

It is important to evaluate observations in the literature about healing of lased tissues based on the power of the laser device, the irradiance, and other parameters such as the use of free-beam versus contact laser systems. Fisher and Frame observed that, within the lased areas the healing epithelium proliferated over the fibrinous coagulum at the perimeter of the tissue defect. This was compared with surgical wounds' healing by secondary intention, in which the new epithelial cells grow along the boundary between the surface coagulum and the underlying granulation tissue. These authors also reported the failure of split-thickness skin grafts over lased tissues,[25] which may be related to surgical technique or the "histology" of the laser wound. Most authors have concluded that skin grafting is not necessary after laser excision of premalignant oral lesions or more extensive oral neoplasms.[35, 36] It should be noted that, as lasers become more sophisticated and result in a non-charred tissue reaction approaching in cell injury that of a sharp scalpel, it has been observed (G.A.C.) that successful split-thickness skin grafts can take over lased tissue beds.

LASER STERILIZATION PROPERTIES

One of the numerous posited advantages of using lasers in surgical procedures is the possibility that laser radiant energy may sterilize the wound site. Moreover, it has been reported that, for indolent infected surgical wounds, the carbon dioxide laser is a more effective sterilizing method than a standard surgical scrub.[37] Surgical lasers have also been compared with routine electrocautery for wound sterilization.[38] Stranc and colleagues noted that sterilization by cautery of infected wounds was observed to be significantly superior to that of the carbon dioxide laser ($P < .005$). Infection was observed in 4% of the cautery-sterilized wounds; in contrast, 12% of the wounds managed with the carbon dioxide laser exhibited infection. Earlier, Luomanen and Meurman commented on the rapid colonization of the damaged tissue by (unspecified) microorganisms following laser irradiation.[29] They speculated that such colonization was enhanced as a result of the dryness of the lased tissue in contrast to the surgical wound, which is always damp owing to tissue fluid infiltration. The mechanism of such colonization remains to be elucidated. Lasers continue to be recognized to result in immediate sterilization of the surgical site, and it is difficult to refute this clinical observation based on the action of the laser on cellular architecture (i.e., virtually instantaneous vaporization and sealing of collateral blood vessels and lymphatics). Moreover, perhaps because of this sealing effect, animal studies have revealed no bacteremia following intraoral lasing, in contrast to conventional methods that result predictably in bacteremia.[39]

PHOTOCHEMICAL EFFECT AND PHOTOCHEMICAL THERAPY

Radiant energy possessing a multitude of wavelengths can be used to treat a host of dermatologic diseases by administering a photosensitizing agent to the patient before application of the light. In this manner, an exogenous photosensitizing agent acting as a tissue chromophore causes an alteration of the lesional tissue and the character of the in vivo photochemistry that has a salubrious effect on target and nontarget tissues. Psoralens (tricyclic furocoumarins) have been used as photosensitizing agents in combination with exposure to UVA radiation (wavelength 320 to 400 nm) to manage such dermatologic entities as psoriasis, mycosis fungoides, vitiligo, and variants of eczema.

Parrish notes that the technology of photochemotherapy may eventually be more influential than any of the current applications of radiant energy for similar purposes observed thus far. Systemic administration of the photosensitizing agent offers convenience, bypasses the barrier to radiant energy alone of the stratum corneum, and may cause a uniform skin concentration of photoagent. Because the photoagent is activated by optical radiant energy, the effects of the photosensitizer are confined to exposed areas and the penetrative action of the radiant energy is limited to the skin. By controlling the intensity of the optical radiation applied, the quantity of blood similarly exposed is also regulated.[40]

Photodynamic Therapy with the Laser

Photodynamic therapy (PDT) using the laser is similar, technologically, to the use of photosensitizers and radiant energy possessing less power and, in most cases, shorter wavelengths. The capability of lasers to emit radiant energy of various wavelengths compatible with specific clinical problems and the versatility of laser technology used in conjunction with fiberoptics and operating microscopes to deliver laser energy to comparatively inaccessible anatomic sites, open the door to a wide spectrum of applications in the head, face, and oral cavity. It is indeed fortuitous that lasers became linked to the application of bioactive chemicals that would concentrate in potential laser target tissue.

Initially, photodynamic therapy used hematoporphyrin derivative (HPD) and red light to treat malignant disease in humans. The foundation of photodynamic therapy is the activation of a local or systemically administered photosensitizing agent by radiant energy.[41] PDT turns on the ability of certain chemicals (dyes) to accumulate in malignant tissues and to be rendered cellucidal if activated by exposure to laser energy in the form of low-intensity visible or near-infrared light. Numerous photosensitive agents have been indentified and studied for use in the management of malignant disease. These effects are observed in vivo and in vitro. Moreover, a range of oral microorganisms responsible for both dental caries and periodontal disease are susceptible to the cellucidal effects of PDT, in some cases using low-level laser energy and even red light.[42, 43] This observation opens a new realm of basic and clinical research in which topically applied photosensitizing agents may be used in the future to treat oral lesions, caries, and periodontal disease differently than by physical laser and mechanical methods.

The HPD and its active moiety dihematoporphyrin ethers (esters), or DHE, have been extensively investigated.[44] In addition to localizing in malignant neoplasms, HPD also concentrates in inflamed tissues. In most earlier studies, a continuous-wave dye laser device pumped with an argon laser with the beam focused into a single 200-micron quartz fiber was used for delivery of the radiant energy component. It was observed that insertion of the optical fiber directly into the substance of the tumor mass permitted deep transfer of the laser radiant energy to the lesion. Photodynamic therapy can be delivered to any neoplasm that is accessible by endoscopes, intravenous catheters, or hypodermic needles. Photoactivation results when tissues in which DHE is preferentially bound are then exposed to radiant energy, typically light with a wavelength of 630 nm, which penetrates to a depth of 5 to 10 mm. Radiant energy of the appropriate wavelength incident upon the DHE molecule causes elevation of DHE from its ground state to its singlet (excited) state. The laser energy increases the electronic and vibrational energies of the DHE, resulting in unstable states of the molecule. DHE in the singlet state can undergo conversion to a triplet state that reacts with the ground state of oxygen (triplet oxygen), causing the formation of a highly reactive species, singlet oxygen $^1O_2$, after which DHE reverts to the ground state, at which point it emits photons, combined with intermolecular and intramolecular energy transfer, which, in addition to yielding singlet oxygen, concentrates other reactive sensitizer radicals and radical ions, which are, in turn, cellucidal (tumorcidal).[45]

Photodynamic therapy thus requires adequate tissue levels of photosensitizer, oxygen, and laser energy. Protofrin II is administered in doses of 1.5 to 2.5 mg/kg 48 to 72 hours before lasing a specific lesion. Following the loading or priming dose of DHE, laser energy within the red spectrum (wavelength 630 nm) is applied for 5 to 15 minutes to accumulate a laser dose of 25 to 250 joules per square centimeter in the malignant lesion. The range of DHE doses for treatment of head and neck malignancies has been about 3 to 5 mg/kg. Reports on the use of PDT to manage malignancies of the head and neck have noted effectiveness in limited malignant disease. Gluckman and colleagues reported some success in the head and neck region when TNM stage-T1 lesions and carcinoma in situ are managed with PDT.[46] At present, photodynamic therapy has been observed to be useful in the treatment of recurrent squamous cell carcinomas. Dougherty reported management of recurrent lingual squamous cell carcinoma by use of PDT with preservation of good muscle function.[47] The additional application of photodynamic principles will be evident in the areas of diagnosis and detection of residual tumor cells and tissue in the intraoperative period. In this latter example, the patient will be administered DHE and then examined preoperatively under Wood's light, allowing the surgeon to visualize fluorescence of the operative field before closing the wound.

Photomechanical Effect (Photodisruption)

Although photodisruption is not a laser application that is sought by oral and maxillofacial surgeons as a way of managing diseased tissues, the future is rife with opportunities for the application of all laser's properties. It is, therefore, included here for completness. Ophthalmologists pioneered many of the early applications of laser energy to human tissue, among them the specific technology of photodisruption. The generation and propagation of nonthermal, photodisruptive tissue effects were designed by ophthalmologists to be directed at transparent or translucent tissue membranes in the eye. The generation of photomechanical effects requires the use of extremely high-power Q-switched or mode-locked ophthalmic Nd:YAG lasers capable of generating ultrashort pulses.[48] The beam thus produced is focused to an extremely small spot size of 50 microns diameter, so even lower energy pulses (millijoules) can result in unusually high irradiances (megawatts per square centimeter). Pulse times briefer than 100 femtoseconds are common. When a tiny volume of tissue is vaporized instantaneously, there is a massive energy density build up (as lightning does in air) or is evolved into so-called optical plasma, which may reach 10,000°C. In an extremely small volume of ocular tissue, then, the laser effects depend on a hydrodynamic shock wave that occurs after the formation of plasma anu that can disrupt tissue. This effect is highly applicable to the semitransparent membranes in the eye. Importantly, the massive radiant energy produced by the Nd:YAG laser is absorbed by the production of the plasma, so *vital structures of the globe are not injured.* The approximate diameter of the disruption of the focused laser beam is 200 to 300 microns, and the extent along its long axis on either side of the focal point, 0.5 mm. Incredibly, the irradiance may be of the order of megawatts or gigawatts per square centimeter; therefore, it is only to generate such power levels possible within an extremely small volume of tissue. It is, therefore, evident that the application of photodisruptive laser functions is effective only in microsurgical techniques. The formation of an optical plasma can be likened to phenomena in the field of particle physics in which "extraterrestial" energies allow fusion of hydrogen atoms to form helium with an extraordinary release of massive energies in billionths of a second.

Clinical studies of photosensitive compounds such as Protofrin II (Quadra Logic Technologies, Vancouver, BC) involved randomized controlled studies assessing its efficacy. Protofrin II is a bovine blood product containing 80% DHE (active) and 20% inactive hematoporphyrin compounds. DHE is avidly lipophilic and, in high concentrations, binds to cell membranes and other cellular organelles. Through electron microscopic studies of the vascular stroma, Gomer and Dougherty have observed fluorescence in macrophages, mast cells, and endothelial cells.[49] Bugelski and associates noted that DHE concentrated within the vascular stroma and had a separating effect on the luminal endothelial cells.[50] This mechanism appeared to cause release of initiators and promoters of coagulation (e.g., thromboxane); this indicates that photodynamic therapy has its critical action on the vascular supply of malignant neoplasms and the resultant ischemia promotes tumor necrosis.

Lasers in Wound Healing

Lasers employing low-level radiant energy have been claimed to produce a positive effect on the biologic and biochemical processes of wound reconstitution. As expected, these claims have been received with healthy skepticism in the surgical community. It has been reported that low-level radiant energy of lasers has accelerated wound healing, reduced pain, and enhanced neural regeneration. Dermatologic investigations have demonstrated more rapid epithelialization, enhanced neovascularization, and increased production of collagen by fibroblasts in vivo by the application of radiation from argon or helium-neon lasers.[51–55] Opposing this sample of supportive claims for the efficacy of low-level laser energy on the healing of surgical or experimental wounds is a significant cohort of reports denying such findings.[56–59] A disturbing finding has been the reports of atypical cellular forms apparently caused by low-level laser radiant energy.[60–62] Moreover, other investigators have reported alterations in normal cells and proliferation of neoplastic cells by low irradiance lasers.[63–65] Bosatra and associates,[51] Mester and coworkers,[54] and others[66–68] reported increased synthesis of collagen and enhanced phagocytic activity of leukocytes after use of low-level laser irradiance of tissues in vitro.

Studies involving the management of chronic and acute pain by low-energy laser devices in the clinical environment have proved contradictory. Some of these investigations included chronic rheumatoid arthritis patients and others, acute pain models involving the immediate (acute) postoperative analgesic effects of lasers after excision of third molars.[69–71] In the investigations on the role of lasers in third molar surgery, although the helium-neon laser produced a statistically significant reduction of trismus after third molar surgery, the authors did not report a significant reduction in pain. Despite the use of low-level radiation for the treatment of open wounds in the former Soviet Union and Eastern Europe for more than 20 years, the acceptance of this clinical practice has been tentative in the United States for the last 10 years and has been viewed with curiosity and skepticism.[72–74] In summary, no definitive investigations either support or refute the use of low-level laser energy to enhance the surgical goals of accelerating wound healing, decreasing pain sensation, and controlling muscle spasm, despite numerous efforts to support such claims. This conundrum invariably involves the inherent complexity of wound healing and the vast

biochemical mediators and cellular factors that modulate the process. Unfortunately, studies that attempt to establish a causal relationship of enhanced or salutary effects as products of low-energy laser application suffer from several disadvantages. It is unscientific to compare results when different lasers are used in the experiments, along with incompatible or uncomparable irradiances, time exposures, varied tissue models (e.g., skin, dermis, mucosa), different animal models, and the choice of various kinds of tissue culture media (these may have light-absorbing chromophores that complicate the accumulation of a database with some validity). At present, the majority of laser wound healing literature has focused on the proliferative phase of wound healing, the period 10 to 14 days after wounding that is characterized by populations of proliferating fibroblasts and the initiation of the synthesis of collagen.

REFERENCES

1. Johnson BE, Daniels F: Lysosomes and the reaction of skin to ultraviolet radiation. J Invest Dermatol 53:85–94, 1969.
2. Kupper TS, Chua AO, Flood P, et al: Interleukin I gene expression in cultured human keratinocytes is augmented by ultraviolet radiation. J Clin Invest 80:430–436, 1987.
3. Mathur GP, Gandhi WM: Prostaglandins in human and albino rat skin. J Invest Dermatol 58:291–295, 1972.
4. Black AK, Fincham N, Greaves MV, et al: Time course changes of levels of arachidonic acid, and prostaglandins D_2, E_2, and F_2 in human skin following ultraviolet radiation. Br J Clin Pharmacol 10:453–459, 1980.
5. Black AK, Henshy CN, Greaves MV: Increased levels of 6-oxo-PGF_1 in human skin following ultraviolet-B radiation. Br J Clin Pharmacol 13:351–354, 1982.
6. Hawk JIM, Black AK, Jaenicke KF, et al: Increased concentrations of arachidonic acid, prostaglandin E_2, D_2, and 6-oxo-F, and histamine in skin following UV-A irradiation. J Invest Dermatol 80:496–499, 1983.
7. Mester E, Sellyei M, Tota GJ: Laserstrahlenwirkung auf das Wachstum des Ehrlichschen Ascitestumors. (The effect of laser radiation on the development of ascites tumor.) Arch Geschwultsforsch 32:201, 1968.
8. Mester E, Szende B, Spiry T, Scher A: Stimulation of wound healing by laser rays. Acta Chir Acad Sci Hung 13:315, 1972.
9. Mester E, Szende B, Tota JG: Die Wirkung über langere Zeit weiderholt verabreichten Laserstrahlung geringer Intensitat auf die Haut und inveren Organe von Mausen. (The long-term effect of irradiation at low-intensity on the skin and internal organs of mice.) Radiobiol Radiother 10:371, 1969.
10. Fuller T: Fundamentals of lasers in surgery and medicine. *In* Dixon, JA (ed): Surgical Applications of Lasers, 2nd ed. Chicago, Year Book, 1987.
11. Kelly DF, Brown SG, Calder BM, et al: Histological changes following Nd:YAG laser photocoagulation of canine gastric mucosa. Gut 24:914–920, 1983.
12. Catone GA: Laser technology in oral and maxillofacial surgery. Part I: Qualitative laser physics. *In* Selected Readings in Oral and Maxillofacial Surgery, vol 3, (No 3). Dallas, University of Texas Southwestern Medical Center, 1993.
13. Pogrel MA, McCracken KJ, Daniels TE: Histologic evaluation of width of soft tissue necrosis adjacent to carbon dioxide incisions. Oral Surg, 70:564, 1990.

14. Pogrel MA, Kwan Yen C, Taylor RD: Thermographic evaluation of the temperatures achieved by carbon dioxide laser on soft tissues and teeth. Thermology 3:50, 1988.

15. Bayly JG, Kartha VB, Stevens WH: The absorption spectra of liquid phase HO, HDO, and DO from 0.7 fm to 10 fm. Infrared Physics 3:211–223, 1963.

16. Roodenburg JLN: CO₂ Laser of Oral Leukoplakia. Thesis with English Summary. Groningen, 1985.

17. Aranoff BL: CO₂ laser in surgical oncology. *In* Kaplan J (ed): Laser Surgery. Proceedings of the 1st and 2nd International Symposium on Laser Surgery, 1975 and 1977 (Reprint), Tel Aviv, OTPAZ, 191–216, 1978.

18. Oosterhuis JW: Tumour Surgery with the CO₂ Laser. Studies with the Cloudman S91 Mouse Melanoma. Thesis, Groningen, Veenstra-Visser, 1977.

19. Strong MS, Jako GJ, Polanyi T, et al: Laser surgery in the aerodigestive tract. Am J Surg 126:529–533, 1973.

20. Tuffin JR, Carruth JAS: The carbon dioxide laser. Br Dent J 149:255–258, 1980.

21. Haywood JK: The CO₂ laser. *In* Oswal VH, Kashima HK, Flood LM (eds): The CO₂ Laser in Otolaryngology and Head and Neck Surgery. Boston, Wright, 1989.

22. Catone GA: Lasers in dentoalveolar surgery. Oral Maxillofac Surg Clin North Am 45–61, 1993.

23. Sawchuk WS, Weber PJ, Lowy DR, et al: Infectious papillomavirus in the vapor of warts treated with carbon dioxide or electrocoagulation: Detection and prevention. J Am Acad Dermatol 101:2141–2149, 1981.

24. Fisher SE, Frame JW, Browne RM, et al: A comparative histological study of wound healing following CO₂ laser and conventional surgical excision of canine buccal mucosa. Arch Oral Biol 28:287–291, 1983.

25. Fisher SE, Frame JW: The effects of the carbon dioxide surgical laser on oral tissues. Br J Oral Maxillofac Surg 22:414–425, 1984.

26. Gabbiani G, Ryan GB, Majno G: The presence of modified fibroblasts in granulation tissue and their possible role in wound contraction. Experientia 27:549, 1971.

27. Ben-Bassat M, Kaplan IA: A study of the ultrastructural features of the cut margin of skin and mucous membrane specimens excised by carbon dioxide laser. J Surg Res 21:77–86, 1976.

28. Mihashi S, Jako GJ, Incze J, et al: Laser surgery in otolaryngology: Interaction of the CO₂ laser and soft tissue. Ann NY Acad Sci 267:263–294, 1976.

29. Luomanen M, Meurman JH: Laser-induced alterations in rat oral mucosa. Scand J Dent Res 94:452–460, 1986.

30. Frame JW: Treatment of sublingual keratosis with the CO₂ laser. Br Dent J 156:243–246, 1984.

31. Squier CA, Johnson NW, Hopps RM: Human Oral Mucosa. Oxford, Blackwell Scientific Publications, 1976.

32. RhysEvans PHR, Frame JW, Branddrick J: A review of carbon dioxide laser surgery in the oral cavity and pharynx. J Laryngol Otol 100:69–77, 1986.

33. Schuller DE: Use of the laser in the oral cavity. Otolarynogol Clin North Am 28:287, 1990.

34. Basu MF, Frame JW, RhysEvans PH: Wound healing following partial glossectomy using the CO₂ laser, diathermy, and scalpel. A histological study in rats. J Laryngol Otol 102:322, 1988.

35. Frame JW, DasGupta AR, Dalton GA, et al: Use of the carbon dioxide laser in the management of premalignant lesions of the oral mucosa. J Laryngol Otol 98:1251–1260, 1984.

36. Carruth JAS: Resection of the tongue with the carbon dioxide laser. J Laryngol Otol 96:529–543, 1982.

37. Al-Qattan MM, Stranc MF, Jarmuske M, et al: Wound sterilization: CO₂ laser versus iodine. Br J Plast Surg 42:380, 1984.

38. Stranc MF, Yang FW: Wound sterilization: Cautery versus CO₂ laser. Br J Plast Surg 45:536–539, 1992.

39. Kaminerm R, Liebow C, Margonone JL, et al: Bacteremia following laser and conventional surgery in hamsters. J Oral Maxillofac Surg 48:45, 1990.

40. Parrish JA: Laser photomedicine: Selective laser-tissue interaction. *In* Dixon JA (ed): Surgical Application of Lasers, 2nd ed. Chicago, Year Book Medical Publishers, 1987.

41. Dougherty TJ, Weishaupt KR, Doyle DG: New methods of cancer treatment. *In* DeVita VT, Hellman S, Rosenberg SA (eds): Cancer: Principles and Practice of Oncology. Philadelphia, JB Lippincott, 1982.

42. Wilson M, Dobson J, Harvey W: Sensitization of periodontal pathogenic bacteria to killing from a low-power laser. Oral Microbiol Immunol 8:182–187, 1993.

43. Burns T, Wilson M, Pearson G: Laser-induced killing of photosensitized cariogenic bacteria. J Dent Res 71:675, 1992.

44. Dougherty TJ: Photosensitization of malignant tumors. Semin Surg Oncol 2:24–37, 1987.

45. Weishaupt KR, Gomer CJ, Dougherty TJ: Identification of singlet oxygen as the cytotoxic agent in photo-inactivation of a murine tumor. Cancer Res 36:2321–2379, 1976.

46. Gluckman JL, Waner M, Shumrick K, et al: Photodynamic therapy. Arch Otol Head Neck Surg 112:949–952, 1986.

47. Dougherty TJ: Photodynamic therapy. *In* Withers HR, Peters LJ (eds): Medical Radiology Innovations in Radiation Oncology. Berlin, Springer-Verlag, 1988.

48. Steinert RF, Puliafito CA, Kittrell C: Plasma shielding by Q-switched and mode-locked Nd:YAG lasers. Ophthalmology 90:1003–1006, 1983.

49. Gomer CJ, Dougherty TJ: Determination of [³H] and [¹⁴C] hematoporphyrin derivative distribution in malignant and normal tissue. Cancer Res 39:146–151, 1979.

50. Bugelski PJ, Porter CW, Dougherty TJ: Autoradiographic distribution of hematoporphyrin derivative in normal and tumor tissue of the mouse. Cancer Res 41:4606–4612, 1981.

51. Bosatra M, Jucci A, Olliaro P, et al: In vitro fibroblast and dermis fibroblast. Activation by laser irradiation at low energy. Dermatology 168:157–162, 1984.

52. Brunner R, Haina D, Landthaler M, et al: Applications of laser light of low power density. Experimental and clinical investigations. Curr Probl Dermatol 15:111–116, 1986.

53. Kana JS, Hutschenreiter G: Effect of low-power laser radiation on healing of open skin wounds in rats. Arch Surg 116:293–296, 1981.

54. Mester E, Nagylucskay I, Tisza S, et al: Stimulation of wound healing by means of laser rays. Investigation of the effects of immune competent cells. Acta Chir Acad Sci Hung 19:163–170, 1978.

55. Averbakh MM, Jorkin MJ, Dobkin BG, et al: The influence of helium neon on the healing of aseptic experimental wounds. Eskp N Khirur: Anestez 3:56–59, 1976.

56. Monfrecola G, Martellotta D, Lembo G, et al: Valutazione dell Irradiazione con Laser He-Ne delle Ulcere de Stasi Venosa. Ann Ital Dermatol Clin Sperimen 36:415–422, 1982.

57. Surinchuk JS, Alago ML, Bellamy RF, et al: Effects of low energy lasers on the healing of full-thickness skin defects. Laser Surg Med 2:267–274, 1983.

58. Jongsma FHM, Bogarrd AEJM, vanGemert MJC, et al: Is closure of open wounds in rats accelerated by argon laser exposure? Laser Surg Med 3:75–80, 1983.

59. Colver GB, Priestley GC: Failure of a helium-neon laser to affect components of wound healing in vitro. Br J Dermatol 121:179–186, 1989.

60. Goldman L: Biochemical Aspects of the Laser: The Introduction of Laser Applications into Biology and Medicine. Berlin, Springer-Verlag, 1967.

61. Goldman L, Richfield DF: The effects of repeated exposures to laser beams: Case report of nine months observation. Acta Dermatol Venerol 44:264–268, 1964.

62. Parr WH, Fisher RS: Aberrant corneal epithelial cells pro-

duced by ruby laser irradiation. Invest Ophthalmol 6:656–663, 1967.

63. Jamison CW, Litwin MS, Lango SE: Enhancement of melanoma cell culture growth rate by ruby laser radiation. Life Sci 8:101–106, 1969.

64. Mims JL: Some effects of low energy ruby and neodymium laser radiation on transplantable subcutaneous mouse tumors. Tex Rep Biol Med, 26:434–435, 1968.

65. Moskalik KG, Koslov AP: Effect of pulsed laser radiation on mitotic activity and DNA synthesis of tumor cells. Dokl Acad Nauk, SSSR 244:206–208, 1979.

66. Lam T, Abergel R, Castel J, et al: Laser stimulation of collagen synthesis in human skin fibroblast cultures. Laser Life Sci 1:61–77, 1986.

67. Abergel R, Lyons R, Castel J, et al: Biostimulation of wound healing by lasers: Experimental approaches in animal and in fibroblast cultures. J Dermatol Surg Oncol 13:127–133, 1987.

68. Mester E, Kosma L, Dudash V: The effect of laser radiation on the phagocytic activity of leukocytes. Dokl Acad Nauk, SSSR, 23:749–752, 1979.

69. Goldman L, Chiapella J, Casey N, et al: Laser therapy of rheumatoid arthritis. Laser Surg Med 1:93–101, 1980.

70. Walker J: Relief from chronic pain by low-power laser irradiation. Neurosci Lett 43:339–344, 1983.

71. Carrillo JS, Catatayud J, Manso FJ, et al: Randomized double-blind clinical trial on the effectiveness of helium-neon laser in the prevention of pain, swelling, and trismus after removal of impacted third molars. Int Dent J 40:31–36, 1990.

72. Mester E, Spiry T, Szende B, et al: Effect of laser rays on wound healing. Am J Surg 122:532–535, 1971.

73. Kleinkort J, Foley R: Laser: A preliminary report on its use in physical therapy. Clin Manag Phys Ther 2:30–32, 1982.

74. Basford J: Low-energy laser treatment of pain and wounds: Hypo, hope or hokum? Mayo Clin Proc 61:671–675, 1986.

CHAPTER 3

Laser Safety in Anesthesia and Oral and Maxillofacial Surgery

EDWARD TEEPLE, MD

Since the 1950s, when lasers were first developed, lasers remained in the realms of the physics laboratories and comic books. The initial research focused on defining what lasers were and how they worked. Comic books heralded the ability of the laser to be used as a weapon. Flash Gordon's ray gun evolved into a nifty hand-held laser pistol. In the 1970s, more practical applications for the laser were defined as new lower power and noninjurious types of lasers were discovered. In the early 1980s, lasers were beginning to be applied to clinical cases. From the mid-1980s until now, wider development and use of more types of lasers has occurred. Laser surgery is still in its infancy. Safety for the laser operator, coworkers, and the patient was and still is a primary concern. The laser as a heat and ignition source poses great challenges to the practitioner. Laser surgery can be done safely, providing that risk patterns are known and steps are taken to prevent or minimize risk.

The goal of this chapter is to define clearly the risk patterns for laser surgery and anesthesia. Special emphasis is placed on the management of the anesthesia for oral and maxillofacial surgery.

PHYSICS OF THE LASER

Laser is an acronym that stands for *l*ight *a*mplification by the *s*timulated *e*mission of *r*adiation. The energy of the laser gradually dissipates as the distance from the beam increases. Energy levels in the beam can be high enough to cause injury in front of and behind the aperture point. Hence, any contact with the beam is to be avoided.

The neodymium:yttrium-aluminum-garnet (Nd:YAG) laser has a fiber-optic source that carries the laser energy. As the laser leaves the source, the beam forms a cone shape. The energy from this laser also decreases with increasing distance from the source. The energy dissipation rate for this type of beam is r4th power, where r equals the radius of the base of the cone formed by the beam.[1, 2]

Although it might appear that the carbon dioxide laser may be more dangerous over a greater distance, this may or may not be true. Different tissues have different energy requirements for injury to occur. The skin may require 5 to 20 watts to create a burn injury, while the retina may require 2 to 3 milliwatts to create a permanent visual field loss. The carbon dioxide laser does not reach the retina owing to its wavelength characteristics, whereas the Nd:YAG laser readily reaches the retina even at low levels of power. With this in mind, the best recommendation is to assume that the *injury range* extends to all parts of the room. The laser can injure anyone within the room where the laser is used. Whenever the laser is in use, all persons in the room must observe all recommended specific precautions for the type of laser being used.

Duration of exposure to the beam's energy is also important. The beam will deliver a steady amount of energy to the surface it impacts on. The longer the exposure, the higher the amount of energy delivered. Certain laser techniques use higher levels of power for very short periods to avoid overheating

45

the tissues surrounding the intended target. Some techniques involve immersion of the operative site in a water stream to keep the tissues from overheating.

There are many types of lasers available that the surgeon can choose to use for a specific task. These lasers differ from each other in their specific wavelengths. The wavelengths vary from the visible light (optical) spectrum to the invisible. The relative danger to a person relates to the type of laser. An example to show the difference between lasers is the type of lens required to protect the eyes of the awake patient and the personnel. Carbon dioxide lasers require clear glass or plastic of a certain density. The type of eyeshield is very specific for each type of laser. Whereas the eyeshields used with the Nd:YAG are goggles with a green tinted lens, the eyeshields used with the argon laser are an amber-orange color. The optical density specifications for the eyeshields should be obtained from the laser company (Fig. 3–1).

OPERATING ROOM SAFETY

Patient Safety

The patient is anesthetized or sedated during the surgical procedure. Therefore, the ability of the patient to warn the surgeon of possible injury is impeded or removed. Hence, all efforts for safety must be directed toward prevention of possible complications. This includes the use of nonflammable materials where possible. Laser-resistant shielding materials are available for the surgical field and for protecting the anesthesia equipment. Certain adjustments in the anesthesia technique may

also decrease the potential hazards. These adjustments are discussed below.

Personnel Safety

Personnel working in the laser environment can be at risk for injury. Similar patterns of injury from the laser occur in the workers as in the patients. However, because the operating room personnel are awake, they should be able to be aware of an injury situation that develops. Once aware, they should correct the problem and thereby prevent or minimize the injury.

Absolute rules for the safety of the personnel are as follows:

1. Post signs that lasers are being used (Fig. 3–2). (See chapter on the Carbon Dioxide Laser.) These signs should
   a. describe the type of laser.
   b. indicate the risk class of the laser.
   c. indicate the required safety equipment for personnel (specific eyeshields).
   d. state that if unprotected personnel enter the area, the laser is to be turned off.
2. Eyeshields must be worn at all times by all personnel.
3. Safety shields must be used (Fig. 3–3).
4. A bucket of sterile water should be immediately available in the operating room.
5. A laser safety officer must be stationed at the laser at all times.
6. Safety orientation for laser use should be required of all surgeons, anesthesia personnel, and operating room staff.
7. Credentialing of surgeons for use of each type of laser and laser apparatus is needed.

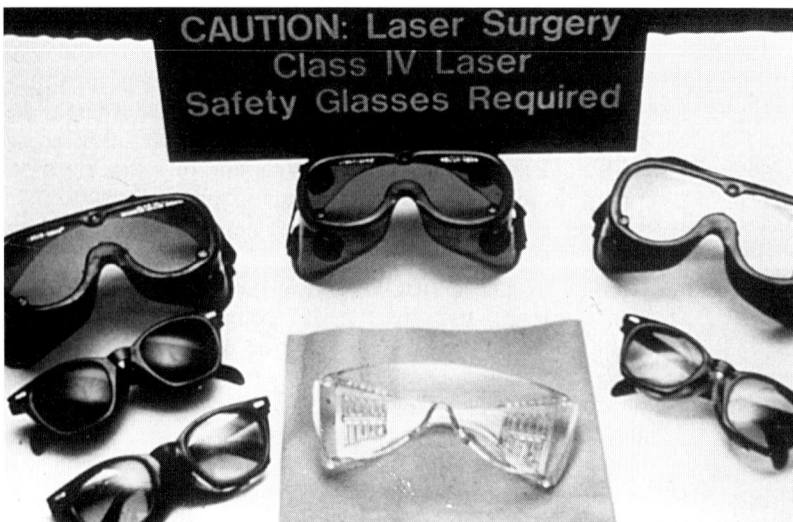

FIGURE 3–1. Example of multiple protective eyeglasses used for each laser, depending on the wavelength of the laser beam. The optical density of the eyeglass lens must shield out the potential damaging effects of the laser beam to the structures of the globe.

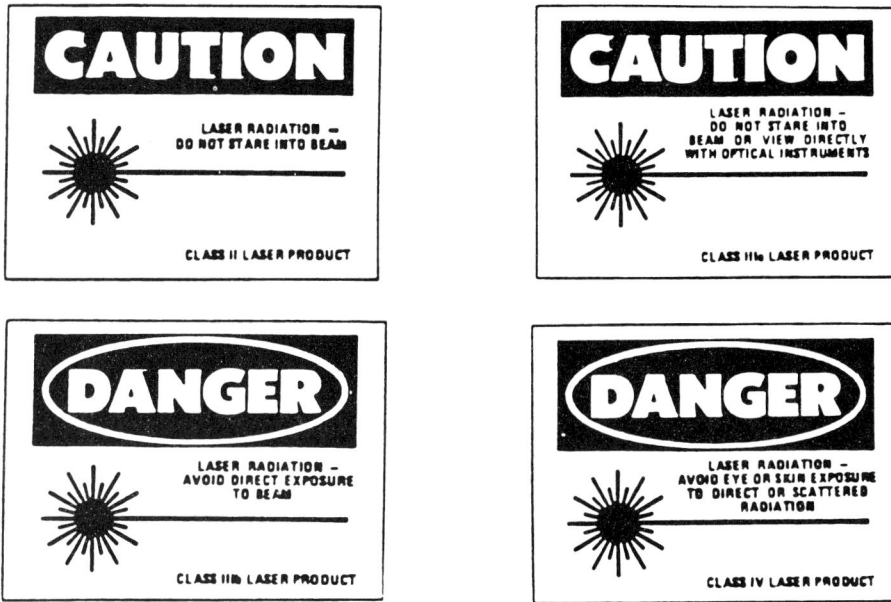

FIGURE 3–2. Types of laser safety signs and labels. These signs are posted at the doorways to the operating room in which a laser is being used. A pair of safety glasses are also hung on or taped to the door to encourage entering personnel to use them.

FIRE HAZARDS

Lasers generate significant heat. This heat presents a fire hazard to all materials near the beam or laser knife. Materials that are used for draping during normal surgical procedures may be completely inappropriate for surgery involving lasers. Cloth is flammable and penetrable. If the laser beam hits the cloth, it could cause a fire, resulting in a severe or lethal burn to the patient. When cloth drapes are used, it is recommended that heavily moistened sterile towels be used in the immediate area of the surgical field. The operating room scrub nurse must maintain the saturation of the towels during surgery because if the towels are dry, they become flammable (Fig. 3–4*A* and *B*).

Drapes

Drapes that are and are not recommended are listed in Table 3–1.

Sterile Field Drape

Paper drapes ignite easily and burn rapidly. Hence, **paper drapes should not be used.** Rapidly

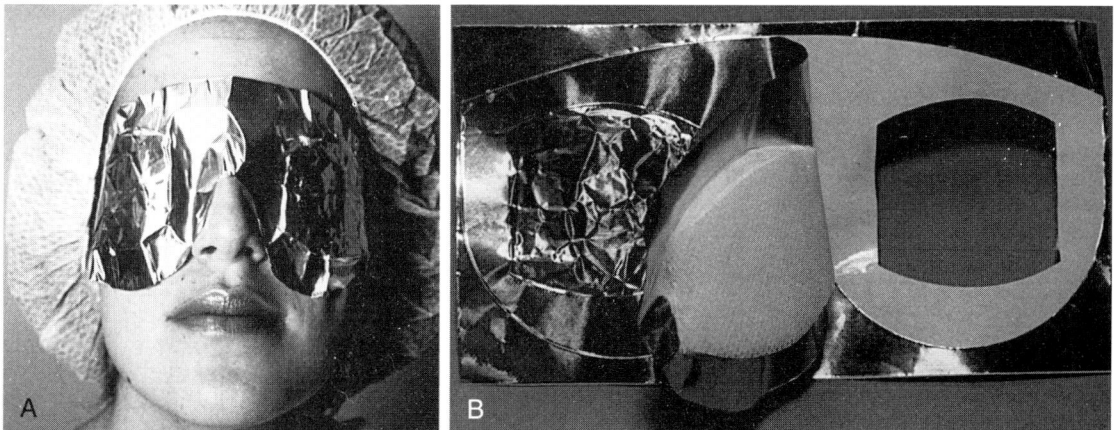

FIGURE 3–3. *A,* Example of self-adhering laser-safe eyeshields that are placed on the patient's eyes durning the laser operation. *B,* Soft foam pads on the undersurface of the eyeshield placed directly on the taped closed eye of the patient.

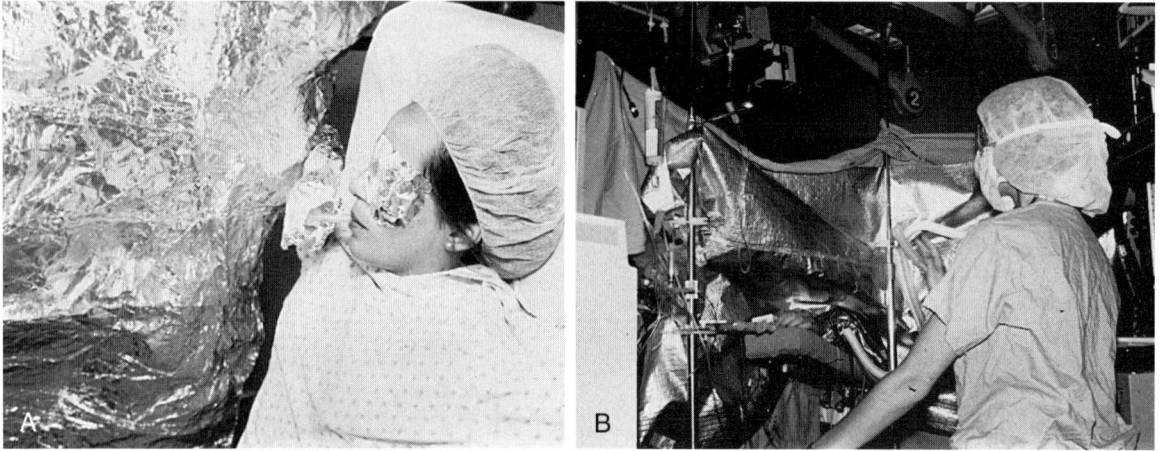

FIGURE 3–4. *A* and *B*, Examples of laser-resistant drapes for the protection of the patient and operating room personnel.

burning materials are very dangerous because they can spread the fire to other objects near the field. The quick spread of the flames also can create a large burn on the patient.[3, 4]

An important point to remember is that certain anesthesia practices and scrub solutions can greatly increase the flammability of the drapes. During anesthesia, oxygen is used to support the patient. If the patient is under general anesthesia, the increased concentration of the oxygen is contained inside the endotracheal tube and anesthesia circuit. If the patient is sedated, the patient is given oxygen supplementation via nasal cannula. The oxygen is used to maintain better arterial oxygen levels and to provide a fresh inspired gas source for the patient while he or she is under the surgical drapes. **As the percentage of oxygen increases near a flame, the rapidity of burning and the ease of ignition increase.** The stage is set for a major disaster if an ignition occurs. This is why it is recommended not to use paper drapes. Still, cloth drapes that are not moistened in a high-oxygen environment will also burn quickly.

In addition to oxygen, nitrous oxide aids burning in the presence of significant amounts of oxygen.[5–7] To avoid this risk, it is recommended that oxygen supplementation be minimized during laser surgery. If general anesthesia is employed, attempts to keep the FIO_2 at or slightly below 0.25 should be made. If intravenous sedation is used, oxygen supplementation should be kept to a minimum or avoided. The surgeon can warn the anesthesiologist to turn off the supplemental oxygen when the laser is activated.

Another important component of possible drape ignition hazard is the use of **alcohol as part of the surgical field preparation.** Alcohol solution to prep the field prior to surgery is appropriate, provided that it is allowed to vaporize completely prior to draping the surgical field. Sometimes plastic drapes are used on the surgical field and alcohol can be trapped under the plastic as a liquid or gas. Alcohol can also be absorbed by cloth drapes when they are applied near the planned incision or field. Alcohol fumes in the presence of a diathermy electric spark, or a laser beam and oxygen can quickly ignite and burn the patient and surgeon. The alcohol also can serve as an ignition source for other flammable materials in the operative field.

Certain companies have marketed flame-retardant and flame-resistant paper drapes for use with lasers. These drapes still present a hazard of penetration by the laser beam and potential patient burn injury. It is not recommended that paper drapes be used.

Laser-resistant drapes are available. These drapes are designed to be **resistant to laser beam penetration as well as being ignition resistant.** The drapes are lightweight and malleable, and they have specified power limits for safety with each type of laser. To ensure laser resistance, these power limits are not to be exceeded. The drapes are designed as personnel shields, anesthesia circuit shields, and eyeshields. There are shields that are sterile for the immediate surgical field area. There are also materials designed to shield the endotracheal tube, which are discussed later.

In summary, lasers can cause fires and injury. All means should be employed to decrease the risk of

TABLE 3–1. Drapes Used in Laser Surgery

Not Recommended

   Paper
   Plastic
   Flame-resistant or flame-retardant materials

Recommended

   Cloth saturated with water around field
   Laser-resistant drapes for personnel, anesthesia circuit, and eyeshields

fires and accidental penetration of the drapes around the surgical field. Remember, too, that operating room personnel are wearing clothing that may ignite or be penetrated. Paper gowns are not recommended for laser procedures. A standing rule should be if any patient or person feels unexplained warmth during a laser procedure, turn off the laser and investigate the cause. One should not wait for an ignition or full penetration to decide that something is wrong.

SPECULAR REFLECTION

Aiming the laser at the surgical field is the obvious goal during laser surgery. However, the beam may be misaligned or altered by a reflective object placed in the beam's path, which can result in the laser's striking unintended objects near or far from the surgical field. The following are safety procedures designed to minimize the chances of specular reflection.

The surgical beam should be tested for alignment prior to each use of the machine. The test involves hitting a target with the beam to test for the alignment of the spot (lower power visible beam) and the surgical laser (higher power and can be invisible). The testing also involves checking the wattage and aperture setting. Lasers can become misaligned during storage if the arm or delivery device is inadvertently struck. With lasers that travel along fibers of a fiber-optic cable, lateral leakage of laser energy can occur if certain fibers are fractured. Laser-resistant sheaths to shield the fiber-optic cables are available. Certain YAG laser machines have monitors to test the fiber-optic cable for power leakage. This test should be performed prior to use. If significant lateral leakage is occurring, then the cable should be replaced.

To avoid the risk of specular reflection from an instrument placed in the path of the laser, certain rules should be followed by the surgical assistant and the operating surgeon. **No instruments are passed across the intended path of the laser.** This is very important, because not only does it decrease the risk of specular reflection but it also inhibits an injury to the surgical assistant or the operative surgeon from the laser beam. Most instruments used in oral and maxillofacial surgery can be anodized by the manufacturer, thus decreasing surface reflectivity of misguided laser beams (Fig. 3–5).

OTHER OBJECTS AT RISK

During oral maxillofacial surgery, the *anesthesia circuit* is very near the field. During procedures involving the oropharynx, the *endotracheal tube* may lie in front of, next to, or behind the surgical pathology. Considerations in the choice of the endotracheal tube are discussed in the next section. However, it must be pointed out that the proximity of the anesthesia circuit to the laser beam and the risks of specular reflection absolutely demand shielding of the anesthesia circuit and the proximal endotracheal tube from the laser. An anesthesia circuit shield is available on the market, and its use does not inhibit access to the surgical field.

During laser surgery at Allegheny General Hospital in Pittsburgh, a specular reflection struck the **sterile plastic drape that is used to cover the carbon dioxide laser microscope.** This fire was

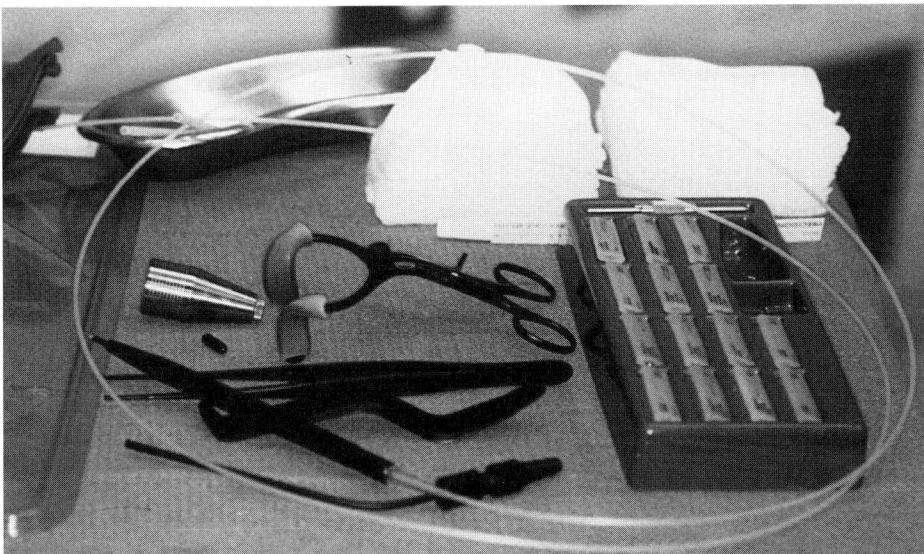

FIGURE 3–5. Examples of anodized instruments for use in oral and maxillofacial surgery.

extinguished without incident, but the plastic microscope drape does present a fire hazard. One must ensure that the sterile plastic drape is always tacked up away from the surgical field (Fig. 3–6).

Management of **eye protection** is discussed later, but it is important to remember that in this type of surgery, the eye is very close to the laser target. Laser-resistant shielding should protect the eye from harm. It must be used for every patient. If the patient is awake, laser safety eyeglasses may be worn, but care must be taken to protect the eye from specular side reflections. It is best to place a laser-resistant shield between the eyes and the surgical field, if it is possible. There are also commercially available laser-safe contact lenses that have variable sizes.

ELECTRIC SHOCK

Lasers develop their high-energy beams by exposing confined gases to **high-voltage electrical current.** The laser device presents a shock hazard to anyone who manipulates the machine. The laser safety officer is instructed in the proper use of the machine. The laser safety officer and the company representative are the only personnel who should service the machine. If other personnel manipulate the laser, they run the **risk of electrical burns, cardiac arrhythmias, or cardiac arrest.**

EXPLOSION HAZARDS

The laser is an ignition source; therefore, if a highly combustible material or gas in a confined space is hit by the laser beam, an explosion can result. In modern operating rooms the use of explosive anesthetics is prohibited; hence, **ether** or **cyclopropane** use is contraindicated during laser surgery. **Alcohol,** used during the skin prepping, can cause an explosion. Also, during gynecologic or colonic laser surgeries, if the laser encounters **methane-containing flatus** in high enough concentrations, flash fires have occurred. These have resulted in burns both to the patient and to the operative surgeon's hands. If flatus is encountered, the laser should not be used until the methane is dissipated. To prevent injury during colonic surgery, the colon is insufflated with a nonflammable gas to wash out the methane-containing hazardous gas.[8]

VIRUS PARTICLES

Lasers are used sometimes to fulgarize pathologies caused by viruses. Venereal warts and circumoral condylomata are examples of this. There have been cases reported in which surgeons have reported facial venereal warts in areas of the cheeks not covered by the face mask during surgery. Culture specimens have been taken of the laser smoke flumes and have produced viral cultures.[9–11] One should assume that the smoke coming from the operative site does contain viral particles. Vacuums to remove the smoke and filters to remove the viral particles from the air should be used at all times. If smoke is escaping from above the vacuum, it must be stopped.

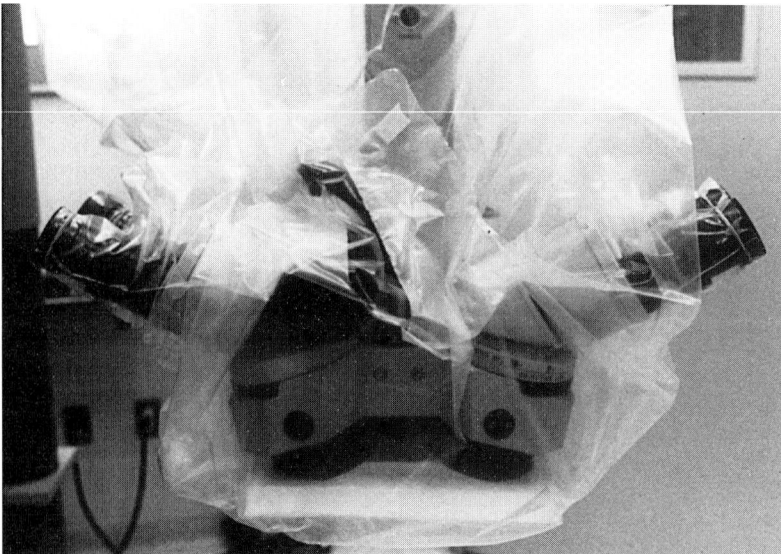

FIGURE 3–6. Vulnerable plastic shield used to create a sterile field during microlaser surgery. This shield is not laser resistant and, therefore, should not be used near a laser handpiece to avoid ignition.

COMBUSTION PRODUCTS

Not only can viral products be carried by the smoke, it has been suggested that some of the **chemicals carried in the laser smoke may be carcinogens.** Hence, the same policy concerning the use of a vacuum and air filtration system should be enforced.[12]

SHIELDING DEVICES

Injury Patterns

The Eye, Sclera, Pupil, Retina, and Eyelid

Each tissue in the human body reacts to the laser differently. Heating, desiccation, cutting, and permanent damage occur at different energy levels. The **eye** and its contents are certainly the most sensitive. Eye structures, when injured, are usually irreversibly harmed. Prevention of exposure must be the ultimate goal (Fig. 3–7).

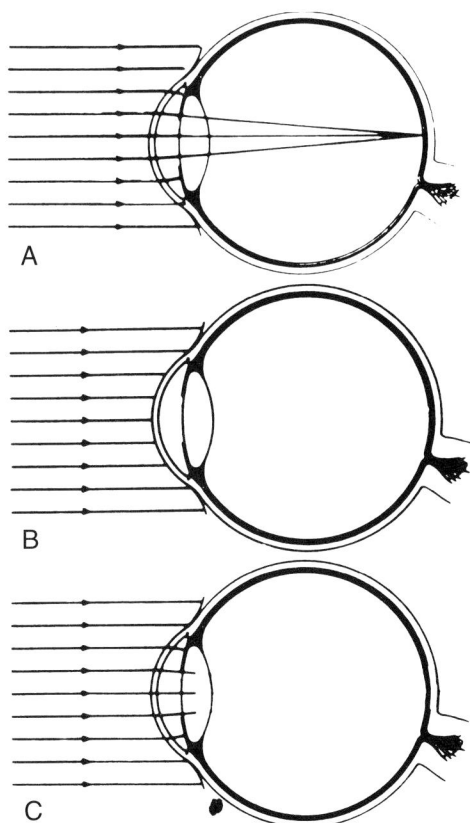

FIGURE 3–7. Examples of various wavelengths and their locus of potential injury to the structures of the eye. *A,* Focused to injure retina—400 to 1400 nm; *B,* injury to cornea and sclera, for example, carbon dioxide laser—3 μ to 1 mm; *C,* near-ultraviolet and midinfrared affecting the lens of the eye.

Each type of laser has different physical effects on the eye. For instance, if the carbon dioxide laser hits the **sclera** or **pupil,** it will cause superficial heating and a burn. As the power and duration of exposure increase, penetration of the eye occurs. Superficial injury of the eye occurs because the mechanism of heating by the carbon dioxide laser is superheating of the water contained in the outermost tissues. YAG lasers penetrate into the deeper structures of the eye because they are conducted readily in the aqueous and vitreous humors. **Retinal damage** occurs readily and with very low wattage levels. The reason for this injury is that the YAG laser energy beam enters the pupil and passes through the lens and is focused by the lens. The result of the focusing is that the energy is concentrated on a specific area of the retina. Permanent damage to the retina results. If the **macular area** is struck, severe deficits of the primary visual field occur.[4, 13]

Closing **the eyelids** decreases some of the risk of injury to the eye. However, injury to the eye can still occur because the eyelids can be easily penetrated, especially if high-power density levels are being used. The eyelids may not be completely shut; hence, the laser could still have a direct impact on the eye. The eyelids themselves could be burned and scarred. Retraction of the eyelid after the burn with secondary exposure of the eye could be a devastating complication.

The following method should be used to prevent injury to the eye. Close the eye, and moisten it, if desired. Only normal saline is to be used. Lacrilube is normally used by anesthesiologists to keep the eye moist under anesthesia. **Lacrilube is petroleum based and can ignite** if struck by a laser beam. Lacrilube should be avoided.[4] The eyelids should be taped closed. Tape is ignitable. The tape should be cut small enough so that it is not visible under the laser-resistant eyeshield. The eyeshield should be placed over the eyes and should extend to the orbital ridge.

Other products used for ocular protection include opaque plastic or metal contact lenses that can be placed by the practitioner to shield the eyes. For the most part, these contact lens shields are for specific applications in cosmetic surgery, where laser procedures may be performed on or near the eyelid. If a plastic contact lens is struck by the beam, it should be removed and examined immediately. If any signs of thinning or penetration of the contact has occurred, then the contact lens should be discarded and a new one used. If the contact lens is penetrated, then the eye should be examined for potential injury (see Chapter 12).

The Skin

The skin is usually a more forgiving organ than the eye. Higher power levels are required to cause injury, and often smaller lacerations or burns may heal with little residual damage. Do not forget, however, that **burns and lacerations occurring in facial areas can easily disfigure** the patient (Fig. 3–8). Hence, care must be taken at all times and with all potentially exposed parts of the anatomy of the patient. Shielding skin areas not involved in the operative procedure is important. Avoidance of flammable surgical drapes, as was discussed previously, is important. **Hair** near the operative site can be ignited, which can result in a severe burn with scarring and disfigurement. Hair should be shielded, kept moistened, or removed, if possible, from the proximity of the operative site.

Teeth

Teeth require very high energy levels to cause significant structural damage. However, etching of the enamel surface of the teeth can occur at lower levels of power. Etching can result in disfigurement of the teeth. Etching can be prevented by shielding the teeth from exposure to the laser beam. Dental splints fabricated from laser-resistant material are commercially available. It is important to use this type of material because a powerful laser beam can cause pitting of enamel or cementum, or both, presumably rendering a tooth more susceptible to caries and pulpitis. However, this is controversial.

The Tracheobronchial Tree and Oropharyngeal Tissues

Mucosa has an injury pattern similar to that of the skin. Burns and lacerations can occur. Burns are less likely to cause disfigurement, but significant structures such as the **vocal cord and epiglottis,** if injured, could cause **swelling and upper airway**

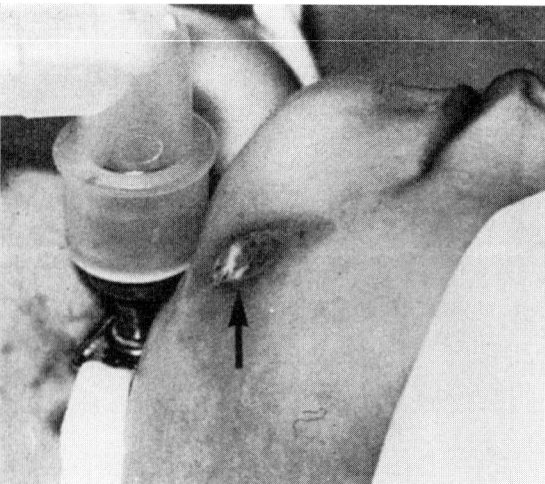

FIGURE 3–8. Potentially disfiguring laser burn of the lower face due to inadequate protection of the skin.

obstruction. Potential chronic dysfunction is also possible. One other potential source of airway and facial burns is heating of metallic endotracheal tubes by the laser beam.[14–16] **Lacerations of the trachea** that resulted from specular reflections off a metallic endotracheal tube have been reported.[17] Subcutaneous emphysema occurs as a complication during the postoperative period.

Although mucosal injury may occur from a direct impact of the laser beam, another potential source of injury is the **ignition of the endotracheal tube or other flammable objects** placed in the oropharynx or trachea during the surgical procedure (Fig. 3–9). The burn that occurs under these circumstances may be caused by thermal energy released from the burning material. The amount of the burn injury reflects the type of material involved, the amount of material burned, and the duration of the burning process. As noted earlier, if oxygen in higher concentrations is present, it may hasten the rate of burning and the release of thermal energy. Also, if the patient is being ventilated through an endotracheal tube, the fresh gas source blowing past the ignition point may act similar to an engine and further speed the burning process (Fig. 3–10).

A burning endotracheal tube can release toxic chemicals during the burning process. The chemicals released may cause further tissue injury to the mucosa. This factor is discussed further in the section on endotracheal tubes used for laser surgery.

In summary, laser surgery involving structures near or in the airway incurs potentially severe complications. Any method should be employed that prevents or minimizes risks of injury.

Methods of Prevention of Injury

The Perioperative Site. The surgeon will learn, as a part of the training for laser surgery, how to minimize tissue damage in the immediate vicinity of the operative site. Remember that the laser will be employed to remove or debulk a lesion, and it is intended to cause complete destruction or removal of the diseased tissue, or both. One of the advantages suggested by proponents of the laser is that it causes minimal injury to adjacent tissue structures. Certain techniques have been developed to achieve this result.[17]

Use the least **amount of power (wattage)** required depending on the laser used. The use of the highest power density that is controllable by the surgeon minimizes the risk of collateral damage. Employing the lowest energy level, such as defocused continuous mode, may increase the risk of heat build-up and injury to other tissues. Higher wattage for short bursts (pulsing) is a method used to avoid heat damage to adjacent tissues by enhancing thermal relaxation time.

Use the **appropriate laser for the job required.**

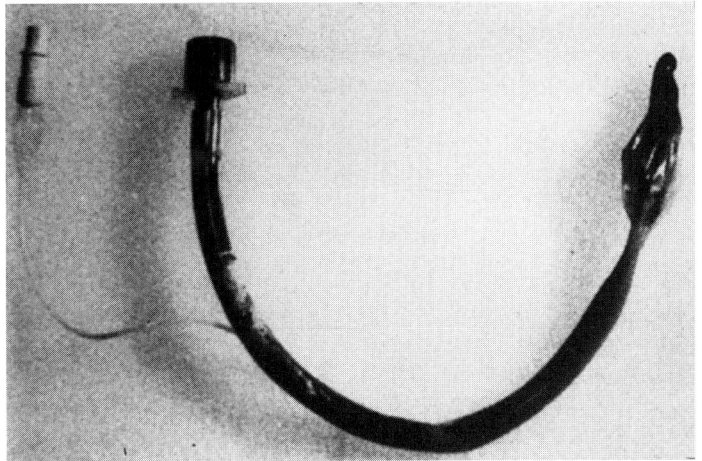

FIGURE 3–9. Charred remains of endotracheal tube after ignition of the tube supported by intraluminal anesthetic gases.

Different lasers have various properties that make them more appropriate for specific applications. During laser orientation courses, the instructors and the materials provided should describe the correct applications for each type of laser and tissue pathology.

Short bursts, intermittent lasing, and changing from one area of the lesion to another sequentially are designed to minimize heat build-up in the target tissue. If continuous lasing is performed, significant amounts of heat can build up in the target tissue and cause temporary or permanent damage. Continuous lasing for long periods of time is not recommended. It is important to keep the laser spot moving in a predetermined pattern.

Use **cooled irrigation to keep tissues from heating** with appropriate laser surgery. However, keep in mind the effect of water on laser (carbon dioxide) penetration of tissues.

Remember the **three-dimensional anatomy of the area being lased.** Important structures may lie in proximity or below the surgical target. If the beam strikes these structures, complications can occur. Some examples of possible complications are the following:

Laceration of an artery with subsequent blood loss.
Laceration of a vocal cord.
Heating of a nerve with subsequent loss of sensation or paresis.

It is very important for the surgeon to anticipate possible structural injuries that might occur. Possible complications and preparation for the management of these complications should be discussed with the **anesthesiologist. A team approach to minimizing risk is very important.**

Finally, as discussed previously, evaluate the operative site for other potential risks. Flammable drapes, either paper or plastic, may ignite. Alcohol used as a part of the prep solution must be allowed to evaporate or dry before covering the site with drapes. If the patient is receiving supplemental oxy-

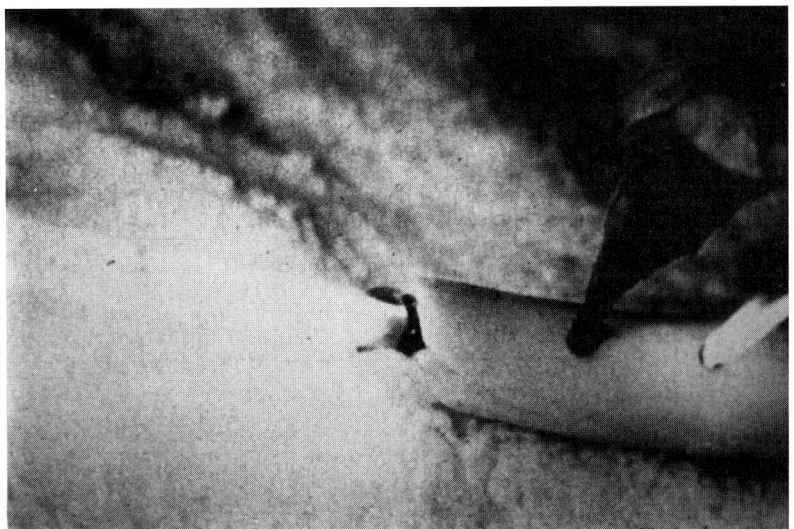

FIGURE 3–10. Blowtorch phenomenon at the distal end of an endotracheal tube perforated by a powerful laser beam.

gen during sedation, remember that the oxygen can build up near the operative site and enhance a rapid ignition of flammable materials. During laser oropharyngeal surgery, some of the anesthesia techniques for general anesthesia may increase oxygen concentrations and risk of ignition.

All potential sites of injury, and all potential sources and components of ignition must be evaluated. If possible, flammable materials should be avoided. If flammable materials are used, then they must be kept moist throughout the procedure, or they must be shielded from the laser beam.

COMPONENTS OF THE ANESTHETIC PLAN

Nonmetallic Endotracheal Tubes

Owing to the fire hazard that exists with lasers, steps must be taken to minimize risk during anesthesia. This is especially true during general anesthesia for surgery involving the oropharynx, facial structures, trachea, and bronchial tree. Avoidance of tubes and instruments made of combustible material during anesthesia would be the ideal solution, but in some situations, this approach is impossible. The discussion that follows mentions most of the suggested methods in the literature. An attempt is made to elucidate the benefits and costs of each approach. The reader must then decide what technique or instrument provides the best and safest method for the clinical situation.

When lasers were first used, the tubes were wrapped in metallic foil—specifically aluminum foil. When sheets of aluminum were applied to the tube, the edges sometimes cut the mucosa, or they unfolded to expose the endotracheal tube to the laser. Some practitioners chose to wrap the tube with **metallic tape of copper or silver.**[18, 19] The tape had to be very carefully wrapped in an axial fashion (Fig. 3–11) and edges had to overlap. Still, there were problems of exposure if the tube bent too much, or the cuff was inflated under the tape wrap. The advantage to the tape was that it added little external diameter to the tube. One potential problem with the tape was the accidental placement of a silver paint tape that was not laser resistant. Hence, painted tape and metallic tape must be labeled and stored in different areas.

A later development in endotracheal tube protection was the creation of a **silver anode** sheet that had a spongy, water-absorbent material on the outside and an adhesive material on the inside.[20] This material formed a double layer of protection against the carbon dioxide laser. Its adherence to the tube also avoided the risks of unraveling that occurred with the taped tubes. This material is still used today when clinicians elect to use nonmetallic endotracheal tubes. This material can be penetrated at higher powers, so again the clinician should refer to the package insert for the safe power limits of this product.

Another strategy for endotracheal tube protection is the **ceramic-coated endotracheal tube by Xomed** (Boca Raton, Florida) to shield against laser ignition and penetration by using a nonflammable coating on the outside of the endotracheal tube.[21] If low powers were used, this ceramic shield worked very well. However, the higher powers of the carbon dioxide laser and lower powers of the Nd:YAG laser were able to penetrate the tube and ignite it. A later ceramic formulation used by Xomed increased the resistance to penetration, but the practitioner must still be careful to shield this tube with moist gauze when it is used. A paper was also published that described the potential risk for ignition of the inside of the tube with hot ignition

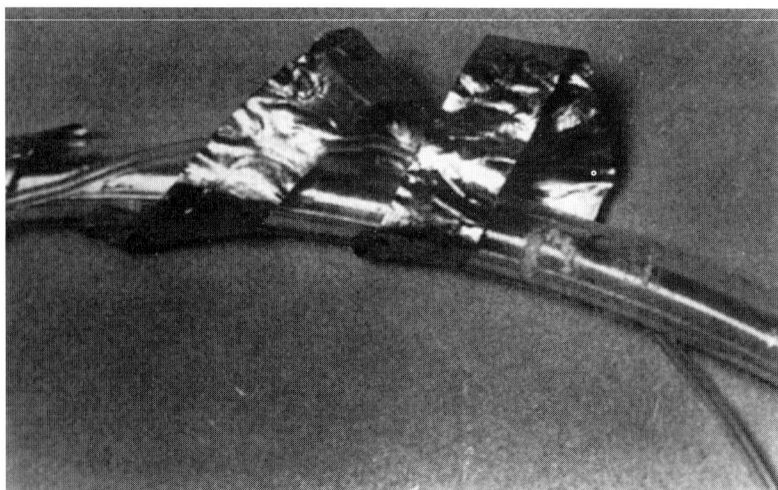

FIGURE 3–11. Polyvinylchloride endotracheal tube is wrapped with metallic foil, taking care to overlap edges of the foil to avoid exposure of the tube to possible penetration by the laser beam.

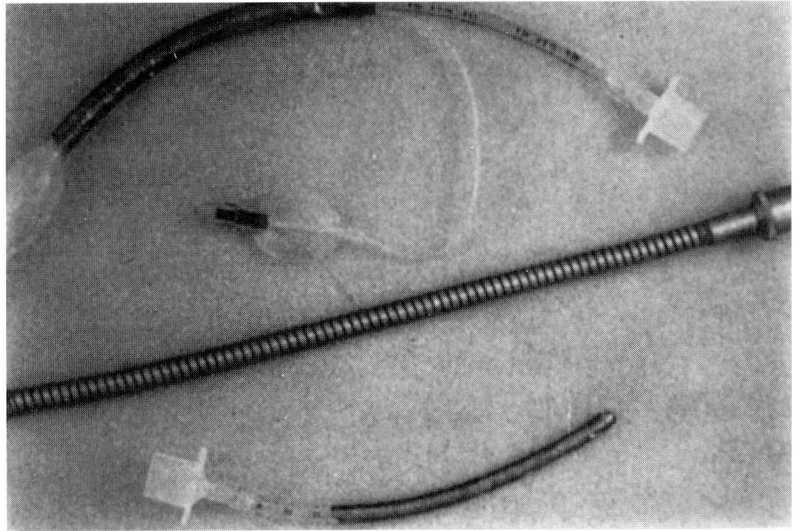

FIGURE 3–12. Nonmetallic and metallic endotracheal tubes. *Top,* Foil-covered polyvinylchloride endotracheal tube with tape wrapped along the longitudinal axis of the tube with overlap of the tape. *Middle,* Standard flexible metal anode tube used for oral endotracheal intubation. *Bottom,* Silver-coated polyvinylchloride endotracheal tube.

products created from the laser-tissue interaction. Hence, this type of tube may not be appropriate for endobronchial YAG laser fiber-optic cable surgery. This tube does have one clear advantage in that it can be passed down through the nose for nasal intubation with less trauma and bleeding than a metal tube. Laser procedures using a carbon dioxide laser involving the oral cavity and tongue are most appropriate for the Xomed tube (Fig. 3–12).

Metallic Endotracheal Tubes

The **Norton** and **Devos endotracheal tubes** and the **Porch tube** can be used during laser surgery on the oropharynx or trachea.[22, 23] These tubes cannot be passed through the nose because they are metal. Also, they are used with orotracheal intubation. The

advantages of these tubes are that they do not contain any combustible materials. The construction of these flexible metal tubes employs a series of thin metal bands that are wrapped to form a central lumen. The tube can be bent a certain amount. The bands are held together at the ends with a proximal and distal circle. There is no cuff provided on the tube; hence, normal anesthetic circuits cannot be used (see the section on anesthesia techniques later). The Norton tube has less flexibility but a larger internal diameter. The Devos tube has a greater number of bands to give it more flexibility, but this is at the cost of the internal diameter of the lumen. The Devos tube has a very narrow lumen (Fig. 3–13).

Often, the surgeon operating on the vocal cords or lower oropharynx requests a small external diameter endotracheal tube to maximize the vision of the

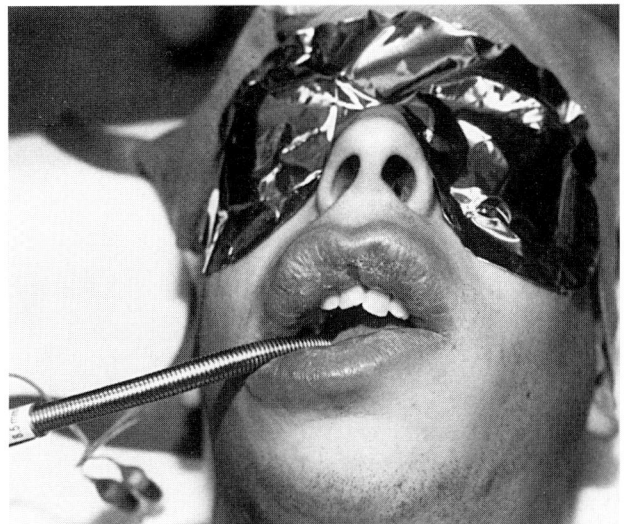

FIGURE 3–13. Flexible metallic endotracheal tube must be used via the oral route and cannot be passed orally. It contains no combustible material and, therefore, is comparatively laser-safe.

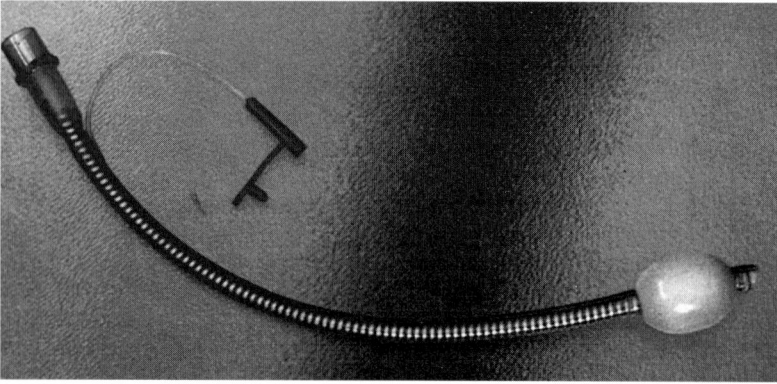

FIGURE 3–14. Example of cuffed flexible metallic endotracheal tube.

surgical field. This is usually accomplished using a 4 to 5 external diameter Devos tube. Use of this tube is combined with either a **jet ventilator or a high-frequency ventilator.**[24–30] These methods do not employ regular anesthesia circuits and are discussed below.

Regular anesthesia circuits could not be employed until the later development of the cuffed metal endotracheal tube (Fig. 3–14). There is still a problem with the cuffed metal tube chosen, because the lumen is small. A size 6 to 7 external diameter tube with a cuff is the best compromise between surgical field view and lumen size. Effective ventilation using an anesthesia circuit in an adult requires an internal lumen size of 6 mm diameter or greater. Some authors have suggested the use of helium in the gas mix. Helium with 30% oxygen is not flammable and has less resistance to flow. Therefore, **helium-oxygen** as a mixture could be employed with tubes of lower internal diameter. However, changeover of the anesthesia machines to carry helium is expensive. Other anesthesia techniques not employing the anesthesia circuit are available and provide acceptable alternatives if a very small external diameter endotracheal tube is required.

Another type of metallic tube that is available is the **straight ventilating bronchoscope** (Fig. 3–15). This tube existed prior to the clinical use of lasers and was adapted to laser use because it is nonflammable. The tube is placed in the trachea between the vocal cords. The gas source is hooked up to the lateral side of the tube, and the patient is ventilated. The surgeon must occlude the end of the tube to ventilate. This technique employs periods of surgery with periods of ventilation, unless the target tissue lies outside the lumen of the tube. In this case, the tube would just be used to ventilate the patient. Often, a jet ventilator is placed on the side of the tube. The tube is used primarily for tracheal lumen lesions or scarring. It can also act as a conduit for a YAG laser fiber-optic cable during endobronchial carcinoma laser surgery.

Jet Ventilation

Previously, it was noted that **jet ventilation can be used to provide ventilatory support** during laser surgery.[28–30] **Jet ventilators cannot be used to provide anesthesia** because the gas outflow

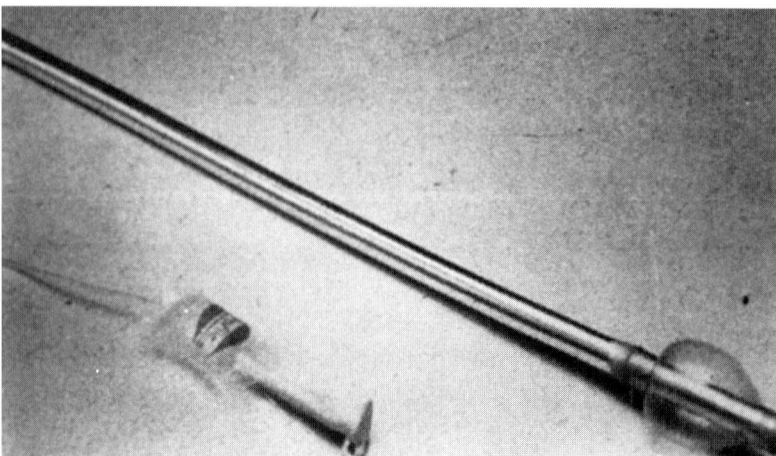

FIGURE 3–15. A straight ventilating bronchoscope (see text).

around the uncuffed endotracheal tube would contaminate the operating room with anesthetic gases. Thanks to intravenous anesthesia, this is not an impediment to providing excellent anesthesia. The choice of using jet ventilation revolves around the location of the operative field and the mechanism involved in exposing the oropharynx and airway. A **ventilating laryngoscope** is commonly employed for posterior pharyngeal, laryngeal, and vocal cord lesions (Fig. 3–16). In some circumstances, a small Devos tube will be used. Commonly, the ventilating laryngoscope has a small **suction catheter welded to its side.** The jet source can be attached to the proximal catheter. In some versions, the distal tip of the jet catheter lies outside the vocal cords. Here, ventilation occurs when positive pressure is built up in the oropharynx and the air moves into the lungs. The possibility of **aspiration** exists in this method from two sources: First, the pressure build-up can push air into the esophagus and stomach, and second, the cords remain open. When this technique is employed, pressure build-up in the oropharynx should be minimized. This can be achieved by using short bursts of jet ventilation. One author places pressure monitors through a second catheter on the ventilation laryngoscope and attempts to keep the pressure below 12 mm H_2O in children and below 20 mm H_2O in adults. Another author describes a suction catheter that slides, which attempts to place the distal tip of the jet source catheter on the tracheal side of the vocal cords.

An important point to remember when using a jet ventilation system is the **risk of barotrauma if a pressure build-up occurs.** Care must be exercised when using the jet to **avoid prolonged bursts of gas** volume because this can cause pressure build-up. Also, a **ready path for gas exit must exist.** If the passage for gas outflow is obstructed, the risk of barotrauma increases greatly. Outflow obstruction can occur if a larger size endotracheal tube is used, and obstruction can occur if the lumen of the tube is kinked. Blocking of gas outflow can also occur sometimes when moist packing is placed around the surgical field in the deep pharynx.

In some circumstances, a **percutaneous catheter (transtracheal jet ventilation)** is placed from the exterior into the distal trachea to achieve ventilation. This is a special circumstance. The patient may be a child, and the operative site size requires the alternate source of gas. Occasionally, the presence of numerous tracheal polyps might require this method. Remember, before giving vigorous bursts of jetted gas, the patency of the outflow path must be ensured.

Another method used to avoid barotrauma risk is **high-frequency jet ventilation.** An oscillating membrane of a high-revolution low-volume pump is used to cause a brownian motion flow of gas in and out of the lungs. It has been shown that satisfactory oxygen and carbon dioxide levels can be maintained with this method. **Oxygen saturation monitors** are absolutely required. At our institution, a **Venturi gas mixer** is employed to control the oxygen percentage. Air and oxygen are mixed to provide a desired oxygen percentage.

Types of Nonmetallic Endotracheal Tubes

Types of nonmetallic endotracheal tubes include red rubber, polyvinyl chloride, and silicon. The

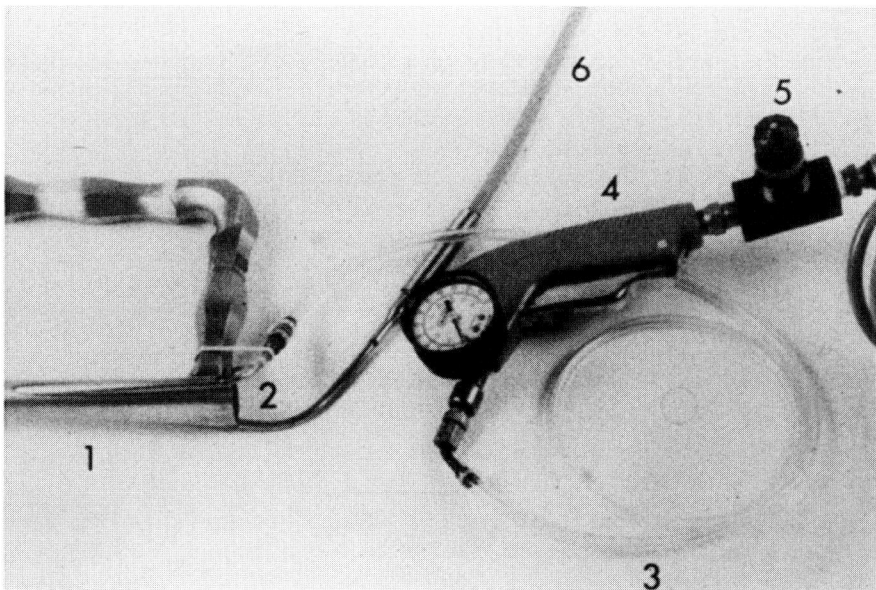

FIGURE 3–16. Example of ventilating laryngoscope (# 1), employed with jet ventilating system.

characteristics of each type of tube are provided in Table 3–2.

As was discussed in the section on metallic endotracheal tubes, avoidance of flammable endotracheal tubes is preferred. However, certain clinical instances exist in which the use of nonmetallic tubes may be required. Therefore, it is appropriate to discuss the flammable characteristics of the three types of commonly used endotracheal tube materials. In Table 3–2, it is obvious that all the tubes can ignite and burn if they are hit by the laser. From the table, it is obvious that **red rubber tubes may be the best overall nonmetallic tube to use. Polyvinyl chloride tubes** are not recommended for two reasons. First, the polyvinyl chloride tube ignites easily and burns quickly. Second, the burning of the polyvinyl chloride tube releases very toxic substances both as a gas and as a carbonaceous residue. These toxic materials can increase the amount of damage to the lung and trachea from the tube ignition. Red rubber tubes burn more slowly, and when they burn, the smoke is less toxic to the lung parenchyma. Red rubber tubes are also slightly more resistant to initial ignition.[4, 31–33]

Silicon tubes were initially thought to be safer, because when they burn, they produce only a white ash residue. However, the white silica ash is large in amount. The ash is difficult to remove from the bronchial tree after the surgery. The silica ash residue may present a long-term hazard from silicosis of the lung. So the initial support for silicon endotracheal tubes has diminished.

The reader must remember that these nonmetallic tubes can ignite and that shielding material must be used with each tube (shielding material is discussed in another section). Also, strategies must be employed so that if an endotracheal tube ignition does occur, then its rate of burning and full ignition will be slowed. These strategies are also discussed later but include using low oxygen concentrations; diluting oxygen with an inert carrier (nitrogen or helium); avoiding nitrous oxide; using volatile anesthetic if the tube is cuffed; and if the tube is uncuffed, using a continuous intravenous anesthesia technique.

Endotracheal Tube Cuffs

Most anesthetic procedures for general anesthesia employ a **cuffed endotracheal tube.** The few exceptions to this approach are pediatric cases and situations in which jet ventilation or high-frequency jet ventilation are used. The cuff is inflated around the endotracheal tube both to create an air seal to allow effective ventilation and to prevent aspiration of fluids from the esophagus and stomach. One might argue that the cuff could also be used to isolate the oxygen away from the surgical field during laser surgery. This is not a valid use, because a nonmetallic tube or cuff could be penetrated and burn, exposing the higher oxygen content and rapidly increasing the rate of burn of objects near the field. In laser surgery, the endotracheal tube cuff can be problematic. The cuff is usually made of flammable material, so it presents a fire hazard. One can choose a metal tube, an uncuffed tube, or a method of ventilation that does not require a cuff to avoid potential problems with the cuff.

The air in the cuff may contain either high oxygen or nitrous oxide concentrations that may increase the rate of burning. To avoid this problem, **water is injected into the cuff** to prevent burning and ignition of the cuff during laser use.[34] Owing to the stiffness of the cuff with water versus air, on removal, the anesthesiologist should take care to extract all the water to avoid damage to the vocal cord or narrowest part of the airway. When a cuff contains water, it will not burn. However, the cuff can be penetrated by the laser beam and leak. The leak can cause a loss of the air seal, and the tube must be replaced. Certain tubes were designed to overcome this problem. The **double-cuffed tube** allowed penetration of the more proximal cuff without loss of the airway seal because the more distal cuff was still intact. A second approach was a

TABLE 3–2. Types of Nonmetallic Endotracheal Tubes and Their Characteristics

	Tube Material		
Tube Characteristics	*Rubber*	*Polyvinyl Chloride*	*Silicon*
Sensitive to carbon dioxide laser	+	+ + +	
Sensitive to Nd:YAG laser	+ + +	+ + +	+ + +
Blowtorch fire			
Easiest ignition	+	+ + +	+ +
Intensity of flame		+ + +	
Residue carbonaceous material	+	+ + +	
Postmortem damage		+ + +	
Residue white silica ash (silicosis)			+

sponge-filled cuff that was filled with water (Fig. 3–17). If the cuff was hit by the laser, the water leaked out but the sponge remained filled and the airway seal remained intact. The danger with the sponge cuff is that if it is filled with air and not water there is a higher thermal mass to burn. Therefore, if the sponge-filled cuff is employed, water must be used.

A French scientist developed **a shield that can protect the endotracheal tube cuff.** The shield folds along the length of the cuff. Once the endotracheal tube is in position and the cuff is up, the loop at the proximal end of the tube is pulled. The metallic shields fold up and hide the cuff from exposure to the laser beam. This tube seems awkward to use and would not be appropriate for use with vocal cord surgery.

Once the tube is placed and the cuff inflated, usually **moistened gauze is placed around the base of the distal tube as it enters the larynx.** The moistened gauze creates a heat sink to protect the cuff from the laser beam. The gauze **must be kept moist** to maintain the protection. This is accomplished by the circulator who must periodically moisten the gauze in the posterior oropharynx. A second alternative for gauze moistening is to place an **epidural catheter inside the gauze** and bring it out through the side of the mouth. A syringe can then be used to moisten the gauze periodically without creating any distraction in the operative field.

Alternative Ventilation Systems—Uncuffed

Most anesthesia gas delivery is accomplished through a cuffed endotracheal tube and an anesthesia circuit system. This system ventilates through positive pressure that moves gas volumes into the patient's lungs. The volumes employed and the rate of delivery of the volumes assume a system pressure sealed by an endotracheal cuff. During laser procedures, the use of a cuff may be impossible, or the cuff's seal may be compromised by the laser. Also, the cuff creates a fire hazard because it is made of flammable materials. Certain adjustments have been made to minimize the risk of the cuff during oropharyngeal laser procedures (see earlier). However, an alternative exists for anesthesia that does not employ pressure-sealed anesthesia circuits or cuffs.

The first part of this discussion describes different methods of gas delivery in uncuffed systems. Each method is described, and then strengths and weaknesses in each method are pointed out.

The first system to be discussed is an older system that was used prior to laser surgery. This is the **ventilating bronchoscope.** This system is usually employed for masses or scarring in the trachea. The anesthesia circuit is attached to an adapter on the side of the bronchoscope. The surgeon and the anesthesiologist take turns. **Apneic periods** occur when the surgeon examines the airway or uses the laser. Then intermittently (every 40 to 50 seconds), the anesthesiologist ventilates the patient. During the ventilation period, the surgeon occludes the proximal end of the bronchoscope to allow the ventilation to occur.[35, 36]

When other systems that do not use a cuff are used, one must first consider how to get the gases into and out of the patient in a manner that will adequately oxygenate the patient and remove carbon dioxide. Without a cuff to seal the system, larger volumes are required and the flow rates have to be faster. **A jet ventilation system can be employed.** The jet will take a gas supply and allow free flow while it is open. At present, most systems employ a tubing with a control mechanism, a trigger, that is hand-held and controlled by the anesthesiologist. The major risk with a jet ventilation system is associated with an obstruction to the outflow

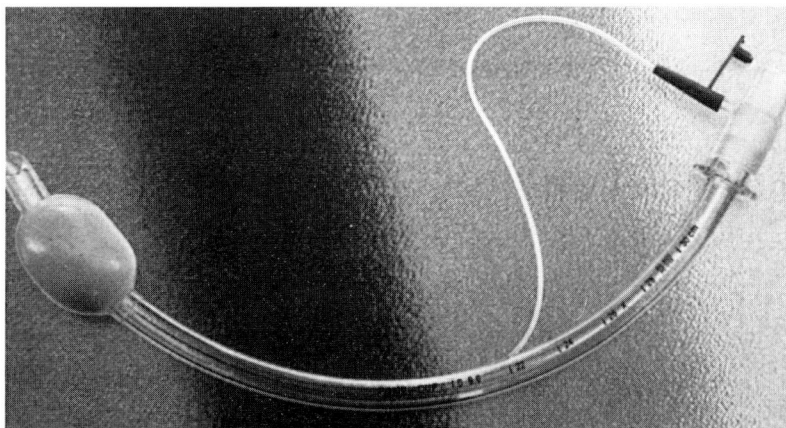

FIGURE 3–17. Endotracheal tube with sponge-filled cuff saturated with water.

of gas. When the obstruction occurs, pressure builds up in the patient's lungs quickly and barotrauma can result. It is important for the anesthesiologist or the surgeon to watch for obstruction and to stop the ventilation immediately if it occurs. The obstruction to gas outflow must be corrected before ventilation is continued. Some causes of outflow obstruction can result from gauze being placed in the oropharynx, or changes in the position of the tube or the head. **To combat this barotrauma risk, some anesthesiologists use only jet systems with a pressure relief valve. The pressure relief valve is in the circuit on the distal side of the trigger mechanism.** The pressure valve is set to 15 mm Hg in children and 30 mm Hg in adults. If the pressure in the distal jet line exceeds these values, the gas is vented to the outside. An operator using this system must watch the patient to ensure adequate ventilation, because normal carbon dioxide monitors of ventilation are not used in this system.

Remember that oxygen must be diluted to decrease the burning risk around the field. With a jet system, the volumes of gas employed to ventilate the patient will flood the operative field. To decrease the oxygen concentration, two methods can be employed. The first is using a **premixed gas cylinder** that contains an oxygen concentration lower than 30%. The second method employs a **Venturi gas mixer** that can adjust the oxygen concentration as desired. The Venturi system using air dilution is probably the least complicated method.

Where the jet injector is placed during ventilation of the patient can also be important. As mentioned previously, certain techniques employed metal suction catheters attached to the gas supply to deliver the gases to the patient. These small metal tubes were placed on the suspension laryngoscope or held in position. The distal end of the metal tube was either proximal to the cords or posterior to the cords in the trachea. This thin metal tube was employed usually to maximize the surgeon's view of the vocal cords or upper trachea. If the metal tube was placed outside the vocal cords, there was an increased risk of aspiration. It would seem better, if possible, to place the tip in the trachea below the cords. In this way, the pressure build-up during ventilation would tend to propel any liquids entering the trachea back into the oropharynx.[37, 38]

One author suggested that if the metal tip is placed in the oropharynx, a pressure monitor should be employed. The pressure monitor would measure the atmospheric pressure in the oropharynx. The anesthesiologist's goal should be not to exceed 12 cm H_2O pressure in the oropharynx in children or 20 cm H_2O pressure in adults. These pressures correlate with the values of the lower esophageal sphincter tone in children and adults.

During the last few years, many anesthesiologists have used cuffed metal endotracheal tubes to provide anesthesia during laser procedures. A common problem with the metal tubes is the small internal diameter that can make the use of a circle system difficult in larger adults. Use of a jet injector with a small uncuffed metal endotracheal tube provides a perfect solution. The small external diameter of the metal tube allows for adequate exhaust of the gases used to ventilate the patient. The rapid delivery of gas via the jet injector allows for satisfactory delivery of the gas to the patient. This overcomes the narrowed internal diameter of the flexible metal endotracheal tube.

The problem that needs to be solved, however, is how one connects the jet source to the metal endotracheal tube. One author has employed a proximal large-bore jet. This is a device that inserts a short plastic or metallic tube into the proximal metallic endotracheal tube to achieve ventilation. There is the possibility of inadequate venting of carbon dioxide because the gas source is proximal in the tube.

This author has patented a **distal extending tip laser endotracheal tube** that provides advantages over other systems. The tube has a distal tip that extends forward into the trachea. During placement, the tip is pulled back into a hockey stick position to facilitate placement. When the tube is positioned in front of the vocal cords, the angle is corrected to fit into the trachea. The distal portion of the tube is extended into the trachea past the vocal cords. The proximal portion of the endotracheal tube is then rotated axially to the right or left depending on the surgeon's needs. The external diameter of the tube is small because the system employs jet ventilation. The tube is uncuffed. The internal diameter of the tube is larger because the tube is flexible in one place and therefore does not need full-length metallic strips to achieve flexibility. On the proximal portion, a universal adapter that fits the end of any metallic endotracheal tube is placed. This tube contains a plastic flexible tube, like a central venous catheter, that is held in position by the universal adapter mechanism. The jet ventilation system is connected to this catheter, and the ventilation of the patient can be easily achieved. The use of the flexible plastic catheter creates a distal gas jet that avoids carbon dioxide retention during ventilation. The plastic catheter is not a significant fire hazard because of its low thermal mass, and if it did ignite, it could easily be removed by pulling off the universal adapter. It is shielded from the laser beam by the projecting distal endotracheal tip.

The use of a high-frequency ventilator can be advantageous. It avoids the risk of barotrauma because it does not use high volume and high pressure to ventilate the patient. Instead, the high-frequency ventilator mechanism counts on brownian motion of the gases to achieve adequate gas exchanges. Rates of ventilation of approximately 50 per minute are adequate. The system works better if the gas source is closer to the distal end of the endotracheal tube; hence, this system works well with the extending tip endotracheal system above. The universal adapter with its central plastic catheter supplies the gas at the distal end of the tube. This set-up tends to minimize carbon dioxide retention.

Anesthetic Gas Mixtures and Techniques

Anesthetic Gases

Laser surgery involving the face, oropharynx, and trachea has created great difficulties for the anesthesiologist. These problems revolve around access to the airway, flammability of anesthetic instruments, and the potential explosive and ignition hazards of various anesthetic gases. Most of the physical access problems and instrument problems have been discussed. The final area to be explored is the territory of which anesthetic agent to use and why. If the wrong agent is employed, then that agent can cause an explosion or create a flash ignition of draping materials or clothing.

Which gas should be used to ventilate the patient? The choices are air (nitrogen 78% and oxygen 21%); nitrox (some mixture of nitrogen and oxygen with an oxygen concentration <30%); 100% oxygen; nitrous oxide and high concentrations of oxygen; and heliox (helium and oxygen <30%).

Compressed air is the cheapest. However, most patients under anesthesia require higher than 21% oxygen to maintain their oxygen saturation at 100%. In older patients or patients with chronic obstructive pulmonary disease, this is certainly true. Hence, air used as a partial dilutent of oxygen is the most commonly applied method. The air is supplied in cuffed systems through a compressed air line installed on the anesthesia machine. In uncuffed systems in which jet ventilators are used, the air is usually added via a Venturi gas mixing apparatus. Adjusting the dial on the apparatus controls the percentage oxygen delivered. Usually, oxygen concentrations between 25% and 30% should be adequate to maintain optimal blood oxygen saturation.

Some authors have suggested the use of **helium and oxygen** during laser surgery involving the airway.[39–41] **Special circumstances including endobronchial tumors or multiple polyps on the vocal cords or in the trachea** may make ventilation difficult. Helium is a light inert gas. It facilitates ventilation in cases of near airway occlusion. Its inert quality and its ability to distribute heat eliminate it as a fire hazard. Helium has three drawbacks.

It requires specific equipment, the equipment can be installed on the anesthesia machine, and it is more costly to use. Finally, it is such a good conductor of heat that it can increase the cooling of the patient during the surgical procedure. In conclusion, in special cases, there can be a clear benefit in the use of helium-oxygen mixtures.

Nitrous oxide is used as a component of most general anesthetics. However, during laser surgery involving the airway, nitrous oxide should be avoided.[4, 42] Nitrous oxide does not burn by itself. However, in the presence of oxygen, it can act to promote the rate of burning. This promotion of burning increases as the oxygen concentration increases. Because intravenous anesthetics can now be used easily to achieve full anesthesia and amnesia, nitrous oxide is not necessary for anesthesia and should not be used.

Volatile Anesthetics

Ether and cyclopropane are explosive and are not used in modern operating rooms. Both agents are not to be considered for use with laser surgery.

Other volatile halogenated anesthetic agents do not burn or increase ignition rates. These agents include **halothane, enflurane, isoflurane,** and **sevoflurane.**[43] These agents can be used during laser surgery. However, their delivery requires a cuffed endotracheal tube system. Therefore, these agents cannot be used with jet ventilator and uncuffed endotracheal tube systems. Avoiding the use of these agents as part of the anesthesia may have presented problems for the anesthesiologist a few years ago. However, with the newer continuous intravenous anesthesia systems available, the avoidance of volatile halogenated anesthetics is not a formidable obstacle.

Anesthetic Technique

Anesthetic technique can be divided into two broad categories for anesthesia involving the oropharynx and trachea. **If the endotracheal tube is a cuffed system,** then regular anesthesia techniques involving air and oxygen (FIO_2 < 30%) and a normal anesthesia machine can be employed. Volatile anesthetics can be used and combined with opioids and benzodiazepines. With volatile anesthetics, the use of neuromuscular blockers is optional; however, when neuromuscular blockers are employed, the patient can be given lower concentrations of the inhaled agent and he or she will recover quicker.[44–55]

If the endotracheal tube or jet system is an uncuffed system, then the jet system will be used to supply adequate oxygenation and ventilation. The anesthesia that is needed is supplied by either **bolus**

administration or **continuous intravenous administration** of the anesthesia. Neuromuscular blocking agents will have to be employed as part of this technique. Monitoring of the level of neuromuscular block is indicated as well.[56-58]

Continuous intravenous anesthesia has progressed rapidly in the past few years. Intravenous pumps that deliver accurate doses of the anesthetic agents make the quality of the technique better. Newer anesthetic agents like propofol achieve good anesthesia while allowing for quicker recoveries. Etomidate can be used for intravenous anesthesia in patients with a history of cardiac disease. Even thiopental can be employed for anesthesia. All of these agents should be combined with an adequate dose of midazolam to ensure amnesia. The use of an opioid decreases the necessary dose of the intravenous general anesthetic agent and provides necessary analgesia.

SUMMARY

After reading this chapter, it should be obvious that laser surgery increases the risk of anesthesia significantly. Knowledge of all available anesthesia methods and instruments is necessary before the laser surgery can occur. Use of correct equipment and the proper anesthesia technique can significantly reduce risk. A team approach must be used. The surgeon, the anesthesiologist, the scrub nurse, and the laser safety officer must all act in unison to minimize the risk of injury. Correct training of all components of the team must occur. Obtaining the correct airway equipment and modifications of the anesthesia machine as necessary must occur far in advance of a specific laser case. Laser surgery is a special circumstance, and normal anesthesia may be completely inappropriate. Venturi gas mixers must be purchased and checked for accurate delivery of specific oxygen concentrations prior to use. Airway- and eye-shielding materials must be obtained. This chapter covers most topics of safety and anesthesia for oropharyngeal and tracheal surgery. The chapter should provide a sound conceptual basis for anesthesia during laser surgery. The referenced material can be reviewed for more specific discussion of various topics that were presented.

REFERENCES

1. Van Der Spek AF, Spargo PM, Norton ML: The physics of lasers and implications for their use during airway surgery. Br J Anaesth 60:709–729, 1988.
2. Council on Scientific Affairs: Lasers in medicine and surgery. JAMA 256:900–907, 1986.
3. Bauman N: Laser drapes fires: How much of a risk? Laser Med Surg News Adv 7:2–5, 1989.
4. Rampil IJ: Anesthetic considerations for laser surgery. Anesth Analg 74:424–435, 1992.
5. Verheecke G: Nitrous oxide and laparoscopy (see comments). Anaesthesia 46:698, 1991.
6. Sosis M: Nitrous oxide should not be used during laser endoscopic surgery (letter). Anesth Analg 66:1054–1055, 1987.
7. Wolf GL, Simpson JI: Flammability of endotracheal tubes in oxygen and nitrous oxide enriched atmosphere. Anesthesiology 67:236–239, 1987.
8. Smith LE: Hemorrhoidectomy with lasers and other contemporary modalities. Surg Clin North Am 72:665–679, 1992.
9. Garden JM, O'Banion MK, Shelnitz LS, et al: Papillomavirus in the vapor of carbon dioxide laser treated verrucae. JAMA 259:1199–1202, 1988.
10. Ferenczy A, Bergeron C, Richart RM: Human papillomavirus DNA in CO_2 laser generated plume of smoke and its consequences to the surgeon. Obstet Gynecol 75:114–118, 1990.
11. Sawchuck WS, Weber PJ, Lowy DR, et al: Infectious papillomavirus in the vapor of warts treated with carbon dioxide laser or electrocoagulation: Detection and protection. J Am Acad Dermatol 21:41–49, 1989.
12. Nezhat C, Winer WK, Nezhat F, et al: Smoke from laser surgery: Is there a health hazard? Lasers Surg Med 7:376–382, 1987.
13. Zheltov G, Glazkov V, Podoltzef A, et al: Retinal damage from intense visible light. Health Phys 56:625–630, 1989.
14. Hanowell LH, Martin WR, Savelle JE, Foppiano LE: Complications of general anesthesia for Nd:YAG laser resection of endobronchial tumors. Chest 99:72–76, 1991.
15. De Vane GG: Laser initiated endotracheal tube explosion. AANA J 58:188–192, 1990.
16. Pahayan AG, Gravenstein N: High incidence of CO_2 laser beam contact with the tracheal tube during operations on the upper airway. J Clin Anesth 1:354–357, 1989.
17. Sosis MB: Which is the safest endotracheal tube for use with the CO_2 laser? A comparative study. J Clin Anesth 4:217–219, 1992.
18. Sosis M, Dillon F: What is the safest foil tape for endotracheal tube protection during Nd:YAG laser surgery? A comparative study. Anesthesiology 72:553–555, 1990.
19. Sosis MB: Evaluation of five metallic tapes for protection of endotracheal tubes during CO_2 laser surgery (see comments). Anesth Analg 72(3):414–416, 1991. Anesth Analg 68:392–393, 1989.
20. Sosis MB, Dillon F: Prevention of CO_2 laser-induced endotracheal tube fires with the laser-guard protective coating. J Clin Anesth 4:25–27, 1992.
21. Sosis MB, Dillon FX: A comparison of CO_2 laser ignition of the Xomed, plastic, and rubber endotracheal tubes. Anesth Analg 76:391–393, 1993.
22. Hawkins DB, Joseph MM: Avoiding a wrapped endotracheal tube in laser laryngeal surgery: Experiences with apneic anesthesia and metal laser–flex endotracheal tubes. Laryngoscope 100:1283–1287, 1990.
23. Hermens JM, Bennett MJ, Hirschman CA: Anesthesia for laser surgery. Anesth Analg 62:218–229, 1983.
24. Gussack GS, Evans RF, Tachi EJ: Intravenous anesthesia and jet ventilation for laser microlaryngeal surgery. Ann Otol Rhinol Laryngol 96:29–33, 1987.
25. Shikowitz MJ, Abramson AL, Liberatore L: Endolaryngeal jet ventilation: A 10-year review. Laryngoscope 101:455–461, 1991.
26. Aloy A, Schachner M, Cancura W: Tubeless translaryngeal superimposed jet ventilation. Eur Arch Otorhinolaryngol 248:475–478, 1991.
27. Aloy A, Schachner M, Spiss CK, Cancura W: Tube-free translaryngeal superposed jet ventilation. Anaesthesist 39:493–498, 1990.
28. Schumacher P, Stotz G, Schneider M, Urwyler A: Laryngospasm during transtracheal high frequency jet ventilation. Anaesthesia 47:855–856, 1992.

29. Giunta F, Chiaranda M, Manani G, Giron GP: Clinical uses of high frequency jet ventilation in anaesthesia. Br J Anaesth 63(Suppl 1):102S–106S, 1989.
30. Rouby JJ, Viars P: Clinical use of high frequency ventilation. Acta Anaesthesiol Scand Suppl 90:134–139, 1989.
31. Mathews WS Jr: A method for determining depth of un-marked endotracheal tubes used in laser surgery (letter). Anesth Analg 79:340, 1990.
32. Sosis MB: What is the safest endotracheal tube for Nd:YAG laser surgery? A comparative study. Anesth Analg 69:802–804, 1989.
33. Sosis M, Dillon F: Hazards of a new, clear, unmarked polyvinylchloride tracheal tube designed for use with the Nd:YAG laser. J Clin Anesth 3:358–360, 1991.
34. Sosis MB, Dillon FX: Saline-filled cuffs help prevent laser-induced polyvinylchloride endotracheal tube fires. Anesth Analg 72:187–189, 1991.
35. Weisberger EC, Miner JD: Apneic anesthesia for improved endoscopic removal of laryngeal papillomata. Laryngoscope 98:693–697, 1988.
36. Hawkins DB, Joseph MM: Avoiding a wrapped endotracheal tube in laser laryngeal surgery: Experiences with apneic anesthesia and metal laser-flex endotracheal tubes. Laryngoscope 100:1283–1287, 1990.
37. Aun CS, Houghton IT, So HT, et al: Tubeless anesthesia for microlaryngeal surgery (see comments). Anaesth Intens Care 18:497–503, 1990.
38. Welty P: Anesthetic concerns and complications during suspension microlaryngoscopy procedures. CRNA 3:113–118, 1992.
39. Torre M, Amari B, Barbieri B, et al: Emergency laser vaporization and helium-oxygen administration for acute malignant tracheobronchial obstruction. Am J Emerg Med 7:294–296, 1989.
40. Pashayan AG, Gravenstein JS, Cassisi NJ, McLaughlin G: The helium protocol for laryngotracheal operations with CO₂ laser: A retrospective review of 523 cases. Anesthesiology 68:801–804, 1988.
41. Torre M, Amari B, Barbieri B, et al: Emergency laser vaporization and helium-oxygen administration for acute malignant tracheobronchial obstruction. Am J Emerg Med 7:294–296, 1989.
42. Wolf GL, Simpson JI: Flammability of endotracheal tubes

43. Paes ML: General anaesthesia for carbon dioxide laser sur-gery within the airway. A review. Br J Anaesth 59:1610–1620, 1987.
44. Keon TP: Anesthetic management during laser surgery. Int Anesthesiol Clin 30:99–107, 1992.
45. Spiess BD, Ivankovich AD: Anesthetic management of laser airway surgery. Semin Surg Oncol 6:189–193, 1990.
46. DeVane GG: AANA journal course: new technologies in anesthesia: Update for nurse anesthetists—lasers. AANA J 58:313–319, 1990.
47. Garry BP, Bivens HE: Anesthetic technique for safe laser use in surgery. Semin Surg Oncol 6:184–188, 1990.
48. Rontal M, Rontal E, Wenokur ME, Elson L: Anesthetic management for tracheobronchial laser surgery. Ann Otol Rhinol Laryngol 95:556–560, 1986.
49. North C, March B, Hirshman CA: Anesthetic management of a patient with reactive airway disease for carbon dioxide laser debulking of a laryngeal tumor. Anesth Analg 65:1225–1226, 1986.
50. Paes ML: General anaesthesia for carbon dioxide laser sur-gery within the airway. A review. Br J Anaesth 59:1610–1620, 1987.
51. Sosis M: Anesthesia for laser surgery. Int Anesthesiol Clin 28:119–131, 1990.
52. Keon TP: Anesthetic considerations for laser surgery. Int Anesthesiol Clin 26:50–53, 1988.
53. Heine P, Axhausen M: Anesthesia and laser surgery of the laryngo-nasal-ear region. Anaesthesist 37:10–18, 1988.
54. Padfield A, Stamp JM: Anaesthesia for laser surgery. Eur J Anaesthesiol 9:353–366, 1992.
55. Gussack GS, Evans RF, Tachi EJ: Intravenous anesthesia and jet ventilation for laser microlaryngeal surgery. Ann Otol Rhinol Laryngol 96:29–33, 1987.
56. Perrin G, Colt HG, Martin C, et al: Safety of interventional rigid bronchoscopy using intravenous anesthesia and sponta-neous assisted ventilation. A prospective study. Chest 102:1526–1530, 1992.
57. Mignone L, Villani L, Zappi L, et al: A ketaler-propofol combination in laser surgery for removal of obstruction from the upper respiratory tract. Minerva Anestesiol 56:821–822, 1990.
58. Jacobs IR, Reeves JG, Glass PSA: Continuous infusions for maintaining anesthesia. Int Anesthesiol Clin 29:1–82, 1991.

CHAPTER 4

Wavelength Conversion Effect—Contact and Free-Beam Laser Surgery

TERRY A. FULLER, PhD

THE PROMISE OF SURGICAL LASERS

The original advantages attributed to the use of surgical lasers included the possibility of a less traumatic, nontouch mode of operation and the ability to produce selective surgical effects on target tissues that were within or behind other healthy nontargeted structures. Some of the most elegant examples of these types of surgical laser applications are to be found in ophthalmology, in which the surgeon can precisely coagulate deep-lying intraocular structures without disturbing the overlying cornea, lens, or sclera.

These advantages, however, brought with them certain limitations and drawbacks. Sometimes, the advantages and problems stemmed from the same phenomena. Many of the earliest laser enthusiasts became discouraged over the technologic complexity and constraints of the new instruments. They found that although lasers did indeed provide valuable new capabilities, their applications were more narrowly compartmentalized than had originally been hoped. Most of the early studies of laser use in the dental, oral, and maxillofacial fields, outside of the open cutting, coagulation, and ablation of soft tissue, failed to lead to practical results.[1]

A nontouch method of delivery of laser energy (often referred to as "free-beam" surgery), although often desirable in selected procedures, frequently requires changes in technique to initially difficult and awkward maneuvers for the surgeon, for whom tactile impressions typically provide an important element of feedback and control. Additionally, owing to the fundamental interactions of light with both tissue and the materials of which surgical instruments are made, a beam of light can be reflected or scattered from tissue or from the instruments, or inadvertently pass beyond the target structures. One example of this limitation is in the cutting of adhesions. After the laser energy cuts through the adhesion, the free beam of light continues beyond the desired target tissue, resulting in damage to underlying healthy tissue. Moreover, uncontrolled or unexpected changes in the distance or angle of incidence (Fig. 4–1) of the laser delivery system to the tissue result in variations in the laser beam shape and power density, and will vary the thermal (clinical) response within the tissue. When fiber optics inadvertently touch tissue during surgery, they can become fouled. The end of the fiber frequently melts or deforms, altering the beam profile and thus its clinical effect. These fibers must be repaired or replaced before the procedure continues to ensure consistent results.

WAVELENGTH DEPENDENCE

An attribute and major limitation of free-beam surgical lasers is the relationship between wavelength and tissue effect. Absorption, in the context of laser surgery, is the transformation of radiant energy into thermal energy when it passes through and is absorbed by tissue. The absorption coefficient of tissue, α, is a measure of the amount of incident

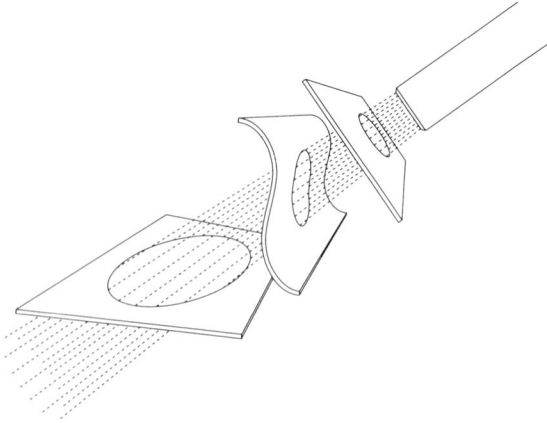

FIGURE 4–1. Divergence of laser energy from a fiberoptic source. Noncontact laser surgery.

radiation absorbed through a given depth of tissue. Certain molecules and biologic structures absorb, in characteristic ways, different wavelengths of laser light.[2] Figure 4–2 illustrates the absorption spectrum of light from the ultraviolet region through the mid-infrared region. This curve shows areas of high and low absorption of light. High absorption of light results in concentration of energy in surface layers of the tissue. Such concentration of energy results in highly elevated tissue temperatures.

In any particular tissue, there are several distinct absorption peaks resulting from the composition, pigmentation, and water content of the tissue. At the subcellular level, the opportunity exists to target specific chromogens, resulting in very precise and unique tissue effects. At the tissue level, however, volume heating predominates.

Laser energy that is absorbed creates two distinct thermal effects. The first is heating of tissue by direct absorption of light. The second is conduction of heat into the surrounding tissue. All lasers or other volume heat sources heat neighboring tissue through the process of thermal conduction.

Temperatures between 60°C and 100°C thermally coagulate and destroy tissue. Tissue proteins are denatured, and the tissue becomes dehydrated and begins to shrink. At these temperatures, tissue is not physically removed at the instant of surgery. Rather, it will slough or be resorbed over time. Temperatures above the boiling point of water (100°C) result in vaporization, that is, the conversion of liquid and solid tissue components into vapor. This results in an instantaneous removal of tissue—the surgical defect. The distribution of the heat and the resulting temperature within tissue are referred to as a temperature gradient. The temperature gradient is the key determinant in defining the nature of the surgical lesion. Temperature gradients in tissue are illustrated in Figure 4–3.

The energy emitted from a carbon dioxide laser, for example, is heavily absorbed by water ($\alpha \cong 100$ cm^{-1}). In tissue, which is predominantly composed of water, this energy is completely transformed into heat within approximately 0.1 mm of the tissue surface. This high absorption of light generates a localized zone of high temperature with a very steep temperature gradient back to body temperature. In consequence, the carbon dioxide laser is most useful for surface cutting and vaporizing, but it is less well suited for coagulating tissue. It is not a very hemostatic surgical device. Owing to its absorption by water, the CO_2 laser emission must be delivered through a gas rather than through an aqueous medium. This has limited its utility in orthopedics and other specialty areas in which aqueous distention of the anatomic site is required.

As a result of its absorption by tissue, the carbon dioxide laser is most commonly used to cut soft tissue. The wavelength of the carbon dioxide laser,

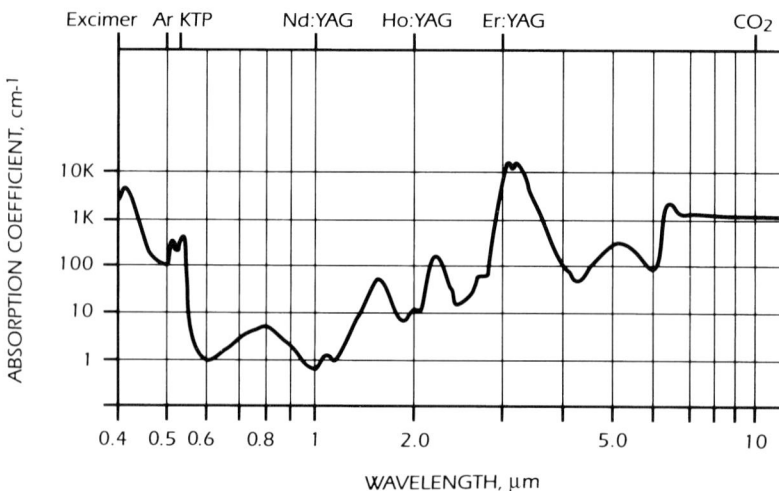

FIGURE 4–2. Composite absorption of tissue. (From Fuller T: Thermal Surgical Lasers: A Technical Monograph. Oaks, Pennsylvania, Surgical Laser Technologies Press, 1993.)

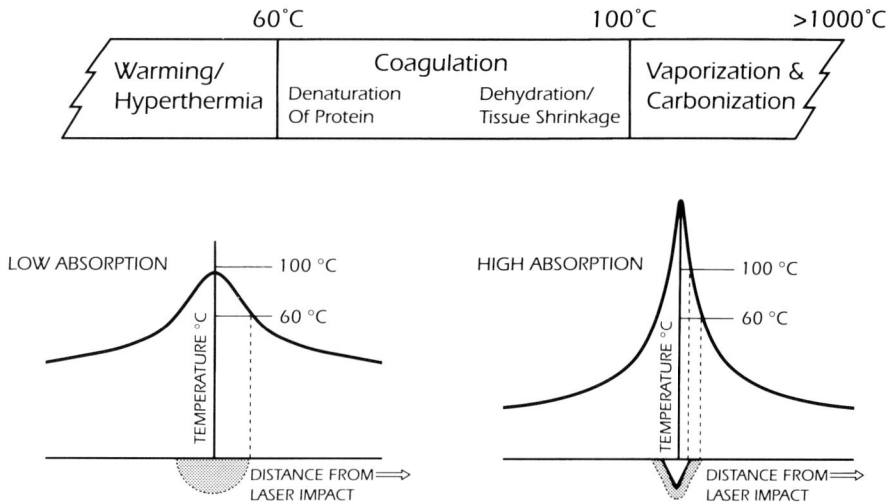

FIGURE 4–3. Temperature gradients in tissue. (From Fuller T: Thermal Surgical Lasers: A Technical Monograph. Oaks, Pennsylvania, Surgical Laser Technologies Press, 1993.)

10,600 nm, is not transmitted by fused silica (quartz) and thus cannot be transmitted through conventional fiber optics. Hollow waveguides (hollow tubes with special optical coatings) are available for transmission of the carbon dioxide laser and provide some degree of flexible laser delivery. The waveguides are limited, however, in the minimum spot size and maximum power that can be achieved. In addition, the bend radius is severely limited. Waveguides have their maximum utility when used in conjunction with straight, rigid endoscopes, in which minimal bending is required.

When tissue is vaporized by the carbon dioxide laser (or any other noncontact heat source), a plume of smoke results. This smoke, which principally contains incinerated tissue components (principally carbon), acts to absorb a portion of the incoming laser energy. This absorption reduces the amount of energy reaching the tissue for therapeutic purposes. Smoke evacuators are frequently used to reduce or eliminate the noxious and interfering smoke. In addition to making the surgery more pleasant, the decrease in smoke reduces the laser energy absorption loss and improves visualization of the surgical site.

Blue-green emission from the argon laser (488 and 514 nm) and the green emission (532 nm) from the frequency-doubled neodymium:yttrium-aluminum-garnet (Nd:YAG) laser are principally absorbed by the pigmented proteins hemoglobin and melanin. In addition to the amount of absorption, the degree of scatter by tissue is an important variable in determining the nature of a lesion created by a laser. Scatter within tissue is inversely proportional to the wavelength, λ, of the light entering the tissue, that is, $1/\lambda^{-4}$. The result of the selective absorption and high scatter of argon and second harmonic Nd:YAG laser by tissue is that the temperature gradients created are broadly distributed and vary from tissue type to tissue type. For example, a hemangioma or a pigmented lesion heavily absorbs green light. Despite the high scatter, the high absorption by the pigmented tissue predominates. The result is shallow penetration with high surface temperatures and a steep temperature gradient. The same wavelengths in avascular tissue penetrate deeply and, as a result of the high scatter, cause lower surface temperatures and a shallow temperature gradient. For these reasons, visible wavelength lasers, which are generally referred to as selective absorbers, result in varying tissue effects.

The Nd:YAG laser emits light in the near-infrared region of the electromagnetic spectrum at 1064 nm. It has a very low absorption coefficient ($\alpha \cong 30$ cm^{-1}) and is heavily scattered on interaction with tissue. As a result, this energy penetrates deeply into tissue, causing a moderate surface temperature rise and shallow temperature gradient throughout the volume of tissue. This shallow temperature gradient makes it suitable for deep coagulation or the ablation of large tissue volumes. Depending on the delivered power and power density, coagulation alone or volume ablation or vaporization can be achieved.

The dependence of surgical effect on the absorption of specific wavelengths of light by particular types of tissue and tissue components is acceptable or even advantageous in certain well-defined applications. However, when the surgeon is faced with the need to create different temperature gradients in tissue in order to perform multiple surgical functions, for example, cutting, ablation, and coagulation, or to work with tissues of varying consistency and pigmentation, it is necessary to have available multiple free-beam lasers, one for each function.

An alternative approach is the creation of the desired thermal profile in tissue with a single laser wavelength in combination with interchangeable delivery systems. Changing the thermal profile in tissue can be accomplished by uncoupling the thermal effect in tissue from the laser wavelength. This uncoupling is easily and efficiently accomplished by use of contact laser technology.

CONTACT LASER TECHNOLOGY

Contact laser[3] technology was developed more than 10 years ago as a means of accurately creating a controlled thermal lesion in tissue. This technology incorporates the use of laser energy in a novel way for open or endoscopic incision, excision, coagulation, or ablation.[4, 5] The key components of the technology are a set of laser scalpels and probes (tips) made of synthetic sapphire or fused silica and apparatus that facilitates conversion of radiant laser energy into thermal energy. The tips are available in many different geometric shapes and sizes that are designed to optically modify the laser beam profile. Used most commonly with the Nd:YAG laser, these delivery elements are either integral or affixed to the end of conventional silica fiber optics.

Owing to the physical properties (melting point, hardness, dimensions) of the contact laser tips, laser beam size and shape can be precisely controlled. As a result, the laser beam profile is not subject to changes due to changes in distance from the delivery system to tissue or in the angle of incidence to the tissue. Such changes dramatically alter the degree of hemostasis and coagulation necrosis and the precision and control of vaporization. The mechanical and thermal properties of the contact laser tips allow direct contact of the delivery system to the tissue while delivering laser power, despite temperatures frequently above 1000°C! The high melting point and mechanical strength of synthetic sapphire permit the design and use of long or slender laser optical scalpels. Such devices consistently deliver laser power to tissue with little change in physical geometry or laser beam profile over the duration of a surgical procedure. The generally shorter and wider fused silica probes are effective for wide-area vaporization or ablation. They have lower melting points and are not as strong as sapphire. However, these probes perform better, and are frequently used within a fluid medium, such as that found in the oral cavity. Fiber optics with shaped tips are also useful for contact laser surgery but principally for short, lower power, less precise applications. This is a result of the small thermal mass and fragile design of the shaped fiber optic tip.

The geometry of the contact laser tips also defines the laser beam profile when the tip is not contacting the tissue. Some contact laser scalpels are designed to provide a beam that is highly divergent in air or other gas, as encountered after the probe tip passes through tissue. This feature is extremely useful in cutting adhesions overlying vital structures. In this instance, the tip in contact with tissue cuts the tissue. After the tip passes through the tissue, the beam rapidly diverges, reducing the laser power density to levels that minimize or eliminate tissue damage. Other contact laser tips are not highly divergent and preserve a beam profile in air that is useful for free-beam coagulation.

Surgeons accustomed to using mechanical instruments to palpate or "feel" tissue find contact laser surgery technique more natural and easier to learn in comparison with free-beam laser applications.

WAVELENGTH CONVERSION EFFECT

Perhaps the most valuable asset of contact laser technology is what is referred to as the Wavelength Conversion Effect. This technology builds on the principles that determine the degree of conversion of radiant energy into thermal energy: the greater the amount of light that is absorbed per unit volume, the greater the surface temperature and the steeper the resulting temperature gradient. Thus, by placing a thin, partially absorbing surface on a contact laser tip, a portion of that laser energy will be absorbed and converted to heat. When the tip is in contact with the tissue, the tissue is heated by both direct absorption of the laser energy and by laser conduction of heat from the probe surface. The use of Wavelength Conversion Effect surface treatments essentially redistributes the site in which energy is transformed from light into heat. This technique makes laser surgery less dependent on the laser

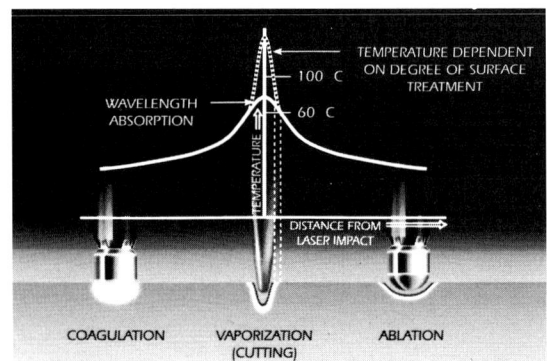

FIGURE 4–4. Changes in temperature gradient and tissue effect by Wavelength Conversion Effect treatments. (From Fuller T: Thermal Surgical Lasers: A Technical Monograph. Oaks, Pennsylvania, Surgical Laser Technologies Press, 1993.)

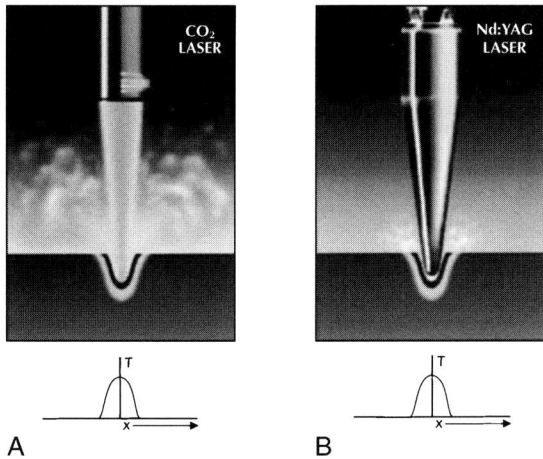

FIGURE 4–5. Different lasers, same effect. (From Fuller T: Thermal Surgical Lasers: A Technical Monograph. Oaks, Pennsylvania, Surgical Laser Technologies Press, 1993.)

wavelength and different absorption characteristics of tissue.

As this heat is generated on the probe surface when in contact with tissue, it is conducted into the surrounding tissue. The conducted heat raises the temperature of the tissue higher than the radiant laser energy alone. Figure 4–4 illustrates the typical temperature gradient created from absorption of energy from an Nd:YAG laser (solid line). Note that, for this example, the maximum temperature is less than $100°C$, and thus the tissue is coagulated. The result of this temperature gradient is shown on the bottom left. By placing a Wavelength Conversion Effect absorbing surface on the probe tip in contact with tissue, the temperature of the tissue is elevated, resulting in a steep temperature gradient (dotted line). The clinical effect is that of cutting or vaporizing tissue, as shown in the bottom center of this illustration. By changing the shape and size of the tip and altering the Wavelength Conversion Effect absorbing surface, the effect of ablation (bottom right) can be obtained.

The Wavelength Conversion Effect technology does not change the wavelength of the laser light; rather, it alters the effect of the wavelength on tissue. This is a powerful technique that permits one wavelength to mimic the effect of many different wavelengths by simply altering or changing the contact laser tips.

Referring back to the carbon dioxide laser example, when absorbed by tissue the energy results in tissue vaporization and a steep temperature gradient (Fig. 4–5A). This same effect can be achieved with an Nd:YAG laser in combination with a contact laser scalpel that has a Wavelength Conversion Effect surface treatment (Fig. 4–5B). By choosing a different probe or scalpel with a different geometry and Wavelength Conversion Effect surface treatment, the surface temperature gradient of a second harmonic Nd:YAG or argon laser can be achieved. A contact laser probe or scalpel with no absorbent surface treatment acts similarly to a free-beam Nd:YAG laser light beam but with the benefits of control in beam diameter, tactile feedback, and improved efficiency.

CONTACT LASER SCALPELS AND PROBES

The combination of different tip geometry and surface treatments places a wide selection of surgical instruments at the surgeon's disposal. Round probes, for example, provide the power density and distribution needed to ablate larger volumes of tissue, as required in the treatment of tumors or oral hemangiomas. A flat probe with no absorbing surface treatment provides the mechanical ability to tamponade bleeding vessels, together with the power density and inherent wavelength of the Nd:YAG laser for deep coagulation. A chisel-shaped probe can hemostatically excise or ablate tissue in linear planes. There are several conically shaped scalpels that are designed to incise lesions with minimal coagulation necrosis (creating a lesion

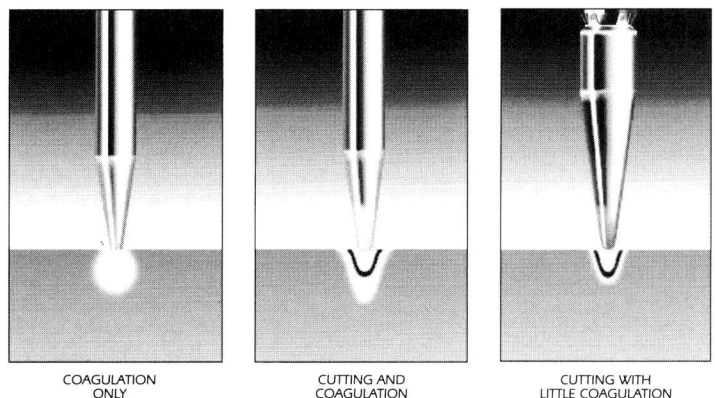

FIGURE 4–6. Same laser, different effects. (From Fuller T: Thermal Surgical Lasers: A Technical Monograph. Oaks, Pennsylvania, Surgical Laser Technologies Press, 1993.)

COAGULATION ONLY

CUTTING AND COAGULATION

CUTTING WITH LITTLE COAGULATION

comparable to that produced by the carbon dioxide laser). These general purpose devices are frequently used to excise polyps or tumors. The clinical results are comparable to those with conventional operative techniques but with a significant reduction in post-operative morbidity.[6]

Laser scalpels and probes are used in direct contact with tissue and, resulting from the Wavelength Conversion Effect surface treatments, require considerably less power to create an effective lesion. This substantially reduces the required power as well as the risk of unwanted damage to neighboring structures. In conclusion, as illustrated in Figure 4–6, contact laser technology permits the use of a single laser in combination with multiple interchangeable tips to mimic the effects of several different laser systems.

REFERENCES

1. Pogrel MA: Application of laser and cryosurgery in oral and maxillofacial surgery. Current Opinion in Dentistry 1:263–270, 1991.
2. Fisher JC: Basic laser physics and interaction of laser light with soft tissue. *In* Shapshay SM (ed): Endoscopic Laser Surgery Handbook. New York and Basel, Marcel Dekker, 1987, pp 31–46.
3. Surgical Laser Technologies, U.S. Patents B1 4, 592, 353, 4, 693, 244, 4, 736, 743, and other U.S. and foreign patents.
4. Galluci JG, Zeltsman D, Slotman GJ: Nd:YAG laser scalpel compared with conventional techniques in head and neck cancer surgery. Lasers Surg Med 14:139–144, 1994.
5. Daikuzono N, Joffe SN: Artificial sapphire probe for contact photocoagulation and tissue vaporization with the Nd:YAG laser. Med Instrum 19:173–178, 1985.
6. Midgley HC: Nd:YAG contact laser surgery: The scalpel of the future? Otolaryngol Clin North Am 23(1):99–105, 1990.

SECTION TWO

CHAPTER 5

Fundamentals of the Carbon Dioxide Laser

TIMOTHY J. ATKINSON, DDS

Developments in the instrumentation used to perform surgery have occurred throughout history, with some form of incising instrument being the focal point of the surgeon's armamentarium. Various forms of the sharp scalpel and the development of diathermy and cryoprobes allowed surgeons to improve the outcome in the treatment of diseases requiring surgery. Laser technology as a surgical scalpel has not replaced the conventional method but possesses advantages over other instrument options. The use of laser technology in nearly all the surgical and invasive medical specialties attests to the fact that this modality has a special place in the treatment of diseased tissue.

Using a laser, the surgeon can precisely perform the necessary surgery for incising or ablating tissue. Choosing the appropriate system, whether carbon dioxide or other laser energy source, is paramount. Each system has inherent advantages and can allow delivery of the radiant energy through either an articulated arm or a flexible quartz crystalline fiber. Various delivery systems are available. A free-beam or nontouch laser system can be chosen that eliminates the direct instrument contact with tissue. Additionally, the contact technique, which uses free fibers or sapphire tips, allows tissue contact similar to a conventional scalpel; however, this technique does not provide the customary tactile sensations. Attaching the laser to a surgical microscope with the use of a micromanipulator, or so-called joystick, is another option. All in all, these systems allow minimal retraction of tissue, resulting in less postoperative pain.

During surgical procedures, lasers have specific advantages over other instrumentation options (Table 5–1). The delivered laser energy appears to be bactericidal and viricidal, creating a sterile surgical site. Wound contraction by cicatrix formation is reduced, especially when dealing with lesions of the oral mucosa at the vestibule, oral commissure, or vermilion. Access to difficult-to-reach anatomic sites, hemostasis, and ablation of diseased tissue, as well as a decreased risk to adjacent anatomic structures, have directed surgeons to select this device.[1-4] As with any type of surgical instrumentation, lasers have limitations and disadvantages (Table 5–2). Operation of this technology requires didactic and clinically oriented instruction, as well as trained ancillary assistants.[1]

HISTORY OF LASERS

During the early 20th century (Table 5–3), the physical principles that define this scientific parameter began to be realized with the introduction of quantum theory by Neils Bohr in 1913. In 1917 Albert Einstein published the paper "Zür Quanten Theorie der Stralung" ("The Quantum Theory of Radiation").[5] Einstein was able to theorize the physics involved in stimulated emission of radiation. In this landmark publication, he described the interaction of atoms with electromagnetic fields and the principle of spontaneous emission. He proposed the possibility of stimulated emission of energy in this same interactive model.

Physicists continued to work with Einstein's theories. The first to report application of the theory was Charles Townes in 1954.[6] He stimulated the emission of microwaves, later to be described as a maser. In 1958, Townes and Schawlow examined the maser principles, which were eventually used

TABLE 5–1. Commonly Known Advantages of the Carbon Dioxide Laser

a. Production of a sterile surgical field, bactericidal, viricidal.
b. Minimal cicatrix formation/wound contraction.
c. Access to difficult to reach anatomic sites by reflection or through waveguides.
d. Ability to coagulate, vaporize, or incise tissue.
e. Good hemostasis.
f. Reduced local tissue trauma and edema.
g. Precise delivery of energy to diseased tissue via microscopes for reduced damage to surrounding structure.
h. Reduced pain by induced neural anesthesia as a function of neuron sealing and decreased pain mediator release.
i. Minimized tumor cell dispersion by lymphatic sealing.

for the conversion of high energy using light from visible and infrared portions of the electromagnetic spectrum.[7] This examination introduced the principles of light amplification by the stimulated emission of radiation, or laser. It was not until 1960, however, that the first laser was developed. In this year, Theodore Maiman successfully stimulated ruby crystals to produce red laser light with a wavelength of 0.69 nm.[8] Within a year, ophthalmologists used this device for photocoagulation. This technique led the way for creation of additional lasers with various wavelengths. The carbon dioxide laser was developed in 1964 by Patel and operated by Bell Laboratories.[9] In 1965, Polanyi was the first to perform a surgical procedure with a carbon dioxide laser.[10] Identification of specific cutting and hemostatic properties of the continuously operating carbon dioxide laser beam was documented in 1966 by Yahr and Strully.[11]

Throughout the 1970s, lasers were used successfully in the treatment of lesions in the oral cavity. This technique was well documented in the otolaryngologic, plastic and reconstructive, and general surgical literature. The excision of a buccal hemangioma of an 8-year-old boy appears to be the first documented case in the American oral maxillofacial surgical literature. Shafir, a plastic and reconstructive surgeon, and his associates reported the procedure in 1977.[12] Carbon dioxide surgical laser research continued, and Sachs and colleagues employed this device to remove recurrent palatal papillomatosis, later reporting the technique in 1981.[13] Researchers have continued to experiment with the carbon dioxide laser and its interaction with biologic tissues since these early days, leading to new applications for this radiant energy.[9, 10, 14] Applying newly developed equipment has expanded the array of novel procedures available today. Among the most recent applications are the laser-assisted uvulopalatoplasty, microscopic treatment of internal de-

rangement within the temporomandibular joint, and adjunctive esthetics and facial cosmetic procedures.[15–21] Despite the late application of this technology in oral and maxillofacial surgery and the inherent disadvantages, lasers do have a place in this field of surgery. Knowledge of the physical properties of light and laser energy is essential for the surgeon to use this armamentarium appropriately. Additionally, the surgeon can competently assess new and broader applications of the laser, as well as the laser's advantages over the use of conventional surgical techniques.

PHYSICAL PROPERTIES OF LIGHT

Light is radiant energy produced by all physical matter, whether it be gas, liquid, or solid. The energy contained in all atomic structures forms an electromagnetic spectrum (Fig. 5–1). This spectrum is an orderly array of a property of energy and light called the wavelength. Release of the energy and light in atomic systems can be accomplished by an uncontrolled discharge, as in a nuclear explosion, or in a controlled fashion, as occurs in the laser.

The term light originally described only the portion of the electromagnetic spectrum that was visible. In 1800, W. Herschel, a British-German astronomer, experimented with sunlight and a prism. He discovered a radiant energy band not visible to the eye that exists beyond the violet portion of visible light. This area was detected by a notable increase in temperature when a thermometer was placed next to the purple color of the visible color spectrum.[22] Later experimentation revealed a similar area adjacent to the red portion of the visible light. These areas became known as the ultraviolet and infrared energy bands, respectively, and were eventually grouped with the visible range of energy and collectively described as light. As x-rays, radio waves, television waves, and other electromagnetic energy discoveries were made, the total spectrum was expanded.

TABLE 5–2. Commonly Known Disadvantages of the Carbon Dioxide Laser

a. Specialized didactic and clinically oriented instruction required for laser use by the surgeon and ancillary assistants.
b. Hazards to patient, operating and assistant team, and anesthesia personnel from misdirected and inadvertent laser radiation.
c. Expense of laser equipment.
d. Specialized wiring and plumbing connection.
e. Maintenance requirements.
f. Fire hazard as related to anesthesia risk.
g. Electrical hazards of laser equipment.

TABLE 5–3. Timetable Reflecting the Development of Laser Technology to the Carbon Dioxide Laser

Year	Contributor	Development
1913	Bohr	Quantum Theory
1917	Einstein	Theory of Stimulated Emission
1955	Townes	Maser Production
1958	Townes & Schawlow	Laser Principles
1960	Maiman	Developed the Ruby Laser
1990	Ball	Ophthalmologic Application of Ruby Laser
1964	Patel	Developed the Carbon Dioxide Laser
1970	Polanyi	Clinically Applied the Carbon Dioxide Laser
1977	Shafir	First Documented Case in the Oral and Maxillofacial Surgical Literature

The traditional view of light is described by two properties. First, light energy can be considered a particle or photon with a mass possessing a velocity. This concept has been advocated since Sir Isaac Newton. Much later, in the 20th century, Bohr and Einstein described light energy as a quantum or a wave traveling through space as packets of energy. This concept is fully described by the theory of light in quantum mechanics.[5] Despite this complex relationship, electromagnetic energy should be viewed as a photon propagating as a continuous wave. This perspective can assist in the comprehension of the electromagnetic spectrum and ultimately the laser. Based on the wave theory, a photon has four characteristics, each specific for the matter from which it was produced. The waves produced have a wavelength, frequency, velocity, and amplitude (Fig. 5–2), which is illustrated by the waves generated when an object is dropped into water.

The wavelength is the distance between two successive crests of the wave. This property determines the color of the light generated. Examining the electromagnetic spectrum, one notes that light has a wavelength ranging from 100 to 10,000 nm. The human eye is able to detect a small portion of this electromagnetic energy. The visible light comprises a small segment of the spectrum between 385 nm (violet light) and 760 nm (red light). Long electrical or radio waves are at one end of the electromagnetic spectrum, which extends to the cosmic rays having a shorter wavelength. The carbon dioxide laser, when compared with other laser types, has a relatively long wavelength of 10,600 nm. It is within the infrared region of the electromagnetic spectrum and is invisible. The number of wave crests passing a given point per second is the frequency of a wave. This characteristic is expressed as Hertz (Hz), or oscillations per second. The wavelength and frequency are inversely proportional to each other and are determinants of the wave's energy as well as its position on the electromagnetic spectrum. Long wavelengths have fewer oscillations per second and

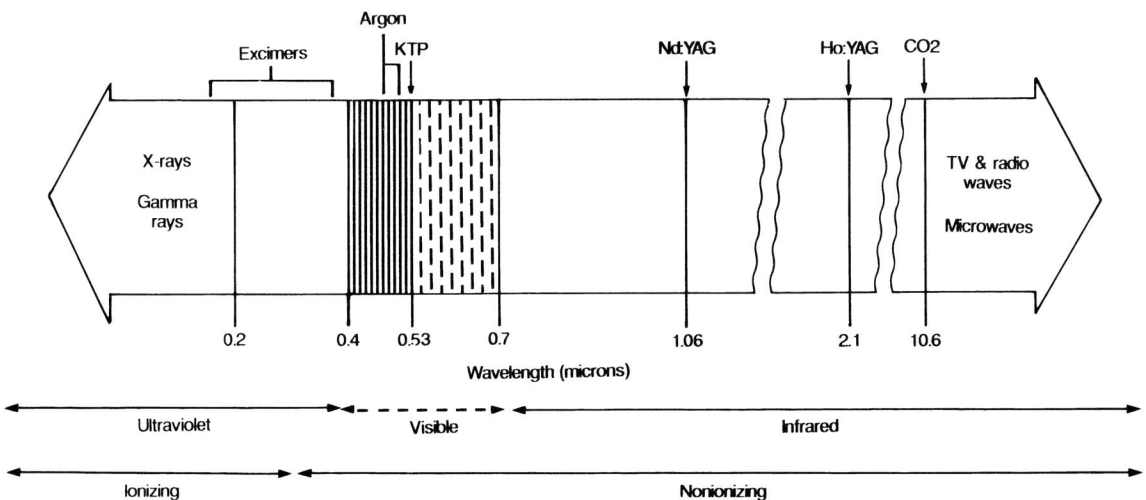

FIGURE 5–1. The electromagnetic spectrum. A well-defined band of visible light with a wavelength between 385 to 760 nm. The carbon dioxide laser is infrared light with a wavelength of 10,600 nm. adjacent to visible light and the long wavelength of television, radio, and microwaves. (Adapted from Trost D, Zacherl A, Smith MF: Surgical laser properties and their tissue interaction. *In* Smith MFW: Neurological Surgery of the Ear. St Louis, Mosby–Year Book, 1992, pp 131–162.)

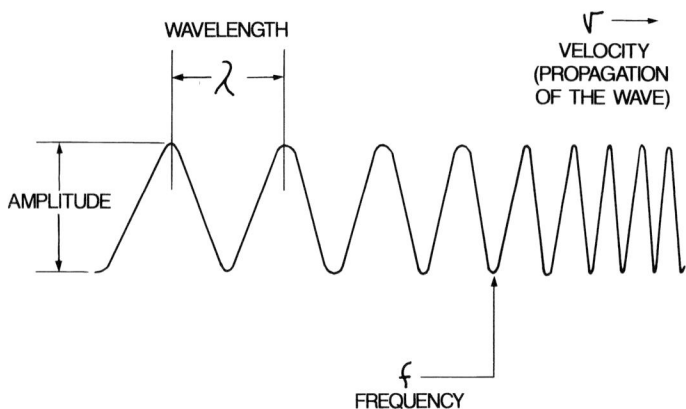

FIGURE 5–2. The basic properties of a wave. Velocity (v) is the speed a wave travels and is constant for light. Wavelength is the distance between two successive crests of the wave. Amplitude is the height of the wave from the crest of one wave to the trough of the next. Frequency is the number of waves that pass a given point in a specific amount of time.

produce lower energy. These waves fall within the infrared light, and include microwaves and radio and television waves. By contrast, short wavelengths have a higher frequency with greater energy, and include ultraviolet light, x-rays, and cosmic and gamma rays. Despite the differences in wavelength and frequency of light, the velocity is constant at 3 $\times$ 10^9 meters/second for all forms of light.

Waves also are described by their amplitude. This parameter is the vertical height of the wave from the peak of one wave to the trough of the next. The amplitude is a measure of the power of the wave. The higher the wave, the greater the power. An analogy between the power and intensity of light can be made with this property whereby higher power produces a brighter light.

LASER LIGHT CHARACTERISTICS

A laser beam that is produced has unique characteristics when compared with light generated by the sun or a light bulb. The coherent, collimated, and monochromatic nature of this artificial light gives rise to its many diagnostic and therapeutic applications.

Light that originates from the ordinary light bulb is composed of many wavelengths radiating in all directions and is known as incoherent light (Fig. 5–3A). This can be compared to the waves generated in a pond when many stones are thrown in a close area. The waves travel haphazardly in all directions. By contrast, laser light is coherent (Fig. 5–3B). The waves of laser light all progress forward at the same rate through space and time. In other words, the peaks and troughs move in synchrony spatially and temporally in the same direction. This coherent pattern can be likened to the gentle lapping of waves onto the shore of a lake. The result of coherency is amplification of the wave with increased power of the light (Fig. 5–4).

Laser light waves travel parallel to each other, with little or no divergence over a long distance whereby each light wave is equidistant. This collimated beam, which minimizes power loss by maintaining the concentration of light to a pinpoint spot, enhances precision during surgical procedures (Fig. 5–5).

Ordinary light consists of wavelengths from a large portion of the electromagnetic spectrum, resulting in white light, which is a mixture of all colors. The laser produces a monochromatic light

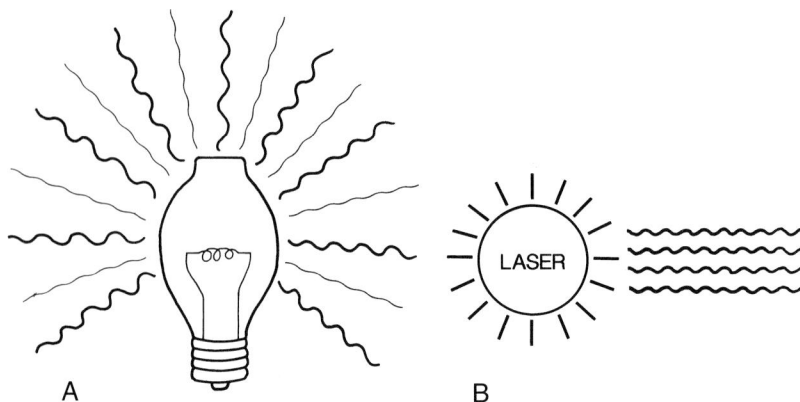

FIGURE 5–3. *A*, Incoherent light has many wavelengths generated in all directions, such as that by a white light bulb. *B*, By contrast, laser light is monochromatic and coherent, having a single wavelength in phase aligning all the peaks and troughs and moving in synchrony in the same direction.

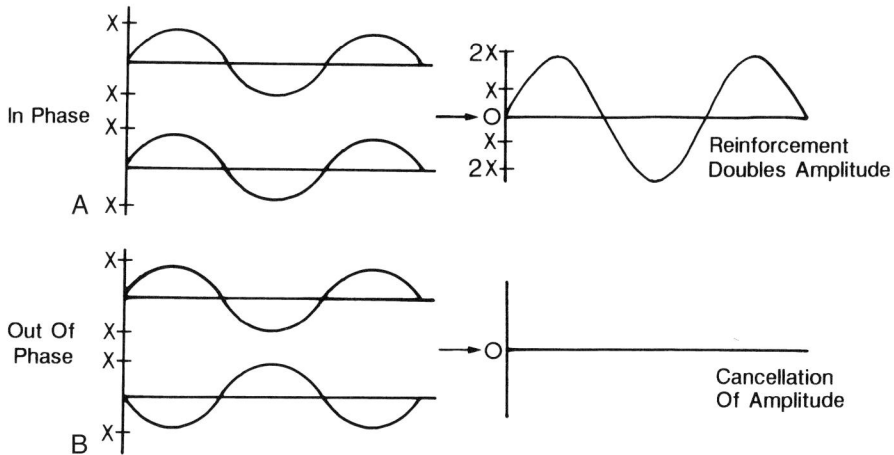

FIGURE 5–4. Coherent amplification. *A,* Waves are in phase when all the peaks and troughs are in alignment. The resultant wave is reinforced to double the amplitude, thus increasing the power and brightness. *B,* Waves are out of phase when the peaks oppose troughs. This results in a cancellation of the waves' power and brightness.

beam that contains a single wavelength (see Fig. 5–3). This monochromaticity is responsible for generating the laser's strength.

QUALITATIVE CARBON DIOXIDE LASER PHYSICS

The most widely used laser in oral and maxillofacial surgery is the carbon dioxide system, which emits an infrared light with a wavelength of 10,600 nm. This laser was the first to be developed for incising and ablating tissue in a controlled fashion. It is characterized by the unique ability to be focused to a small spot size, with relatively high power and near-complete absorption by most biologic tissues.

The generation of carbon dioxide laser light is accomplished by applying Einstein's theory of stimulated emission of radiation. The functional unit of

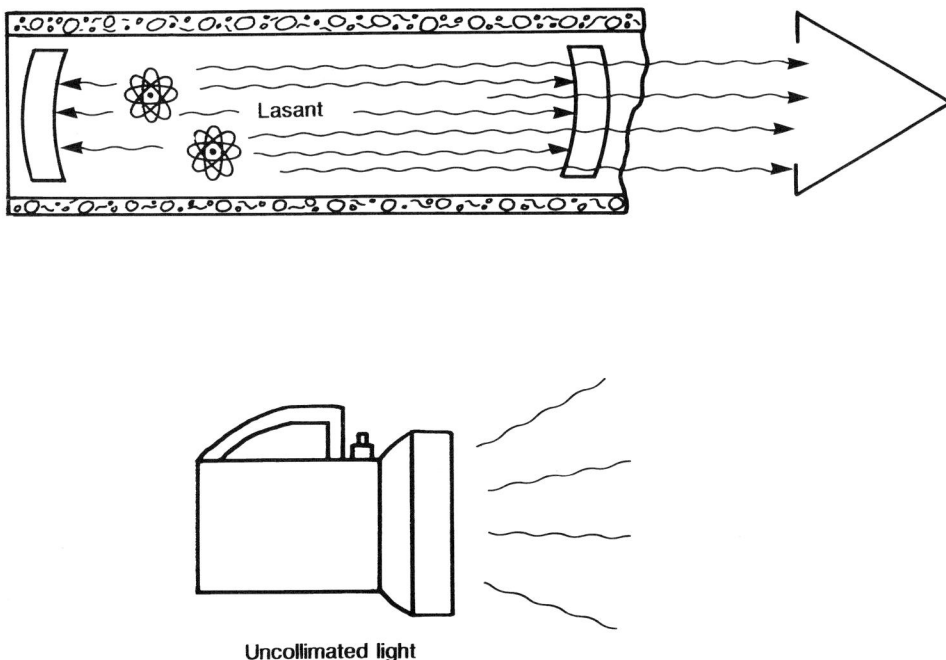

Uncollimated light

FIGURE 5–5. Collimated light does not diverge on exiting from its source when compared with an uncollimated light such as from a flashlight. The collimated laser light maintains the focus of the beam, minimizing power loss.

the laser is a chamber called an optical resonator
(Fig. 5–6). The active medium, or lasant, is confined
within the chamber. The medium is a mixture of
gases consisting of 10% to 15% carbon dioxide,
10% to 20% nitrogen, and the remaining 65% to
80% helium at a pressure of 6 to 15 mm Hg, which
is a near vacuum.

The carbon dioxide laser, being a molecular laser,
has energy levels involving the nitrogen and the
carbon dioxide molecules responsible for laser light
production. The remaining constituent atoms are
not involved in the production of the energy levels
to be described.

Neils Bohr explained the emission and absorption
spectra of atomic systems. Electrons that are contained in every atom possess certain energies that
define discrete energy states of the atom. These
energy states can be likened to stair steps, where
the atomic energy is at either one energy level or
another. There are no levels in between, just as it is
impossible to stand between steps. Unlike steps,
these systems do not have equal spacing between
the energy levels.

The movement of an electron "down the stair
step" to a lower energy level emits light. This
emission occurs as a burst of energy called a photon. The energy within the photon is equal to the
amount of energy released by the electron during
the change from one energy level to the other. On
the other hand, absorption of a photon of energy in
the correct amount causes an electron to move to

a higher energy. This is similar to going up the
stair steps.

To summarize, absorption of a photon produces
an electron transition from a lower to a higher
energy level. By contrast, emission of a photon is
due to a similar but reversed movement of the
electron from a higher to a lower energy level.
The energy levels described are different for each
chemical element. Therefore, the emission and absorption spectrum is unique for each element.

The processes of absorption and emission of photons are based on three radiative transitions within
atoms. These three processes are stimulated absorption, spontaneous emission, and stimulated emission. Within the laser's resonator chamber, the three
processes are occurring simultaneously, but stimulated emission is what creates the uniquely characteristic laser light.

Figure 5–7 demonstrates an atomic model with
two energy levels: E^1 and E^2. When the atom is in
its resting state, the lower energy level (E^1) contains
the electron. Stimulated absorption occurs when a
photon containing a specific amount of energy equal
to $E^2 - E^1$ elevates the electron to a higher energy
level (excited state). This higher energy level is
unstable, and the electron spontaneously emits a
specific photon of energy, again equal to $E^2 - E^1$,
transferring to a lower energy level. When the atom
is excited and in its higher energy state (E^2), there
is a predetermined lifetime prior to its spontaneous
decay to a lower energy state. When this occurs, a

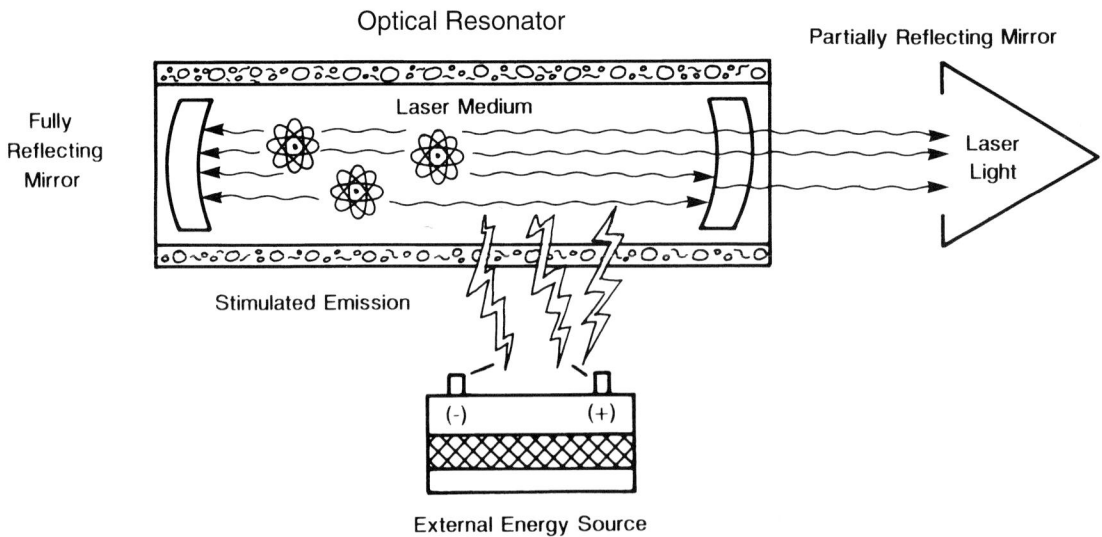

FIGURE 5–6. Optical resonator. The laser chamber is a tube that contains a lasant, the active
medium. An external energy source excites the molecules in the medium which spontaneously
degrade to their resting state. The resulting emitted photon can interact with another excited
molecule and cause the release of two identical photons that traverse between a fully reflective
mirror and partially reflective mirror. During travel, these photons can stimulate other excited atoms
to produce an increasing population of identical photons. Eventually, a certain number of photons
are released through the partially reflective mirror. The laser beam is focused and transmitted to the
interactive site.

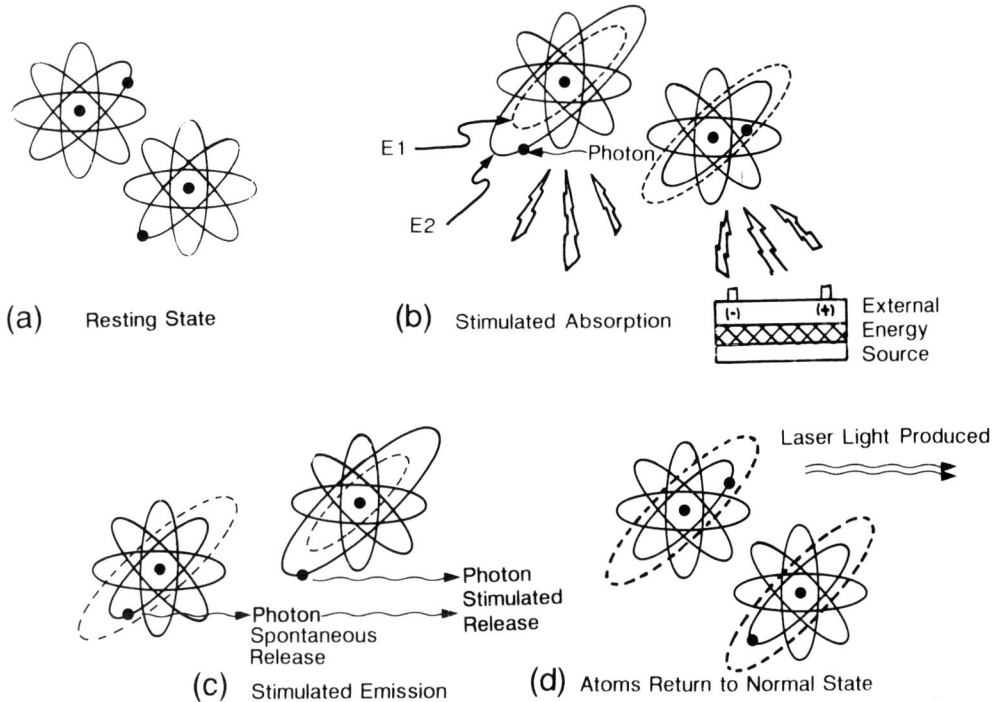

FIGURE 5–7. Atomic structure. *A,* Depicts the atom in the resting state, E_1, in which electrons orbit closest to the nucleus. *B,* When an atom absorbs external energy, an electron moves to a higher energy orbit, E_2, and is excited. Excited atoms are unstable and spontaneously emit energy as a photon, allowing electrons to return to the resting state, E_1. *C,* Stimulated emission occurs as a photon passes near an excited atom, causing release of the energy and producing an identical energy level photon and, *D,* laser light. (Adapted from Trost D, Zacherl A, Smith MF: Surgical laser properties and their tissue interaction. *In* Smith MFW: Neurological Surgery of the Ear. St Louis, Mosby–Year Book, 1992, pp 131–162.)

photon of light is created by spontaneous emission. If an identically energized photon courses past the excited atom before the spontaneous emission, the photon causes a resonance to occur between itself and the excited atom. In doing so, the atom decays from a high energy level to a lower level, emitting an identical photon. Both photons possess the same energy, wavelength, phase, and direction. This stimulated emission is what creates the laser beam with monochromatic, collimated, and coherent light.[23–25]

Molecules can possess energy in specifically defined amounts or discrete energy levels similar to atoms. By contrast, however, the energy level transitions of the nitrogen and carbon dioxide molecules are a result of vibrational and rotational movement about their molecular bonds and their axis of symmetry. This motion creates the absorption and emission spectra unique to the carbon dioxide laser.

The carbon dioxide molecule is excited by the pumping mechanism of the laser resonator. Carbon dioxide is a "linear triatomic molecule with three nondegenerated modes of vibration."[26] The vibrational-rotational modes are

1. Symmetric stretch mode—opposing forces

aligned 180 degrees to each other and parallel to the long axis of the molecule.

2. Bending mode—torsional forces perpendicular to the long axis of the molecule and opposing a central force.

3. Asymmetric stretch mode—partially opposing and partially attracting forces parallel to the long axis of the molecule.

These modes account for the energy levels in molecular systems defined by the stretching and bending of their molecular bonds (Fig. 5–8).

Electrons that form the electric current supplying a laser are released from the cathode and accelerate toward the anode. Electrons collide with the nitrogen molecule, increasing the vibrational energy levels. The energized nitrogen molecules transfer the vibrational energy to the carbon dioxide molecule, causing asymmetric stretching through stimulated absorption. This creates a population inversion with an excessive number of high-level metastable molecules through stimulated absorption. Photons are produced from the spontaneous emission occurring as the molecule reverts to the lower level symmetric stretch or bending mode from the higher level

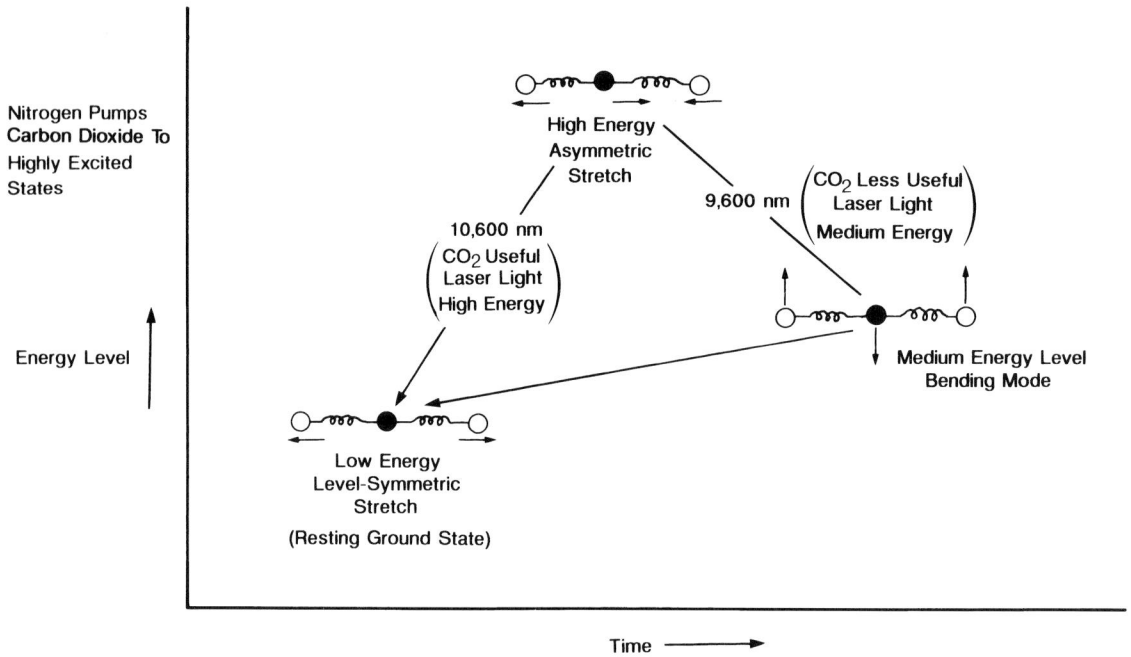

FIGURE 5–8. The three vibrational modes of the carbon dioxide triatomic molecule. The diagrammatic scheme of stimulated absorption by nitrogen molecules and emission creating 10,600 nm. Laser light by degradation to the resting ground state. Adapted from Dorros G, Seely D: Understanding Lasers: A Basic Manual for Medical Practitioners Including an Extensive Bibliography of Medical Applications. Mount Kisco, NY, Futura Publishing Company, Inc., 1991, pp 37–62.

asymmetric stretch. The characteristic carbon dioxide energy necessary to form laser light occurs with photon emission as relaxation occurs between the asymmetric stretch and symmetric stretch modes.

Creating laser light requires a resonator chamber, an external excitation source, a lasant, and a delivery system. The mixture of carbon dioxide, nitrogen, and helium is confined within the resonator of three typical laser systems. The difference lies in the design of the laser tube and the method employed to generate the laser light. A longitudinal free-flowing gas system (Fig. 5–9) is an open resonator tube, which is connected to a high-volume vacuum pump and carbon dioxide mixture supply cylinder. The laser converts the alternating current supplied by the standard hospital electrical outlet (110 volts) to a higher voltage (20,000 to 30,000 volts) of direct current. Strategically located electrodes within the tube stimulate the nitrogen and carbon dioxide molecules to produce laser light, as previously described. This reaction dissociates the carbon dioxide molecules to carbon monoxide as the light is produced. Removal of the "spent" fuel from the tube, particularly the carbon monoxide, with continual replenishing to prevent contamination is accomplished by the vacuum pump. The carbon dioxide gas supply cylinders have reserves for only a few hours of operation and then require replacement. Heat produced by the dissociation process is removed by diffusion to the water-cooled

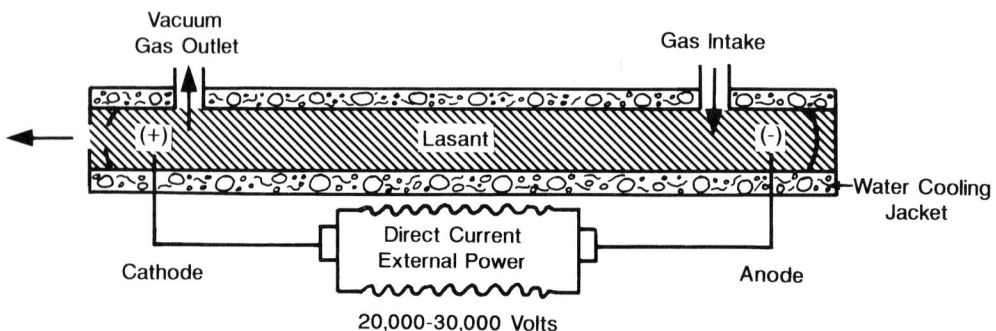

FIGURE 5–9. Longitudinal free-flowing gas system. The external energy supply source is high voltage with electrodes inside the chamber to interact with the active medium. A vacuum pump continuously replenishes the gas mixture lasant within the chamber.

walls of the chamber. The maximum power output that can be produced per chamber length is 50 to 60 watts per meter.

In actuality, the laser system output is dependent on two associated factors. First is the diameter of the resonator. Owing to heat production in the dissociation process, larger diameter resonators have greater difficulty in diffusing thermal energy to the water jacket surrounding the resonator. Second, the heat itself limits the production of the inverse population of excited carbon dioxide molecules. In an attempt to overcome the limitations caused by heat production, the resonator optimal diameter is kept small. The use of helium with high thermal conduction within the resonator increases cooling of the carbon dioxide by facilitating transfer of heat to the resonator walls.

This type of laser system, in addition to being costly and noisy to operate, is bulky owing to the added vacuum pump and carbon dioxide cylinders.

A variation of this system uses electrodes within the resonator and a sealed tube design. The mechanics are similar, except there is no vacuum pump or carbon dioxide gas supply cylinder. The lasant is sealed within the tube along with a catalyst, which functions to reassociate the carbon dioxide molecules as they break down during laser light production. This is accomplished by the addition of a small amount of water (1%) to the lasant. The distinction between this product and the free-flowing system is the longevity of the resonator, which requires replacement after extended use of several thousand hours or every couple of years. This technology contributes to a more compact design, decreasing the laser's cost of production and operation. In addition, it eliminates the added dangers of the external gas cylinders.

When higher power outputs with more rapid frequency of delivery became more desirable, these designs fell short of supplying the surgical demands. The limitation was a combination of gas dynamics creating overheating and erosion of electrodes called sputtering, which causes metallic deposition onto the internal optics of the resonator. As overheating and sputtering occur, the power output and pulse frequency are limited, thereby hindering the laser's performance. A radio frequency design (Fig. 5–10) precluded the need to have electrodes in contact with the laser tube's carbon dioxide gas. This lack of internal electrodes eliminated the sputtering. Additionally, the external power supply was reduced to 200 to 300 volts. This factor benefited the system by producing less heat, allowing delivery of higher pulsed energies with adjustable width frequencies.

The carbon dioxide lasers commercially available for surgery range in power from 8 watts to 100 watts, with peak power outputs of 500 watts. Portable office units produce 25 watts or less and usually are of the sealed tube design. Lasers used in a pulsed mode can deliver much higher peak powers with each pulse. The average power, including the time between each pulse, however, is similar to that produced by the continuous-wave lasers.

Photons created by spontaneous emission from the carbon dioxide molecule radiate in all directions. The majority of this radiation dissipates as heat to the walls of the resonator. A small number of the photons released traverse the laser chamber, paralleling the long axis, and reflect between two mirrors inside the resonator. The laser mirrors are made of glass but do not have the same reflective surface as those used every day. The rear mirror is totally reflective and usually is made with copper and nickel. A coating layer of gold is used to increase the reflectivity. Occasionally, a multilayered germanium dielectric mirror is used (Fig. 5–11). The front mirror or outlet coupler is multilayered germanium. The multilayered construction is one quarter wavelength thick and alternates between high and low refractive material. Photons incident on these surfaces may undergo phase changes equal to one half wavelength. This process ensures that all waves are reflected in phase to each other. Other variable incident wavelengths traversing the long axis of the chamber that do not undergo construc-

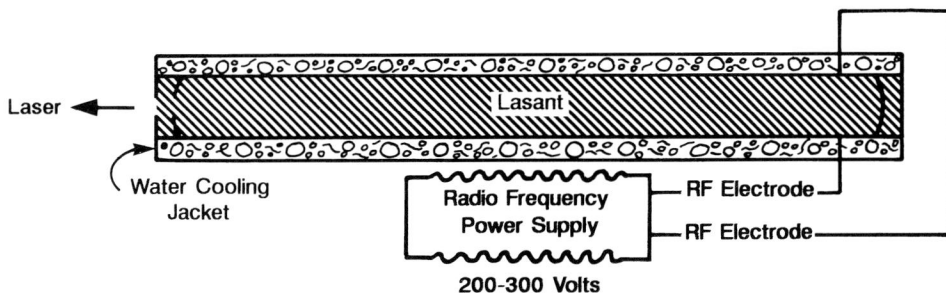

FIGURE 5–10. Radiofrequency resonator. By the use of a low voltage radiofrequency external energy source, there are no electrodes in direct contact with the active medium. Sputtering is eliminated, increasing the efficiency of the laser.

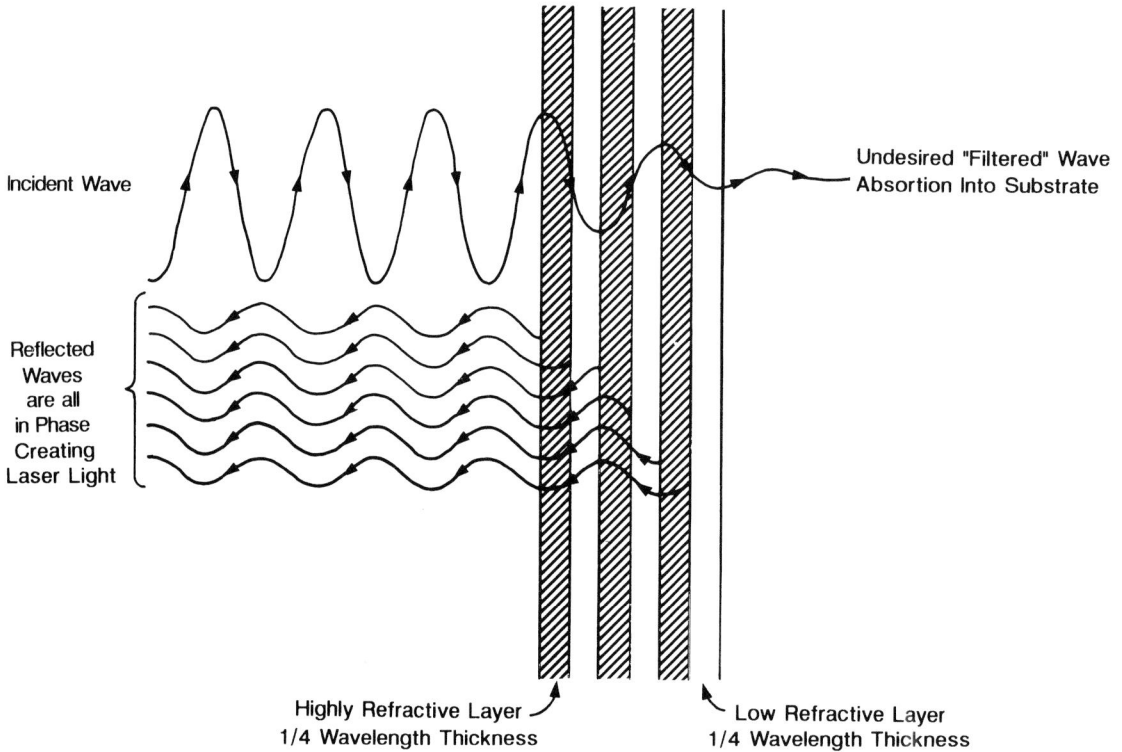

FIGURE 5–11. A dielectric mirror constructed with alternating layers of high and low refraction. This pattern produces constructive interference which ultimately produces a monochromatic and coherent laser beam. (Adapted from Dorros G, Seeley D: Understanding Lasers: A Basic Manual for Medical Practitioners Including an Extensive Bibliography of Medical Applications. Mount Kisco, NY, Futura Publishing Company, Inc., 1991, pp 11–20.)

tive interference as they strike the mirrors are filtered by transmitting their energy into the chamber walls as heat.

The reflectance of the dielectric mirror depends on the number of layers. Approximately 100% reflectance is obtained with 20 layers or more. As the photons are continually reflected between the two mirrors, they course past carbon dioxide molecules in a state of asymmetric stretch. The photon's near passing or collision with these molecules causes the other photons of identical energy, wavelength, and temporal spacing (phase) to be released. This stimulated emission continues and produces the energy necessary to create the laser light.[23, 24, 26] As photons are allowed to exit the output coupler, they are transmitted through an articulated arm via a reflecting mirror to a focusing lens (Fig. 5–12). The articulated arm design requires meticulous care during transportation and use to prevent shocks or impacts, or both, to the device from disrupting the alignment of the mirrors and subsequently the laser beam. The wavelength of the carbon dioxide laser does not allow it to be transmitted through a flexible fiber. Recent developments have enabled this laser energy to be conducted through flexible cables mounted to waveguides.[1]

The console houses the various laser components (Fig. 5–13). In addition to the resonator head, excitation source, and delivery arm, a cooling system is included. This is necessary due to the laser's inefficiency at converting the input energy to laser light. Operating efficiencies range from 0.01% to

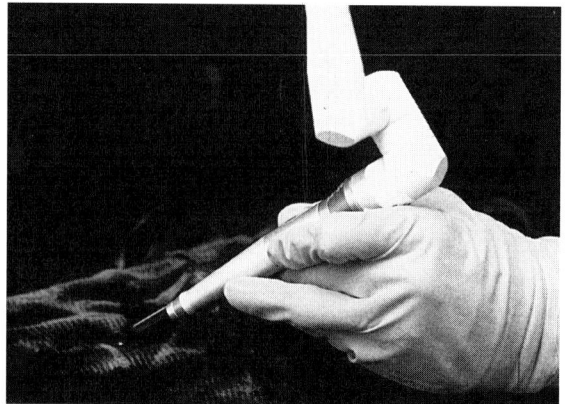

FIGURE 5–12. Articulated arm delivers the carbon dioxide laser beam from the source to the surgical site by a series of articulations and precisely aligned mirrors. The arm is attached to a suitable delivery device for surgical procedures.

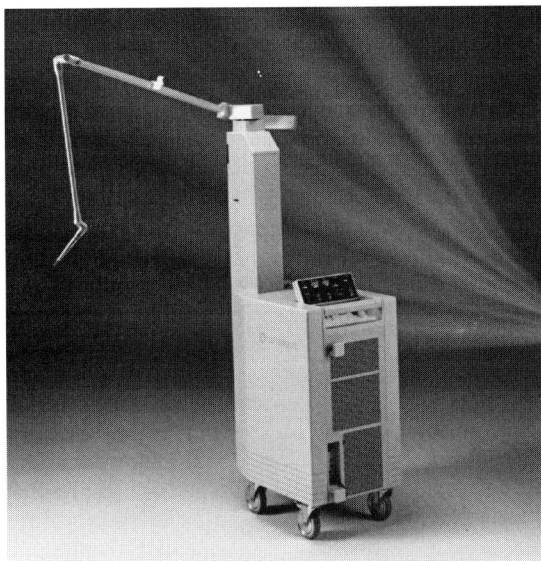

FIGURE 5–13. The console contains the complete apparatus to produce and deliver the laser beam. (Courtesy of Coherent Medical Group, Palo Alto, California.)

greater than 30%, with most operating below 1%. Therefore, with the majority of this input energy producing heat, special cooling systems are required to prevent overheating. This can be accomplished by water from an external source freely circulating through the system. A constant, uninterrupted supply of water must be connected with each relocation of the laser. To reduce the risk of water pressure fluctuations or improperly connecting the water supply, some models have been equipped with a radiator and a fan in a closed system similar to that used in an automobile.

Carbon dioxide produces an invisible laser beam of relative high power. A visible low-power beam is generally operated coaxially as a visual reference.

This is created by a helium:neon laser coupled to the carbon dioxide system. This combination allows the surgeon to focus the laser beam accurately onto the correct area of the target tissue.

It is important for both the operating surgeon and laser nurse to be completely familiar with the control panel (Fig. 5–14). The settings of wattage, timing, delivery mode, on and off, and standby must be properly communicated and set to allow the laser to function with the expected power output and surgical outcome. The parameters are chosen by the surgeon, who directly informs the laser nurse to adjust the laser appropriately. This request is reiterated back to the surgeon to ensure programming accuracy.

CONTINUOUS-WAVE AND CONTINUOUS-PULSED LASERS

Carbon dioxide lasers can be operated through various modes. The photothermic energy generated can be delivered to the target tissue in a continuous wave or by single or multiple phases. The continuous-wave lasers operate on a gated principle. This method allows the low-power continuous wave to be transmitted in short and discreet bursts. The energy achievable by this method is significantly different from that created by a pulsed laser. The laser system produces much higher energy delivery, and each pulse typically lasts less than 1 millisecond. By operating a carbon dioxide laser in chopped pulse or chopped mode, the radiant energy is delivered automatically in an incremental fashion.

The laser tube is pumped or induced with high levels of direct current or radio frequency at short intervals. The released high-energy pulses of laser energy, which last for microseconds, are adjustable and have peak power levels two to nine times

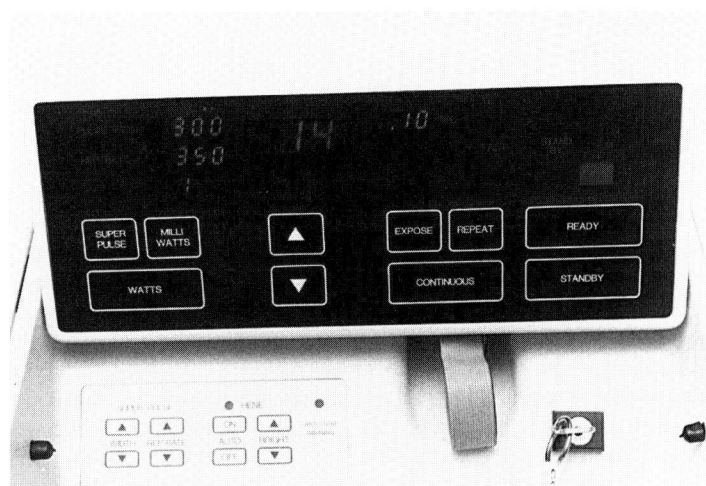

FIGURE 5–14. The control panel contains the switches that are used to calibrate the parameters controlling the laser beam power and timing. On/off/stand-by switches are included. (Photograph courtesy of Coherent Medical Group, Palo Alto, California.)

greater than that obtained during continuous-wave operation. By receiving the photothermic energy in the high-powered fashion, target tissue is instantly vaporized, with minimal conduction of heat to adjacent tissue. The delay between pulses (short interval) allows heat to radiate away from the impact site prior to the next pulse of laser energy delivery. Various manufacturers have been able to achieve high-powered delivery for extremely short periods of time to "achieve the cutting or ablating process with minimal thermal damage to adjacent underlying tissue."[24] This is accomplished by single-pulse ablation.[25] A single pulse instantly boils cellular fluid into vapor, and the resultant cellular burst allows a plume to transport the cellular debris and heat into the atmosphere. This technique minimizes thermal destruction of tissue margins ranging from 100 to 200 micrometers, allowing the pathologist to examine specimens accurately.[27–29] Clinically, there are reduced areas of blanching and less char production. Efficient performance during rapid superpulsed modes requires each pulse to vaporize all the tissue at the target site. Once the energy delivered is greater than the threshold level, a larger spot can be used, reducing the surgical exposure time and thus minimizing radiant heat energy to adjacent tissue. Again, a surgical learning curve is involved for the surgeon to choose the appropriate power for the spot size, with experience playing an important role in performing the procedure efficiently.

LASER AND TISSUE INTERACTION

The power density is the most important factor for effective laser operation. It determines the laser's ability to coagulate, vaporize, or excise tissue. The power density is defined as watts per square centimeter and is, therefore, directly proportional to the wattage and is inversely proportional to the area of the spot size. Power density is calculated by using the following formula[30]:

$$PD = 100 \text{ W/d}^2$$

The W is equal to the power on the console in watts, and d is equal to the measured diameter in millimeters of the imprint left on a moistened tongue depressor using a 10-watt, 0.1-second pulse. An increase in power output results in only a linear effect on power density. A reduction in spot size produces a quadratic increase in energy intensity at the impact site.

To obtain a power density of about 1000 W/cm², power output should be turned to the maximum level, with a defocused beam. For instance, a 100-W beam defocused to a 3.2-mm spot and a 10-W beam defocused to a 1-mm spot deliver the same power density of 1000 W/cm². When both of these parameters are set and the speed of hand movement is constant, the resultant depth of crater formation is the same. The focused 10-watt beam increases the thermal energy by a factor of 10 compared with the unfocused 100-watt beam.[31]

Guidelines for cutting with the carbon dioxide laser are simple. Spot size should be reduced to a minimum. This results in a two-dimensional rather than a three-dimensional incision. Power density is tailored by adjusting the power output to the same speed of hand movement required for the conventional scalpel.

The wavelength has a significant effect on the rate at which thermal energy is absorbed into the surrounding tissue. Carbon dioxide radiation is rapidly absorbed and dissipated, having a minimal depth of penetration (0.02 mm). This results in a system that produces a precisely accurate effect. This minimal penetration allows for greater precision of the beam with less adjacent tissue destruction during application. Not only is the depth of penetration dependent on wavelength, color, and tissue type but the surgeon must note that it is equally dependent on the power of the laser and spot size used during the application.

The carbon dioxide laser and tissue-interactive phase has been well studied since its inception. Even today, it continues to dominate many areas of research. There are four basic laser tissue interactions, which are known as absorption, scattering, transmission, and reflection (Fig. 5–15). By far, absorption is the most evident in the operative field and is the primary interactive effect sought by the surgeon. The absorption of laser photothermic energy causes tissue temperature to elevate. As temperature rises, the surgeon meticulously adjusts tissue effects between ablation and coagulation to create the desired treatment outcome.

Carbon dioxide laser light has a long infrared wavelength, which is nearly 20 times that of visible light. The majority of the carbon dioxide laser light is rapidly absorbed by water, which is the predominant component of the body. Absorption occurs more slowly in areas with decreased water content, such as osseous tissues. The surface is not the only area affected by the application of a laser beam. A portion of this photothermic energy is transmitted into deeper layers before it is absorbed by cellular fluid. The amount of tissue medium that can absorb a constant percentage of light is defined and can be calculated through Beer's law of absorption. Absorption length commonly describes the depth to which light must travel to be absorbed by 63%. It is also the depth to which laser heats tissue. By contrast, extinction length defines the distance a wavelength travels in the medium before it is absorbed by 90%. The residual 10% of the laser

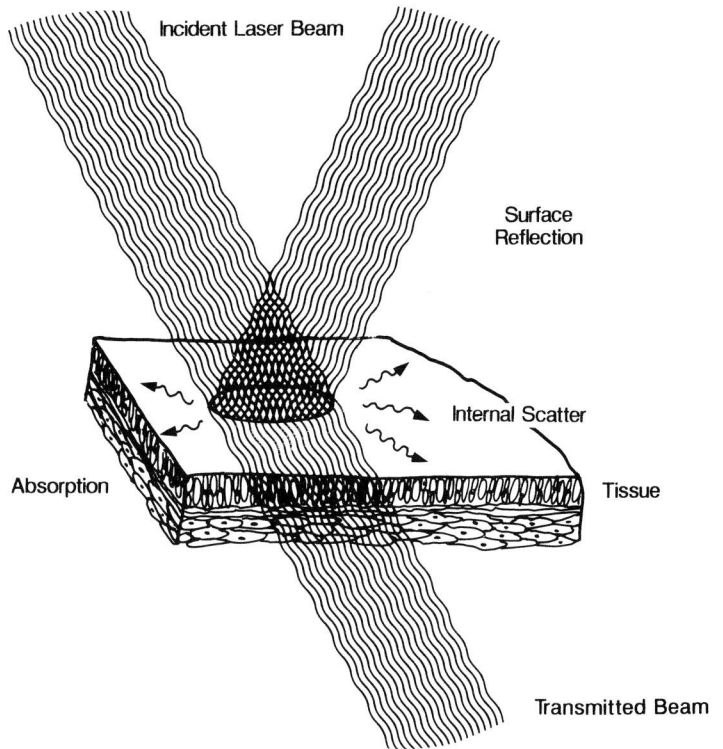

FIGURE 5–15. The four primary interactions of laser light with tissue occur when light strikes the tissue surface. A small amount of light is reflected at the surface level. As the light beam traverses the tissue, some is scattered by cellular components and structures or intracellular and extracellular fluids. As the light continues through the tissue by scattering or an uninterrupted beam, the tissue absorbs the light energy. Light is transmitted through the tissue if it is not totally absorbed. (Adapted from Trost D, Zacherl A, Smith MF: Surgical laser properties and their tissue interaction. *In* Smith MFW (ed): Neurological Surgery of the Ear. St. Louis, Mosby–Year Book, 1992, pp 131–162.)

power continues to penetrate the tissue for each extinction length, decreasing the remaining power by a factor of 10 (i.e., 10%, 1%, 0.1%). Mathematically derived, there are 2.3 absorption lengths per extinction length. Carbon dioxide's absorption length is 10 mm in water and 20 mm in tissue, regardless of pigmentation. This type of laser can heat and vaporize surface tissue leaving surrounding tissue unaffected and can dissipate thermal energy into the fluid of adjacent tissue. As a result, the

carbon dioxide laser provides consistent and predictable outcomes.

As the laser beam traverses tissue, some light is scattered, causing it to travel in various directions prior to being absorbed and heating tissue. Depending on the wavelength and mode of delivery, this thermally affected tissue can be cylindric, hemispheric, or conical (Fig. 5–16). Operating the carbon dioxide laser in the continuous-wave mode creates a hemispheric shallow zone of thermally

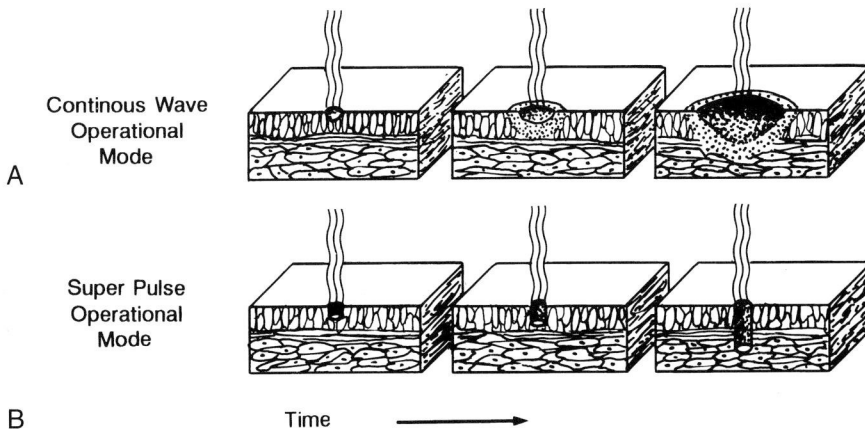

FIGURE 5–16. Hemispheric, conical, and cylindric vaporization due to absorption and internal scatter by varying quality laser beams. *A,* Continuous wave creates a hemispheric or conic zone of thermal injury. *B,* Super-pulse modes cause thermal tissue injury in a cylindric shape. (Adapted from Anonymous: Clinical effects of pulsatile carbon dioxide laser delivery. Health Devices 20[7–8]:305–309, 1991.)

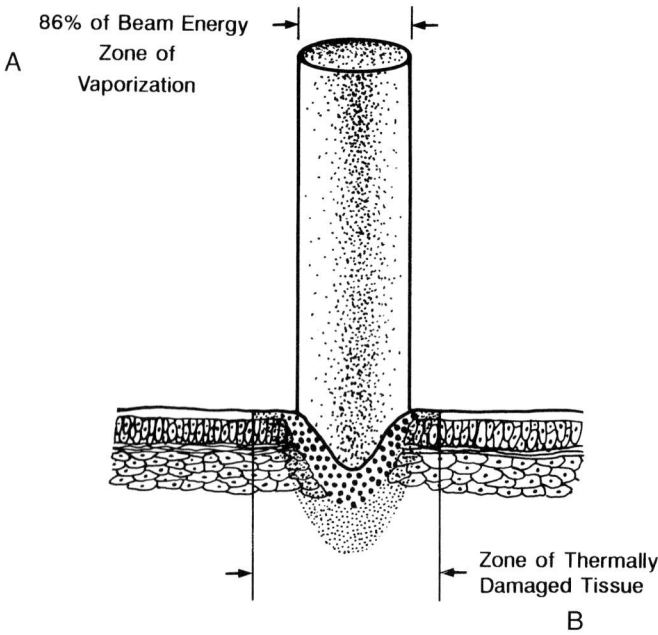

FIGURE 5–17. *A,* The effective spot size is the area of the laser beam that contains 86% of the photothermic energy. The average power density is calculated using this diameter and the definition of the spot size. The actual power density is greater centrally and is diminished as the periphery is approached. *B,* Impact size is the area of vaporized tissue plus the surrounding area of the thermally damaged tissue. (Adapted from Trost D, Zacherl A, Smith MF: Surgical laser properties and their tissue interaction. *In* Smith MFW (ed): Neurological Surgery of the Ear. St. Louis, Mosby–Year Book, 1992, pp 131–162.)

damaged tissue owing to the strong absorption of the wavelength by water and internal scatter. This pattern is altered to a cylindric shape when a superpulsed mode with higher power densities is used.[29, 32, 33]

A mathematic calculation of the laser beam diameter, which contains 86% of the energy when focused onto tissue, is the spot size (Fig. 5–17).[34] This depicts the visual area for the location of the laser beam. By contrast, the impact size is a measure of the crater left after applying laser energy. The resultant defect, taking into consideration absorption and scatter, is the zone of thermally damaged tissue (see Fig. 5–17).

When a carbon dioxide laser beam strikes a surface, a percentage of the light is reflected. Diffuse reflection or backscatter occurs when the light reflected is scattered in many directions (Fig. 5–18). This happens when the beam strikes tissue or an instrument that has an irregular surface or has been anodized. The energy is dispersed, reducing but not eliminating the risk to the surrounding tissue, the anesthesia apparatus, and the operating personnel. Specular reflection is the reflection of a laser beam without loss of power (Fig. 5–19). As the beam strikes a polished surface, the angle of incidence equals the angle of reflection, keeping the light intact. This characteristic of laser light can benefit the surgeon by allowing access to difficult areas and is actually the process by which the laser beam is transmitted through the articulated arm. On the other hand, an errant, specularly reflected beam has potentially destructive consequences if it strikes an unintended location, which poses a safety hazard.

Laser light is converted into heat instantly once

it is absorbed by tissue. The dissipation of heat into the surrounding tissue over time is described as heat conduction. Thermal relaxation is the time necessary to diffuse heat through soft tissue and is proportional to the square of the distance traveled. If heat contacting a surface is brief enough, surrounding tissue conducts the energy away from the contact point, producing minimal or no damage. On the other hand, if the contact time is increased and conduction cannot spread the thermal energy to surrounding tissue, damage occurs. Conduction continues and extends the burn beyond the immediate contact point once a critical temperature is attained.

Various biologic tissues react differently to laser

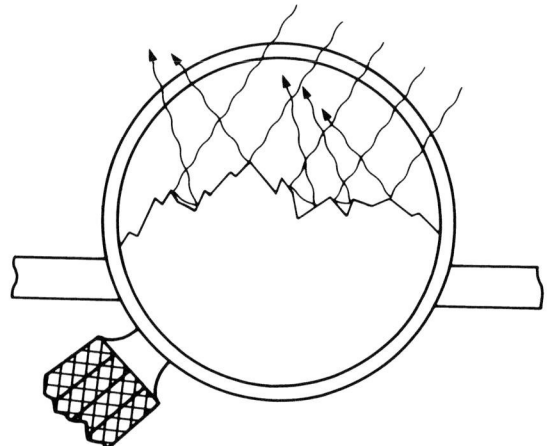

FIGURE 5–18. Diffuse reflection is also known as backscatter. The laser beam is reflected into many directions such as when light strikes an irregular surface.

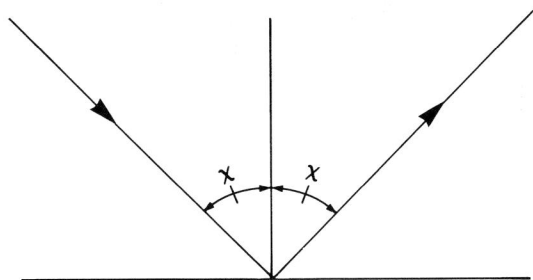

FIGURE 5–19. Specular reflection is the change in direction of a laser beam on impact with a highly reflective surface such as a mirror or polished instrument. The angles of incidence and reflection are equal.

radiation. The carbon dioxide beam is strongly absorbed by water independent of color. The greater the cellular water volume, the greater the tissue absorption of energy. The surgical effect produced by the laser is a photothermic energy transfer to target tissue, causing coagulation and vaporization. Other physiologic effects caused by photothermic energy may be discovered and biomechanically applied in the future.

Biologic photothermic effect (Table 5–4) begins between 37°C and 60°C despite the lack of visual change. Physiologically, at 42.5°C, malignant cells are irreversibly damaged and die, with the same process occurring at 44°C for normal tissue cells. Visual tissue changes begin, with blanching of the surface becoming apparent at 60°C. Additionally, cellular collagen helices uncoil reversibly, allowing tissue to be welded. Protein denaturization starts at 65°C, with resultant coagulation and shrinkage of the surface topography. Application of focused laser energy continues to elevate the tissue temperature to greater than 100°C (Fig. 5–20).[35] If this temperature increase occurs rapidly, cellular water boils instantly and can attain temperatures greater than 700°C. All cellular contents are destroyed, with a rapid overexpansion of cellular volume leading to isobaric vaporization. Clinically, an incision or volume of ablated tissue is noted on the surface, with the

production of a cloud of steam called a plume. This plume not only carries water vapor and cellular debris but also transfers laser-generated heat into the atmosphere, decreasing thermal conduction and damage in adjacent tissues. The surrounding tissue further conducts the laser heat to minimize thermal injury.

LASER APPLICATIONS IN SURGERY

Communication

A laser is a precise and technical device that requires equally precise attention to communication and safety protocols. In the operating theater, the surgeon is responsible for maintaining the protocol to prevent unnecessary harm not only to the patient but also to the ancillary staff, anesthesia personnel, and himself or herself. The actual function of the laser is communicated between the operator and the laser nurse by expressing four phrases. "Laser on" instructs all personnel that the laser is activated and prepared for energy delivery on depressing either the foot pedal or the finger switch. The laser nurse verifies this operational mode by stating "laser ready." "Laser standby" indicates that the unit is on safety; the mechanics are prepared, but no lasing energy can be delivered. Finally, "laser off" indicates that the unit has been deactivated, with all energies and lasing parameters having been discharged.

Laser Preparation

The preoperative protocol is a rational approach when preparing the laser for activation. The protocol encompasses technical and safety evaluations of the system, as well as verification that personnel comply with the safety recommendations. Once the laser and all necessary equipment are brought into the room, this process commences as follows[27]:

1. Obtain the laser key.

TABLE 5–4. The Visual and Biologic Effects on Tissue as a Function of Temperature Change

Temperature	Visual Change	Biologic Change
42.5°C	None	Malignant cells are functionally damaged and die
44.0°C	None	Normal cells are functionally damaged and die
60°C	Blanching	Warming, welding
65°C	Hemostasis	Coagulation
65–90°C	Tissue coloration to white or grey	Protein denaturization
90–100°C	Topographic shrinkage	Desiccation of tissue
100°C	Water vaporization, smoke plume	Vaporization of tissue, ablation
300°C	Char formation	Burning tissue
700°C	Iridescence	
3652°C	Smoke plume	Carbon sublimation

2. Place the appropriate "laser in use" sign at all entrances into the room. This sign should include the laser type, wavelength, and need for protective eyewear (Fig. 5–21).

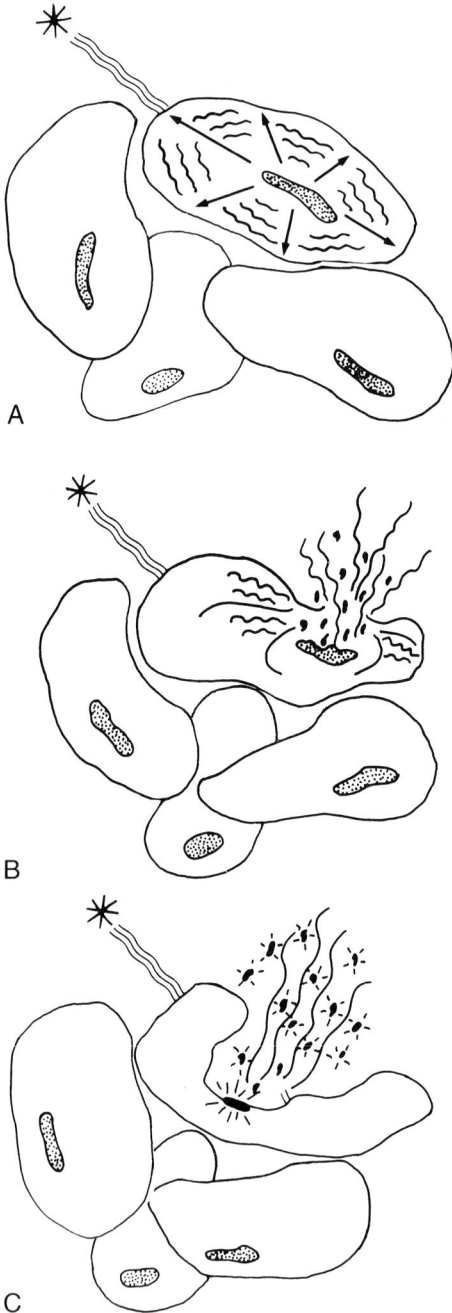

A

B

C

FIGURE 5–20. Cellular vaporization. *A,* Laser energy is converted into heat and rapidly superboils the intracellular fluid, increasing the intracellular pressure. *B,* The cell explodes, with water vapor, cellular debris, and heat released into the atmosphere. *C,* The debris from this process is carbonized by the laser energy and is removed by plume evacuation or deposited onto the surrounding tissue. (Adapted from Absten and Joffe: Laser interactions. *In* Absten GT, Joffe SN: Lasers in Medicine. London, Chapman and Hall, 1989, p 19.)

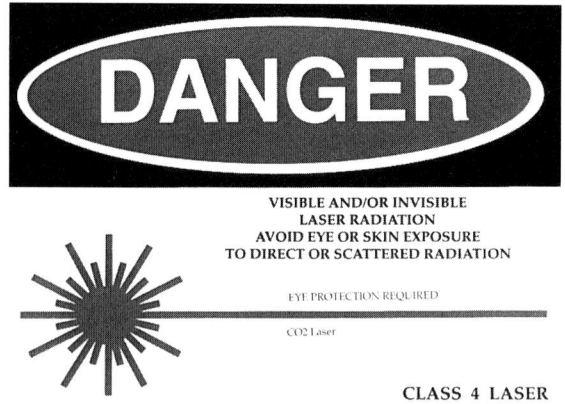

FIGURE 5–21. A "Laser-in-Use" sign depicting the type of laser, wavelength, and need for protective eyewear should be posted at each entrance into a surgical suite.

3. Place protective eyewear at all entrances to the room for incoming personnel to don prior to entering.
4. Verify that a fire extinguisher is present.
5. Connect the power cord to the supply outlet, verify that the manual safety shutter is closed, and unfold the articular arm.
6. Verify that all personnel are wearing protective eyewear of the correct optical density.
7. Open the control panel, insert the laser key, and turn the laser on.
8. Allow the control panel to illuminate, and check for fault codes.
9. Engage the "emergency off switch," and verify that the laser has power off by the lights on the control panel being extinguished.
10. Turn the laser back on.
11. Verify beam alignment between the aiming beam and the carbon dioxide laser beam (Fig. 5–22). This is accomplished by the following steps:
    a. Attach the handpiece-focusing lens and pointing blade to the articulating arm.
    b. Verify that all personnel have the appropriate protective eyewear in place.
    c. Mark an X on a water-moistened tongue depressor (see Fig. 5–22A).
    d. Select settings of continuous-wave mode, 10 watts, 0.1 second, and single exposure on the control panel.
    e. Open the manual safety shutter.
    f. Place the laser into ready mode.
    g. Touch the pointing blade to the tongue depressor, aligning the aiming beam with the center of the X (see Fig. 5–22B).
    h. Depress the foot switch to lase the tongue depressor, then return the unit back to standby.
    i. Observe the burn spot.
    j. Verify that the burn spot lies within the

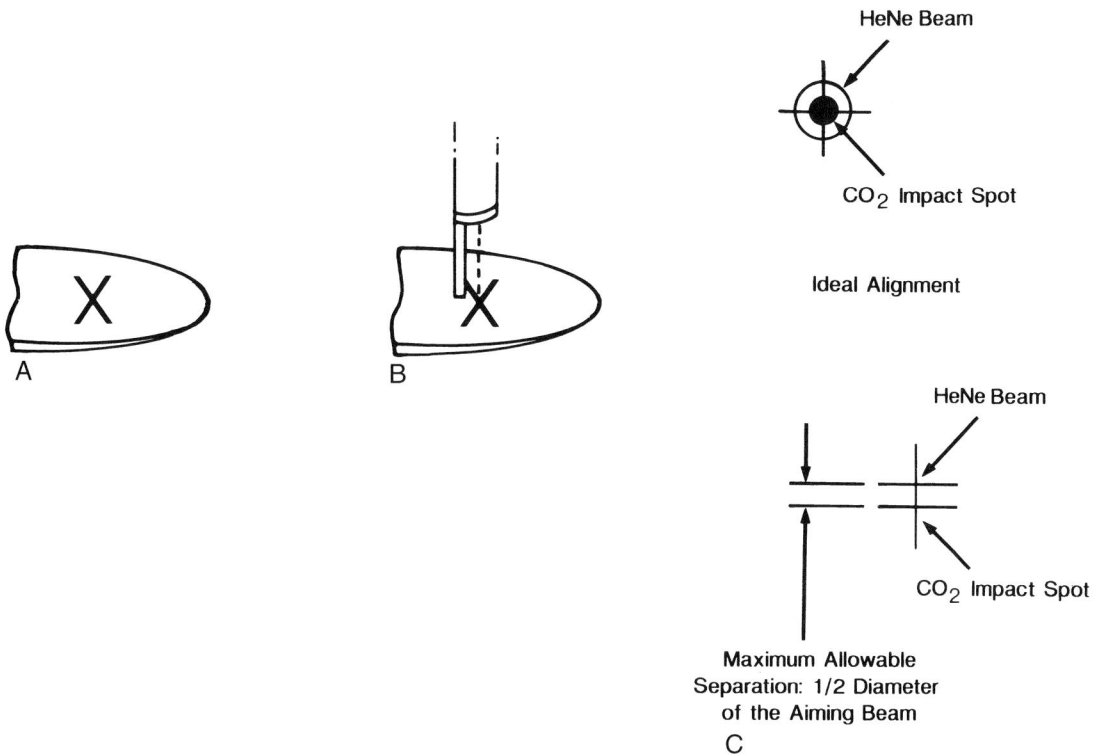

FIGURE 5–22. The beam alignment check is accomplished by *A,* placing an "x" on a moistened tongue blade; *B,* aligning the aiming beam on the center of the "x" and test firing; *C,* examining the impact site to determine whether it aligns within one-half of the aiming beam. (Adapted from Ultrapulse Carbon Dioxide Laser Operator Manual. Palo Alto, California, Coherent Medical Group, Inc., 1993.)

area of the aiming beam. The maximum allowable separation between the centers of the carbon dioxide impact site and the helium:neon beam is one half the diameter of the aiming beam (see Fig. 5–22C).

   k. If the burn is not within one half of the diameter of the aiming beam, check the handpiece for proper connection to the articulated arm. Repeat the alignment check.

12. After it is determined that all systems and safety equipment are performing satisfactorily, the patient can be brought into the operating theater and prepared for the surgical procedure.

Once the patient enters the room and is anesthetized (regional or general), and the surgery is ready to commence, procedural and safety protocols continue. The method to prepare for the actual surgery can vary to some degree but overall the necessary steps include the following:

1. Verify that the patient and all personnel in the room have donned the proper eye protection for the specific laser used. Placement of moistened eye pads, gauze, or towels can be used instead of glasses or goggles for the patient.

2. Drape the patient in such a fashion as to protect him or her from harm that can be caused by an errant laser beam. Areas that require protection include the following:

   a. Teeth can be protected with either aluminum foil conformed to the surface or the use of a prefabricated guard.

   b. Oral soft tissue, lips, and face are shielded with moistened gauze and towels.

   c. The endotracheal tube can be wrapped with protective film, isolated with moistened gauze, or a commercially available endotracheal tube, which is laser-beam protected, can be used.

   d. Keep a basin of water available for dousing a fire in an emergency.

3. Position the laser delivery system near the patient. The articulating arm should be free to maneuver to the operative site without stress to the arm joints or forcing the arm to reach the anatomic field.

4. Position the plume evacuator, and connect the power supply. The unit is self contained with filters. This prevents repeated use of the standard hospital or office general wall suction, which can lead to eventual clogging, down time, and costly repair. Additionally, the filters minimize atmospheric organic contamination.

5. Turn the laser system power on and place in standby mode. Open the manual safety shutter.

6. Select the laser mode and power, which vary according to the procedure being performed and the surgeon's preference. The operator

communicates the desired parameters to the laser nurse, who programs the necessary data on the laser control panel.

7. When the laser treatment is ready to begin, the operator communicates "laser on." The laser nurse turns the laser on and replies "laser ready." When the foot switch or the finger switch (controlled by the operator) is depressed, laser energy is delivered, tissue interaction occurs, and the plume is evacuated. Between each interval of laser treatment, the operator tells the laser nurse "laser on standby," whereby the nurse positions the laser in "standby" and communicates this action back to the operator.

8. The operator and the laser nurse are responsible for ensuring that all safety and procedural protocols are followed.

9. At the completion of the laser treatment, the operator (surgeon) issues the request "laser off" and appropriate documentation is recommended to describe the area treated, laser parameters used, and safety measures implemented. A laser log in duplicate allows one copy to be kept with the patient's record and the other with the laser use documentation manual (Fig. 5–23).

10. The laser is finally disconnected, cleaned, and prepared for storage or the next use.

Delivery Systems

The delivery system of the nontouch carbon dioxide laser transmits the beam to the target tissue through a suitable device. One delivery instrument is the handpiece (Fig. 5–24). Most carbon dioxide

---

GEISINGER MEDICAL CENTER
Danville, PA 17822

LASER LOG

Date: _____ Physician: _____

Procedure: _____

Laser Type/GMC Asset # : _____

Patient Protection: ☐ Moist Eye Pads   ☐ Goggles   ☐ Moist Sponges, etc.

Physician Eye Protection: ☐ Goggles   ☐ Eye Safety Filter

Personnel Eye Protection: ☐ Goggles

Smoke Evacuation System: ☐ Smoke Evacuator   ☐ None

Fire Extinguisher Available: ☐ Yes   ☐ No

Water Available: ☐ Yes   ☐ No

Warning Signs Posted at Each Entry: ☐ Yes   ☐ No

Laser Tested by: _____

Power Range: _____

Wattage: _____

Duration: _____

Area Treated: _____

Comments: _____
_____
_____
_____
_____

Signature/Title: _____

FIGURE 5–23. Laser log. A part of the patient's permanent record that lists biographic information as well as the laser type, wavelength, power, duration of use, area lased, safety precautions implemented, and complications that may have occurred. A second copy is placed within the laser use documentation manual. (Courtesy of Geisinger Medical Center, Danville, Pennsylvania.)

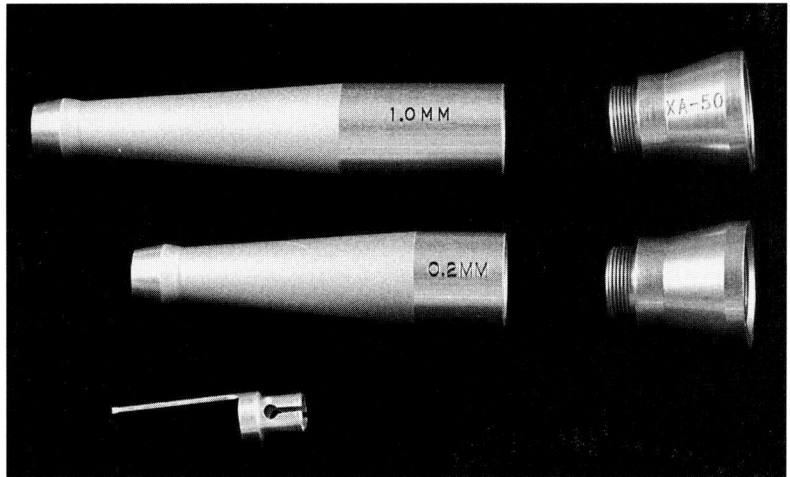

FIGURE 5–24. Laser handpieces are used to deliver the laser beam to the target tissue. The carbon dioxide laser has the handpiece attached to the articulated arm. A focusing lens within the handpiece produces a specified spot size when coupled with the pointing guide.

lasers have a fixed focal length of 125 mm built into the handpiece. This focal length forms a spot size of 0.2 mm, which increases precision during the surgery. A pointing blade attached to the distal end of the handpiece ensures the constant delivery of the photothermic reaction at a specific diameter when the blade tip rests against the tissue surface. Various focal lengths that change the source-to-target distance and spot size are available. A larger surface interaction ablating a broader area is caused by defocusing the beam. This occurs as the pointing blade is withdrawn from the tissue surface. As the beam is defocused, the power density is decreased, thus reducing the cellular response to the laser beam.

Removing the pointing blade and placing an angled mirror specularly reflects the beam either 90 or 120 degrees. These mirrors improve access to areas of the oral cavity such as the anterior palate and floor of mouth. The operating surgeon is left with the task of determining the spot size and focus of the laser beam when these mirrors are used.

The carbon dioxide laser can also be attached to a microscope. The interfacing connector is a micromanipulator constructed with specialized co-axial mirrors and shutters (Fig. 5–25). Connecting the laser to the microscope requires matching the focal length of the laser focusing lens and the microscope's objective lens. Generally, a 300-mm focal length is incorporated to allow a suitable working zone between the microscope and the target tissue. This distance permits the microscope to be outside the mouth, providing enough room for the surgeon to maneuver the instruments necessary while maintaining precision with a 0.6-mm spot size. Through the use of a manual joy stick, the laser beam is maneuvered to the critical target site and activated by a button on the micromanipulator.

Focusing the microscope causes the laser beam

to be focused in front of the visual impact site on the target tissue. This is useful in debulking and coagulating tissue or when using low power. It is important to consider the location of the focal point and be aware of structures deep to the surface impact point. As the laser is operating, tissue penetration is faster with greater temperature production as the focal point is approached. This may lead to inadvertent injury to deep structures beyond the intended impact site.

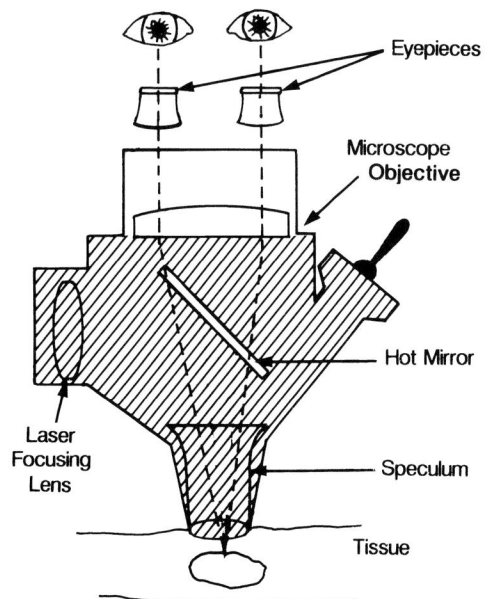

FIGURE 5–25. Micromanipulators provide the interface between the carbon dioxide laser and microscope. With specialized optics, the laser beam and an aiming beam are projected through the microscope onto the target tissue. The micromanipulator control allows the surgeon to locate precisely the laser beam at the surgical site and change the spot size for the desired effect. (Adapted from Clearspot Micromanipulators. Product Bulletin. Palo Alto, California, Coherent Medical Group, Inc., 1992.)

The combination of microscope and laser also can be used in the defocused mode. The focal point of the laser is above the target tissue and provides a diffuse impact site. This technique facilitates coagulation of vascular tissue and, with high-power settings, broad areas of tissue vaporization.

Waveguides are devices that extend the application of the carbon dioxide laser to endoscopic procedures (Fig. 5–26). This apparatus provides delivery of the laser beam to restrictive anatomic sites. These rigid, hollow, highly reflective, straight or slightly curved tubes are made from metallic or ceramic substances. Waveguides are attached to the articulating arm via a coupler. To secure the coupler, it must be threaded securely to the articulated arm so it does not become loose during the surgical procedure. A gas purge hose should also be used and attached to the lure fitting on the laser coupler. A sterile drape can be placed over the coupler and articulating arm after the gas purge hose has been connected.

Waveguides generate a spot size of 0.4 mm, which is not as small as that which can be produced by the handpiece but is functional. Waveguides should not be used in areas that cannot be directly visualized. During surgery, the waveguide has to be brought close to the surgical site and may obstruct the surgeon's view. Care must be taken to isolate the field appropriately to minimize misdirected transmission. This instrument provides delivery of the laser beam to restricted anatomic sites. Cutting

and vaporization of intra-articular tissues within the temporomandibular joint has been accomplished.

The type of delivery unit chosen depends on the nature of the surgery. In general, the oral and maxillofacial surgeon incorporates the hand-held unit into practice for surface lesions and waveguides for arthroscopic surgery. Once there has been a decision to perform surgery with the carbon dioxide laser, additional understanding of its biologic tissue effect is necessary for appropriate applications.

Photocoagulation

Ninety-eight percent of the photothermic energy produced by the carbon dioxide laser is absorbed within 0.17 mm of tissue penetration. This is due to the high absorption coefficient of water, and soft tissues are comprised of 80% to 90% water. The zone of coagulation necrosis produced is, therefore, minimal with the use of the carbon dioxide laser when a cutting mode is applied. The nontarget adjacent tissue has radiant thermal energy histologic changes consisting of a narrow zone of carbonized tissue, an underlying desiccated tissue necrosis zone, and a peripheral zone of edematous reversibly damaged tissue (see Fig. 5–17).

During the incision of tissue, the carbon dioxide laser can concurrently coagulate blood vessels of up to 0.5 mm diameter. Larger vessels, up to 2

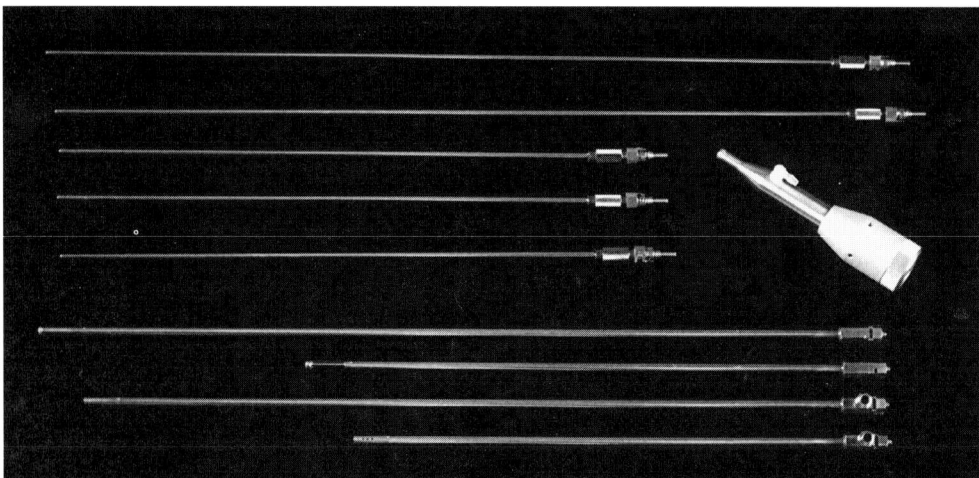

FIGURE 5–26. Hollow waveguides extend the capability of carbon dioxide laser surgery through endoscopic and arthroscopic instruments. They have the disadvantage of requiring close proximity to the target site, which occasionally obstructs the view. Rigid waveguides provide a way of delivering a relatively small beam through an endoscope or arthroscope, extending the capability of carbon dioxide laser surgery. The end of the waveguide is brought into close contact with the tissue. Rigid waveguides typically do not provide spot sizes as small as those achieved with a micromanipulator, but they can gain access to tighter spaces. However, there is some tendency for the end of the waveguide to obstruct the field view. (Photograph courtesy of Coherent Medical Group, Palo Alto, California.)

mm, require interruption of the incising process and defocusing of the laser beam to cause coagulation (Fig. 5–27). The defocused beam is systematically activated circumferentially around the vessel, creating diminished blood flow through adjacent tissue edema, tissue necrosis, and carbon deposition.

Prolonging the exposure allows heat to be conducted to greater depths, until the temperature reaches a critical level for coagulation to occur. Essentially, coagulation cannot result unless lateral thermal conduction and damage take place. By operating with a combination of low power, large spot size, and a pulsed mode, hemostasis is more likely to be produced.

The surgeon must realize, however, that the carbon dioxide laser is not the sole nor primary coagulating instrument. When necessary, for persistently bleeding vessels, use of a bipolar or diathermic coagulator or ligating suture should be substituted.

Incision

The carbon dioxide laser can be used easily to create surgical incisions without tissue contact. This is accomplished by focusing the laser beam onto the tissue surfaces with the smallest spot size possible, which possesses the highest power density. The precise incision that results has minimal lateral thermal conduction injury or thermodistortion limited to 100 to 200 micrometers when generated by a 0.2-mm spot size. The margins of a specimen obtained in this fashion can, therefore, be accurately examined. Additionally, the surgical site is relatively dry, with the surrounding vessels and lymphatics sealed.[2]

When the laser beam is systematically applied, removal of a soft tissue specimen can be accomplished (Fig. 5–28). This is attained by employing the carbon dioxide laser in a rapid superpulsed mode with a focused beam. For skin and mucous membranes, set the laser from 10 watts to 20 watts. The laser energy is directed perpendicular to the tissue surface, and an outline is made circumferentially around the lesion, incorporating normal and altered tissue.

A trough is created when radial traction is applied. Adequate margins of all borders should be included and consistent with sound clinical practice. The handpiece can be angulated to remove a wedge of tissue, or a tissue margin can be lifted and retracted, with the laser beam incising beneath the lesion, parallel to the tissue surface. Blood vessels that are less than 2.0 mm in diameter and continue to bleed can be coagulated by using a defocused continuous-wave beam. Larger vessels may require conventional ligation techniques to arrest the hemorrhage. At the discretion of the surgeon, the excised tissue can be forwarded for histopathologic review.

Incisional biopsies are performed in an identical fashion. As with conventional methods, a margin of

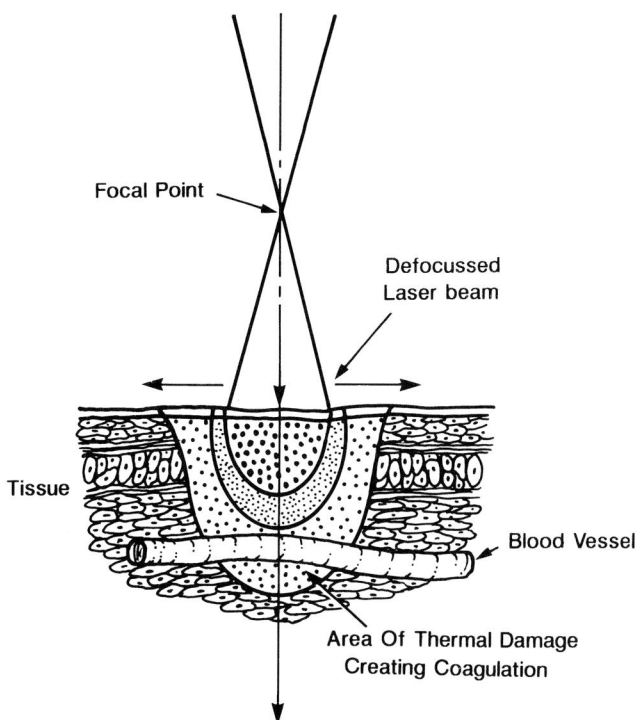

FIGURE 5–27. Defocusing the laser beam decreases the power density and increases thermal conduction and coagulation capability.

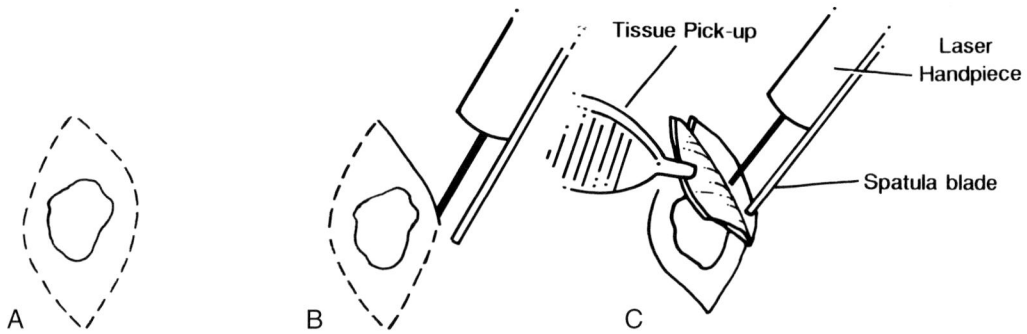

FIGURE 5–28. Excisional and incisional biopsies can be performed. *A,* First, an outline is made with adequate margins around the altered tissue to be excised, with the laser beam perpendicular to the surface. *B,* A forcep is used to elevate a margin and the specimen is raised ahead of the laser beam thus excising the lesion. Larger vessels (up to 2.0 mm) that continue to hemorrhage can be coagulated by defocusing a continuous-wave laser beam. *C,* The resultant wound can be left to granulate secondarily or closed primarily in a routine fashion. (Adapted from Pick R, Pecaro BC: Use of CO_2 laser in soft tissue dental surgery. Lasers Surg Med 7:207–213, 1987.)

normal tissue is included for diagnostic purposes. The resulting wound can be closed primarily or allowed to granulate. This is determined by the dimension of the defect and the surgeon's judgment.

Vaporization or Ablation

Another effective method for removal of diffuse soft tissue lesions is vaporization or ablation. This process allows high-power densities to be applied for brief periods with a defocused method. When combining high power and short exposure, the surgeon is able to work at a slower pace without the risk of great thermal damage to contiguous structures. Once the lesion is vaporized, there is no tissue available for microscopic examination. Therefore, an important consideration prior to vaporizing a lesion is whether to obtain a tissue diagnosis to confirm the clinical impression. Strategically placed punch biopsies are adequate to allow histologic identification preoperatively and confirmation of complete removal of the lesion postoperatively.

The pulsed laser, which delivers a high-power laser beam for a preset duration, maximizes tissue ablation with minimal thermal elevation in surrounding tissue. The amount of power delivered per pulse to produce a char-free, thermally unaffected surgical area must be high enough to vaporize all the tissue at the impact site. The vapor, debris, and residual heat are carried by the plume and evacuated 1 to 2 inches from the interaction site.

When diffuse skin and mucous membrane lesions require vaporization, using a defocused 15- to 20-watt beam and repeated crosshatching of the surgical area, with occasional wiping of accumulated debris from the surface for improved visibility, removes the lesion (Fig. 5–29). Cells coming in con-

tact with a laser beam are immediately vaporized. This vaporization seals the lymphatic channels, minimizing the seeding of malignant cells and the spread of infectious bacteria or viruses. Such spread of infectious agents occurs more readily with a scalpel, diathermy, or cryoprobe.

Vaporization depends on the rate of heating of the target tissue to a critical temperature. With the use of higher laser energies, heat remains localized with a faster rise in cellular temperature. The result is an increased rate of vaporization, even though coagulation in deeper tissue does occur. Maximizing tissue ablation with a minimal contiguous zone of thermal damage depends on the power density. For the carbon dioxide laser, this critical value is 50 watts/mm² and has a corresponding 0.02-mm absorption length.[31] The carbon dioxide laser operating at this power density vaporizes tissue efficiently. The rate of tissue removal can be increased by raising the power. To minimize the zone of thermal damage when debulking large volumes of tissue, another factor to consider is the duration of the exposure. High-power densities allow shorter exposure times, which increase heat conduction through vaporization into the atmosphere and decrease the conduction into the tissue. It has been recommended, therefore, to operate the laser at the highest power setting with which the surgeon is

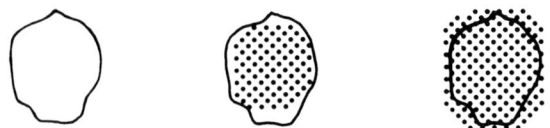

FIGURE 5–29. Laser vaporization/ablation is accomplished by first achieving the critical power density, which is 50 watts/cm². Using a pulsed mode in a crosshatch pattern, the lesion is removed with minimal thermal damage to adjacent tissue.

comfortable and can manage safely. The expertise to make this decision is "developed through training and experience" using surgical lasers.[36]

Anhydrous carbon formation on the adjacent soft tissue is known as black char. This material represents carbonization of cellular protein caused by relatively slow heating of tissue and drying until it is overheated. There is some vaporization of cellular fluid, but heat is significantly retained in the surrounding tissue rather than conducted away by a plume. The remaining carbonized tissues continue to absorb laser energy with further conduction to surrounding areas. This process occurs when a laser beam is used with less than the critical power density necessary to perform ablative techniques. Understanding the theory of power density and its application during surgery is necessary to minimize charring and the zone of thermal damage.

Operating at a low power to decrease the risk to adjacent structures can actually have the opposite effect, risking injury by increasing thermal conduction. This is more noticeable during continuous-wave operation. By contrast, pulsed modalities can perform slow and precise tissue ablation with minimal thermal conduction and less char formation.

Wound Healing

Both clinical and laboratory studies demonstrated that the carbon dioxide laser produces wounds that heal differently from those made by a scalpel.[37] Scalpel wounds contracted significantly and developed rolled margins that remained present 42 days later. Laser wounds also developed the rolled borders, but flattening occurred 28 days after lasing.[38, 39] Histologically, there are fewer myofibroblasts present, which appears to be responsible for less scar contraction.[37–42] In addition, less collagen formation is noted, and the epithelial regeneration is delayed. The regeneration from the epithelial margins appears to extend over the fibrinous coagulum rather than proliferating beneath the granulation tissue, as when wounds heal by secondary intention. Reepithelialization appears to be complete in 6 weeks, with the original wound outline visible. There is minimal scarring, and the overlying surface remains palpably soft. It is important to note that ductal orifices incorporated into the lased field do not demonstrate stenosis on healing.[37] Later studies, however, refute this finding. Basu and colleagues have demonstrated large populations of myofibroblast in healing glossectomy wounds in rats.[43]

Sterilization of the surgical wound also has been studied. Literature demonstrates more effective wound sterilization with the carbon dioxide laser than with the use of a standard surgical scrub.[44] By contrast, when comparing the carbon dioxide laser with electrocautery, the authors found significantly improved sterilization with the use of routine electrocautery.[45] Despite these controversies, lasers are still considered to produce sterile surgical sites based on instant vaporization of tissue and adjacent vascular and lymphatic sealing. Furthermore, studies have reported that no bacteremias occur following intraoral lasing when compared with conventional surgical techniques.[46]

Laser-produced wounds are thought to produce less postoperative pain. The vaporization of cellular structure, organelles, and cellular chemical mediators, as well as sealing of nerve endings, is considered responsible.[37] Basu also noted that nerve endings were not sealed, contradicting earlier hypotheses for this lack of pain.[43]

CONCLUSION

Not to be forgotten, the carbon dioxide laser is a surgical instrument that can be used interchangeably with various other devices. The treatment modality chosen by the surgeon depends on his or her knowledge, training, and comfort level; equipment availability; procedure amenability for use with specific technologies; desired outcome; patient's demands; and cost. The device does not cure the disease. The appropriate use and surgical selection based on sound clinical judgment are responsible for elimination of disease processes.

As with most new products developed either for medical use or as general consumer goods, the cost of a laser is high. To expand its use in the future, it may be necessary for the industry to produce less expensive, smaller models that are amenable to office use. Building a laser with computer software that could be programmed to perform specific tasks with minimal human interaction may be generations away but is not unlikely. By integrating microprocessors, thermocouples, imaging, and diagnostic processes, a smart laser with feedback control could be developed. This system would function reliably to excise lesions through ablation and coagulate blood vessels and lymphatic channels with precision, causing minimal thermal damage to surrounding tissue.

On the horizon, however, advancement in laser technology could allow for the delivery of a carbon dioxide laser beam through a flexible fiber. Small hand-held models are being developed, and these will be used to treat dental disease effectively without pulpal damage.

REFERENCES

1. Catone G: Laser Technology in Oral and Maxillofacial Surgery, Part 1. Principles. Selected Readings in OMS 3(4), 1993, pp 1–37.

2. Bailin PL: Lasers in dermatology. J Dermatol Surg Oncol 11:3, 1985.
3. Fisher SE, Frame JW, Browne RM, Tranter RM: A comparative histological study of wound healing following CO_2 laser and conventional surgical excision of canine buccal mucosa. Arch Oral Biol 28(4):287–291, 1993.
4. Smith TA, Thompson JA, Lee WE: Assessing patient pain during dental laser therapy. J Am Dent Assoc 124:90–94, 1993.
5. Einstein A: Zur Quanten Theorie Der Stralung. Physikalische Zeitschrift 18:121, 1917.
6. Gordon JP, Zeigler HJ, Townes CH: The MASER—new type of amplifier frequency standard and spectrometer. Physiol Rev 99:1264, 1955.
7. Schawlow AL, Townes CH: Infrared and optical red masers. Physiol Rev 112:1940, 1958.
8. Maiman TH: Stimulated optical radiation in ruby. Nature 187:493, 1960.
8a. Ball KA: Lasers, the Perioperative Challenge. St. Louis, C. V. Mosby, 1990, pp 19–41.
9. Patel CKN: Interpretation of CO_2 optical laser experiments. (Letter.) Physiol Rev 12:588, 1964.
10. Polanyi TG, Bredemeier HC, Davis TW: A CO_2 laser for surgical research. Med Biol Eng Comput 8:541, 1970.
11. Yahr WZ, Strully KJ: Blood vessel anastomosis and other biomedical applications. J Assoc Adv Med Instrum 1:28, 1966.
12. Shafir R, Slutzki S, Bornstein LA: Excision of buccal hemangioma by CO_2 laser beam. Oral Surg Oral Med Oral Pathol 44(3):347–350, 1977.
13. Sachs SA, Borden GE: The utilization of carbon dioxide laser in treatment of recurrent palatal papillomatosis. Report of Case. J Oral Maxillofac Surg 39:299, 1981.
14. Clayman L, Fuller T, Beckman H: Healing of continuous wave and rapid superpulsed CO_2 laser–induced bone defects. Oral Surg 36:932, 1978.
15. Wennu OC, Olsson P, Flisberg K, Paulson B, Luttrup J: Treatment of snoring—with and without carbon dioxide laser. Acta Otolaryngol Suppl 492:152–155, 1992.
16. Grontved A, Jorgensen K, Petersen SV: Results of uvulopalatopharyngoplasty in snoring. Acta Otolaryngol Suppl 492:11–14, 1992.
17. Icamami YV: Laser CO_2 for snoring. Preliminary results. Acta Otorhinolaryngol Belg 44(4):451–456, 1990.
18. Carenfelt C: Laser uvulopalatoplasty in treatment of habitual snoring. Ann Otol Rhinol Laryngol 100(6):451–454, 1991.
19. Babitz JB, Catone GA, Happel MB, Heine RD: Comparison between CO_2 microsurgical laser and conventional meniscectomies in sheep: A preliminary report. J Oral Maxillofac Surg 47(4):383–385, 1989.
20. Bardach J, Panje W: Surgical management of the large cavernous hemangioma. Otolaryngol Head Neck Surg 89:792, 1981.
21. Kaplan I, Ger R, Sharon U: The CO_2 laser in plastic surgery. Br J Plast Surg 26:359, 1973.
22. Rockwell Laser Manual II-1. Cincinnati, Ohio, Rockwell Laser Industries, 1990.
23. Dorros G, Seeley D: Understanding Lasers: A Basic Manual for Medical Practitioners Including an Extensive Bibliography of Medical Applications. Mount Kisco, NY, Futura Publishing Company, Inc., 1991.
24. Dixon JA: Surgical Application of Lasers. Chicago, IL, Year Book Medical Publishers, Inc., 1987.
25. Fuller TA: The physics of surgical lasers. Lasers Surg Med 1:5, 1980.
26. Svelto O: Principles of Lasers. New York, Plenum Press, 1989.
27. Ultrapulse Carbon Dioxide Surgical Lasers Operator Manual. Palo Alto, CA, Coherent, Inc., 1993.
28. Ultrapulse Carbon Dioxide Slide Presentation, Coherent Medical Group. Palo Alto, CA, Coherent, Inc., 1992.
29. Duncavage JA, Ossoff RH: Use of the carbon dioxide laser for malignant disease of the oral cavity. Lasers Surg Med 6:442–444, 1986.
30. Catone GA: Lasers in dentoalveolar surgery. Oral Maxillofac Surg Clin North Am 5:45–61, 1993.
31. Grossenbacher R, Sutter R: Carbon dioxide laser surgery in otorhinolaryngology: Pulsed beam versus continuous wave beam. Ann Otol Rhinol Laryngol 88(97):222–228, 1988.
32. Reid R: Physical and surgical principles governing carbon dioxide laser surgery on the skin. Dermatol Clin 9(2):297–315, 1991.
33. Fuller TA: Laser tissue interaction: The Influence of power density. *In* Baggish MS (ed): Basic and Advanced Laser Surgery. Norwalk, CT, Appleton-Century-Crofts, 1985, pp 51–60.
34. Lanzafame RJ, Nalm JO, Rogers DW, et al: Comparison of continuous wave, chop wave, and superpulse laser wounds. Lasers Surg Med 8(2):119–124, 1988.
35. Anonymous: Clinical effects of pulsatile carbon dioxide laser delivery. Health Devices 20(7–8):305–309, 1991.
36. Trost D, Zacherl A, Smith MF: Surgical laser properties and their tissue interaction. *In* Smith MFW (ed): Neurological Surgery of the Ear. St. Louis, Mosby–Year Book, 1992, pp 131–162.
37. Fisher SE, Frame JW: The effects of the carbon dioxide surgical laser on oral tissues. Br J Oral Maxillofac Surg 22:414–425, 1984.
38. Fisher SE, Frame JW, Browne RM, Tranter RMD: A comparative histological study of wound healing following CO_2 laser and conventional surgical excision of canine buccal mucosa. Arch Oral Biol 28:287, 1983.
39. Ben-Bassat M, Kaplan IA: A study of the ultrastructural features of the cut margin of skin and mucous membrane specimens excised by carbon dioxide laser. J Surg Res 21:77, 1976.
40. Gabbiani G, Ryan GB, Majno G: The presence of modified fibroblasts in granulation tissue and their possible role in wound contraction. Experientia 27:549, 1971.
41. Frame JW: Treatment of sublingual keratosis with the CO_2 laser. Br Dent J 156:243, 1984.
42. Rhys Evans PHR, Frame JW, Branddrick J: A review of carbon dioxide laser surgery in the oral cavity and pharynx. J Laryngol Otol 100:69, 1986.
43. Basu MK, Frame JW, Rhys Evans PHR: Wound healing following partial glossectomy using the carbon dioxide laser, diathermy, and scalpel: A histological study in rats. J Laryngol Otol 102:322, 1988.
44. Al-Qattan MM, Stranc MF, Jarmuske M, Hoban DJ: Wound sterilization: CO_2 laser versus iodine. Br J Plast Surg 42:380, 1989.
45. Stranc MF, Yang FW: Wound sterilization: Cautery versus CO_2 laser. Br J Plast Surg 45:536, 1992.
46. Kaminer R, Liebow C, Margonome JL, Zambon JJ: Bacteremia following laser and conventional surgery in hamsters. J Oral Maxillofac Surg 48:45, 1990.
47. Absten GT, Joffe SN: Lasers in Medicine. Chapman and Hall, London, 1989.

CHAPTER 6

Laser Management of Intraoral Surface Lesions

GUY A. CATONE, DMD

Many of the host of lesions that occur on the surface of the oral mucosa are easily controlled with laser energy. Excluding vesiculobullous diseases, ulcerative conditions, pigmentations, and angiodysplasias, the vast majority of these lesions appear white in color or have an opaque surface. With the exception of premalignant variants such as dysplastic leukoplakia, sublingual keratosis, and so-called speckled erythroplakia, these entities exhibit a benign course and, in most instances, are not treated. White lesions share their common clinical appearance with other similar lesions in the colorless family, owing to their ability to scatter incident light and to obscure the underlying color of the lamina propria by the nature of their altered mucosal layer. Mucosal changes that lead to an opaque surface appearance may be caused by a thicker layer of the stratum corneum, an increase in the cell population of the stratum malpighii, or intracellular edema of epithelial cells. A variety of causes can be implicated in the development of white lesions. Chronic irritation or physical trauma, genetic anomalies, tobacco habits, dermatologic or mucosal diseases, and inflammatory reactions are usually related to such mucosal changes. Although many entities may render the oral mucosa opaque or white looking, only conditions that are manageable by the laser are discussed here; the reader is referred to any comprehensive textbook of oral pathology for more details of similar-looking lesions and related differential diagnoses.[1]

INCISIONAL AND EXCISIONAL BIOPSIES

When tissue specimens are required from more massive unknown lesions, a laser may offer advantages for cutting or incising. In such cases, the biopsy site usually does not require coaptation and all the advantages of the surgical laser will be apparent, such as enhanced hemostasis, less pain, precise tissue cutting, good access to comparatively inaccessible areas of the oral cavity, and reduced vulnerability to infection, among others. The carbon dioxide laser can be used in a pulsed mode, either superpulse or UltraPulse (Coherent Laser, Palo Alto, Calif.), and the site of specimen harvest can be outlined initially by a series of pulses to include normal and altered tissue. With the laser in a focused rather than a defocused mode for skin or mucosa and the power set at 10 to 20 W for superpulse and 5 to 10 W for UltraPulse, the beam is directed to the lesional and nonlesional tissue to be excised and a wedge of tissue is excised. In this case, the beam is approximately perpendicular to the tissue surface. The beam can then be angulated after penetrating the surface and picking up a corner of tissue to reveal the underlying subcutaneous or submucosal layer. In excising a biopsy specimen the laser beam can thus be angled early in the procedure so that an edge of the lesion is lifted and retracted in front of the laser beam. The surgeon simply moves the laser beam from side to side, tactilely sensing the tissues of the lesion as they gradually fall forward. During this process, the laser is kept focused; however, if bleeding is encountered, the beam can be pulled away into a defocused mode, thus increasing the size of the focal spot and changing the wave timing to continuous wave and thus enabling the surgeon to coagulate bleeders smaller than 1 mm in diameter.

The contact Nd:YAG laser can be applied for incisional and excisional biopsies, especially for

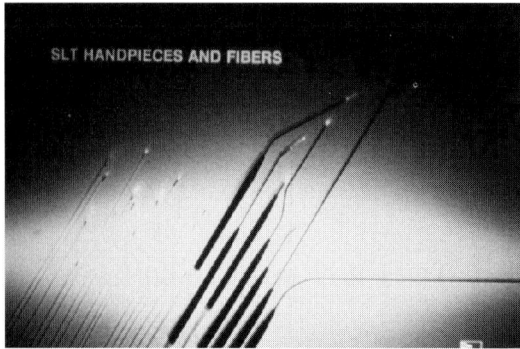

FIGURE 6–1. Multiple shapes and sizes of contact probes available from Surgical Laser Technologies, Oaks, Pa. Handpieces are also available that have a finger trigger or button on the handpiece itself, which facilitates control of switching the power on and off, thus preserving the contours of the tip. (Courtesy of Surgical Laser Technologies, Oaks, Pennsylvania.)

lesions of the mucous membrane (Fig. 6–1). Contact scalpel probes can be used, setting the power at 10 to 20 W. The scalpel tip is placed at an angle of approximately 90 degrees and is drawn across the surface. The tissue is excised by moving the contact tip under the retracted tissues. The target tissues to be biopsied or excised are easily removed using the contact YAG as the tissues are grasped by forceps under tension (Fig. 6–2). Any bleeding is controlled with the contact tip by tapping the tip directly on smaller bleeders (those smaller than 3 mm), and by touching the tissues surrounding larger vessels. This latter maneuver causes edema around the vessel, which reduces the rate of blood flow, eventually occluding the lumen.

By using the free-beam or waveguide type of carbon dioxide laser (the latter simulating the contact probe and the Nd:YAG contact system) the surgical pathologist can easily examine the margins

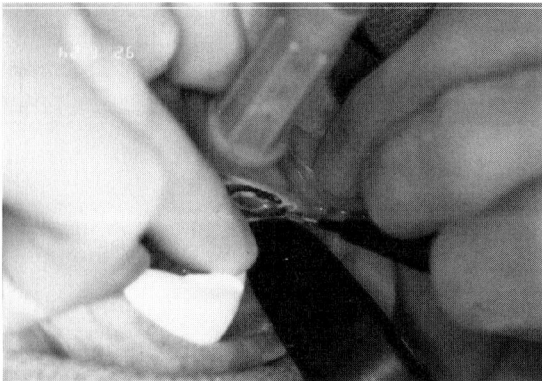

FIGURE 6–2. Contact laser scalpel probe used to excise lesion of buccal mucosa. It is important when using the contact probe to place target tissues under tension. This appears to facilitate the cutting properties of the probe tip.

of the specimen, as they are not altered appreciably during the lasing process. For example, with the free-beam carbon dioxide laser there is approximately 50 to 200 microns of thermal injury in the target tissue margin as a result of a 0.2-mm spot size in a focused mode. About 500 microns of reversible thermal change is observed in the contiguous nontarget tissues (Fig. 6–3).

FOCAL HYPERKERATOSIS (FRICTIONAL HYPERKERATOSIS)

Focal hyperkeratosis is indistinguishable clinically from idiopathic leukoplakia. It is often referred to as a traumatic lesion, having arisen from chronic irritation, as from an intraoral dental appliance. The lesion is seen in areas that are subjected to repeated oral trauma (i.e., lips, linea alba, or occlusal interface with the buccal mucosa, lateral borders of the tongue, and on the crest of the edentulous ridges or on the vestibular mucosa in areas of overextended denture flanges). The lesions are usually asymptomatic but may enlarge to a degree that places them more in harm's way, resulting in gross injury or ulceration, followed in some instances by secondary infection (Fig. 6–4A and B).

On biopsy, the chief finding is the obvious hyperkeratosis with marginal round cell infiltration in the underlying lamina propria. Conservative observation, or resection in the case of chronic injury and pain, is usually warranted, as usually there are no dysplastic alterations in the epithelial tissues. Because the lesion cannot be distinguished clinically from premalignant lesions and for patients who have no history of trauma but a history of predisposing habits such as tobacco or alcohol abuse associated with a positive family history, biopsy of the lesion should be performed. This approach is supported by extensive retrospective studies by Poswillo, Burkhardt, and Roodenburg in which approximately 10% of intraoral leukoplakias have to be considered premalignant entities.[2–4] The management of hyperkeratotic lesions that present with an obvious cause should be expectant observation. If the repeated trauma or the habit pattern of the patient is controlled, then the lesion should either disappear or shrink. Diminution of the lesion may reveal underlying intraepithelial changes that may warrant biopsy or excision. Any white lesion on the surface of the oral mucosa that cannot be scraped away, does not yield to protective measures by the patient, or is observed in a patient at risk because of long-term tobacco or alcohol abuse should be biopsied and managed according to histopathologic findings. For biopsy of a suspicious hyperkeratosis the method described in Chapter 5 is used (see Fig. 5–28). To excise smaller questionable lesions the

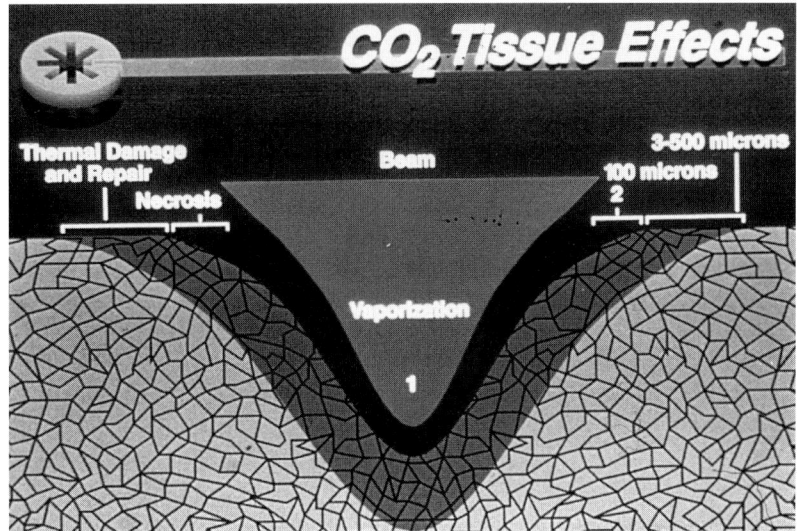

FIGURE 6–3. This is a typical injury profile when tissues such as mucous membrane and skin are lased by a free-beam carbon dioxide laser in a focused mode and using a 0.2-mm spot size. There is total vaporization at #1 in the diagram, from 0 to 50 to 100 microns in all directions, following a gaussian thermal distribution. At about 50 to 200 microns, there is a variable necrosis of tissue. At about 500 microns (#3 in the diagram), there is a reversible thermal tissue injury. (Courtesy of Coherent Laser, Palo Alto, California.)

carbon dioxide laser with a 0.2-mm spot size is applied perpendicular to the elliptical outline surrounding the lesion. The laser can be set at 10 to 20 W of power and the UltraPulse mode. A trough is made around the periphery of the lesion, recognizing that a margin of 50 to 200 microns will be distorted by the thermal effects of the beam. After the outline is created around the lesion, an edge or corner of the tissue can be lifted up by anodized tissue forceps and the underlying tissues thermodissected with the laser beam at a slight angle. The lesion can then be removed easily and sent for pathologic examination with a note to the pathologist on the method of dissection. The base of the lesion can be undermined and closed or left to heal by second intention.

SMOKELESS TOBACCO–INDUCED MUCOSAL WHITE LESIONS

A more insidious lesion that has become increasingly prevalent among young persons is the white patch caused by the use of smokeless tobacco. Interestingly, although women display an obvious lesion caused by smokeless tobacco approximately a decade later, they are more prone to have moderate to severe epithelial dysplasia than men. Epidemiologic, clinical, and in vitro studies have implicated smokeless tobacco in the potential development of oral malignancy. The reaction of the oral mucosa to this form of tobacco use can be related to the tobacco itself as well as to additives. Nitrosonornicotine, a known carcinogen, has been isolated from

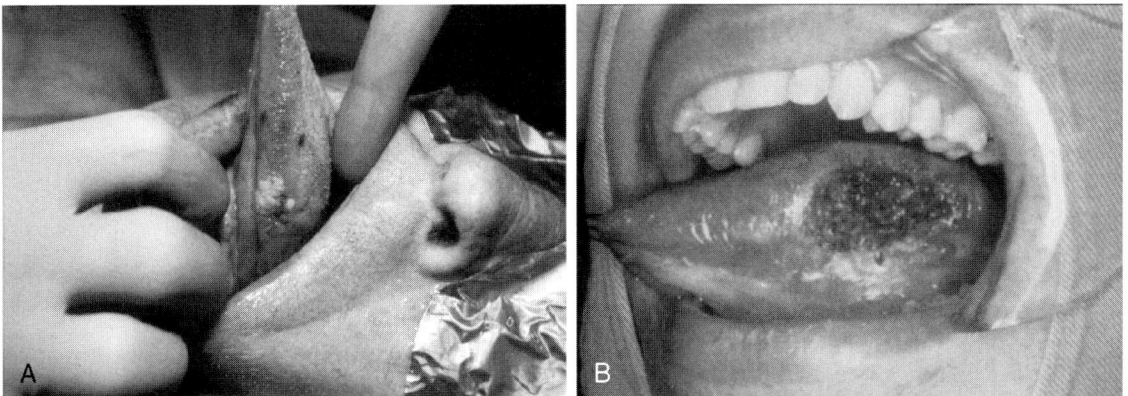

FIGURE 6–4. *A,* Typical lesion of focal hyperkeratosis. This patient had a habit of biting the tongue when under stress. Because there is no induration or any other risk factor, such as alcohol, tobacco, or hereditary history, it was elected to vaporize the lesion to eliminate any defect that would have occurred if conventional modalities were used. *B,* An example of a vaporized keratotic lesion of the lateral border of the tongue immediately after lasing. Note excellent hemostasis and carbonaceous surface.

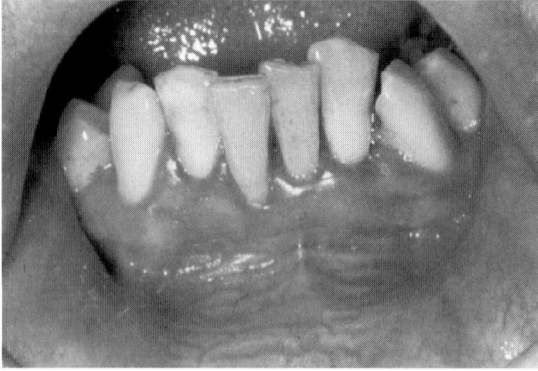

FIGURE 6–5. Clinical appearance of usual site for the intraoral use of snuff in the anterior mucolabial fold. Note the white color of the lesion with a typical folding of the surface. See text for treatment.

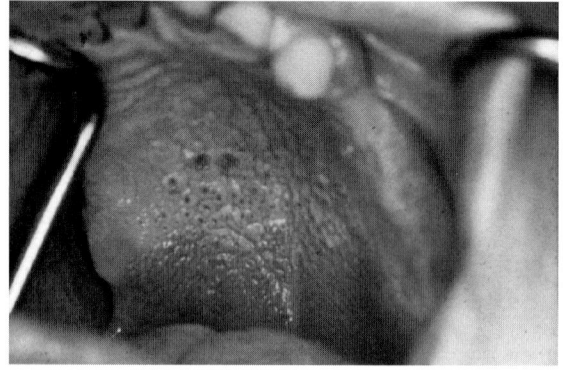

FIGURE 6–7. The usual appearance of nicotinic stomatitis of the palate. Note the random red dots surrounded by the elevated halo of white keratin.

chewing tobacco and snuff. Extracts of smokeless tobacco appear to inhibit DNA synthesis in lympho-kine-activated killer lymphocyte activity, which may be related to mucosal carcinogenesis.

The lesions of smokeless tobacco are usually accessible to the laser, occurring in the mucolabial or mucobuccal fold of the mandible (Figs. 6–5 and 6–6). A period of abstinence is usually all that is needed to produce disappearance of the lesion in several weeks. Those that persist after close observation should be biopsied, especially those lesions that exhibit an erythroplakic surface or develop frank ulceration. In these cases, a small punch biopsy can be used to take specimens of suspicious areas for frozen section examination. If a significant dysplastic change is seen, the lesion can be excised with the laser in a focused mode. The specimen can be oriented and mounted on a piece of cork. The margins can then be examined more precisely by the pathologist.

NICOTINIC STOMATITIS

Nicotinic stomatitis is a form of keratosis that is associated with pipe and cigar smoking, although more severe forms have been seen in countries that have a tradition of reverse smoking in which the lit end of the cigarette is placed in the mouth (Figs. 6–7 to 6–9). Over time, there is gradual formation of an erythematous reaction and, eventually, increased keratinization. The lesion appears as a random collection of red dots surrounded by an elevated halo of white keratin. The red appearance of the lesion is apparently due to an inflammatory reaction of the ductal systems of the palatal minor salivary glands, which may exhibit various stages of obstruction. In most cases of nicotinic stomatitis, the prognosis is excellent, except in persons who engage in reverse smoking, which is more likely to produce malignant change of the palatal mucosa.

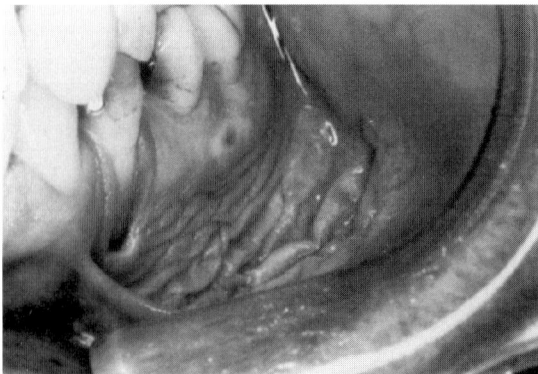

FIGURE 6–6. The usual site for the use of chewing tobacco as opposed to snuff, although snuff is also used less frequently at this site. Note color and folding of surface.

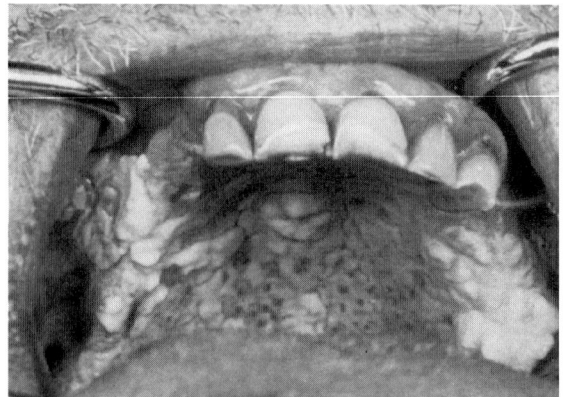

FIGURE 6–8. The appearance of nicotinic stomatitis of long duration. Note the frank leukoplakic plaques with involvement of the crestal alveolar tissues and extension into the mucobuccal vestibule. This lesion proved to have areas of dysplasia on punch biopsy and, therefore, was both vaporized and in some suspicious areas excised down to the submucosal tissues.

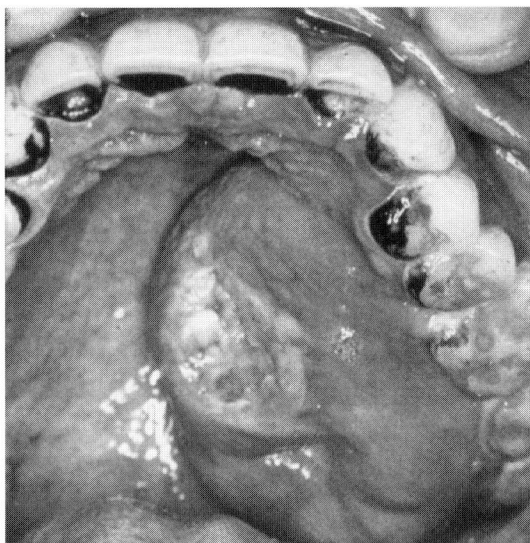

FIGURE 6–9. The appearance of an extensive squamous cell carcinoma of the palate that began as typical nicotinic stomatitis but became markedly aggressive in a patient who engaged in so-called reverse smoking (see text). Because the lesion is well beyond a T1 classification, a combination of conventional surgery involving a hemimaxillectomy and use of a carbon dioxide laser (free beam) in an adjunctive role can be used to manage this entity.

Because the general prognosis for the lesion is good, an attempt at nonsurgical care should be made, especially placing the patient in a smoking reduction or elimination program. The lesion itself should alert the surgeon to explore the patient for other potential sites of carcinogenesis, such as the lungs.

If the patient has symptoms of pain, burning, and ulceration of the palatal tissues, the surgeon may elect to eradicate the lesion using a laser. Surface lesions such as nicotinic stomatitis are usually vaporized after multiple strategic punch biopsy specimens have been taken. The carbon dioxide laser can be set in a continuous-wave mode and defocused using 10 to 20 W of power. Vaporization is achieved by holding the laser handpiece perpendicular to the palatal surface and lasing the length of the longitudinal axis of the lesion and then positioning the beam at right angles to the original strokes and crosshatching the length of the lesion. In most instances, the lesion is wiped with a saline- or hydrogen peroxide–moistened sponge to remove the lased surface to reveal any nonlased surfaces. In finishing the lasing process, the surgeon may leave the carbonaceous final surface layer undisturbed to act as a barrier to protect the underlying healing surface. This can be followed by a prefabricated palatal splint to enable the patient to protect the lased surfaces during eating and drinking. The Nd:YAG contact round surgical probe can be used

in a similar fashion to the carbon dioxide laser by placing the probe against the surface and lasing with 15 to 25 W of power. The probe tip is stroked across the lesion slowly, attempting to avoid adherence of the probe to the tissue surface. Power to the contact tip is controlled by turning off power to the tip while the probe remains in contact with the target tissue. Keeping the power on after having removed the tip from the target tissue could deform the probe tip owing to the development of excess heat in air.

SOLAR CHEILITIS

Solar or actinic cheilitis represents an important premalignant lesion affecting the vermilion portion of the lips and almost exclusively the lower lip. The lesion occurs secondary to regular and prolonged exposure to sunlight and is seen preferentially among whites with fair skin. Exposure to wavelengths of light in the range of 290 to 320 nm is responsible for this lesion, among other degenerative dermatologic lesions caused by infrared radiation. The lesion has been shown chemically and ultrastructurally to be composed of subepithelial deposits of elastin rather than collagen, as was previously thought.

Prolonged exposure of the lips to sunlight causes the vermilion to assume an atrophic, pale to silvery gray, glossy character with inconsistent appearing fissuring and wrinkling at right angles to the mucocutaneous interface. This latter interface can appear to be irregular or missing and the vermilion variably coated by epithelium. There can also be scaling, cracking, and ulceration with eschar formation of the vermilion (Fig. 6–10). Importantly, if the lesion is neglected and evolves into a squamous cell carcinoma, it metastasizes into the regional lymph nodes in about 11% of cases, whereas actinically induced malignancies on other skin surfaces metastasize in fewer than 1% of cases (Fig. 6–11). Multiple modalities, including chemical peeling with 50% trichloroacetic acid, fluorouracil treatment, electrosurgery, cryosurgery, and lip shave with a scalpel have been compared longitudinally with laser management. Laser control has been found to be equal to or better than other management vehicles while offering its own inherent advantages. Using the carbon dioxide laser under microscopic control appears to allow for removal of defined areas of the lip at greater depth. The use of the laser, as compared with other surgical maneuvers, is not associated with postoperative neuropathies, excessive cicatrix formation, hematomas, and lip distortions or esthetic compromise. Laser ablation, of course, does not result in a specimen for pathologic analysis, but studies have yielded no clinically evident neoplastic

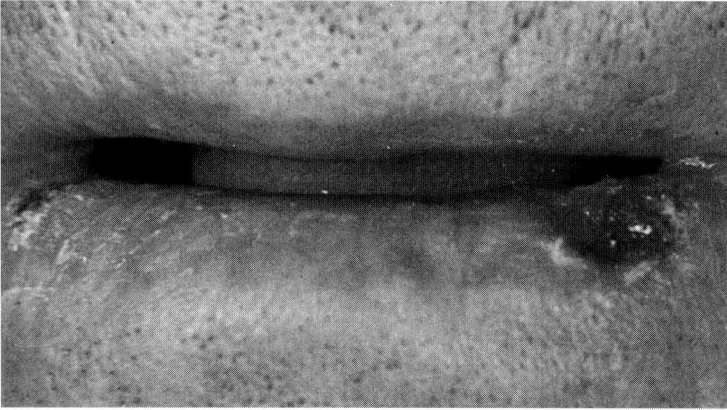

FIGURE 6–10. The typical appearance of actinic-induced cheilitis. The vermilion surface of the lower lip assumes a pale, atrophic, silvery gray, glossy nature with fissuring and wrinkling perpendicular to the mucocutaneous junction. In this case, there is cracking, eschar formation, and on the left side, ulceration. This latter finding makes the lesion more worrisome and a biopsy at the site of the ulcer formation is important.

alterations at the surgical site for as long as 4 years after use of the laser.

The lip lesion can be laser ablated by a simple technique used even in an office setting. The vulnerable areas of contiguous facial skin and eyes are protected by moist drapes and towels and eye shields, and the teeth are shielded by moist gauze and/or preformed splints. Bilateral mental nerve blocks with local anesthetic solution are used, followed by injection of sterile saline into the submucosal tissues to stretch the mucous membrane. The carbon dioxide laser can be set at a focused spot size using a power setting of 5 W. UltraPulse mode with the Coherent laser is ideal to outline the lesion by passing between the vermilion and the hair-bearing skin of the anterior lip surface, extending the laser trench transversely to the commissures and posteriorly toward the labial vestibule, including at least 2 to 3 mm of normal-looking mucosa within the target tissue. Following the outlining procedure,

the laser is held more than one focal length above the tissue at 4 to 6 cm, and a crosshatching pattern is produced with the laser beam in this defocused mode. Depending on spot size and power (in watts), 200 to 250 joules of irradiance is used. As in dealing with other surface lesions of the oral cavity, the carbonized surface tissue is removed layer by layer using a moistened gauze sponge after the target tissue surface area is completely lased. Following lasing, the lased surface is coated with antibiotic ointment, and a nonadherent pad is taped to the surface. Patients are instructed to cleanse the lip with sterile saline and to reapply the antibiotic ointment. Reepithelialization is complete in 14 to 30 days. After reepithelialization, the lip can be protected when at risk in sunlight by a lip balm containing the sunscreen agent para-aminobenzoic acid (PABA). Sun-blocking opaque creams supplement the action of the balm; one such is Ti-silk (Humatech Corporation, Boca Raton, Fla). It is important to arrange for periodic follow-up appointments with the patient because of the observation that an invasive carcinoma can occur after a latent period of as long as 20 to 30 years.

PRECANCEROUS MUCOSAL LESIONS (DIFFUSE)

When a hyperkeratotic-looking lesion of the mucous membrane exhibits histopathologic findings of various degrees of cellular atypia on biopsy, it is no longer considered causally as a frictional type of hyperkeratosis but is a lesion that could easily be a precursor to oral malignancy. One of the most common lesions in this category is oral leukoplakia, which is simply a white patch of the oral mucosa not removable by scraping. True leukoplakia (removing the term from its Greek roots and assigning a histopathologic meaning) is diagnosed in lesions containing hyperorthokeratosis, parakeratosis, and/or acanthosis. An important part of the definition of

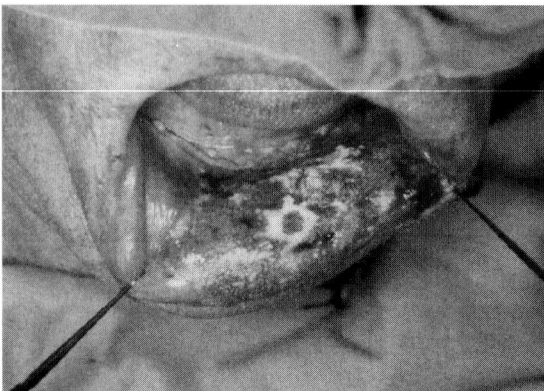

FIGURE 6–11. The appearance of neglected solar cheilitis. Keratinization of the surface is prominent and there are multiple areas of dysplastic change. A more aggressive approach using the laser is warranted; such as lasing the submucosal tissues after strategic biopsies in this area. Note the partial epidermization of the lip and the extension of the lesion into the mucolabial fold.

leukoplakia is the description of varying degrees of dysplasia or atypia—none, mild, moderate, or severe. An important characteristic of potentially malignant lesions that may antedate or accompany such changes is the appearance of erythroplakia, or red stippled surfaces on the lesions. Moderate to severe dysplasia is a predictor of a more dangerous or aggressive course, characteristically seen in patients who have a history of alcohol or tobacco abuse.

Location of the lesion within the oral cavity (e.g., floor of mouth [sublingual keratosis] and lateral tongue) may be an indicator of the likelihood of future malignant transformation (Fig. 6–12*A* and *B*). The anatomic site may dictate to the surgeon the choice of extirpation (i.e., excision or vaporization). To sum up, mucosal leukoplakia is a surface lesion; that is, it exists within the epithelium superficial to the basement membrane. Removal of the lesion with a carbon dioxide laser down to the basement membrane encourages regeneration of new, healthy epithelium.

Leukoplakia must be considered premalignant or malignant until a final pathology report is filed. The surgeon can get an idea of the potential activity of a lesion by staining it with a vital stain such as toluidine blue. Concentration of the stain in one or more areas of the lesion is indicative of significant DNA activity or cell division and therefore points the way to management. If a given lesion is discrete or small (within the range of 2 to 3 cm), excisional biopsy can be performed. For larger, more diffuse lesions one may take multiple small specimens, especially in areas of the oral cavity deemed at risk for malignant transformation. Small, discrete lesions can be removed with a focused carbon dioxide laser with a 3- to 4-mm margin. For diffuse lesions it is important to maintain good control

of lesional tissue, and distortion is prevented by mounting and orienting with descriptive sutures. In this latter instance, once the nature or aggressiveness of the lesion is known, definitive laser treatment can be instituted.

The decision of the surgeon to excise or vaporize a given lesion is often based on personal preference. The epithelial surfaces of the oral cavity vary in texture and thickness—and, therefore, in vulnerability to laser vaporization. Thickened, hyperkeratotic lesions contain little water and are therefore more resistant to laser vaporization. These lesions, depending on their character and anatomic location, can be excised along with a variable quantity of underlying connective tissue, especially in very suspicious lesions. The elimination of this deeper layer may decrease the probability of recurrence. Studies on the role of the subjacent connective tissue in oral squamous cell premalignancy and malignancy have shown that the subepithelial tissues may play a role in the induction of these lesions. It is apparent that in such instances vaporization could be too superficial and fail to ablate the deeper layers, resulting in recurrence of the lesion. In specific isolated lesions, especially erythroplakia, excision rather than vaporization may be indicated when the histopathology is unknown. In view of the higher statistical probability of malignant transformation in erythroplakia to T1 squamous cell carcinoma, the surgeon should perform laser excision.

Diffuse lesions are difficult to manage by excision and can result in severe disability (Fig. 6–13*A* to *E*). In such diffuse lesions, the carbon dioxide laser can be used in a defocused mode at 15 to 20 W of power using a cross-hatch method. The significant downside of vaporization is the inability to generate a specimen for the pathologist so the histology of the undersurface of the lesion cannot

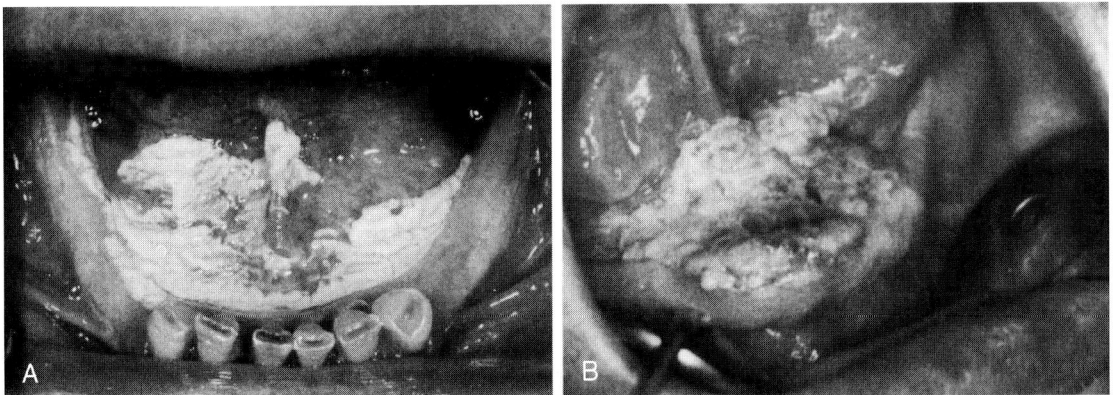

FIGURE 6–12. *A*, A typical worrisome sublingual keratosis. This lesion has a higher incidence of malignant transformation than keratotic lesions at other oral sites with the exception of the lateral tongue. *B*, A significant keratotic lesion of the lateral tongue that revealed induration on palpation but proved to be dysplastic rather than frankly malignant. The lesion was managed by an excisional laser procedure rather than a vaporization technique.

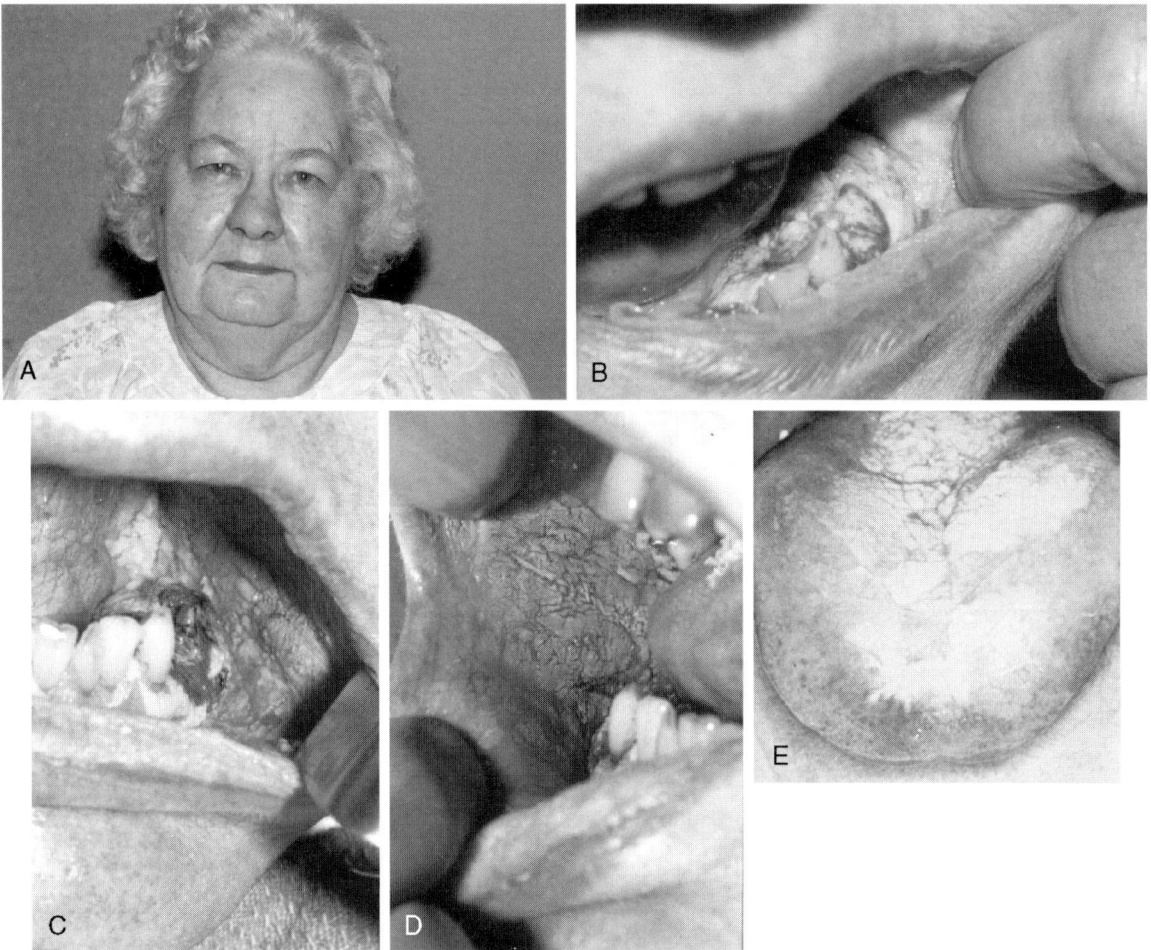

FIGURE 6–13. *A*, A 72-year-old schoolteacher with significant cigarette habit (two to three packs per day). The teacher would spend hours correcting papers while continuously chain smoking. The apparent result was a panoral diffuse leukoplakia involving *B*, the retromolar, parapharyngeal, and sublingual surfaces; *C*, the left buccal mucosa; *D*, the right buccal mucosa; *E*, the dorsal tongue surface.

be determined. The advantage of vaporization is the resulting dry superficial wound, which is covered by a carbonaceous surface layer. The advantages of a carbonized surface layer are the subject of controversy. In some instances, which appear to be dependent on the specific anatomic location in the mouth, the contiguous normal tissue reacts to this layer of carbonaceous—now foreign—matter. The result can be the development of exuberant granulation or polypoid tissue, often associated with tongue lesions, which may obscure recurrence or the appearance of a new lesion. In both excisional and vaporizational techniques, no suturing is necessary. The patient is not administered antibiotics except in some instances when intravenous antibiotics are given just before the laser procedure. The patient is instructed in the use of over-the-counter or prescription analgesics, depending on the extent of the surgery. Oral hygiene is also assisted by the use of

chlorhexidine mouth rinses. For patients whose large, diffuse lesions involving a significant surface area of oral mucosa are vaporized, the author recommends the use of proteolytic enzymes, which can be compounded conveniently by competent pharmacists. These enzymes are effective locally by using an intraoral troche. Impressive elimination of necrotic lased tissue and cellular debris plus enhancement of healing will be noted by the laser surgeon and appreciated by the patient.

Those leukoplakic lesions that appear benign and are comparatively inaccessible can be managed by use of the microscope with a coaxial laser and micromanipulator (Fig. 6–14). More suspicious lesions, such as erythroplakias, can easily be excised using the microscopic technique following the use of vital staining with toluidine blue. Excisional techniques are usually coupled with an attempt to include a portion of the underlying lamina propria,

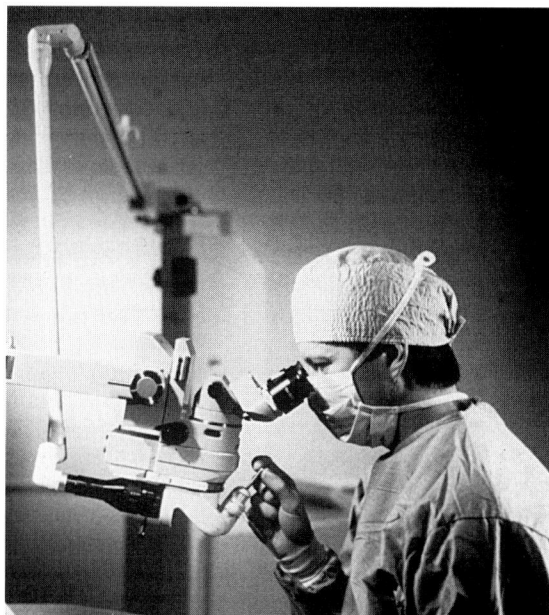

FIGURE 6–14. Use of the carbon dioxide free-beam laser coupled with a microscope and micromanipulator. This set-up enhances access to oral lesions and promotes precision while lasing. A coaxial helium-neon (HeNe) laser may be built into the microscopic system, further enhancing lasing of target tissue, resulting in only marginal nontarget tissue damage. (Courtesy of Coherent Laser, Palo Alto, California.)

consistent with the observation that subepithelial tissues may be critical in the primary or recurrent induction of these lesions. The choice of the laser for the surgical management of erythroplakias and T1 carcinomas is as oncologically appropriate as other surgical approaches. Given that the laser offers local and regional management advantages, its ability to alter the comparatively strong tendency of the T1 lesion to metastasize has not been confirmed.

ERYTHROPLAKIA

Erythroplakia should be reviewed separately because of its greater proclivity to exhibit cellular changes that can lead to true malignancy (Fig. 6–15). The lesion may occur de novo or evolve naturally from one of the premalignant leukoplakias. The term *erythroplakia* has Greek roots and simply refers to a red-looking patch on the surface of the oral mucosa. In many instances, the lesion is a white patch with speckles of red on the surface. In the author's experience, these lesions are more apt to be aggressive. In view of its potential behavior, it is accepted that the lesion has a common origin with squamous cell carcinoma. Thus, the generally accepted factors and cofactors that presumably result in malignant change (i.e., chronic mucosal mi-

crotrauma, alcohol, tobacco, altered nutrition) are associated with the appearance of erythroplakia.

Erythroplakia is much less common than other similar surface lesions with a patchy, white distribution. Generally, the lesion is more worrisome than other intraoral surface keratoses, owing to its potential. In most instances, rather than having margins that disappear into normal-looking mucosa, the lesion of erythroplakia possesses a well-circumscribed margin. Erythroplakia may be seen at any intraoral anatomic site but favors the floor of the mouth and retromolar regions. Middle-aged men or women are equally affected, and lesions are commonly diagnosed between age 50 and 70 years. On clinical examination, palpation reveals a velvety, supple surface in early lesions with induration in late or infiltrative varieties. The lesion can be biopsied as discussed earlier (see Chapter 5) for histopathologic diagnosis. Importantly, on microscopy, the lesion reveals at least severe dyplasia in 90% of cases. It is also observed that 50% are invasive squamous cell carcinomas, 40% of which possess severe dysplastic alteration or carcinoma in situ. The color of the surface of erythroplakia is due to the decreased production of keratin by the keratinocytes and enhanced vascularity.

Erythroplakia is managed by surgical excision and can easily be removed by the carbon dioxide laser. The laser is set on UltraPulse at 10 to 20 W in a pulsed mode to outline the entire lesion. A so-called laser moat is then created by using the laser in a focused mode with a continuous beam. It is important to excise the lesion widely rather than necessarily deeply, because of the superficial nature of dysplastic and in situ lesions. Equally important

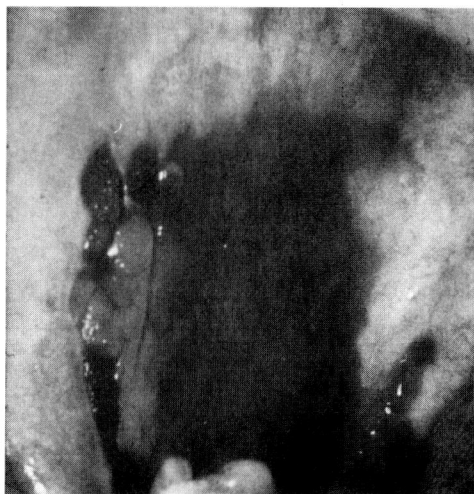

FIGURE 6–15. The lesion of erythroplakia in the buccal mucosa. In contrast to white nonspeckled leukoplakias, the lesion is characterized by a definitive border or margin rather than a diffuse blurred margin seen in other similar surface lesions.

is the realization on the part of the laser surgeon that the changes appearing in the epithelial layer may involve the deeper minor salivary gland excretory ducts in the lesional area. Therefore, the upper portion of the lamina propria should be included in the specimen and multiple deep biopsy samples of the submucosal tissues should be taken to rule out infiltration. The oral pathologist should be asked to perform multiple serial microscopic sections to seek possible salivary duct changes.

KERATOACANTHOMA

Although the lesion of keratoacanthoma rarely appears on the surface of the oral mucosa, it does occur on sun-exposed facial skin and can be detected at the mucocutaneous junction of the lip. Skin lesions are seen to arise from the pilosebaceous system, and intraoral lesions may originate from ectopic sebaceous glands often seen within the buccal mucosa (Fordyce's granules). Multiple causes beside sunlight have been implicated in the development of keratoacanthoma—trauma, carcinogenic compounds, viruses, autoimmune mechanisms. No one factor is regarded as the sole cause. The lesion is seen by oral and maxillofacial surgeons when it appears on the face, vermilion border of the lip, and rarely, inside the mouth. A small erythematous macule will appear that soon evolves into a firm papule. The papule or nodule rapidly becomes larger over a period of weeks and contains a central core of keratin surrounded by a peripheral border of skin or mucous membrane. The course of the lesion is spontaneous regression without treatment; however, this regression can result in a shallow depression in the skin or mucocutaneous junction when the keratin mass is exfoliated. This phenomenon is associated with surrounding cicatrix formation, which may be comparatively disfiguring, especially on the lip.

The lesion is significant in its clinical course, which may leave a residual cosmetic defect, but, more importantly, it has a histopathologic similarity to a well-differentiated squamous cell carcinoma. Through a definitive set of histopathologic criteria, the oral pathologist is able to differentiate between the keratoacanthoma and the malignant markers of squamous cell carcinoma; however, a final diagnosis of keratoacanthoma is difficult to make on the basis of microscopic changes alone, so careful follow-up should be made on a regular basis. If there is any doubt, the lesion should be excised; this is accomplished with limited scarring with the carbon dioxide laser. The author approaches the lesion from the mucosal surface in cases of lip lesions, and a modified shield excision is performed. This is accomplished by setting the laser at 15 to 20 W

with a pulsed mode using UltraPulse to outline the lesion; then, with protection of the surrounding skin and mucosa and using the laser with the beam perpendicular to the margin of the lesion, a full-thickness wedge is removed. The resection can be conservative, because there appears to be no appreciable tendency of the lesion for lateral spread. In this instance, the defect can be closed with appropriate sutures, with careful attention to aligning the vermilion margins.

VERRUCOUS CARCINOMA

Verrucous carcinoma is included here as a distinctive mucosal surface lesion and because of its excellent prognosis in view of its high degree of differentiation and rarity of distant metastatic spread. Moreover, its troublesome local recurrence may make it an excellent lesion to manage by using laser technology because the inherent advantages of laser surgery and the enhanced ability of the patient to tolerate multiple laser operations than of a similar number of procedures using conventional instrumentation (Fig. 6–16*A* to *D*).

Intraoral verrucous carcinoma is usually associated with the use of tobacco in all forms, but in the author's experience chewing tobacco and snuff appear often to be involved. There is also speculation that human papillomavirus (HPV) may be either an initiating or a secondary factor or a cofactor. Apparently, HPV DNA in neoplastic cells and in situ DNA hybridization lend support for this viral etiologic hypothesis. Verrucous carcinoma must be differentiated from several other entities, the most important of which is papillary squamous carcinoma, which has a similar clinical appearance but proliferates more rapidly and is characterized by a much more infiltrative nature. Histopathologically, the typical lesion of verrucous carcinoma exhibits no cellular atypia and, overall, a benign microscopic appearance. This is rather misleading, and the lesion may recur repeatedly so the risk of disabling function or disfigurement is significant. Therefore, early diagnosis is critical, as is excision of the lesion in toto with an acceptable margin and resection of underlying submucosal tissue.

In general, verrucous carcinoma usually presents as an exophytic lesion and can be readily resected with the carbon dioxide laser or the Nd:YAG contact laser using an excisional technique, especially including the base of the lesion. It is easy to have an inappropriately lower index of suspicion in view of past reports in which the approach was to obtain multiple biopsy specimens, many of which proved benign or contained moderate degrees of dysplasia. A current approach, especially in the management of sessile lesions, is to excise a wide margin around

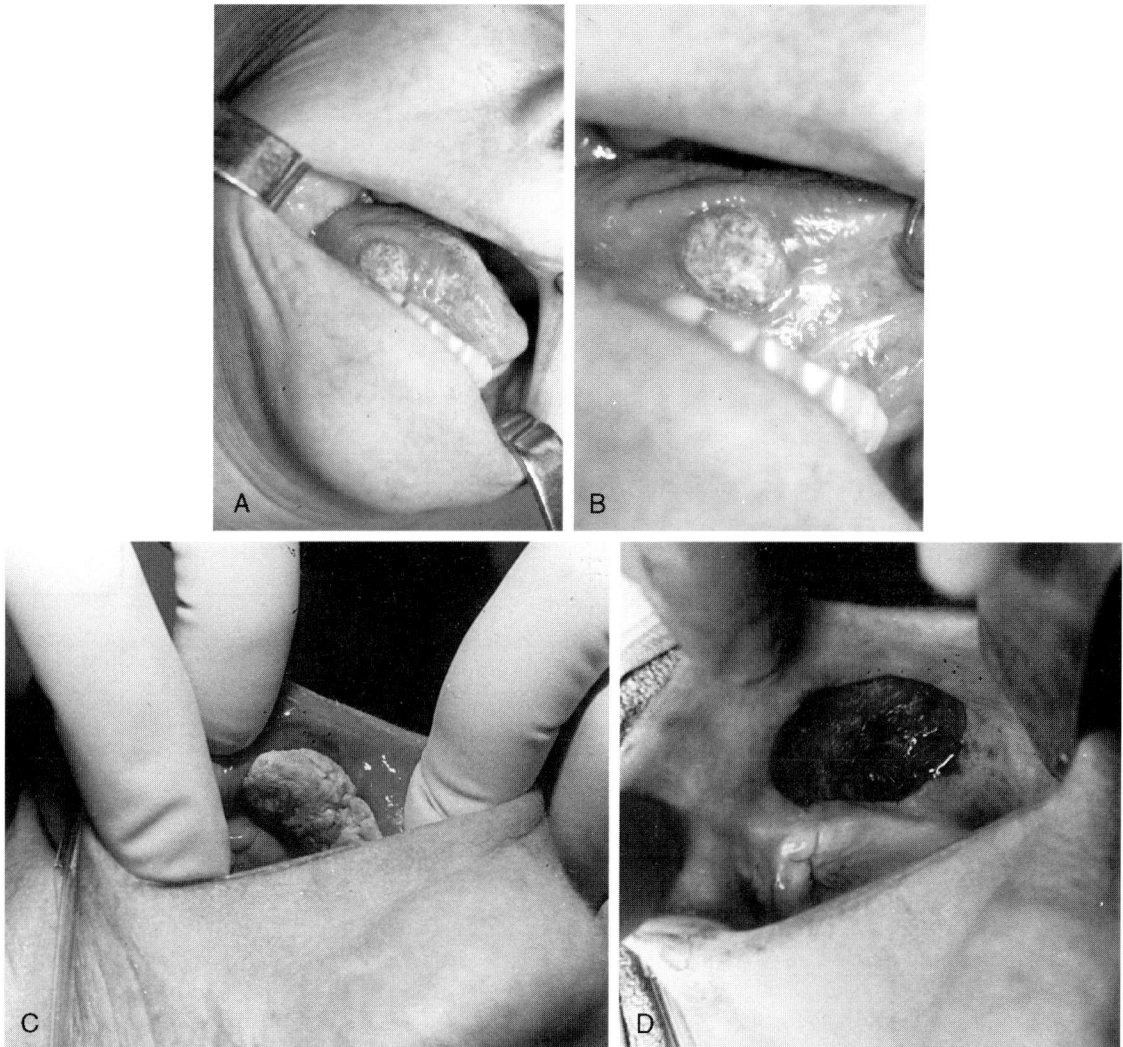

FIGURE 6–16. *A*, Verrucous carcinoma of the lateral border of tongue. The lesion is a sessile mass, which is readily amenable to laser excisional techniques. *B*, Close-up of lesion in *A* with the obvious appearance of villi or folds on the surface. This surface appearance, with the lack of induration, heralds the relatively less aggressive nature of this entity. *C*, Large verrucous carcinoma of the maxillary alveolar process and mucolabial and buccal fold. *D*, Appearance after laser excision in toto down to the submucosal tissues.

the lesion and include Mohs'-type frozen sections of the base of the tumor. The carbon dioxide laser can be used with the handpiece and a focal spot of 0.1 mm with 15 to 20 W of power and the laser on UltraPulse mode.

A wide range of cure rates have appeared in the literature for standard oral leukoplakia using traditional surgical techniques.[5, 6] Other observations using such methods as cryosurgery report a range between 75% and 87%.[7] The results of cryosurgical applications to leukoplakia that report lower cure rates could be related to a continuous etiologic variable or longer periods of observation. Lesions treated with cryosurgery occasionally exhibit recurrence at the margins of the areas exposed

to the cryoprobe.[8–10] Conventional, diathermic, and cryosurgical techniques to manage oral leukoplakia cause destruction of healthy nontarget tissue and the inevitable development of unwanted cicatrix formation; in contrast, especially with carbon dioxide laser energy, the precision of the beam and the vaporization of the target tissues decreases cicatrix formation.

Whether or not the laser holds long-term value in the control of oral leukoplakia remains to be investigated fully. A limited number of reports in the laser surgical literature furnish needed longitudinal studies. Horch and colleagues, however, reported a 78% cure rate using the carbon dioxide laser and handpiece.[11] These results could be attributed to the use of the laser integrated with the handpiece itself or to other related variables. It is well documented that the microscopically controlled carbon dioxide laser, at least in preliminary observations, appears to offer better control and precision and may eventually promise improved outcomes. Lasers used to *control* oral leukoplakia lesions are thus an increasingly useful method of *ablation*, especially for diffuse or so-called panoral lesions in which traditional surgical modalities could be disabling (Fig. 6–17; see also Color Plate 1). The laser advantages have been evident to the author: good hemostasis, precision, control of depth and extent of vaporization, limited damage to collateral tissue, and rapid, comparatively pain-free, and enhanced healing without unwanted cicatrization. Moreover, the surgeon can perform carefully controlled oral procedures in a dry field with appropriate double suction and smoke evacuation while the patient receives intravenous (conscious) sedation. This method virtually eliminates the potential life-threatening laser-associated problems when general endotracheal anesthesia is used (see Chapter 32). Finally, it is important to cite a report by Jones and colleagues, who reported a squamous cell carcinoma that developed in an area where leukoplakic lesions were treated with a carbon dioxide laser.[12] It was noted that an exophytic lesion arose within an area of lased leukoplakia. This mass was shown histopathologically to be a well-differentiated entity, but it did invade the submucosal tissues. The original lesion may already have evolved to a malignant one before lasing, so it is difficult to impugn the laser definitively. It does, however, point out the importance of strategic punch biopsy of suspicious diffuse lesions. Further, it could be speculated that the observation of the development of extensive, exophytic granulation tissue after lasing procedures involving the lateral border of the tongue should be thoroughly investigated histopathologically. Moreover, one could postulate that the laser may have a more specific photobiologic effect on epithelium or lamina propria in inducing proliferation of the keratinocytes, thus multiplying the statistical chances of dysplastic or malignant change, as not only does cell turnover accelerate but the nature of the basilar cellular DNA could also be altered in the generations of cells proceeding to the surface.

ORAL PAPILLOMATOSIS

Papillomatosis or palatal hyperplasia can appear white or colorless as a surface lesion, but it is usually associated with an inflammatory reaction and therefore appears erythematous (Fig. 6–18). Long-standing palatal lesions may undergo some atrophy and scarring, and therefore appear as pebbly white surface lesions as they age. The lesion is disproportionately common under removable prostheses; thus, a causal relationship has been posited by oral pathologists. It is thought that the fungal organism *Candida albicans* is a cofactor in the development of the lesion, in association with an ill-fitting prosthesis that gives rise to continued mucosal trauma.

Less worrisome lesions are commonly confined to the palatal vault. When the alveolar process or palatal incline is involved, especially when the lesion advances to cover the alveolar crest and migrates to the vestibule, the possibility of dysplastic alteration or premalignancy should be entertained. Usually, the lesion presents as multiple erythematous and edematous fine pedunculated projections (villi) that are seen to be closely aggregated, not

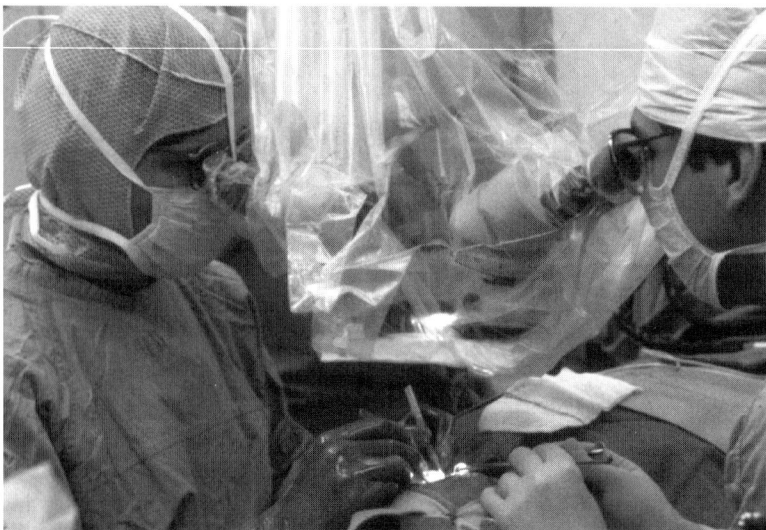

FIGURE 6–17. The use of the microscope with a built-in laser and coaxial soft target laser beam. In this instance, the surgeon and the assistant can see the operative field without distortion of the image for the assistant, thus enabling the assistant to be much more effective. Once again, as in the single-operator microscopes with coupled carbon dioxide lasers, the beam is controlled with the index finger of the operator. The area, direction, and sweep of the beam are controlled with the thumb and index finger of the surgeon. (See also Color Plate 1.) (Courtesy of Dr. Edward Halusic, Mount Pleasant, Pennsylvania.)

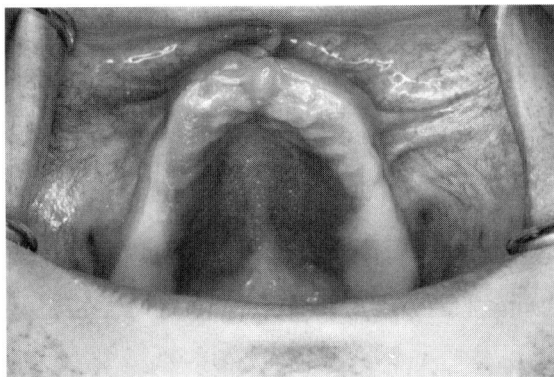

FIGURE 6–18. The typical appearance of palatal papillomatosis; the lesion is confined to the palatal vault and is caused by an ill-fitting prosthesis. When the papillomatous tissue appears or becomes atrophic and white, and involves more of the maxilla than the palatal vault, it may be an indication of a more aggressive underlying histopathologic appearance.

unlike a verrucous granuloma possessing a granular or pebbly surface. In some instances the erythema and villous characteristics are observed to be a tight aggregation of villi without their usual fiery red color. These cases may thus represent a form of pebbly leukoplakia that is more evident when extension over the alveolar ridge has occurred.

Oral papillomatosis, especially those lesions described that migrate to the vestibule, are managed well with carbon dioxide (both free-beam and waveguide units) and with contact Nd:YAG lasers. Sachs and Borden may have been the first surgeons to use the carbon dioxide laser to treat this entity, which was characterized by recurrence.[13] These authors used the operating microscope with the laser set at 30 W with 200-millisecond pulses and a 2-mm spot size to lase the lesion. Diffuse, benign- or premalignant-looking palatal papillomatosis can be vaporized by the carbon dioxide laser after selective punch biopsy specimens are taken. At present, the carbon dioxide laser with the handpiece is set at 10 to 20 W in a continuous-wave mode and applied in a defocused manner using a crosshatching maneuver to cover the area of the lesion. After each laser pass, the lased tissue residue is wiped off with a saline- or hydrogen peroxide–soaked sponge to enable the operator to assess the depth and overall results of the selected power density. The contact Nd:YAG laser using a round probe with the laser set at 15 to 25 W can also be used to eliminate the lesion by touching or stroking its surface in a similar continuous crosshatched manner without lifting the tip of the probe from the surface of the lesion. Using both lasers, the hemostasis is excellent, and if a larger vessel is encountered that is resistant to laser control, the diathermy unit can be used. Finally, a prefabricated palatal splint or the patient's

prosthesis can be relined with tissue conditioner and a collagen-thrombin material placed in it, if necessary, for persistent low–flow rate oozing.[14]

LICHEN PLANUS

Lichen planus is an unusually common mucosal surface lesion. Controversial evidence points to an immune-mediated mechanism. The target tissue of this purportedly autoimmune phenomenon is the basal keratocyte layer of the mucosal epithelium. It is thought that antigens within Langerhans cells and macrophages within the epithelial layer are processed intracellularly and this information is relayed to T lymphocytes; then, after a period of lymphocyte proliferation, T8 lymphocytes are in some manner rendered cytotoxic to the keratinocytes. Presumably, after antigenic interaction within the epithelium the T lymphocytes are attracted to the site by interleukin-1 (IL-1). IL-1 causes the T lymphocytes to produce IL-2, which stimulates proliferation of T cells. The proliferating lymphocytes produce interferon-gamma, which causes the basal cells to express class II histocompatibility antigens (HLA-DR) and increase their rate of differentiation, resulting in hyperkeratosis. It seems apparent that, if the basal cells are stimulated to produce HLA-DR antigen, the lymphocytes that usually express the HLA-DR antigen may contact the epithelial cells. A result of this contact is the inappropriate transfer of epithelial antigenic information. What follows is the formation of self-antigens, which may be processed as nonself, the basic phenomenon of an autoimmune reaction.

A variety of lichen planus lesions are expressed clinically. Most common is the reticular form, which is identified by multiple intersecting keratotic lines (Wickham's striae). Although the lesion can be found virtually anywhere on the oral mucosal surface, typically it is seen on the buccal mucosa. In erosive lichen planus, there are areas of ulceration, usually centrally located. This ulcer is always seen in various stages of healing, typically covered by a fibrinous coagulum. Patients do not complain of unusual pain from most of the manifestations of the disease; however, in the erosive form the patient does complain of pain, burning, thermal sensitivity, and sensitivity to spicy foods. The treatment of lichen planus generally has involved local—and in some cases systemic—steroids. Other agents have been preparations and drugs such as vitamin A analogues (retinoids), cyclosporine, dapsone (diaminodiphenylsulfone; for the erosive variety). Dapsone appears to assist in controlling the lymphocyte-specific process of the disease by modulating the release of cytokines for neutrophils or mast cells, which cause chemotaxis and inflammation.

More recently, one of the editors (G.A.C.) used a specially compounded slurry of misoprostol, which is essentially metabolized to prostaglandin F analogues and has antisecretory properties in the gastrointestinal tract and inhibits prostaglandin synthesis. It thus has been found to protect the mucosal surface during chronic anti-inflammatory drug therapy and, in the editor's opinion, provides a similar protective effect for the oral mucosal surface. Misoprostol is actually compounded by the pharmacist to a 0.0024% mouth rinse⁻ To make 100 ml of rinse, twelve 200-μg misoprostol tabs are pulverized and mixed in purified water (to 100 ml) containing 50 mg sodium saccharin, 200 mg potassium sorbate, 5 ml propylene glycol, 5 ml 95% alcohol, flavoring (creme de menthe), and 20 ml 1% methylcellulose gel.

Erosive lichen planus does not appear to be completely controlled by the laser, but it certainly appears to be palliated. The carbon dioxide laser should be used as adjunctive therapy along with selected local and systemic medications. Usually, the carbon dioxide laser, at a power setting of 10 to 15 W and using a continuous mode and a defocused application, is adequate to treat most lesions with the usual crosshatched lasing pattern. The contact Nd:YAG with a round probe using 10 to 15 W of power is also an alternative. What is seen is not a "cure" but a subjective report from patients of a reduction in burning sensations from the lesion and enhanced tolerance of spicy foods. Hong-Sai[15] reports an "improved" histopathologic appearance; with less intense features in the epithelium, rete pegs, and basilar layer, and decreased accumulation of round cell infiltrate in the subepithelial tissues.

CONDYLOMA ACUMINATUM

Condyloma acuminatum is recognized as an infectious process that, although ordinarily observed in the anogenital area, may also involve the oral mucosal surfaces (Fig. 6–19). This lesion has seen an increase in prevalence in human immunodeficiency virus (HIV)–infected patients and presumably is related to the immunocompromised state; thus, it is classified as an opportunistic infection. The lesion appears as a verrucous or papillary mass and is reported to have an etiology related to HPV subtypes 6 and 11. The natural histories of the subtypes of HPV are similar in the oral and genital mucous membranes. The lesion usually begins as a collection of pink nodules that increase in size and eventually coalesce. The lesion then appears as a sessile papillary mass, which may or may not be keratinized. The diagnosis of condyloma acuminatum is difficult because of its clinical similarity to multiple intraoral verrucae, which are essentially similar lesions. To differentiate more precisely, a good history of the patient's sexual activity and a good biopsy specimen that can rule out other entities are the initial measures. It may be necessary to perform in situ DNA hybridization studies to classify the lesions definitively. Condyloma acuminatum is treated by conventional and laser modalities. Depending on the patient's history and the possibility of underlying HIV infection, the patient might be encouraged to accept an HIV test and to follow through with multiple strategic punch biopsies. The carbon dioxide laser can be used in a free-beam system to excise intraoral lesions. This is accomplished by setting the laser on an excisional mode

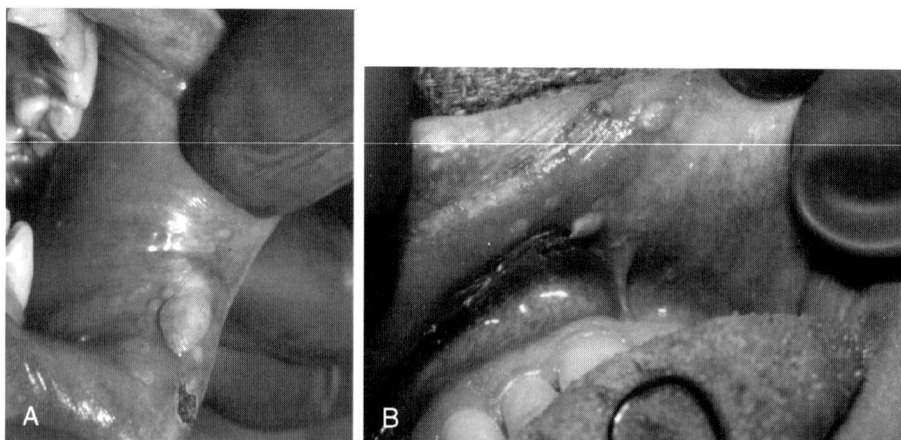

FIGURE 6–19. *A,* Condyloma acuminatum appearing at the commissure of the lip. The importance of this lesion is in the possibility of an undiagnosed human immunodeficiency virus (HIV) positivity and, thus, may represent an opportunistic infection. *B,* The same lesion as it appears early in diagnosis. Several smaller lesions will appear, followed by eventual coalescence. Laser vaporization is dangerous not only for possible infection of the surgeon with localized condylomata but also the threat of HIV infectivity. Therefore, it is mandatory that all operating room personnel, as well as housestaff and nurses, be protected with the knowledge of the HIV status of the patient.

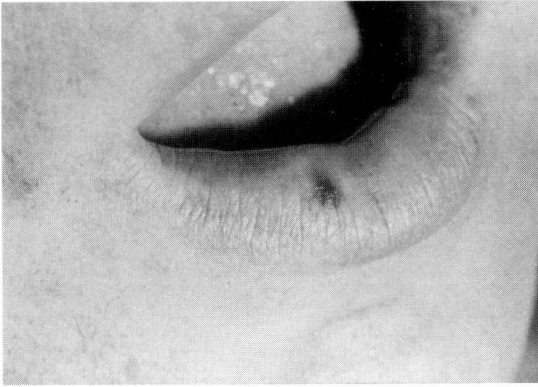

FIGURE 6–20. Oral melanotic macule appearing on the lower lip. Because there is no real way of differentiating these benign entities from more serious neoplastic melanotic lesions, an excisional laser biopsy is advised.

at 15 to 20 W UltraPulse and focusing the spot literally to excise the lesion with a 3- to 5-mm margin. The base of the lesion can be lased using the laser in a defocused mode. It is suggested that lesions in the circumoral region and within the margin of the vermilion border, be vaporized, if possible, to decrease disfiguring tissue loss. Diligent attention to smoke evacuation should accompany the lasing procedure, because condylomas can be contracted by the laser surgeon and the skin lesions can even appear around the surgical mask.

ORAL MELANOTIC MACULE

The term *oral melanotic macule* describes several entities that appear as oral mucosal surface pigmentations. These macules may refer to an intraoral freckle, an idiopathic pigmentation, pigmentation

that follows inflammation (as in lichen planus or after trauma or surgery), and the macular spots that are part of the systemic inherited or acquired entities of Peutz-Jeghers syndrome and Addison's disease, respectively. Although the lesions can occur anywhere on the oral mucosal surface, typically they are observed on the lip vermilion and gingiva (Fig. 6–20). There is no way to differentiate these lesions from other, more worrisome entities such as the early superficial melanomas. Therefore, they can be biopsied with the carbon dioxide laser using the mode for excisional biopsy described above. When extensive or numerous pigmented macules appear confined to the perioral region, one may consider laser resurfacing as a management tool if the cosmetic defect is unacceptable to the patient (Fig. 6–21A and B); however, there is little support in the literature for such a surgical maneuver, except for similar cases in which the laser has been used for resurfacing. At the very least, it is understood that there will be some recurrence, but in cases of extensive, unsightly lip mucosal macules one can control the laser device accurately, thus limiting radiant exposure. Moreover, the process is relatively benign and can be repeated with little expectation of extensive scarring.

CONCLUSION

As one can see, a host of intraoral surface lesions can be managed by using any one of several lasers (Fig. 6–22A to E). By and large, oral and maxillofacial laser surgeons have employed a limited number of these devices to treat mucosal surface lesions. Thus, in the specialty of oral and maxillofacial surgery the carbon dioxide laser has proved a predictable, reliable instrument that has offered repro-

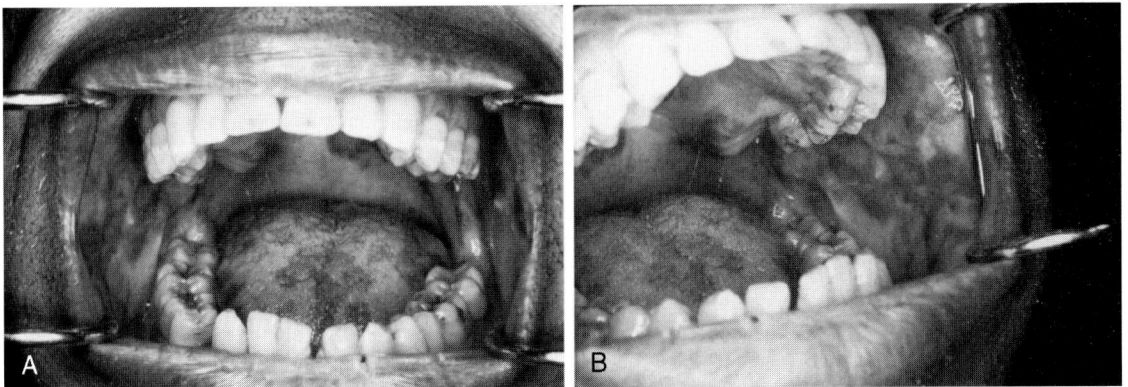

FIGURE 6–21. *A,* Benign multiple mucosal pigmented lesions, frontal view; *B,* appearance of the buccal mucosa. These areas of mucosa hyperpigmentation are entirely benign, and the patient may need to be reassured. In those cases in which there are multiple pigmentations appearing within the perioral or circumoral vermilion and skin, it may be of value to consider laser resurfacing methodologies if the patient complains of significant cosmetic disfigurement.

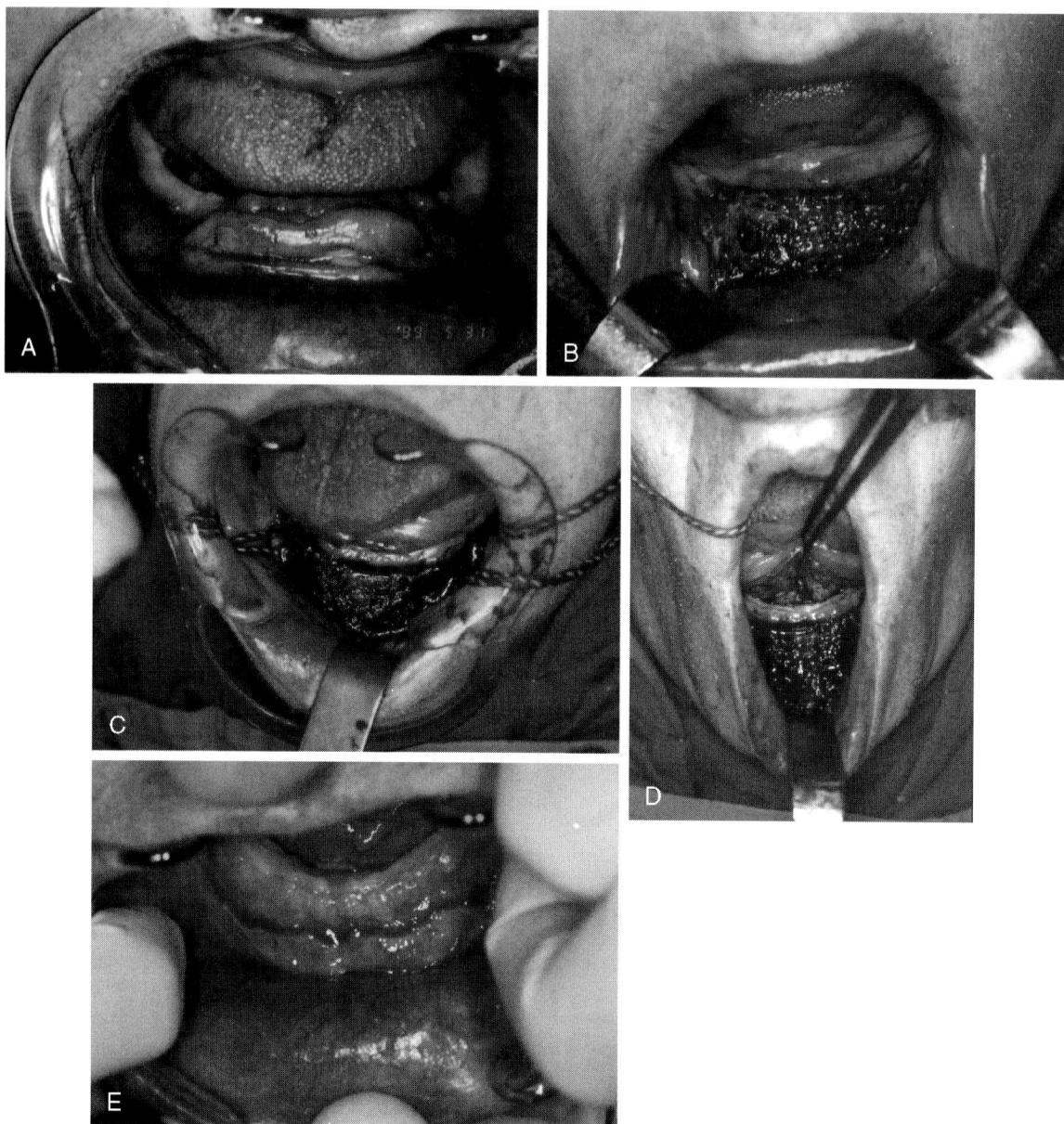

FIGURE 6–22. *A,* The appearance of moderate-sized granuloma fissuratum of the anterior mandible. *B,* After carbon dioxide vaporization of lesion; note charring. *C,* Laser dissection is complete, and the carbonized surface residua is left intact. *D,* View showing protection of mental nerves and the lingual laser mucosal dissection. *E,* Two weeks after lasing with fibrin coagulum still present. Note: Use of a surgical stent or splint is advisable, as in split-thickness skin or mucosal grafting. One can consider grafting, especially using the nonchar technique or device. (Courtesy of Coherent Laser, Palo Alto, California.)

ducible results for the tasks for which it has been chosen. Power outputs for most maxillofacial procedures have been more than adequate, and there has been a movement toward smaller sealed lasers used in office settings. The technologies of pulsing and auto-repeat functions will improve the capability of the carbon dioxide laser to cut and vaporize with a charless field. Controlled power output, pulsing characteristics, and variability of spot size will con-

tinue to make the carbon dioxide laser an important part of the armamentarium of the oral and maxillofacial surgeon. In recent years, the development of waveguides or flexible fibers to deliver the 10.6-micron wavelengths of the carbon dioxide laser has broadened the scope of use of this device to the arena of endoscopy (e.g., sinus surgery), albeit along shorter distances than smaller-wavelength lasers (Fig. 6–23).

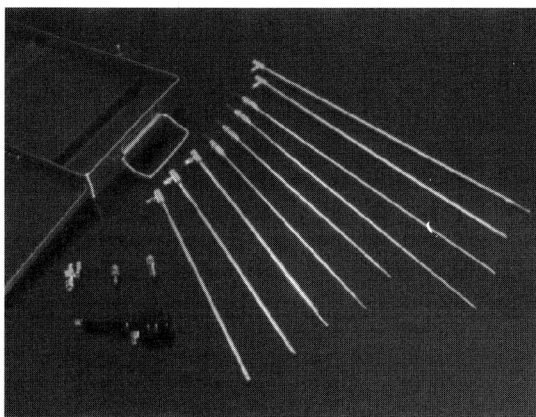

FIGURE 6–23. Carbon dioxide laser infraguides (waveguides). (Courtesy Coherent Laser, Palo Alto, California.) (See Chapter 7 for examples of newer waveguides.)

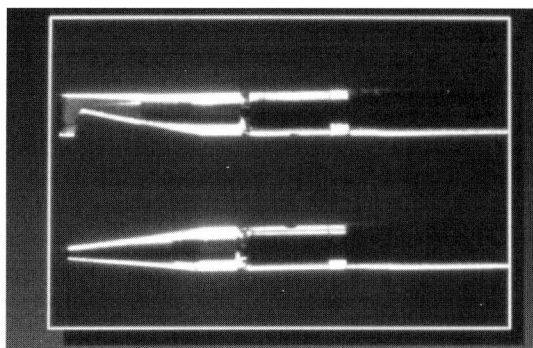

FIGURE 6–24. Example of specialized contact laser probe, an adhesiolysis probe. (Courtesy of Surgical Laser Technologies, Oaks, Pennsylvania.)

The Nd:YAG free-beam laser appears not to be recommended for most intraoral surface conditions, but its advantages in the treatment of deeper or more extensive angiodysplasias are apparent. Its promise in oral and maxillofacial surgery is through its application with sapphire and diamond contact probes mounted on the distal end of quartz fibers conducting Nd:YAG radiant energy and via the newer concepts of the Wavelength Conversion Effect (Surgical Laser Technologies, Oaks, Pa.; see Chapter 4). Used in the contact manner, the total output power required of the Nd:YAG is less, usually between 5 and 20 W, in contrast to powers of 40 to 70 W employed with the exposed fiber. The contact probe enjoys excellent thermal and mechanical properties and is available in a number of shapes and sizes with newer probes shaped for evermore specialized services (e.g., adhesiolysis

probe, Surgical Laser Technologies, Oaks, Pa.; Fig. 6–24). There is a rapid drop-off of irradiance from the contact probe, owing to its containment of radiant energy at its tip and the inherent high refractive index of the sapphire; therefore, there is less inadvertent tissue penetration and less collateral damage. In contrast, the depth of penetration of the bare quartz fiber or free beam is not as controlled, and the exposed fiber is rapidly degraded by contact with tissue. Contact laser technology thus appears to offer some advantages for oral and maxillofacial surgery for the forseeable future, when a clearly defined goal is formulated by the surgeon. For example, when the surgeon requires a significant degree of hemostasis, as in dealing with highly vascular lesions (Fig. 6–25). The use of Nd:YAG and carbon dioxide laser energy during the same operation has led to the development of laser equipment that combines the two laser types.

The importance of the use of radiant energy for biopsy and vaporization of extensive, diffuse, in-

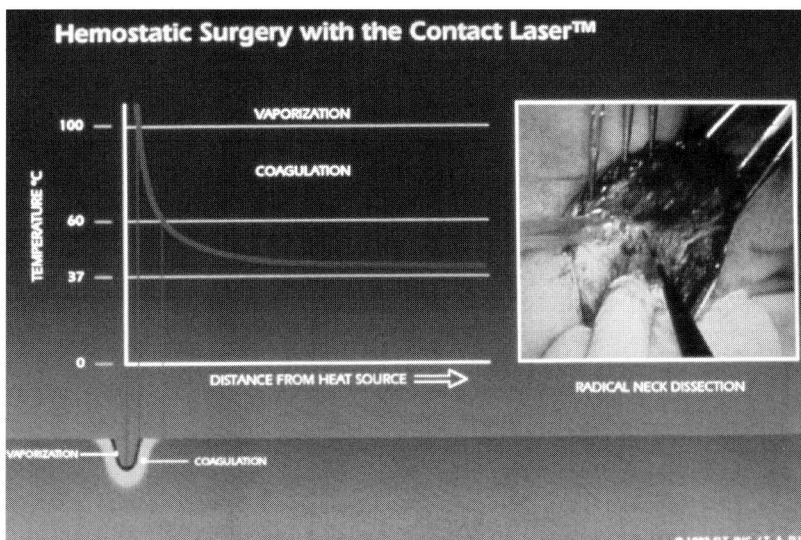

FIGURE 6–25. The use of the contact laser system to affect significant hemostasis. The temperature is plotted against the distance from the heat source with resultant vaporization and coagulation. (Courtesy of Surgical Laser Technologies, Oaks, Pennsylvania.)

traoral surface lesions lies in the incomparable speed, efficacy, and overall tolerability compared with other surgical modalities. The mucosa of almost the entire oral cavity can be vaporized without significant patient morbidity or major consequences in feeding and hydration when the patient is discharged from the hospital.

REFERENCES

1. Regezi JA, Sciubba J: Oral Pathology, Clinical-Pathologic Correlations, 2nd ed. Philadelphia, WB Saunders, 1993.
2. Poswillo DE: Electrosurgery and cryosurgery. *In*: Cohen B, Kramer IRH (eds): Scientific Foundations of Dentistry. London, Heinemann Medical, 1976.
3. Burkhardt A: Der Mundhoblenkrep und seine Vorstadien. Stuttgart, Fischer, 1980.
4. Roodenburg JLN, Vernez A: Die Behandlung der oberflechlich liegenden Abwerchungen der oralen Mukosa mit dem CO_2-Laser. Dtsch Z Mund-Kiefer-Gesichts-Chir 7:36–39, 1983.
5. Pindborg JJ, Jolst O, Renstrup G: Studies in oral leukoplakia: A preliminary report on the period prevalence of malignant transformation in leukoplakia based on a follow-up study of 248 patients. JADA 76:767–771, 1969.
6. Silverman S, Gorsky M, Lozada F: Oral leukoplakia and malignant transformation. Cancer 53:563–568, 1984.
7. Gonglof RK, Samit AM, Greene GW, et al: Cryosurgical management of benign and dysplastic intraoral lesions. J Oral Surg 38:671–676, 1980.
8. Poswillo D: Evaluation, surveillance, and treatment of panoral leukoplakia. J Maxilloface Surg 3:205, 1975.
9. Hausaman JE: The basis, technique and indication for cryosurgery in tumors of the oral cavity and face. J Maxillofac Surg 3:41, 1975.
10. Sako K, Marchetta FC, Hayes RL: Cryosurgery of intraoral leukoplakia. Am J Surg 124:482, 1992.
11. Horch HH, Gerlach KL, Schaefer HE, et al: Erfahrungen mit der Laserbehändlung oberflachlicher Mundschleimhauterkrankungen. Dtsch Z Mund-Kiefer-Gesichts-Chir 7:31–35, 1983.
12. Jones GM, Shepherd JP, Scully C: A case of squamous cell carcimona arising in an area treated with a carbon dioxide laser. Br J Oral Maxillofac Surg 25:57–60, 1987.
13. Sachs SA, Borden GE: The utilization of the carbon dioxide laser in the treatment of recurrent papillomatosis: Report of a case. J Oral Surg 39:299, 1981.
14. Catone GA: Lasers in dentoalveolar surgery. Oral Maxillofac Surg Clin North Am 5:45–61, 1993.
15. Hong-Sai: Initial experience with CO_2 laser for minor and major oral surgery. *In* Yamamoto H, Atsumi, K, Kusakari H: Lasers in Dentistry. Tokyo, Japan, Elsevier Science, 1989.

CHAPTER 7

Laser Management of Discrete Lesions

ROBERT A. STRAUSS, DDS

Benign lesions are a common entity managed by oral and maxillofacial surgeons in the course of daily practice. When defining this entity, however, one must consider a wide variety of pathologic conditions. Benign lesions may be flat, sessile, or pedunculated; they may be small, moderate, or large; they may be inflammatory, developmental, or neoplastic; and finally, they may be easily accessible or totally inaccessible. Because of the wide diversity of clinical presentation, the management of benign lesions is, by necessity, equally varied and complex. Treatment techniques for the management of benign lesions may include incisional biopsy, excisional biopsy, ablation, or wide excision. The choice of treatment, of course, should always be founded on the basic principles of pathology and sound surgical judgment.

Just as there are many techniques for management of these lesions, so, too, are there several modalities of treatment. Surgical steel, electrocautery, cryotherapy, and lasers have all been used in the past with varying degrees of success. The ideal modality would allow a bloodless field, require no anesthesia, allow histologic examination without distortion, provide a precise and controlled cut, enable a painless postoperative period, and cause no collateral damage to adjacent tissues.

Unfortunately, no such modality exists today. Electrosurgery and cryosurgery both cause extensive collateral damage, significant postoperative pain and swelling, and make precise histologic evaluation of close margins difficult or impossible. Even scalpel surgery is not without its problems. Although scalpel excision does allow for a precise incision with minimal (although not negligible[1]) collateral damage and excellent histologic margins, it also usually necessitates working in a bloody field and does little to decrease postoperative pain and swelling.

Lasers have several distinct advantages over the other modalities for the removal of benign lesions and a few disadvantages as well. Because of the extent of lateral thermal coagulation (approximately 300 to 500 microns for the carbon dioxide laser and 500 microns to 3 mm for the neodymium:yttrium-aluminum-garnet [Nd:YAG] laser, depending on the delivery system), vessels smaller than this size are sealed as the beam cuts across them. This creates a virtually bloodless field in most cases.[2] It is also theorized (although the actual mechanism is unclear) that because of the same effect on nerve endings, pain is diminished or eliminated in the immediate postoperative period. Using small handpieces and fibers, focal spots from 0.1 to 0.25 mm are typically possible, making thin, precise cuts with either laser simple. Finally, although some collateral tissue damage may interfere with histologic examination, it is a relatively small zone (this varies with the wavelength of the laser and the delivery system used, but it is generally equal to or slightly greater than with a scalpel and considerably smaller than with electrosurgery[1]) and is easily compensated for by the surgeon and an informed pathologist. This aspect will be discussed later in this chapter.

Of course, the use of the laser to remove discrete and benign lesions has some disadvantages as well. There is, of necessity, a significant investment in both training time and equipment costs that must be considered in this day and age of cost containment in health care. Using a laser may, in some cases, prolong the operation rather than shorten it (although the other advantages of laser use often still make the laser the treatment of choice). Using some lasers also removes the sense of tactility that most surgeons have come to rely on. While in many cases this is a distinct advantage rather than a disadvantage of laser use, it may be disconcerting to the novice laser surgeon. Finally, there is the issue of distorted pathologic margins previously mentioned.

It is clear that lasers have both many advantages and a few disadvantages when used for excision of discrete and benign lesions. It would, therefore, seem prudent for the wise practitioner to assess each lesion individually and decide which surgical modality is best suited for that specific purpose and for the level of his or her skills. In fact, a combination of modalities is sometimes appropriate. An occasional lesion, for example, may lend itself best to scalpel surgery, but the laser may be used secondarily for its hemostatic effect.

In general, the basic principles of surgical pathology should always take precedence when managing any lesion, regardless of the modality used; this is as true with lasers as it is with scalpels. This axiom is *especially* important when using lasers, which provide the oral and maxillofacial surgeon with sophisticated techniques for lesion elimination not previously readily available, such as direct tissue ablation. It is incumbent on the surgeon, therefore, to use the laser's many surgical advantages while always keeping in mind the inherent rule of pathology surgery. If one is unsure of the nature of a lesion, it should be adequately biopsied prior to definitive treatment, unless excision in toto with histologic evaluation is indicated as the treatment method of choice. Once the lesion is qualified as definitely benign, the surgeon may choose any method of removal as necessary and appropriate, including surface vaporization or surgical excision. This choice of treatment options may differ from the management of malignant lesions and premalignant lesions, in which treatment must be geared toward complete surgical removal with margins for histologic examination. With benign lesions, the method of elimination (e.g., excision versus ablation) allows greater discretion on the surgeon's part and should be based on several factors, including the need for and ease of closure in a particular anatomic area, adjacent vital structures, size of the lesion, and the depth of the desired removal. Each of these considerations are discussed later in the chapter as use in particular anatomic areas is covered.

LASER PHYSICS REVIEW

It is imperative when using any new medical technology, and is especially true for lasers, that an understanding of the science (in this case physics) is paramount to understanding the clinical uses of the device.[3] Because many lasers are used in a noncontact fashion and no tactile sensation is felt by the surgeon, controlling the extent of incision and ablation is based solely on several interacting factors related to the type of laser used, the intended target tissue, and the basic parameters of how the laser energy is being directed and controlled (i.e., power, spot size). Even contact lasers may cause tissue damage at levels considerably deeper than the depth achieved with the contact tip itself due to incomplete attenuation of the laser beam and subsequent deep tissue penetration. The basic physics of lasers is covered in Chapter 1; however, a review and clarification of these principles as they apply specifically to the removal of benign and discrete lesions is warranted.

Power Density

Carbon dioxide, Nd:YAG, holmium (Ho):YAG, argon, erbium:YAG, excimer, and other lasers are considered to be surgical lasers (as opposed to athermal, or soft, lasers). As with the majority (but not all) of surgical lasers available, they function primarily by producing a thermal effect to cut or ablate tissue. This effect requires that the laser energy be absorbed by the intended target tissue. Surgical lasers primarily work by using one of three principles: incision, vaporization/ablation, or hemostasis. Which effect is produced is primarily dependent on the amount of laser power applied to, and absorbed by, any given area of the tissue. This is defined as the *power density* (or fluence) and is measured by the following formula:

$$\text{Power density} = \text{watts/cm}^2 \text{ or } \frac{\text{watts}}{\pi \, r^2}$$

The net effect of power density is essentially to control the depth of the cut made by the laser. The higher the power density (i.e., the more power per unit area), the deeper but thinner the cut into tissue (Fig. 7–1). In order to produce an incision deep enough to perform a moderately rapid biopsy or surgical excision, one needs a fairly high power density, in the range of 1000 watts/cm^2 or greater. Power density is dependent on two factors: (1) power output and (2) the spot size of the beam used. Surgical lasers have the ability to variably control the power output of the machine incrementally up to the maximum capabilities of that particular device. It should be remembered that maximum power outputs vary widely among the different wavelengths used and even between machines using the same wavelength (carbon dioxide lasers gener-

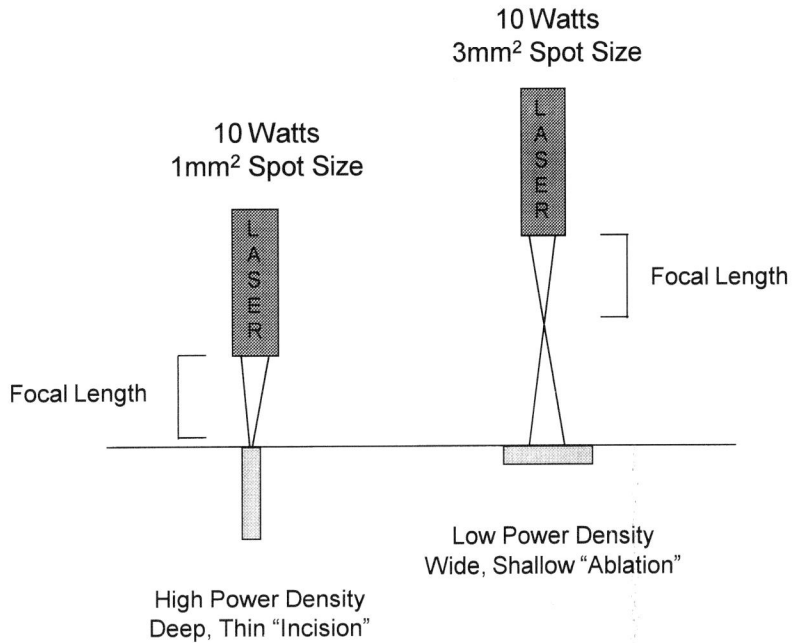

10 Watts
3mm² Spot Size

10 Watts
1mm² Spot Size

Focal Length

Focal Length

Low Power Density
Wide, Shallow "Ablation"

High Power Density
Deep, Thin "Incision"

FIGURE 7–1. Power density. This diagram indicates that when the same power is applied to a smaller spot size, the resultant increase in power density causes a deeper but thinner cut tissue when compared with a larger spot size.

ally range from 20 to 120 watts, whereas Nd:YAG lasers range from 3 to 35 watts). Also, one should keep in mind that, unlike continuous wave lasers, which have average powers that equal their maximum powers, pulsed lasers are reported as mean power output (i.e., the average power over a given time period) even though each pulse might generate peak power on the order of at least one magnitude higher than the average power (Fig. 7–2). Therefore, the surgeon should not compare powers from one wavelength machine to the next. Each wave-

length should be considered individually as to the appropriate power levels needed for a particular surgical use.

Spot size capability also varies widely among machines and is also generally adjustable for each given surgical need. As the beam is widened, the power per unit area drops and the power density falls geometrically according to the inverse square law. The end result is a shallower and wider cut. Therefore, increasing power changes the spot size of the laser beam and has the greatest effect on

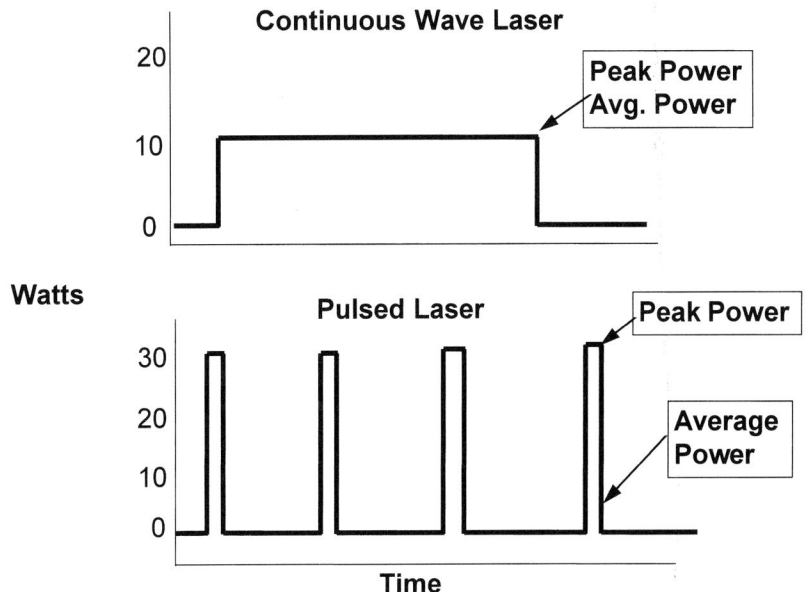

Continuous Wave Laser

20

10

0

Peak Power
Avg. Power

Watts

Pulsed Laser

Peak Power

30

20

10

0

Average
Power

Time

FIGURE 7–2. Continuous-wave versus pulsed lasers. Continuous-wave lasers have peak powers and average powers that are the same, whereas pulsed lasers have peak powers much higher than their low average powers but for very short pulse durations.

depth of tissue destruction and must be carefully considered. In noncontact lasers, this is accomplished by lengthening the distance from the laser and allowing some divergence of the beam. The process of moving the laser closer or farther from the target tissue to change the spot size is called focusing (at or near the focal point for highest power densities) and defocusing (beyond the focal point for lower power densities. See Figure 7–3A and B). Incisions and excisions use the focused, or cutting, mode. The defocused mode is primarily used for vaporization or ablation of the surface layers of larger, more superficial lesions.

Energy Density

As might be expected, the longer the laser is applied to the tissue, the greater the thermal effect to both the intended target tissue and the adjacent normal tissues. *Energy density* represents the *total* amount of energy imparted to the target tissue. It is essentially the power density multiplied by the time the laser is actually on the tissue and reflects the total amount of tissue damage. It is measured in joules (watt-seconds)/cm² and is annotated by the following formula:

$$ED = \text{power density (watts/cm}^2) \times \text{time (seconds)/cm}^2$$

Assuming complete tissue absorption has occurred (i.e., no transmission, reflection, or scatter), the energy density is generally reflective of the total amount of controlled tissue damage to the surgical site and the surrounding tissues. Obviously, when removing benign lesions, it is the goal of the surgeon to adequately and precisely remove the affected tissue while limiting the energy density to

the lowest level possible in order to minimize damage to adjacent tissue. Thus, having a thorough understanding of the appropriate variations in power, time, and spot size for planning and managing any particular lesion is imperative if the surgeon is to provide the best and safest possible surgical therapy.

Coagulation Necrosis

As laser energy is absorbed into the target tissue, the heat released by the photothermal process is used mainly to cause intracellular and extracellular vaporization, with resultant cellular explosion and tissue ablation. If given enough time, however, some of the heat will be absorbed laterally into the adjacent tissues. Assuming homogeneous tissue composition, this occurs in a series of concentric circles around the target tissue, each representing lessening degrees of thermal damage as the heat is dissipated within the tissue. *Coagulation necrosis* is the area surrounding the intended target tissue that is reversibly or irreversibly damaged by the thermal effects of the laser (Fig. 7–4A and B). The longer the laser is applied, the greater the zone of coagulation necrosis. This increase in damaged tissue can lead to prolonged healing and a larger wound site than intended.

Although usually noted for its negative effects, coagulation necrosis also has a positive effect. Any vessel smaller in diameter than the area of coagulation necrosis is sealed. This process provides hemostasis during surgery and is one of the main advantages of laser surgery. Without some area of adjacent coagulation, the surgical site would likely bleed and make surgery more difficult. This is especially important when removing benign lesions, in which small margins are often used and visualizing

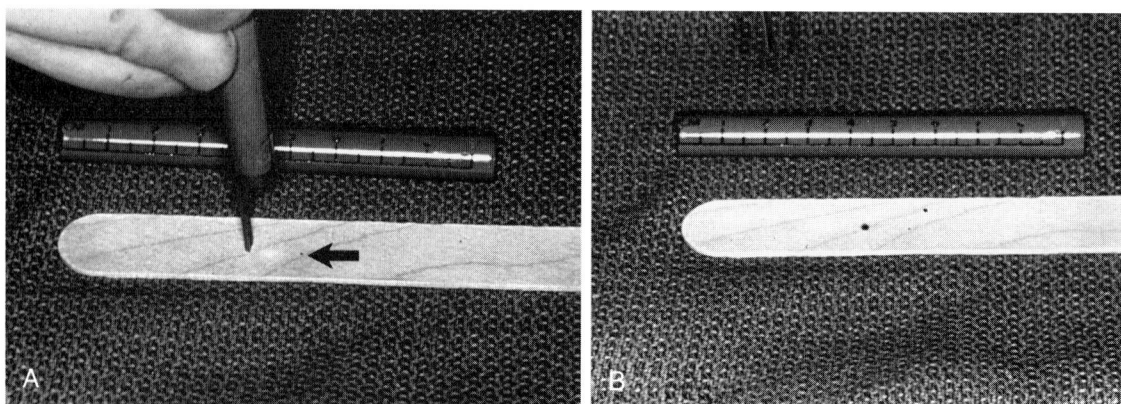

FIGURE 7–3. Focusing and defocusing. A, At the focal length of the laser, the resultant spot size is very small and the power density very high. B, As the handpiece is moved further from the target, the spot size increases and the power density drops.

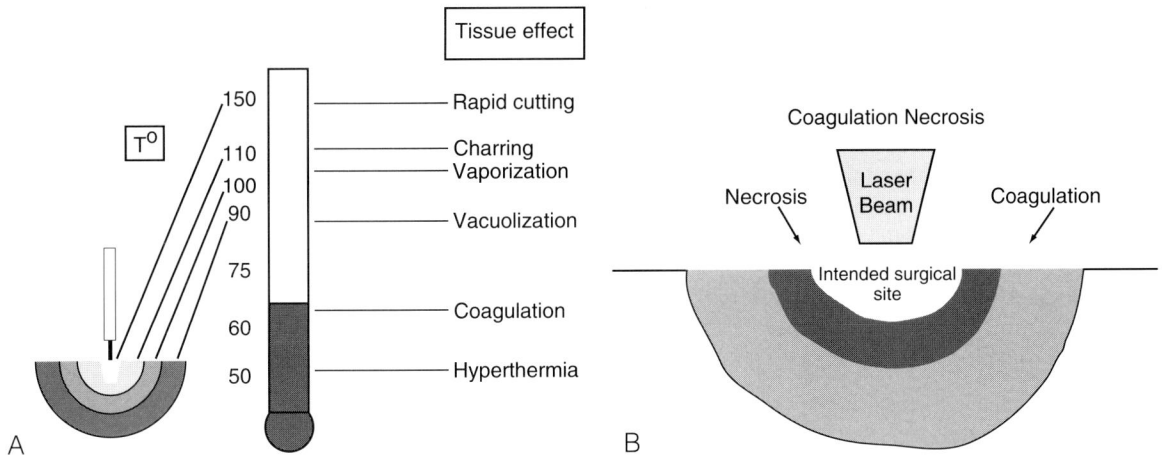

FIGURE 7–4. Coagulation necrosis. *A,* As the laser strikes the target, there is a series of concentric circles formed within the tissue as the heat dissipates laterally. *B,* The zone of coagulation necrosis represents the area surrounding the surgical site that is reversibly or irreversibly damaged by thermal conduction.

the junction of normal and abnormal tissue becomes vital. The loss of tactile sensation also contributes to the difficulty in differentiation.

A final consideration when discussing lateral thermal conduction into adjacent tissues is the effect on the histologic margins of a pathologic specimen. An incisional or excisional biopsy has a border of necrotic and coagulated tissue that may make histologic identification difficult or impossible (Fig. 7–5). The pathologist should be informed that the biopsy was performed with a laser and an additional 500 micron margin should be included in the pathology specimen to account for this coagulated border. Although it is paramount for the surgeon to remember this axiom, an experienced pathologist can easily accommodate for this effect as long as

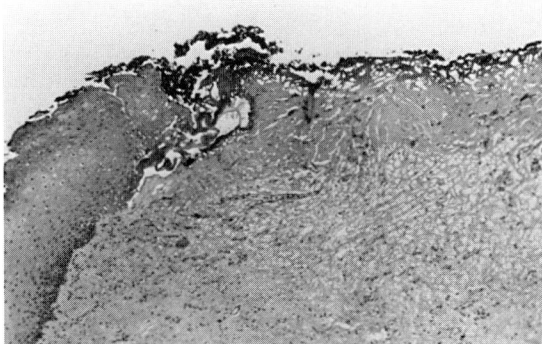

FIGURE 7–5. Coagulation necrosis. A 500-micron zone of coagulation necrosis surrounds the intended biopsy material. This area demonstrates loss of cellular orientation and nuclear staining, eosinophilia, hydrophilia, vacuolization, and surface carbonization. This zone must be taken into consideration when taking the biopsy specimen.

he or she is informed of the laser's use on the pathology form.

Thermal Relaxation Time and Fluence Rate

Coagulation necrosis is based on the lateral spread of heat effect from the point of impact of the laser beam into the surrounding tissues. In order for this to occur, however, the laser impact must last long enough for absorption into the lateral tissue to occur. Each tissue requires different amounts of time for this lateral transmission to occur. The amount of time necessary for a particular tissue to absorb and laterally transmit the thermal effects of a specific wavelength of laser energy is called the *thermal relaxation time.*

For this reason, some lasers are pulsed or superpulsed rather than being used in a continuous-wave fashion. Pulsing or superpulsing allows a laser to provide high-peak powers but very short pulse durations. Some continuous-wave lasers are incapable of true pulsing (e.g., carbon dioxide lasers) and are either superpulsed (an electronic method of pulsing the beam and increasing the peak powers), or gated, a mechanical chopping of the beam, which although it does not increase the peak powers, does allow a shortening of the pulse duration to a limited degree. A laser pulse that is of a duration less than the thermal relaxation time of the tissue will limit its damage to the impact site and demonstrate no spread to adjacent tissue. Once again, although this method limits the area of tissue damage and improves healing, with certain lasers, it may also negate the hemostatic effect that is so helpful and important in the removal of benign lesions.

This effect is of primary importance when dealing with pulsed lasers that permit extremely high powers and very short pulse durations (in the range of the thermal relaxation time of certain tissue). Most continuous-wave carbon dioxide and Nd:YAG lasers do not approach the thermal relaxation time of either oral mucosa or skin and, therefore, cause some adjacent tissue damage. Other types of true pulsed lasers can and do approach the short pulse duration necessary, but depending on the wavelength, they may not provide adequate hemostasis due to the limited adjacent tissue effect.

I have previously defined the total amount of energy (and hence, tissue damage) applied to the tissue as the energy density. It is important to consider, however, the speed with which that energy is imparted as well. As mentioned previously, if the energy is applied very quickly, there is little time for absorption, and therefore, a less damaging lateral tissue effect will result. A slower application allows increased tissue absorption time and maximizes adjacent tissue effect and damage. The speed with which the energy density is applied is called the fluence rate.

As a graphic example to help explain this concept, consider a metal rod at 10,000°F swiped across the side of your hand for 0.1 second and a similarly sized hot (200°F) cup of coffee applied to the same hand for 5 seconds. Experience and common sense would tell us that the 10,000°F would cause more damage to the hand, but, in reality, they both impart the same total energy density (assuming a 1 cm² rod and cup, ED = 1000 cm², i.e. 10,000 × 0.1 or 200 × 5). Despite this, the *total area of damage* will actually be greater for the hot cup of coffee because there is sufficient time for the heat to spread laterally into the hand and cause actual tissue destruction, whereas the metal rod is applied so quickly that there is too little time for lateral absorption, and hence, minimal thermal damage to adjacent tissues occurs (Fig. 7–6).

This factor has important implications in limiting adjacent thermal damage to nearby vital tissues and is, once again, mostly related to pulsed lasers, which allow high powers but extremely short pulse duration times. Although this factor is of importance in oral and maxillofacial surgery in some cases (e.g., when using the laser in close proximity to the lingual nerve for dermatologic uses), it is of vital importance in other areas of surgical practice, such as neurosurgery.

Focusing Techniques

As was mentioned in previous chapters, lasers produce collimated, coherent beams of light that carry tremendous amounts of energy. This energy is absorbed by the target tissue, and the heat that is subsequently produced in the cells causes water vaporization, cellular disruption, and eventually, the loss of organic cellular material and tissue volume that is seen clinically as an incision or area of tissue ablation. Although lasers already carry high energy levels directly as they leave the machine, this effect can be magnified many hundreds of times by focusing the beam down to a much smaller spot size (i.e., beam cross-sectional surface area) and thus, dramatically increase the power density. This is similar to the effect of placing a magnifying lens in front of the sun and focusing the sun's relatively weak rays down to a small but much more energy-

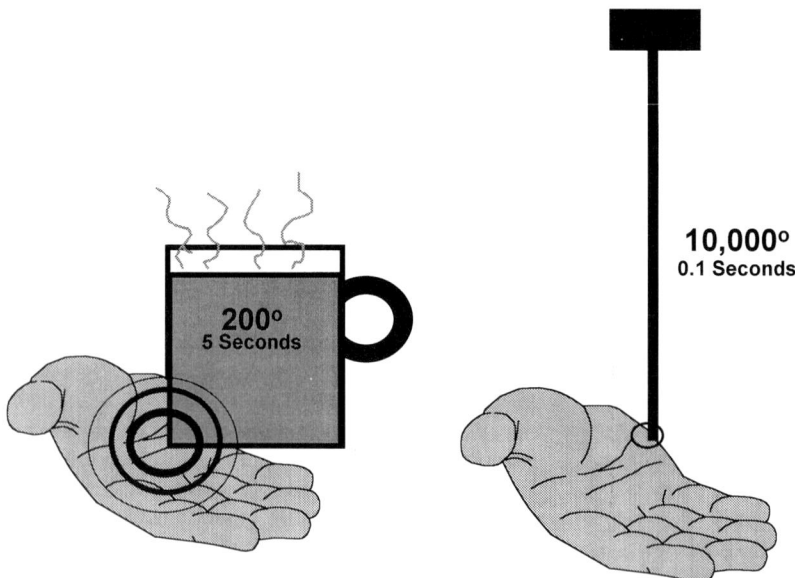

10,000°
0.1 Seconds

200°
5 Seconds

FIGURE 7–6. Fluence rate. The conduction of heat laterally into tissue is time related. A 10,000-degree rod when applied for 0.1 second and a 200-degree cup of coffee applied for 5 seconds impart the same total energy, but the rod's time period is too short for heat to spread laterally into the tissue.

dense spot size. Different lasers use a variety of techniques to focus down the laser beam and carry it to its final destination, the target tissue.

Laser energy may be transmitted and focused by a variety of mechanisms and these are described extensively elsewhere in this book. In general terms, the three most common techniques are articulating arms, fiberoptics, or hollow wave guides (Fig. 7–7A to C). The specific mechanism is usually determined by the wavelength of the laser, because only wavelengths in the visible or near-visible spectrum can be transmitted by fiberoptics (although much research is being done in this area to extend this ability to other areas of the electromagnetic spectrum). The carbon dioxide and erbium:YAG lasers are traditionally transmitted by an articulated arm or hollow waveguide, whereas the Nd:YAG, argon, and Ho:YAG lasers are transmitted by fiberoptics. Each of these systems represents a different way of not only carrying the energy but also of limiting and controlling the desired spot size.

Articulating arms are a series of rigid hollow tubes with articulated mirrors (called knuckles) at the end of each tube that eventually reflect the laser energy down to a handpiece. This is usually a difficult way to manipulate the laser for removal of

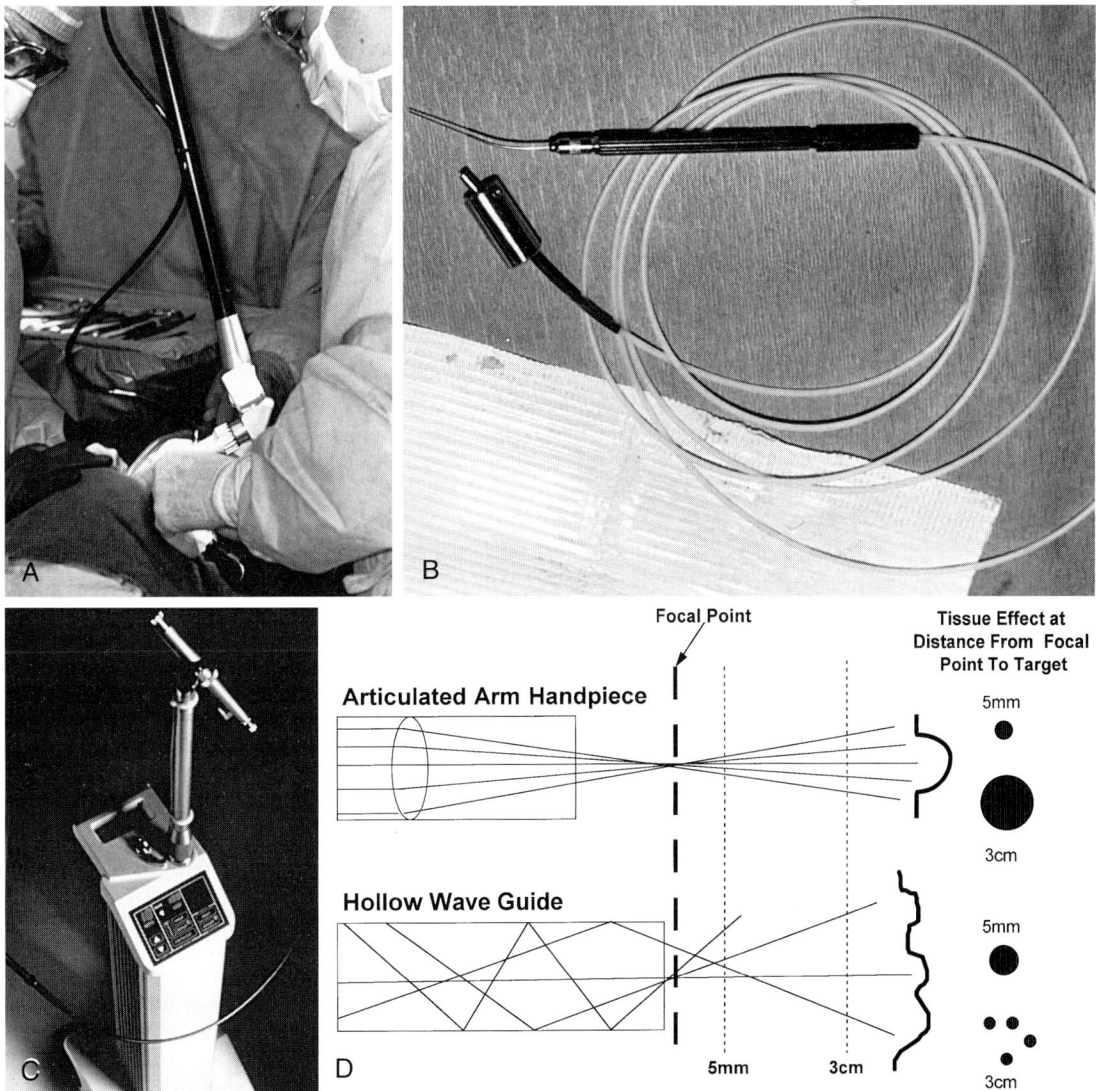

FIGURE 7–7. Methods of transmission. A, Articulated arm systems use a series of hollow metal tubes connected by mirrored knuckles to deliver the energy to a handpiece. B, Fiberoptic systems use flexible fibers to deliver the energy directly to the tissue. C, Hollow wave guides use a hollow, internally reflective metal tube as the delivery system. D, The uniform nature of the beam from articulated arm systems allows extended defocusing. The beam from the hollow wave guide diverges rapidly from the end of the handpiece and quickly degenerates into individual beams.

discrete lesions within the oral cavity because of the sometimes awkward three-dimensional maneuverability of the articulations. The system has the advantage of being adaptable to a surgical microscope for increased precision, as well as better and more homogenous defocusing ability because of its inherent ability to maintain its transverse electromagnetic mode (TEM_{00}) configuration (i.e., single bullet-shaped beam) over long distances, as compared with a hollow waveguide, for example (Fig. 7–7D). Within the handpiece is a type of focusing lens that converges the laser beams down to a small spot size. The distance from the focusing lens to the point of maximum convergence (i.e., the smallest spot size) is called the focal length and varies from about 100 mm with most handpieces (which actually puts the focal spot about 1.5 cm from the tip of the handpiece) to about 400 mm with many surgical microscopes (Fig. 7–8). The smallest spot size in most commercially available medical lasers ranges from about 0.1 mm to about 1 mm. Because the beams are no longer parallel once they extend beyond the focusing lens, the beams converge and diverge rapidly but predictably, allowing for excellent focusing and defocusing ability. When the beam is focused, the small spot size produces a very high-power density and provides superb cutting or incising abilities such as those used in an incisional or excisional biopsy. When the beam is defocused, however, the lower power density but larger surface area provides for surface ablation such as is used to sculpt down a large soft tissue tuberosity or remove a large but superficial leukoplakia (Fig. 7–9).

Fiberoptic guides carry the laser energy directly to the tissue in either a contact or noncontact mode. The minimum spot size is essentially determined by the size of the fiber itself. Fiberoptic guide sizes range from 300 to 1000 microns. When used in the contact mode (which is the preferred method, as discussed in Chapter 4), the effect in tissue is caused by the thermal effect of the tip itself, which is heated up by absorption of the beam by the buildup of tissue on the end of the fiber. This attenuation of the beam by tissue or artificial sapphire on the end of the fiber causes the material to be heated up. This is used to gain the surgical effect with decreased tissue penetration by the Nd:YAG beam itself and then to decrease unwanted deep tissue effects.[4]

Because the effect is essentially the same as a thermal cautery, there is less ability to defocus the laser. Surface ablation is produced by lowering the power to the tip, thereby decreasing power density despite the same target size, and covering the entire surface of the lesion with the tip in contact. In the noncontact mode, one may defocus the fiberoptic tip in the same manner as with the articulated arm or hollow waveguide and cover a wider area with decreased power densities. It should be remembered, however, that the actual effect on, and in, the tissue will be determined not only by the power density and energy density but also by the wavelength and its relative absorption into the specified tissue. With the Nd:YAG wavelength, for example, any laser energy that exits beyond the fiber (even with a contact tip there is undoubtedly less than 100% attenuation of the beam) will penetrate into oral tissues 3 to 4 mm before being totally absorbed by the various chromophores. Thus, unwanted tissue damage may occur.[5] Because of their attenuating effect on the beam, contact fibers can greatly decrease, but may not always eliminate, this consequence. Nevertheless, incisional and excisional biopsies and small areas of vaporization may be easily carried out with fiberoptic lasers.[6] Because of the extreme mobility of fiberoptic handpieces, however, ease of use and access to all areas of the oral cavity are enhanced with their use. Finally, fiberoptic handpieces cannot be connected to microscopes for

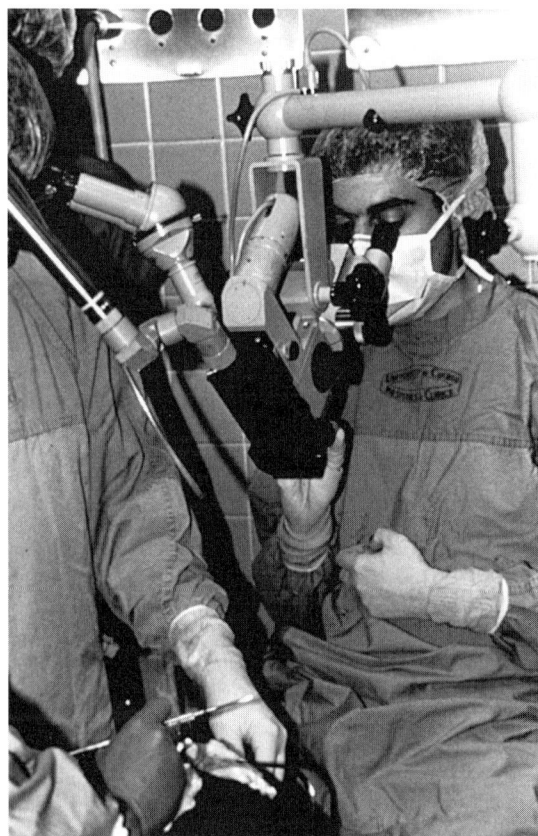

FIGURE 7–8. Microscopic capabilities. The articulated arm may be connected directly to an operating microscope. This allows for extremely accurate surgery under magnified conditions. Control of the beam, which has a focal distance of approximately 400 mm, is obtained by the use of a joystick.

FIGURE 7–9. Focusing. When the laser is placed at its ideal focal length (i.e., the focal plane), maximum power density is obtained and a deep, thin cut is produced. When the handpiece is pulled away from the focal plane, power density falls and a wider, more shallow ablation occurs. Putting the laser closer than its focal length could theoretically, with some wavelength lasers, lead to focusing within the tissue and unwanted extensive subsurface destruction.

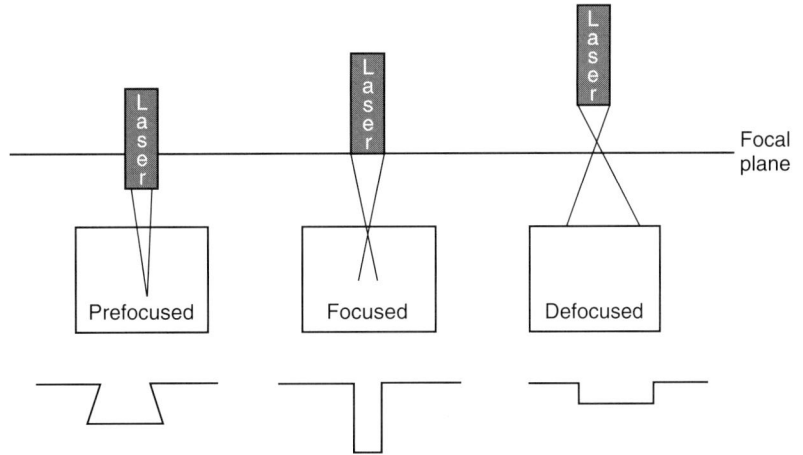

increased precision but can be passed through endoscopes and used for distant endoscopic procedures.

Hollow waveguides are bendable hollow metal tubes that have an internally reflecting surface that allows transmission of the laser beams down the tube to the target tissue. At the end of the handpiece, depending on the manufacturer, a metal or ceramic tip may be used to continue carrying the beam to the target tissue in a more precise fashion (Fig. 7–10). Because there is no focusing lens and the beam is no longer parallel inside the wave guide, the focal point of the beam is at the end of the waveguide, and divergence, and hence defocusing, occurs from this point (see Fig. 7–7D). Some of the smaller metal tips are also internally reflective, and divergence of the beam does not begin until the end of the tip rather than the waveguide fiber itself. The ceramic tips and larger metal tips may allow some internal divergence prior to exiting

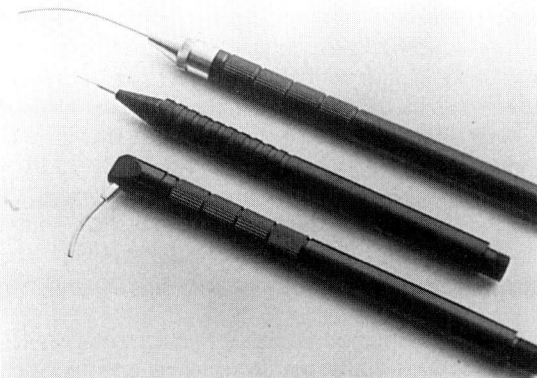

FIGURE 7–10. Hollow waveguide delivery. Unlike articulated arm handpieces, which use mirror extensions on the handpiece to angle the beam, hollow wave guide extensions that fit into the handpiece and come in a variety of sizes may be curved or straight to allow access to remote areas of the oral cavity.

the tip, where divergence continues. The beams lose their collimation once they enter the tube, and therefore, there is no advantage to using a focusing lens at the end of the tube. The beam diameter is set by the size of the waveguide and the tip used in the handpiece. Minimum spot sizes for hollow waveguides typically range from about 0.25 mm to about 1.0 mm and may be effectively defocused to a beam size of approximately 2.0 to 2.5 mm with a 20-watt machine (higher powers are necessary at this diameter in order to maintain a power density that will perform the desired functions). This wide range of minimum spot sizes allows the hollow waveguide to be used for any incisional, excisional, or ablative procedure, irrespective of the size of the lesion. As mentioned previously, fiberoptic delivery has some advantages when operating in remote or difficult areas, but only lasers in the visible and near-infrared spectrum can be transmitted by fiberoptics at the present time. Although the flexibility of the hollow waveguide is generally not as great as a fiberoptic guide, it is still usually far greater for those wavelengths not transmittable by fiberoptics than articulated arm systems and is usually more than adequate to reach all areas of the oral cavity and face. This is also aided by a series of available handpiece designs that include straight, contra-angle, and 360-degree rotatable heads. Hollow waveguides generally cannot be connected to microscopes (although most hollow waveguide machines have an initial articulation that could be fitted for this purpose), or passed through an endoscope, but they do provide an excellent compromise between the need for the outstanding tissue interaction properties of the carbon dioxide laser and the flexibility and access afforded by fiberoptic guides used for other less suitable wavelengths in oral and maxillofacial surgery.

It should be noted that the technology for transmitting laser beams is constantly changing. New fiberoptic materials are being developed that will increase the transmission efficiency for those wavelengths that use fiberoptic technology and will allow fiberoptic transmission for those wavelengths not able to use this technology because of the great power loss seen within the fiber (such as with carbon dioxide lasers). Also, there are several unique transmission devices or techniques that are used specifically for particular surgical procedures or anatomic areas, and these devices or techniques used are discussed later in the chapter.

PRINCIPLES OF INCISIONAL AND EXCISIONAL BIOPSY USING THE LASER

Using the principles of physics described earlier in this chapter and armed with a basic knowledge of surgical pathology, one can easily incorporate the many advantages of lasers into techniques of surgical biopsy. As mentioned previously, the incision, excision, or vaporization of discrete and benign lesions of the oral cavity and face is relatively simple and straightforward.[7, 8]

Incisional Biopsy

The laser is an excellent tool for incisional biopsy for a variety of reasons. Primary among these is its ability to provide a bloodless field in which to work. This affords the surgeon far greater visualization of the biopsy field than with scalpel techniques. Since, by definition, incisional biopsy necessitates violation of the lesion, this is of greatest importance when performing incisional biopsy on lesions with high vascularity or blood loss potential such as pyogenic granuloma, Kaposi's sarcoma, or hemangioma. Another major advantage relates to the fact that the use of lasers often obviates the need to suture the wound following the biopsy. This is made possible due to the decreased scarring seen with laser surgery, the lack of postoperative bleeding, and the lack of postoperative pain, all of which are the prime reasons for closing wounds. Most benign lesions, therefore, would not require suturing unless a significant cosmetic or functional deformity is created (e.g., after laser wedge excision of a lip hemangioma). These lesions may be sutured in the routine fashion, although the sutures should be left in place slightly longer than usual to compensate for the minor delay in healing seen with laser wounds.

There are two caveats that must be remembered when performing incisional biopsy with the laser. First, the lateral zone of thermal coagulation must be accounted for during the biopsy. This zone, measuring 500 microns or less with the carbon dioxide and contact Nd:YAG lasers, is the area

surrounding the incision site that is damaged by lateral heat conduction into the tissues. Failure to accommodate for this area may make histopathologic diagnosis difficult or even impossible and may necessitate a second procedure. Because there are many factors that affect this zone of lateral necrosis, they must be taken into account prior to the biopsy so the surgeon may minimize this effect and the pathologist may accurately interpret the biopsy specimen. It should be remembered that the zone of thermal effect includes not only irreversibly damaged necrotic tissue but also a zone of reversibly thermally damaged tissue as well. Both of these areas of tissue may affect the pathologist's interpretive abilities. Factors that affect the lateral zone of necrosis include

1. The wavelength of the laser: The carbon dioxide and the contact Nd:YAG lasers have similar zones of necrosis in oral mucosa (500 microns or less), whereas the noncontact Nd:YAG has a distinctly greater extent of effect (Fig. 7–11).
2. The target tissue: The zone of thermal necrosis depends on the varying ability of different tissues to absorb and transmit the thermal effect. This is measured by the time necessary for lateral spread of heat in any particular tissue and is represented by the thermal relaxation time (i.e., the minimum time necessary for lateral conduction).
3. The energy density applied: The longer the laser is applied, the greater the total energy density and, hence, the extent of lateral damage.
4. The spot size: Obviously, to have the least *total* width of thermal effect on the surface, one should minimize the initial spot size. This is accomplished by using the smallest spot size possible when making incisions.

Accounting for the lateral zone of necrosis when doing incisional biopsy is relatively simple. The important aspect of an *incisional* biopsy usually is not the periphery but the center of the biopsy specimen. To ensure an adequate specimen, plan the biopsy to include a margin of excess tissue equal in amount to the expected zone of lateral thermal damage (about 0.5 mm with the carbon dioxide and contact Nd:YAG lasers) in addition to the desired width of the biopsy specimen. Thus, a desired 3-mm wide specimen requires a 4-mm wide initial incision with the laser to allow for 500 microns of thermal damage on either side of the margins (Fig. 7–12).

The second caveat is that incisional biopsy, even with a laser, usually requires mechanical elevation of the biopsy specimen with a forceps or a hemostat. This diminishes one of the advantages of laser use, that is, the ability to perform so-called hands-off surgery. Of course, it also adds a degree of tactile sensation back to the surgery, because the

FIGURE 7–11. Tissue interaction depth. The carbon dioxide and contact Nd:YAG lasers both have tissue interaction depths of 500 microns or less. The wavelength of the carbon dioxide laser is absorbed in the first 0.1 mm of oral soft tissue owing to its excellent absorption by water in the surface cells. The noncontact Nd:YAG wavelength, with absorption by water being much lower, must pass through 3 to 4 mm of tissue before being totally absorbed by its tissue chromophores, although its clinical effects may be seen only at the surface.

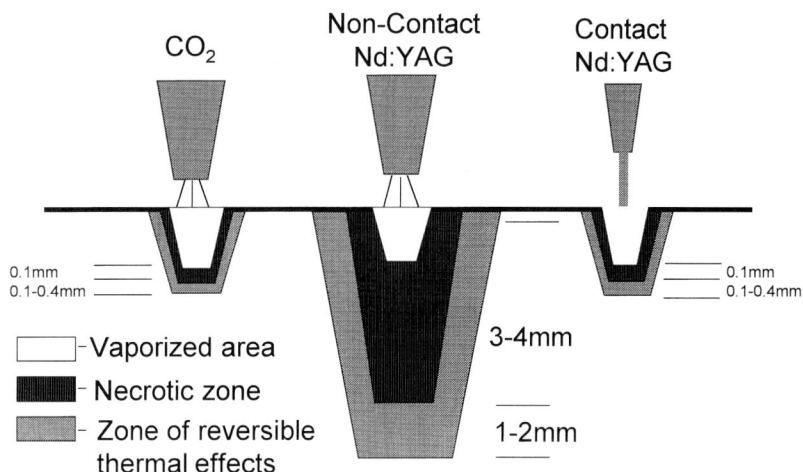

Non-Contact Nd:YAG

CO_2

Contact Nd:YAG

0.1mm
0.1-0.4mm

3-4mm

1-2mm

0.1mm
0.1-0.4mm

☐ - Vaporized area

▓ - Necrotic zone

▒ - Zone of reversible thermal effects

surgeon can feel the specimen separating from the underlying tissues and can adjust the laser power and spot size accordingly. Care must be taken to minimize mechanical tissue trauma in these cases so that the pathologist may make an easier diagnosis.

Incisional Biopsy Technique
(Fig. 7–13A to E)

1. *Provide local or general anesthesia as indicated.* Because, by definition, incisional biopsy involves cutting into the depth of a lesion, local anesthesia is generally required. When possible, local anesthesia should be administered by neural block or deep infiltration rather than by the superficial infiltration technique commonly used for this purpose. If injected superficially into the tissue to be incised, the differential water content in the tissue caused by the anesthetic solution may, in some cases, lead to inconsistent tissue cutting.

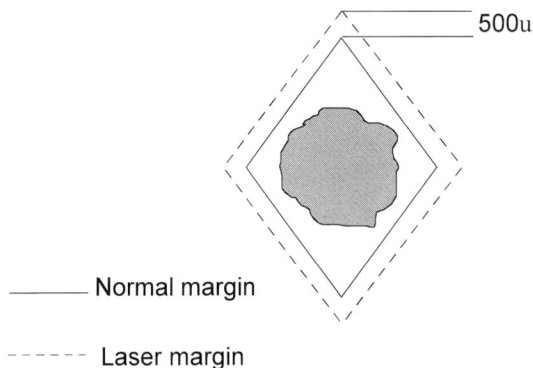

500u

Normal margin

- - - - - Laser margin

FIGURE 7–12. Biopsy margins. Because the 500-micron zone of thermal coagulation can interfere with histologic examination of the margins, an additional 0.5 mm of tissue excision should be added to the normal margin around the biopsy site. This will allow pathologic inspection of the originally planned tissue edge.

2. *Outline the area to be incised.* It is good practice to outline the biopsy area in a slow, controlled fashion. Because lasers are capable of cutting tissue rapidly, it is best to examine the lesion carefully and mark the intended surgical cuts. As mentioned previously, when submitting a specimen for histologic examination, it is advisable to include an additional 0.3-0.5 mm around the intended biopsy site to compensate for the zone of adjacent thermal coagulation. It is advisable to do the marking using a single-pulse or slow repeat mode (e.g., gated mode at 2-10 pulses per second) for increased visibility and control. Using the carbon dioxide laser, 4 to 6 watts in focused mode (usually 0.1 to 0.4-mm spot size, depending on the machine) provides a visible but not too deep outline.

3. *Connect the outlined marks.* Increase the power to the initially desired level for the tissue involved, and connect the outlined marks made previously. Specific power densities for each tissue are discussed by anatomic region later in this chapter. This incision should be carried into the tissue to the desired depth of the biopsy. This, of course, varies by the nature of the lesion being biopsied and should be the same as if a scalpel were being used. When using a small spot size, it is sometimes useful to separate the incision by gently applying tension on the adjacent tissues with a forceps, periosteal elevator, or other suitable instrument. This approach opens the incision site and allows precise deepening of the incision. Failure to do this sometimes results in burning of any char in the incision site, build-up of heat in adjacent tissues, and little productive increase in depth. Occasionally, if charring does occur, a moist gauze or wet cotton-tipped applicator may be used to wipe the char away and allow access to deeper, fresh tissue. It should be remembered that unless the laser tip is inserted further into the incision line as it is being deepened, the beam will begin to diverge and defocus at the

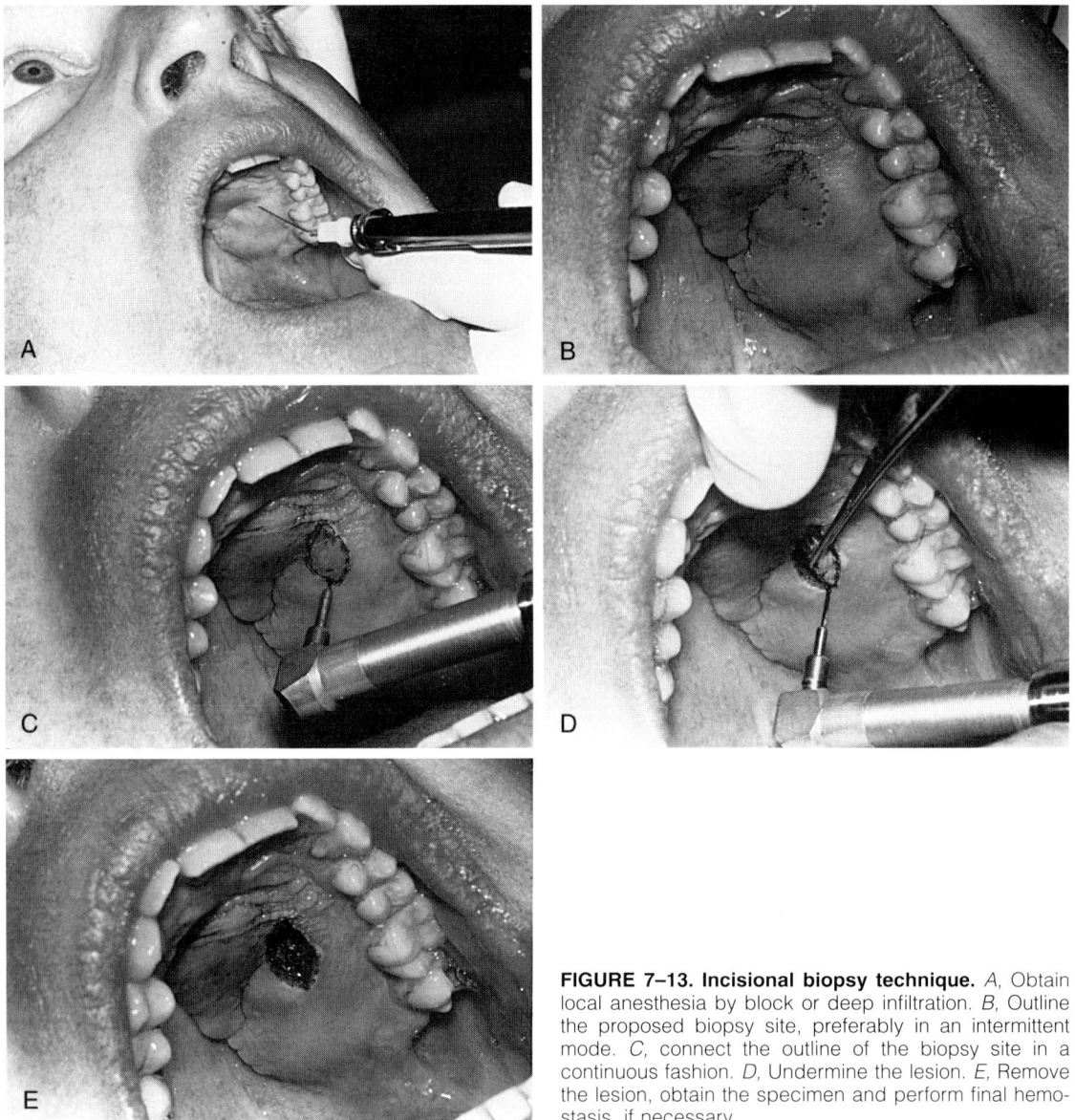

FIGURE 7–13. Incisional biopsy technique. *A,* Obtain local anesthesia by block or deep infiltration. *B,* Outline the proposed biopsy site, preferably in an intermittent mode. *C,* connect the outline of the biopsy site in a continuous fashion. *D,* Undermine the lesion. *E,* Remove the lesion, obtain the specimen and perform final hemostasis, if necessary.

depth of the incision and will exhibit decreased power density and diminished cutting effects.

4. *Excise the specimen.* Gently hold the edge of the biopsy specimen with a forceps and using the laser in focused mode, undermine the specimen along its entire length by directing the laser into the margin at an angle parallel to the base of the lesion. Be careful as the specimen is being removed to protect the surrounding tissues from inadvertently aimed laser beams. This is accomplished by always aiming the beam toward the center of the lesion.

5. *Obtain hemostasis, if necessary.* In a few cases, some bleeding may occur during the procedure, despite the intrinsic hemostatic effect of the laser. This is more likely with the carbon dioxide laser than with the Nd:YAG or argon laser and is usually

related to vessels greater than 0.5 mm or too-rapid movement of the laser handpiece, not allowing enough time for lateral thermal diffusion and coagulation. This problem may be alleviated by slightly defocusing the laser and releasing the involved vessel.

6. *Consider the need for suturing.* As mentioned previously, many of the indications and reasons for suture closure are obviated by the use of the laser. Because incisional biopsy is usually followed by secondary excision anyway, suture closure is mostly unnecessary. In those rare cases in which suturing is desired, appropriate undermining (which may be done very nicely with the laser) and suturing in layers may be performed in the usual manner, if necessary.

7. *Consider tagging the biopsy margins.* As is usual for pathologic specimens, the margins may be tagged for orientation by the pathologist.

Excisional Biopsy

For the same reasons as were cited for incisional biopsy, the laser is often ideally suited for excisional biopsy. Its precision, speed, and hemostasis make lesion excision faster and easier in many cases.

Just as with incisional biopsy, however, there are caveats that must be considered. Vessels larger than the zone of thermal coagulation (about 500 microns for the carbon dioxide laser) will still bleed and will need to be electrocoagulated or ligated. Although in the oral cavity this is rarely necessary, it is more likely to occur during deep surgical excision of a lesion than during superficial biopsy.

The zone of thermal coagulation must be considered as well in aiding the pathologist in determining surgical margins. When margin examination is considered vital, an additional peripheral area matching or exceeding the zone of thermal coagulation should be added. Of course, this margin is usually small (0.5 mm or less) and presents no additional morbidity for the patient or the surgeon.

As opposed to incisional biopsy, when performing excisional biopsy, greater consideration must be given toward protecting adjacent vital structures. Although the laser is often a better, or even an ideal, tool for protecting nearby anatomic features, judiciousness should be exercised near ducts, vessels, nerves, commissures, teeth, and bone. This consideration is covered extensively later in this chapter.

The technique for excisional biopsy varies according to the type of tissue being excised, the anatomic location, and the need for closure. It is in this last respect that laser excision differs so greatly from scalpel surgery, in which closure is usually mandated. Traditional indications for wound closure include hemostasis, coaptation of the margins for faster and more cosmetic healing, and decreasing postoperative pain from wound exposure and trauma. Because of the wound healing, hemostatic, and neural ''sealing'' properties of the laser, closure of the wound often is not necessary.

It has been questioned whether or not the use of the laser actually contraindicates primary closure owing to the negative effect of vascular occlusion and decreased collagen production on wound healing. These effects, generally considered to be two of the main advantages of laser surgery (for their hemostatic and decreased scarring properties) would, theoretically, prevent healing and cause the wound margins to separate if the sutures are taken out at the usual 1 week postoperative visit. In fact,

this has not proved to be true. As mentioned previously, however, it is advisable to leave sutures in place for at least an extra day or two to allow for the slightly delayed epithelialization and healing expected. Although it is delayed, the tensile strength of laser wounds eventually reaches the same strength as that of scalpel wounds.[9]

Finally, skin grafting after laser excision has been shown to be both unnecessary and ineffective due to the sealing of the superficial recipient site vessels and the subsequent lack of imbibition and graft failure.[10, 11]

Excisional Biopsy Technique
(Fig. 7–14*A* to *H*)

1. *Provide local, topical, or general anesthesia, as indicated.* Unless the lesion to be excised is small and pedunculated, for which topical anesthesia is sometimes sufficient, local or general anesthesia is warranted. When possible, local anesthesia should be administered by neural block or deep infiltration rather than by the superficial infiltration technique commonly used for this purpose. If the anesthetic is injected superficially into the tissue to be incised, the differential water content in the tissue caused by the anesthetic solution may, in some cases, lead to inconsistent tissue cutting.

2. *Outline the area to be excised.* It is good practice to outline the area to be excised in a slow, controlled fashion. Because lasers are capable of cutting tissue rapidly, it is best to examine the lesion carefully and mark the intended margins. As mentioned previously, when submitting a specimen for histologic examination, it is advisable to include an additional 0.5 to 1.0 mm around the lesion to compensate for the zone of thermal coagulation. It is also advisable to do the marking using a single-pulse, slow repeat, or gated mode (2 to 10 pulses per second) for increased visibility and control. Using the carbon dioxide laser, a wattage of 4 to 6 watts in focused mode (usually 0.1 to 0.4 mm depending on the machine) provides an outline that is visible but not too deep.

3. *Connect the outlined marks.* Increase the power to the initially desired level for the tissue involved, and connect the outlined marks made previously. Specific power densities and techniques are described later in this chapter, organized by anatomic region. This incision should be carried to the desired depth into the tissue that is mandated by basic pathologic principles and the anticipated depth of the lesion. For superficial lesions of the oral cavity, this depth usually is 2 to 4 mm. When using a small spot size, it is sometimes useful to separate the incision by gently applying tension on the adjacent tissues. This opens the incision site and allows precise deepening of the wound.

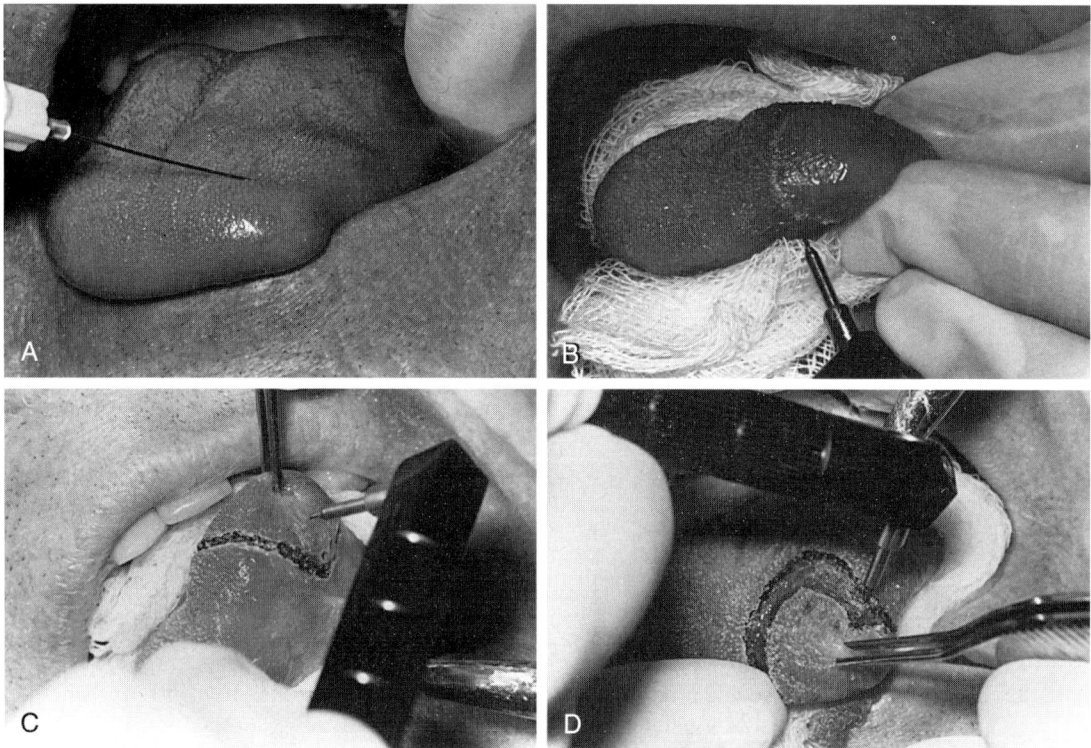

FIGURE 7–14. Excisional biopsy technique. *A,* Obtain local anesthesia by block or deep infiltration. *B,* Outline the proposed biopsy site, preferably in an intermittent mode. *C,* Connect the outline of the biopsy site in a continuous fashion. *D,* Undermine the lesion.

4. *Undermine the lesion.* Gently pick up an edge of the lesion with a forceps and, using the laser in focused mode, undermine the lesion along its entire length. Remember that as you undermine, you must continue to move the laser along the long axis of the lesion, otherwise, you will defocus the laser and vaporize the margins rather than incise them. As you reach the far end of the lesion, the laser should be redirected to always be aiming into the wound. This approach will prevent accidental lasing of adjacent normal tissue beyond the far extent of the lesion.

5. *Obtain hemostasis, if necessary.* In a few cases, some bleeding may occur during the procedure, despite the intrinsic hemostatic effect of the laser. This is more likely with the carbon dioxide laser than with the Nd:YAG or argon laser and is usually related to vessels larger than 0.5 mm or to too-rapid movement of the laser handpiece, not allowing enough time for lateral thermal diffusion and coagulation. Releasing may be tried, or an electrocautery may be used.

6. *Consider the need for suturing.* As mentioned previously, many of the indications and reasons for suture closure are obviated by the use of the laser. Suturing should clearly be undertaken, however, when an uncosmetic defect would be left behind if

the lesion were not primarily closed. Appropriate undermining and suturing may be performed in the usual manner in these cases.

7. *If desired, leave a light char layer.* Some laser surgeons like to leave a light char layer on the surgical bed to act as a physiologic bandage. This may be accomplished by defocusing the laser to a spot size of 1.5 to 2.0 mm and quickly covering the entire surface of the surgical bed at a power setting of 4 to 6 watts. The clinical effect of this maneuver has yet to be proved, and it is believed by some surgeons that the charred tissue merely acts as a foreign body and prolongs the healing time. It would seem prudent, therefore, for each surgeon to assess his or her individual results using this technique in different clinical situations.

Traditionally, the definitive management of discrete and benign lesions has relied on excisional biopsy. Although this technique does provide a pathologic specimen and remains as the most common technique for these lesions, it does have disadvantages that must be considered. Despite the laser's improved healing capabilities, excision may leave an uncosmetic vertical defect, and suture closure for cosmesis may require a larger incision to allow tension-free coaptation. Excision is also more likely to injure underlying structures.

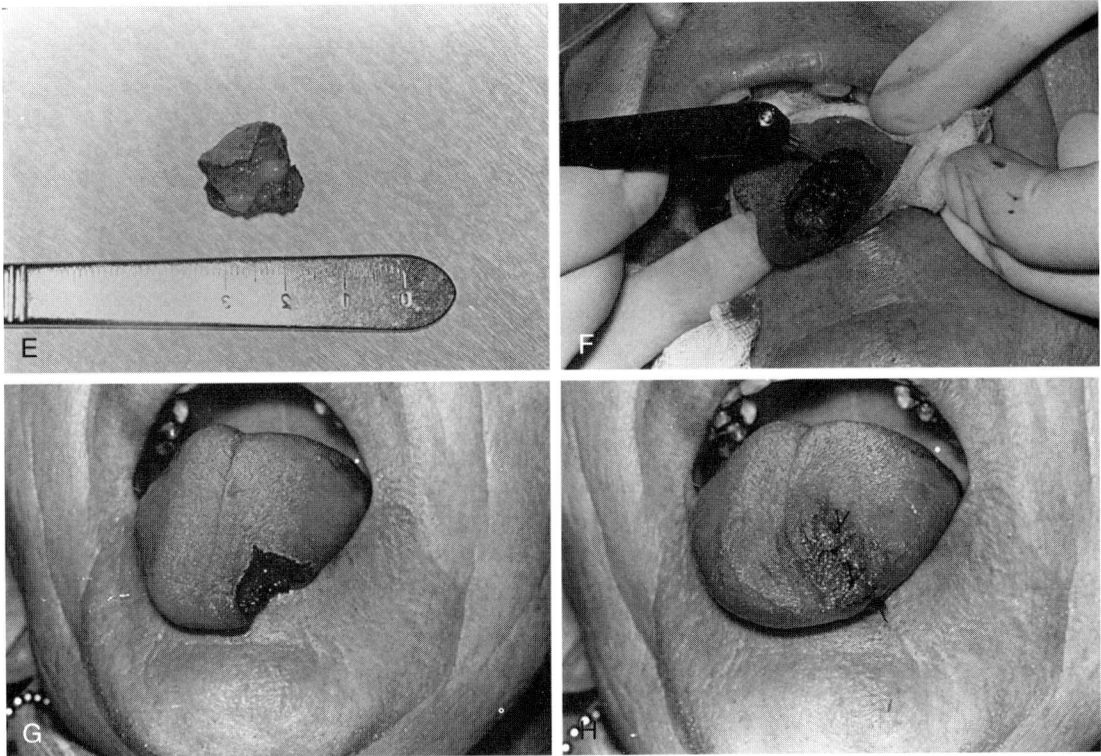

FIGURE 7–14 *Continued E* and *F,* Remove the lesion, and obtain the specimen, and conduct final hemostasis, if necessary. *G* and *H,* Depending on anatomic and functional location, suturing may be performed, if desired.

An alternative to excision is vaporization. Primarily used for premalignant mucosal lesions such as epithelial dysplasia, vaporization may also be used effectively for benign and discrete lesions, provided, of course, that a pathologic specimen is not deemed necessary or when adequate presurgical incisional biopsies have been performed and no additional biopsy is needed.

There are several advantages to the use of vaporization for eradication of benign lesions. Lesion ablation allows conservative sculpting of the tissue without excessive tissue removal at the base of the lesion. In addition, vaporization has been shown to lead to a better preservation of the elasticity of oral mucosa than has scalpel excision when used for ablation of surface lesions.[12] This can be of importance when scar contracture or postsurgical tissue rigidity might present a functional problem, such as in a wound near the commissure or on the ventral surface of the tongue. Finally, for smaller lesions, excisional conservatism may be greatly improved with the use of vaporization in a slow-pulsed mode. Small benign dermatologic lesions that are removed strictly for cosmesis are excellent examples of lesions that may be easily removed by laser vaporization, with minimal scarring, discomfort, and damage to adjacent tissue.

The principle of vaporization is based on defocusing the laser (moving the laser away from the target and beyond the focal point of the laser) to obtain a lower power density and a wider spot size. This causes a wider and more shallow destruction than does the focused mode, in which the higher power density causes a deeper but thinner cut. When ablating large mucosal epithelial lesions, the spot size is kept big (1 to 3 mm) to vaporize a large but shallow area, allowing rapid coverage of the entire mucosal lesion. When vaporizing smaller but discrete lesions, the laser is defocused to a spot size between the focused and defocused modes (0.5 to 1.5 mm). This allows individual beam eradication to the depth of the lesion, a large enough spot size to facilitate the removal of most small lesions, and enough power density to ablate the vertical volume of tissue involved.

Once again, it is imperative to remember that the lesions most amenable to vaporization are those that are being removed electively for cosmesis or functional improvement, or those that have undergone biopsy and for which it has been determined that conservative ablation without the need for absolute margin control is acceptable. Total excision of a large lesion with adequate margins can be more difficult and time consuming but allows for histologic examination of the entire lesion. Vaporization provides a quicker and safer mechanism for removal of some lesions but eliminates the possibility of histologic examination. Although this factor is of less importance for benign lesions than for premalignant and malignant lesions, it must still be considered.

It must also be remembered that with any type of surgery, including laser surgery, some scarring is inevitable. This does not, of course, present a problem for intraoral surgery, in which cosmesis is not usually an issue. Although scarring following ablation of small facial lesions is usually acceptable, it is wise in the case of multiple lesions to remove one in an inconspicuous spot and then, if the result is beneficial, continue with the rest of the lesions. Keeping the ablation in the papillary dermal layer will allow epithelial remnants and adnexal structures to provide a basis for excellent reepithelialization.

The technique for vaporization of discrete lesions is as follows:

1. Examine the lesion to determine its approximate size and depth. This is important to determine the needed power and spot sizes. For smaller lesions, the spot size may be increased from focused

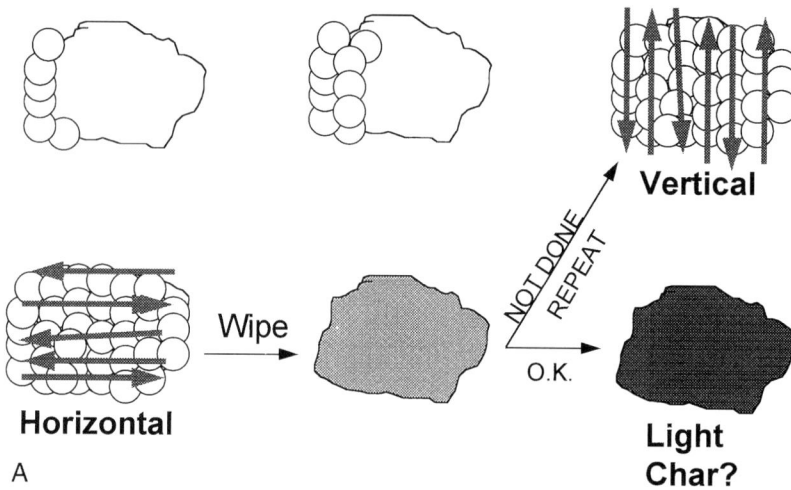

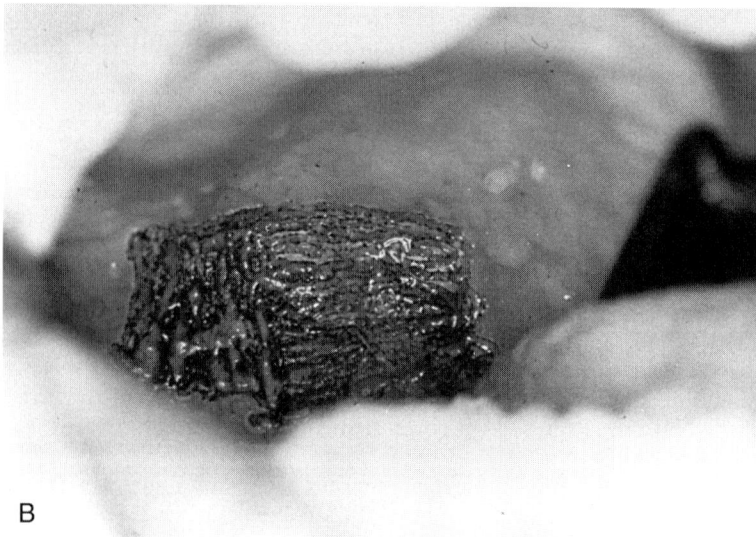

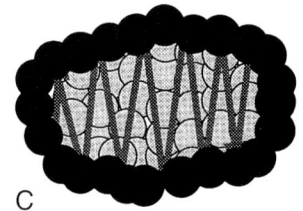

FIGURE 7–15. Ablation technique. *A,* Proper technique involves using vertical, horizontal, and oblique passes over the lesion. After gently wiping the char layer, further depth of ablation may be obtained by repeating the passes as needed. A final light char layer may be placed, if desired. *B,* Clinical example demonstrating the vertical and horizontal passes during ablation of soft palate lesion. *C,* using continuous L-shaped motions, rather than a series of Vs, prevents deep troughing in the periphery of the lesion.

size to 0.5 to 1.5 mm. The power levels for these lesions must be high enough to allow rapid cut to depth but low enough to allow accurate control without overextension laterally or at depth, generally 5 to 8 watts for the carbon dioxide laser. For larger lesions, the spot size may be increased to 1.0 to 2.0 mm and the power increased accordingly to maintain or slightly increase the power density, generally 6 to 10 watts.

2. For larger lesions, the standard technique for vaporization of mucosal lesions may be applied. This technique involves performing a criss-cross pattern on the lesion extending laterally only to the extent of the lesion. The procedure should be performed using a series of overlapping vertical, horizontal, and oblique rows so that the entire lesion is covered in a homogeneous fashion (Fig. 7–15A and B). It should also be remembered that the rows should not be done in up and down Vs but rather in a continuous motion, with no stopping at the top or bottom of the rows. To do otherwise will create a groove around the extent of the lesion as the energy density is doubled by the increased time spent at the top and bottom of each stroke (Fig. 7–15C). The continuous mode is usually used, but it may be performed at a high-repetition mode (10 to 20 pulses per second) if available on the machine used. If a pulsed or gated beam is used, care should be exercised to ensure homogeneous and even coverage because there may be areas between the pulses that are not being lasered. After each set of vaporizational strokes, any resultant char should be removed with wet gauze to prevent burning (since the char contains no water for the carbon dioxide laser to affect, it will essentially just heat up and

burn, causing increased postoperative pain and prolonged healing) (see Fig. 7–15B). Further layers of vaporization may be performed as necessary until the lesion is eradicated to the desired depth. It is always a good idea to outline the area to be ablated prior to definitive vaporization. This is best performed at low power in a rapid pulsed mode (10 to 20 pulses/second) but one that allows slow and precise controlled outlining.

3. For smaller or cosmetically important lesions, a slightly different technique is used. When absolute accuracy is needed, such as for small nevi, tissue tags, or other facial lesions, the smaller spot size is used in a slow repeat (1 to 5 pulses per second) or single-pulse mode to progressively chip away at the lesion. This is accomplished by moving the beam spot over the lesion in slightly overlapping circles until the entire surface has been covered and the lesion has been vertically lowered. This is continued in layers until the lesion has been removed to the level of the surrounding surface (for cosmetic removals) or the depth of the lesion (for benign neoplasms) as desired and necessary (Fig. 7–16).

4. Dress the wound, if desired. By definition, vaporization of the lesion precludes suture closure. Facial lesions may be covered with a thin layer of antibiotic ointment and a sterile bandage but this is generally unnecessary except for temporary cosmesis.

Hemostatic Technique

Hemostasis is an important primary benefit of the laser during surgery. There are times, however, when an alternative technique to laser surgery may

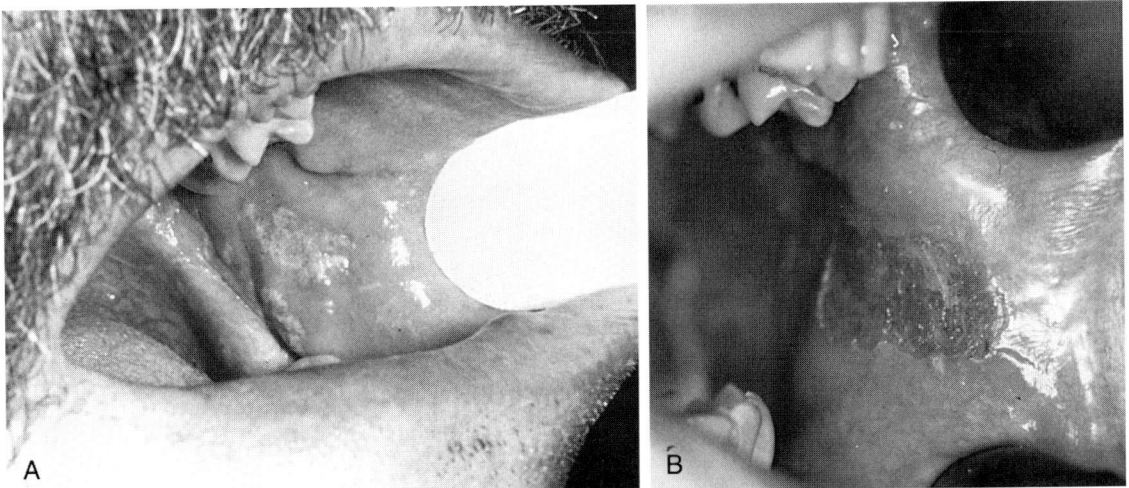

FIGURE 7–16. Ablation depth. Clinical example of ablation of a mild dysplasia of the buccal mucosa just into the submucosa. *A* and *B,* The depth of ablation is easily controlled by changing the parameters of power and spot size. Additional depth may also be obtained by repeating the vaporization procedure as needed.

be indicated for the primary management of the lesion. In these cases, during or after definitive scalpel surgery, the laser may be used to obtain secondary hemostasis (Fig. 7–17A to F). Laser hemostasis is particularly useful in areas of difficult access such as the soft palate or on soft tissue graft donor sites. This simple technique is accomplished as follows:

1. *Remove the lesion by whatever sharp means is deemed appropriate* (e.g., scalpel or scissors).

2. *Obtain initial hemostasis by direct pressure.* It is important that there not be brisk, active bleeding if the carbon dioxide laser is to be used because the water content of the blood will readily and ineffectively absorb the energy and coagulation of the vessel will not be gained. Remember, it is the vessel and surrounding connective tissue that are lased, not the blood.

3. *Slightly defocus the laser.* The laser should be backed up to a spot size of 1.5 to 2.0 mm. Because no cutting effect is desired, the power density

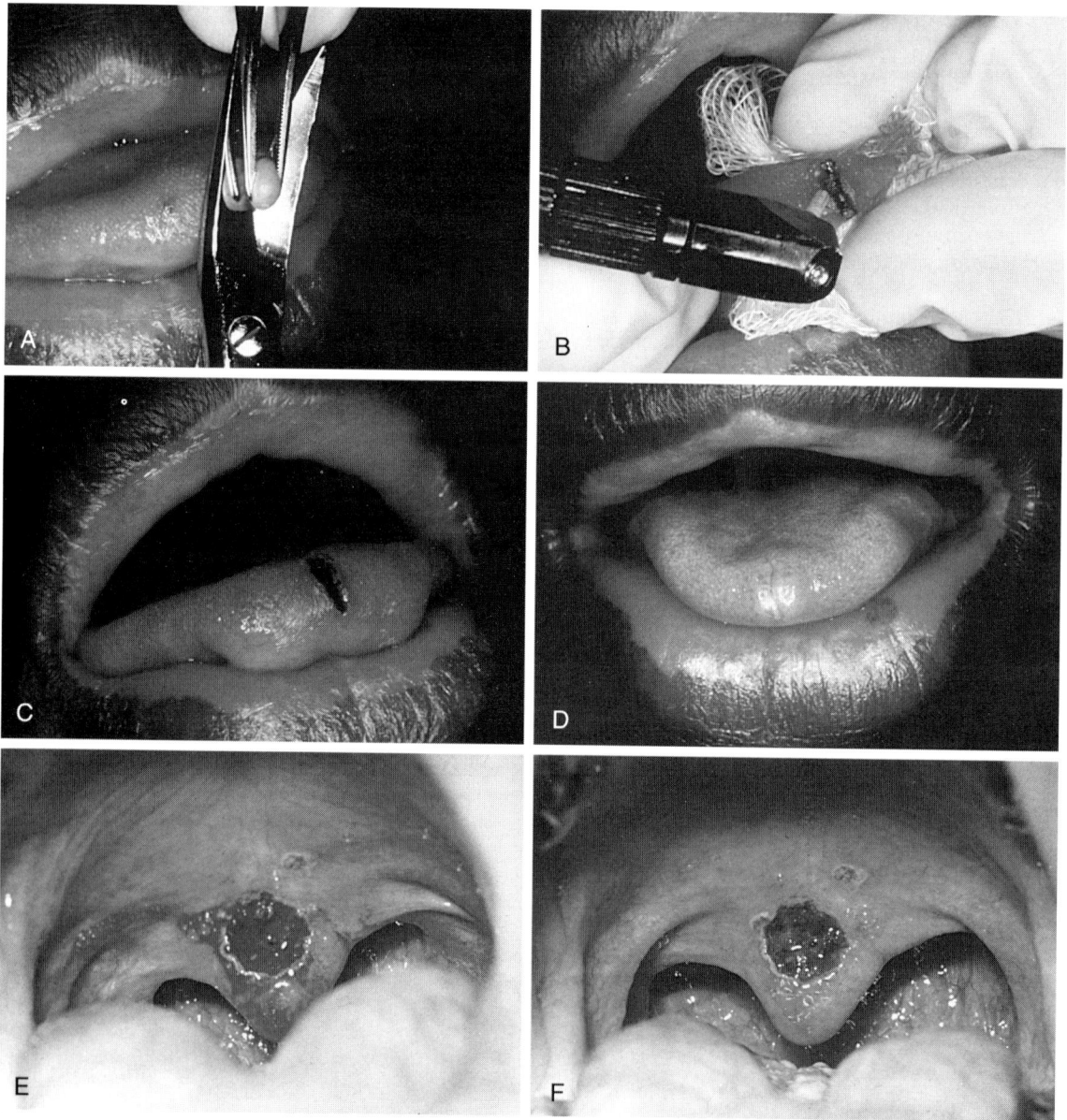

FIGURE 7–17. *A to D,* Fibroma of the tongue removed by sharp excision. The laser is then slightly defocused and used at low power to coagulate the biopsy site. Some initial hemostasis should be obtained by direct pressure prior to using the laser. *E,* Soft palate bleeding after tissue removal with biopsy forceps. *F,* Immediately following this procedure, laser hemostasis is performed using 4 watts in slightly defocused mode.

needed is relatively low and can be obtained with power levels in the range of 4 to 5 watts.

4. *Sweep the bed of the wound.* The wound can be lasered in the standard criss-cross pattern (as one would do for a lesion ablation) for a generalized hemostatic effect, or the beam can be aimed at a specific bleeding area for direct hemostasis. Either of these methods may be performed in continuous fashion or any repeat mode. Repeat the lasering as needed to obtain satisfactory hemostasis. Continued bleeding indicates a vessel larger than 500 microns (which requires an alternative hemostatic technique), too-rapid lasering to allow coagulation, too low a power density, or excessive blood in the lasing field.

Finally, although the carbon dioxide laser is the most common wavelength used in oral and maxillofacial surgery owing to its excellent absorption by water-containing tissues such as mucosa and skin, when working on large lesions with significant vascularity, such as a hemangioma, consider a laser wavelength that is more specific for the hemoglobin chromophore and has deeper tissue penetration than does the carbon dioxide laser, such as the argon, Nd:YAG, or KTP:YAG laser.

PITFALLS OF LASER INCISIONAL, EXCISIONAL, AND VAPORIZATIONAL TECHNIQUES

The use of the laser for incisional and excisional biopsy is generally safe, reliable, and predictable. There are, however, a few complications that can result from improper or careless use of the machine, violation of standard safety rules, ignorance of the basic principles of pathology management, or lack of forethought.

Some of the complications include

1. *Injury to adjacent tissues.* Because of the often confined area involved in incisional biopsy or small lesion excision, injury to adjacent uninvolved tissue may occur. It must be remembered that the laser can travel several millimeters if unimpeded by an appropriate tissue or other chromophore. The magnitude of this effect depends on the type of delivery system used and the power being applied and can be prevented by surrounding the lesion or biopsy site with wet gauze (Fig. 7–18*A* and *B*). In addition, the laser should always be aimed at the center of the lesion or biopsy site, never toward the adjacent tissues.

2. *Inadequate lateral margins.* If the biopsy width is too small, lateral thermal damage to the specimen may make histologic diagnosis difficult. This problem can be prevented by taking at least an additional 0.5 mm on either side of the specimen, as mentioned previously. This also makes physical delivery of the specimen easier.

3. *Impingement on the lesion.* It is the natural tendency for the surgeon to angle the head of the laser handpiece to allow direct visualization of the incision. Because of the nontactile nature of laser surgery, it is possible for the beam to unintentionally impinge on the lesion at its deep aspect. This is easily prevented by keeping the beam perpendicular to the surface until the desired depth of incision is obtained (Fig. 7–19).

4. *Inadequate deep margin.* After incising to the desired depth laterally, the specimen is undermined and removed. If this undermining is not kept at the same depth along its distance, accidental impingement on the deep aspect of the specimen may occur. This is usually the most common margin error in lesion excision and must be carefully considered when performing surgery (Fig. 7–20).

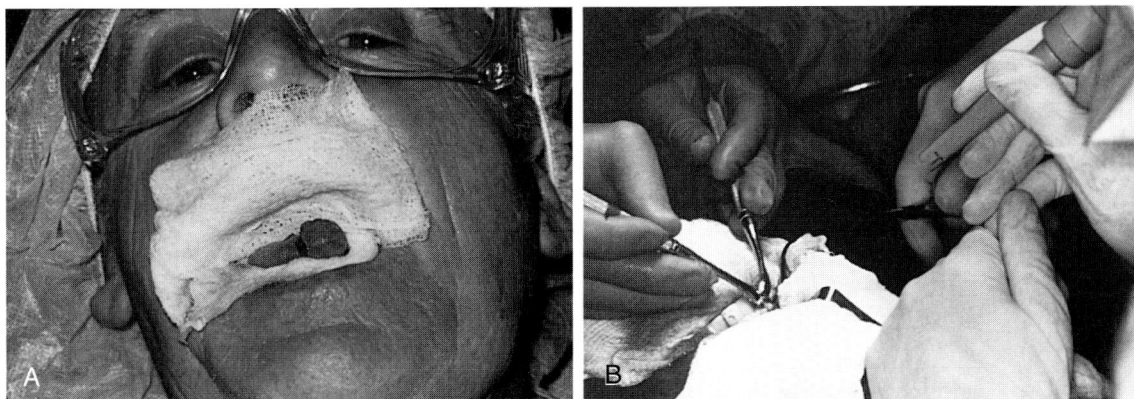

FIGURE 7–18. *A* and *B,* Wet gauze may be used to isolate the laser surgical site. The water absorbs any stray carbon dioxide laser energy. Wet neurosurgical patties, plastic teeth protectors, Freer or periosteal elevators, and wet tongue blades may also be useful to protect adjacent structures from damage and safely retract tissues.

5. *Excessive heat generation.* Some charring of tissue is inevitable with the carbon dioxide laser (although this may be diminished by superpulsing, ultrapulsing, or other special techniques). The problem with charring is that the carbon dioxide laser functions primarily by vaporization of cellular water. Lasering the charred area, which is the dehydrated organic matrix left behind after cellular water vaporization, merely leads to burning of the tissue (even to the point of incineration) and excessive heat generation. This is easily corrected, however, by limiting the exposure time and removing the char by wiping the area with wet gauze intermittently during the procedure.

6. *Excessive defocusing of the laser.* Owing to the peculiar multimodal cross-sectional distribution of hollow wave guide beams, excessive defocusing of the laser leads to the beam being split into several small spots rather than a single beam spot, which can lead to inconsistent vaporization and ablation. This problem varies widely depending on the size of the hollow waveguide and the delivery tip but begins at approximately 1.5 to 2.0 cm beyond the focal point for most hollow waveguide systems (see Fig. 7–7D). This is not as great a problem with articulated arm systems, which usually have a uniform cross-sectional beam configuration (i.e., TEM_{00}). Articulated-arm systems generally just lose power density as they are defocused, but the beam will not break apart. It is also not a

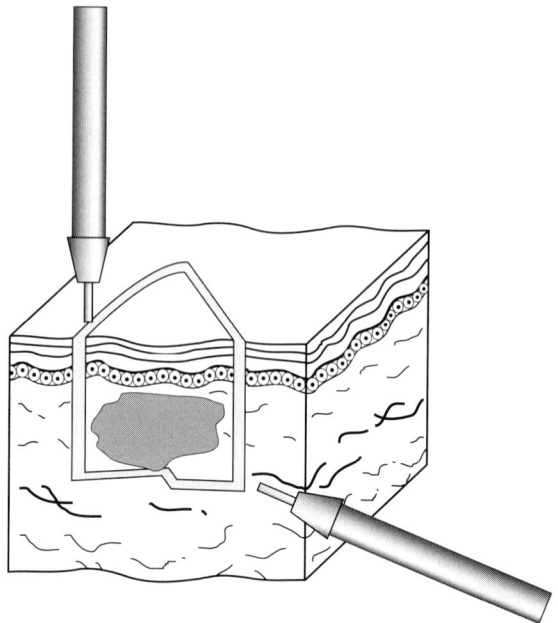

FIGURE 7–20. Because the laser provides no tactile sensation, undermining a lesion must be done with great care to stay in a level plane. Failure to maintain this plane could result in accidental impingement on the deep aspect of the lesion.

problem with contact Nd:YAG lasers, with which significant defocusing is not usually performed.

7. *Accidental defocusing.* When using the laser for incisional or excisional biopsy it is generally used in the focused mode to maintain the smallest spot size. It should be remembered, however, that as the incision is deepened, the laser is progressively moving farther from the base of the incision and, therefore, is defocusing at the same time. This will result in wide ablation and loss of power density at the base of the incision rather than precise cutting. In order to maintain the smallest possible spot size, the laser must be inserted into the incision as the wound is deepened.

LASER MANAGEMENT OF DISCRETE LESIONS BY ANATOMIC REGION

Tongue

There are few anatomic areas where the use of the laser is more suited than the tongue. The tongue's high vascularity and sensitivity to electrical stimuli make the laser's hemostatic and nonelectric nature invaluable in treating benign, premalignant, and malignant lesions.

Although premalignant lesions of the tongue are often treated using vaporizational techniques, benign lesions are most often treated by excision. This

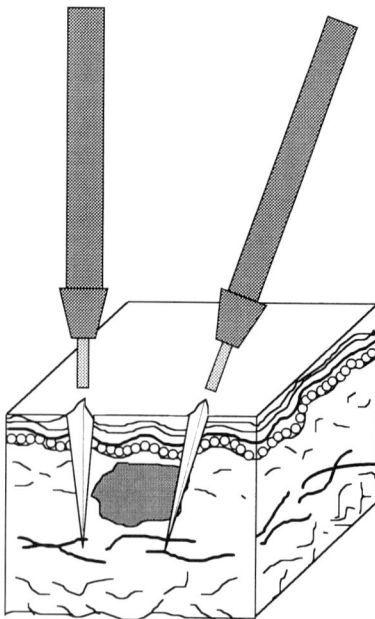

FIGURE 7–19. Just as with a scalpel, holding the laser at an angle to the tissue may result in unexpected impingement on the lesion at its deep lateral aspect. This can be prevented by always holding the laser perpendicularly to tissue.

is due to the fact that benign tongue lesions are usually discrete, pedunculated, or sessile, and often show extension toward the tongue musculature. This clinical presentation is more quickly and efficiently excised than ablated. Small lesions, however, may be effectively treated by either technique.

Benign lesions of the tongue amenable to laser treatment include

- Fibroma
- Papilloma
- Granular cell tumor (granular cell myoblastoma)
- Lingual thyroid nodule
- Hemangioma
- Lymphangioma
- Lingual tonsil
- Pyogenic granuloma
- Lipoma
- Aphthous ulcer

The tongue responds well to the laser, and powers in the range of 6 to 8 watts are usually adequate for most procedures (at a 0.35-mm spot size). For deeper lesions of the tongue, higher powers (i.e., 8 to 10 watts) speed up the procedure and are justified as long as control of the excision is maintained. Bleeding is well controlled with the laser in this region, and the tongue musculature is not stimulated by the beam.

Healing of tongue wounds is rapid, and suture closing is most often unnecessary. In fact, the sutures are often more distressing to the patient than the open laser wound. Even large, deep tongue wounds heal well with minimal deformity, scar contracture, or functional impairment of tongue movement. The management of aphthous ulcers in this region with carbon dioxide laser irradiation has been previously documented,[13] and its use in extensive ulceration secondary to chemotherapy mucositis is also being examined.

CASE HISTORIES

1. **Figure 7–21:** A 15-year-old with hemangioma of the left dorsum of the tongue. The lesion was first outlined with the carbon dioxide laser at 6 watts, 10 millisecond pulses, and 10 pulses per second. Continuous lasering at 6 watts was then used to deepen the outline to below the depth of the lesion and then to undermine and remove the lesion. Note the lack of bleeding. No sutures were placed. This patient had no postoperative discomfort or swelling and was discharged from the clinic immediately after surgery.

2. **Figure 7–22:** A 60-year-old woman 6 weeks after excision of squamous cell carcinoma of the tongue with a small area of nodular growth. Excisional biopsy of the lesion was car-

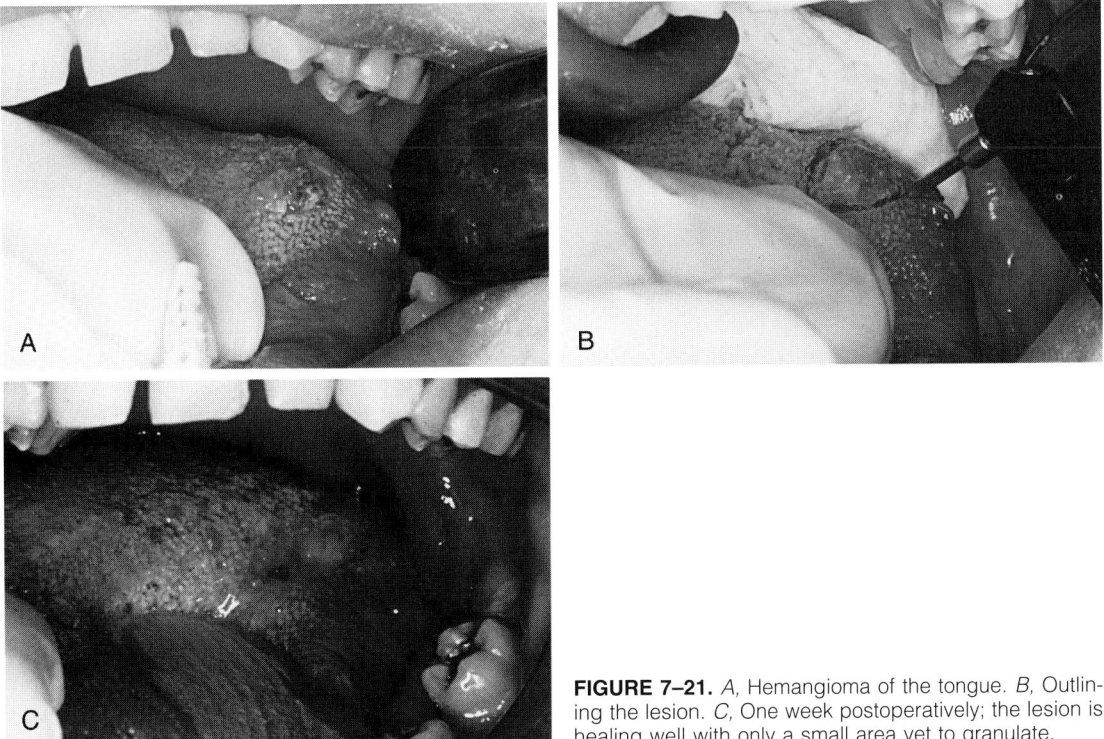

FIGURE 7–21. *A*, Hemangioma of the tongue. *B*, Outlining the lesion. *C*, One week postoperatively; the lesion is healing well with only a small area yet to granulate.

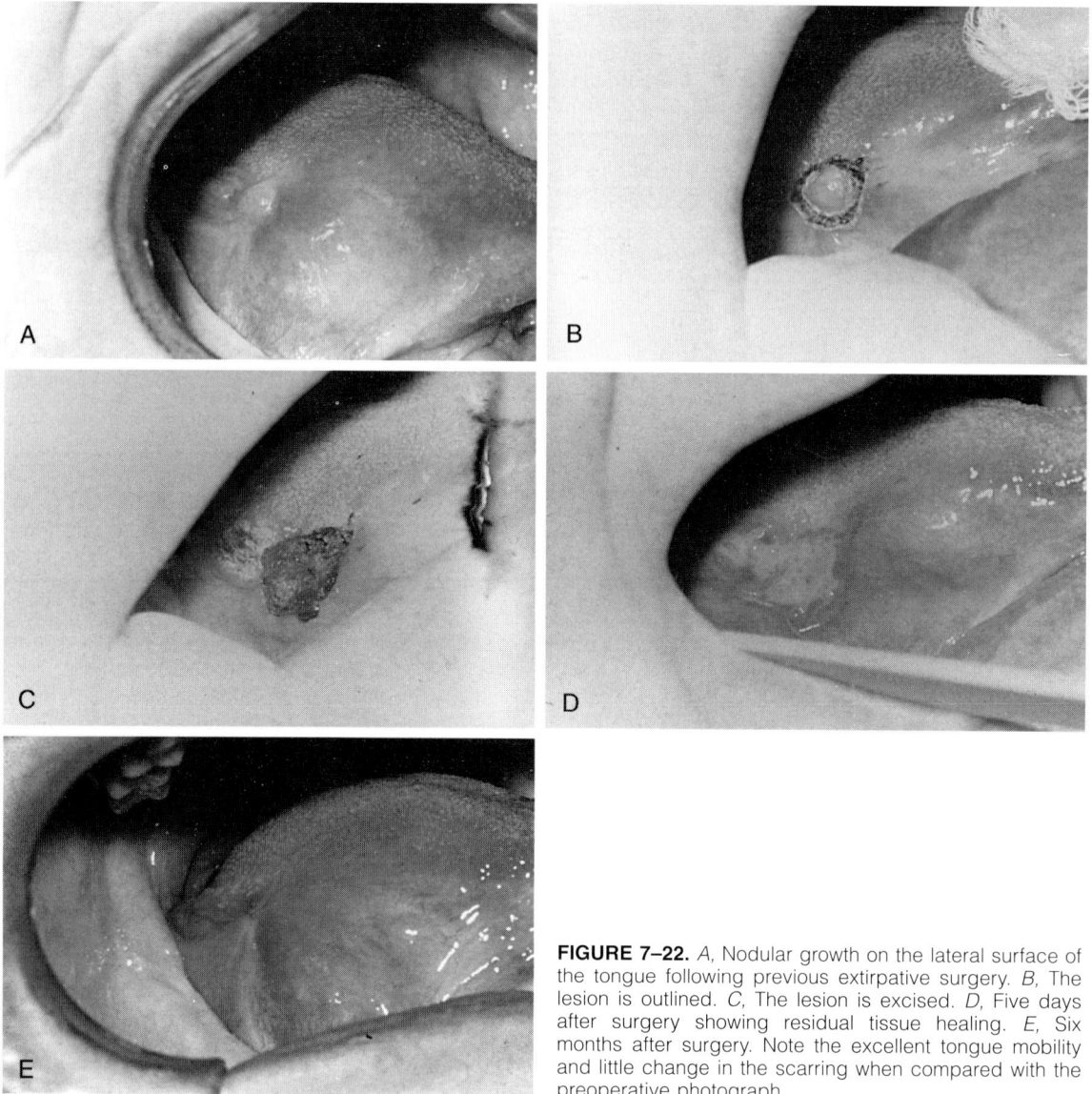

FIGURE 7–22. *A,* Nodular growth on the lateral surface of the tongue following previous extirpative surgery. *B,* The lesion is outlined. *C,* The lesion is excised. *D,* Five days after surgery showing residual tissue healing. *E,* Six months after surgery. Note the excellent tongue mobility and little change in the scarring when compared with the preoperative photograph.

ried out with the carbon dioxide laser using 8 watts of continuous power after outlining the lesion with intermittent pulses of 20 milliseconds each. The lesion was identified as a pyogenic granuloma, and healing ensued uneventfully.

3. Figure 7–23: A patient with a painful ulcer of the tongue. The lesion was anesthetized with topical anesthesia and lasered continuously at 2 watts in a slightly defocused mode. After lasing the entire surface lightly, the patient's discomfort improved significantly, although healing of the ulcer was unaffected.

Lips

Because there is direct access to the lips, they are easily treated by laser surgical procedures. De-

pending on the type of lesion, both excisional and vaporization techniques may be used, and specific consideration must be given to each case. Because of the esthetic importance of the lips, the discrete anatomic borders such as the vermilion border, and their functional importance, the use of lasers for treatment in this region has some important benefits. The use of conservative vaporization, where appropriate, may dramatically enhance the cosmetic and functional result of pathology surgery by decreasing the size of the wound and by obviating the need in many cases for traversing across the ever-important anatomic borders with the wound margins. This is seen most dramatically for treatment of actinic cheilitis of the lip. The traditional treatment using the lip shave procedure is often bloody, painful, and cosmetically challenging. The laser may be used

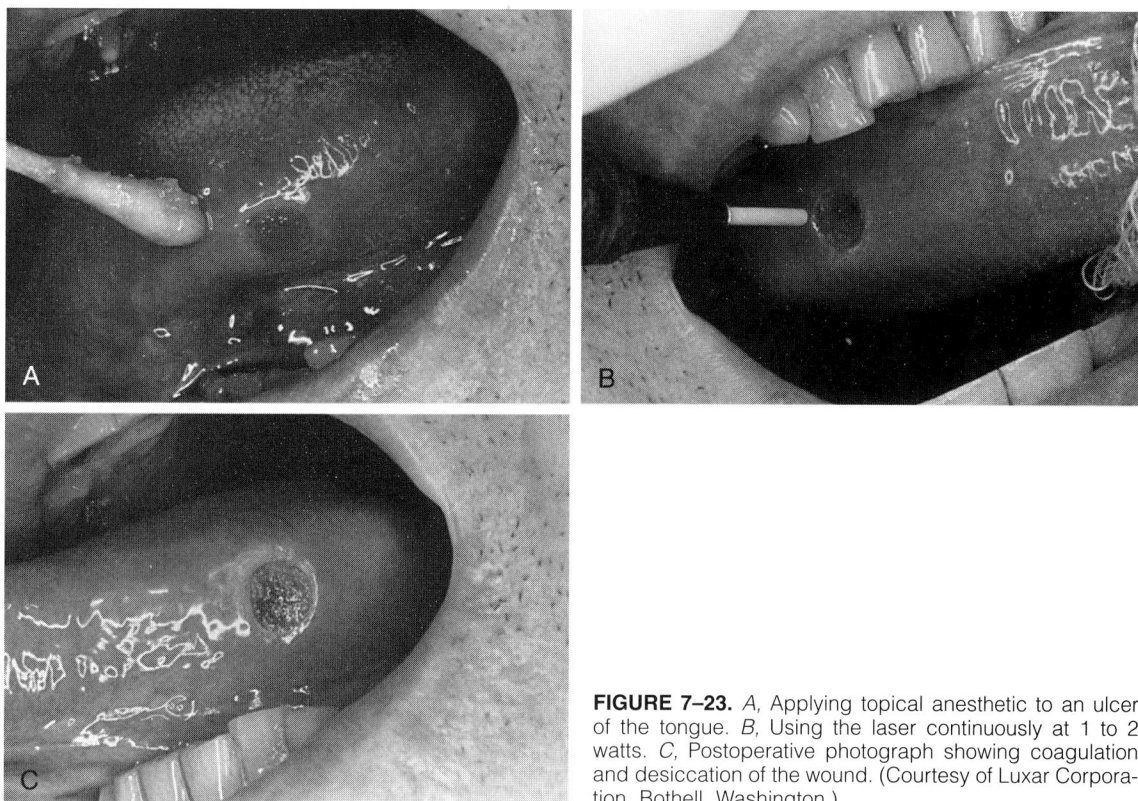

FIGURE 7–23. *A,* Applying topical anesthetic to an ulcer of the tongue. *B,* Using the laser continuously at 1 to 2 watts. *C,* Postoperative photograph showing coagulation and desiccation of the wound. (Courtesy of Luxar Corporation, Bothell, Washington.)

for a laser peel of the lip when biopsies indicate that removal of the epithelium is adequate.[14]

Care should be exercised when operating with the laser on the lips owing to the differential effect on the tissues anterior and posterior to the wet line. Slightly higher power and energy densities may be required in the drier areas to prevent uneven effects across the two types of tissue. Although this difference is usually small, it is a good point to remember.

Some lesions of the lips amenable to laser surgery include

- Mucocele
- Pyogenic granuloma
- Fibroma
- Actinic cheilitis
- Hemangioma
- Aphthous ulcers

Because of the obvious cosmetic deformity that can result from large excisions of lip lesions, suture closure may be indicated in these cases. This is necessary when excision approaches the vermilion border, and an obvious wedge defect is created. Suture closure in this region is usually more cosmetic and is therefore often indicated. Conversely, when ablative procedures are used, scarring and

cosmetic deformity are minimized and no sutures are necessary.

CASE HISTORIES

1. Figure 7–24: A 16-year-old boy with a mucocele of the lower lip. This may either be excised with the gland or the surface and the gland may be vaporized. This lesion was undermined and excised using 6 watts of continuous power after outlining the lesion with 6 watts of power, 10 millisecond pulses, and 10 pulses per second. The lack of bleeding made visualization and dissection of the mucocele easy.

2. Figure 7–25: Hemangioma of the tongue treated by excision with the carbon dioxide laser and sealing of the feeding vessels. This is accomplished in exactly the same fashion as the mucocele in Figure 7–24. This lesion would also have been amenable to treatment by ablation techniques using the Nd:YAG or argon lasers. In this case, cosmesis was an issue and suturing was performed without difficulty.

3. Figure 7–26: Small hemangioma of the lip. In this case, it was decided that the lesion was small enough to vaporize at 6 watts, 200 millisec-

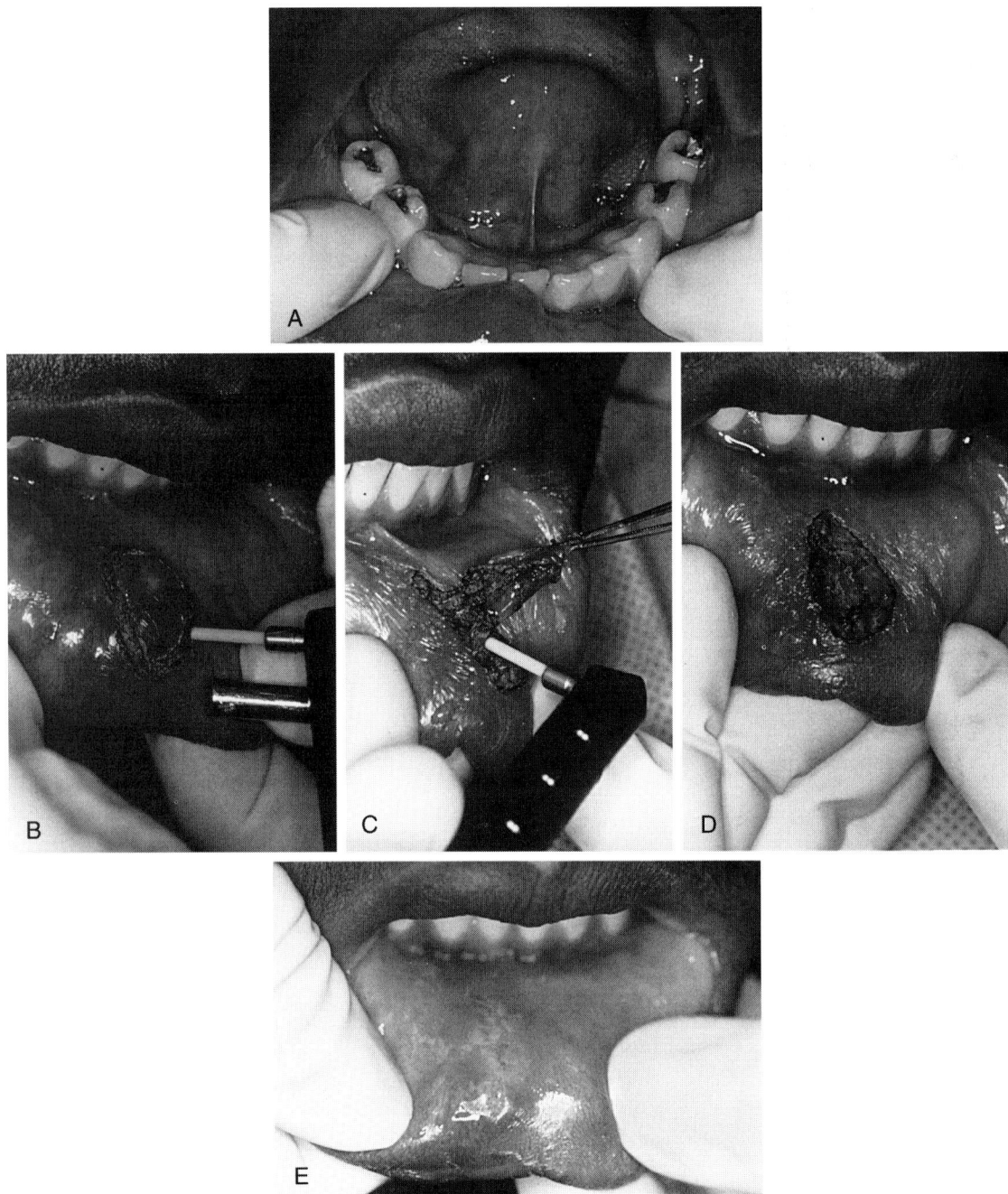

FIGURE 7–24. *A,* Mucocele of the lower lip. *B,* Outlining the lesion. *C,* Undermining the lesion. Note the visibility of the mucocele wall and the mucus draining from the lesion. This is possible due to the bloodless nature of the field. *D,* The lesion excised. *E,* 1 week postoperatively.

ond pulses, and two pulses/second, and to secondarily coagulate the bleeding vessels at the base of the wound. This technique should be reserved for small lesions only. Laser hemostasis was obtained by controlling bleeding initially with pressure and then coagulating the vessel itself in a slightly defocused mode using 4 to 6 watts of power.

Buccal Mucosa

The main advantage of the laser in treating lesions of the buccal mucosa is its ability to manage extremely large lesions without significant deformity. Either vaporization or excisional techniques may be used effectively for the management of benign lesions in this region. Because of the high

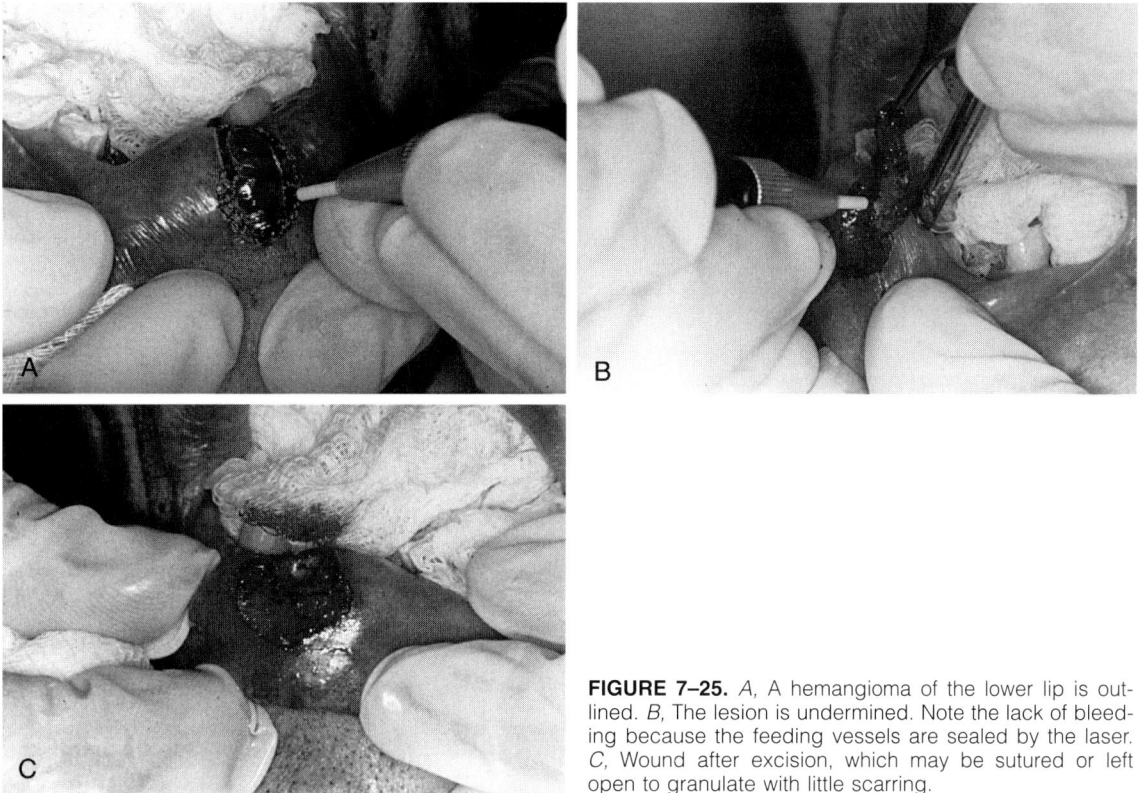

FIGURE 7–25. *A,* A hemangioma of the lower lip is outlined. *B,* The lesion is undermined. Note the lack of bleeding because the feeding vessels are sealed by the laser. *C,* Wound after excision, which may be sutured or left open to granulate with little scarring.

water content of these tissues, low-power densities in the range of 4 to 6 watts with spot size of 0.35 mm or less for excision and 4 to 6 watts with a spot size of 1 to 2 mm for ablation are usually sufficient for treatment. When treating larger lesions using an articulated arm delivery system, larger spot sizes are possible and may facilitate speedy and homogeneous treatment. Using right-angle handpiece tips for the hollow waveguide or right-angle mirror attachments for the articulated arm systems aids in obtaining accurate incisions and ablations in the superior, inferior, and posterior aspects of the buccal mucosa, where direct-line access may be difficult.

Lesions of the buccal mucosa treatable with the laser include

- Hyperkeratosis/dysplasia
- Fibroma
- Pyogenic granuloma
- Hemangioma/lymphangioma
- Salivary gland tumors
- Hyperplastic tissue, scar tissue
- Lichen planus

Although the great distensibility of the buccal mucosa allows for simple closure of even the largest of lesions, there is usually no need for closure at all. Because cosmesis generally is not an issue in this case, closure usually only prolongs the surgery

and increases the possible problems caused by the closure. In addition, suturing near the commissure or Stensen's duct may cause postsurgical deformity and subsequent functional disturbance. Laser wounds of the buccal mucosa commonly heal with little or no contractile scarring, and lasering in this region generally causes no impairment in parotid salivary flow or distortion of the commissure. Lichen planus, a dermatologic disease, is generally treated only when it is erosive or symptomatic. Recurrence may occur, of course, owing to the systemic nature of the disease, but treatment is often useful in decreasing number and the severity of the symptoms and in excising a particular area of erosive lichen planus (which may have a higher incidence of malignant conversion).[15]

CASE HISTORIES

1. Figure 7–27: A 60-year-old woman with a long history of betel nut chewing and a firm, fibrotic buccal mucosa. Incisional biopsy with the carbon dioxide laser was performed for diagnostic reasons. The lesion was outlined in the usual fashion at 6 watts, 2 to 10 pulses per second, and 10 to 20 milliseconds per pulse. Continuous lasering at 8 watts was then used to deepen the outline and undermine the lesion for removal.

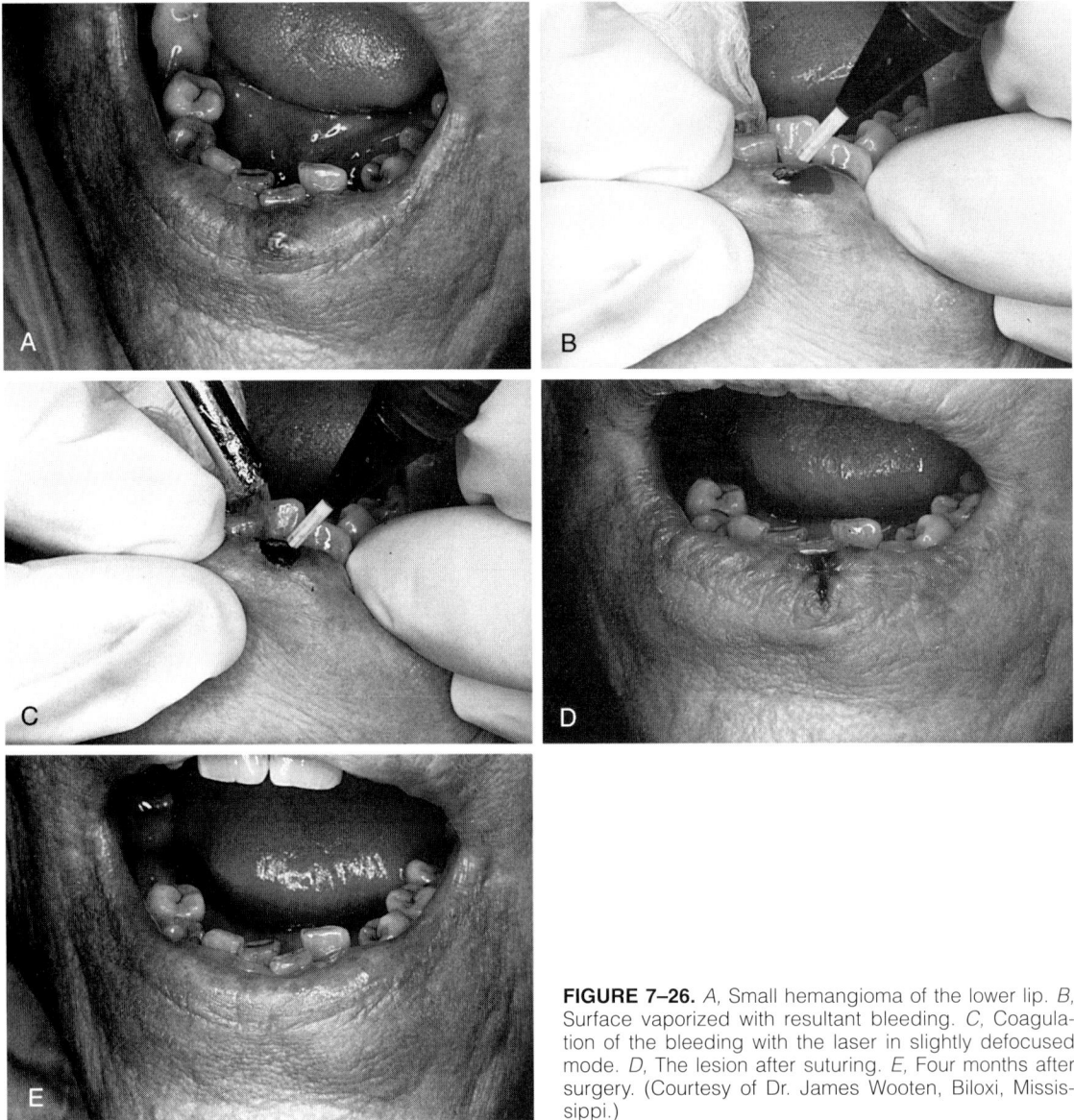

FIGURE 7–26. *A,* Small hemangioma of the lower lip. *B,* Surface vaporized with resultant bleeding. *C,* Coagulation of the bleeding with the laser in slightly defocused mode. *D,* The lesion after suturing. *E,* Four months after surgery. (Courtesy of Dr. James Wooten, Biloxi, Mississippi.)

Although this would normally only require approximately 6 watts to accomplish, the fibrotic nature of the mucosa, with its decreased water content, necessitates the higher power density for adequate cutting ability. The lesion was left unsutured and healed well. As is typical in laser wounds, some scarring may be evident, but it is usually soft, pliable, and noncontractile. The diagnosis of submucous fibrosis was confirmed.

2. Figure 7–28: A 52-year-old woman with a fibroma of the buccal mucosa at the commissure. The lesion was outlined and excised in the routine fashion and left unsutured. The patient had no postoperative discomfort or morbidity despite the sensitive location. Because of the minimal scarring, lesions near important functional struc-

tures, such as the commissure, can be treated easily without fear of causing undue cosmetic or functional effects. Although advocated by some authors, in this case (and in most cases by this author's choice), no light char layer was placed on the final wound bed.

Floor of Mouth

Difficult access, prominent vascularity leading to vision-obstructing bleeding, and extreme tissue distensibility often make scalpel surgery of the floor of the mouth a tedious and difficult task. The hemostasis and nontactile surgical nature of the laser, therefore, favor its use in this anatomic region.

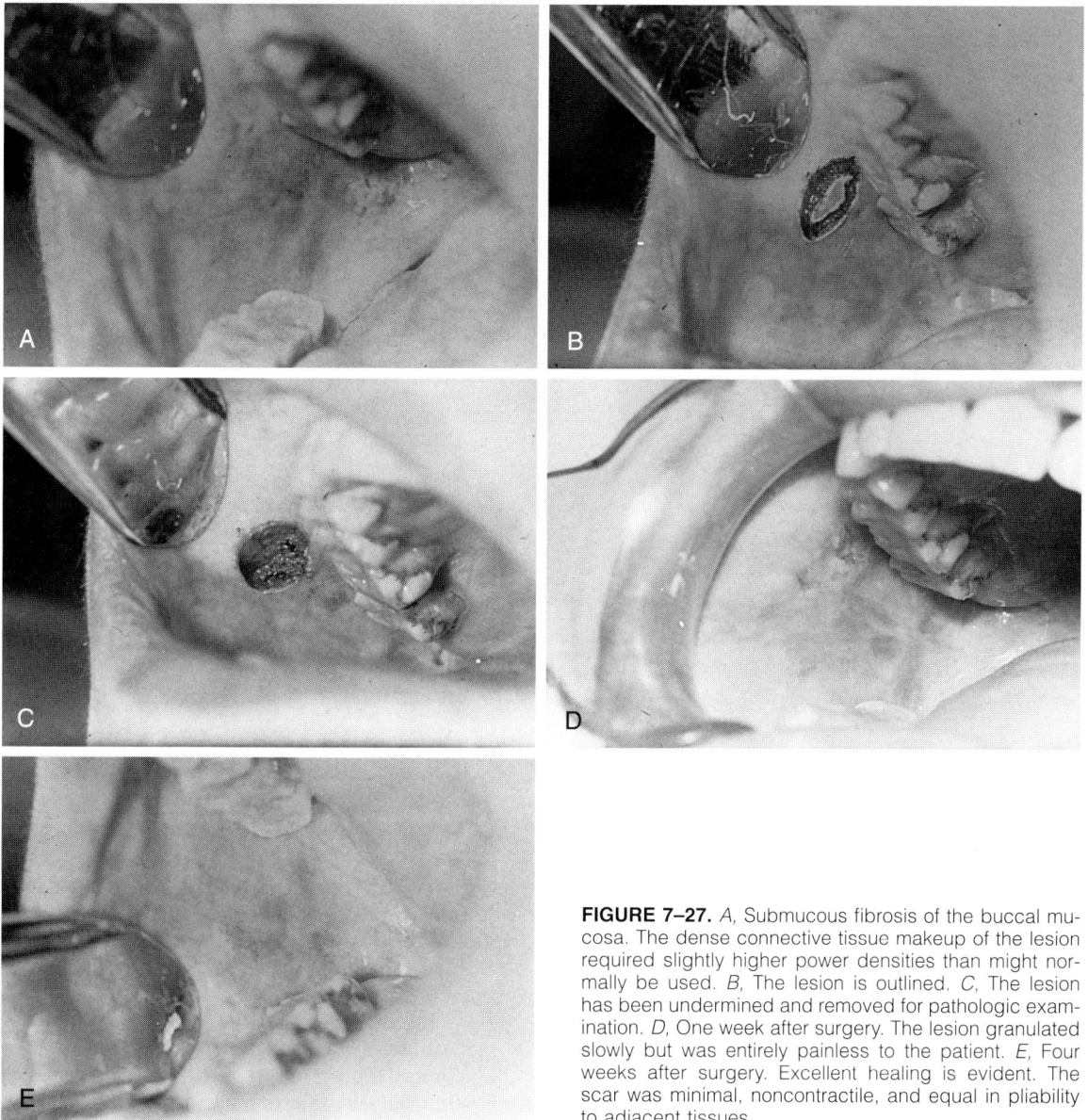

FIGURE 7–27. *A,* Submucous fibrosis of the buccal mucosa. The dense connective tissue makeup of the lesion required slightly higher power densities than might normally be used. *B,* The lesion is outlined. *C,* The lesion has been undermined and removed for pathologic examination. *D,* One week after surgery. The lesion granulated slowly but was entirely painless to the patient. *E,* Four weeks after surgery. Excellent healing is evident. The scar was minimal, noncontractile, and equal in pliability to adjacent tissues.

Carbon dioxide hollow waveguide handpieces with contra-angle heads or curved guide tips, or fiberoptic Nd:YAG handpieces make surgery in this area simple. Articulated-arm carbon dioxide lasers may require a right-angle mirror attachment to allow access to the floor of the mouth; however, not all articulated-arm machines have such attachments, and straight handpieces are sometimes difficult to use for this purpose.

The thin nature of the tissues in this region and the nonkeratinized surface suggest that modest power densities should be used. Powers in the range of 4 to 6 watts of carbon dioxide energy in focused mode (0.1 to 0.35 mm) or 6 to 8 watts in defocused mode (1.5 to 3.0 mm) are usually sufficient for excellent cutting and ablating effects, respectively.

A major area of concern in the floor of the mouth is the proximity to underlying anatomic structures, such as the submandibular duct and lingual nerve. Although the laser's unique ability to ablate rather than excise selected appropriate lesions minimizes the danger, and its hemostatic properties afford excellent visibility and avoidance of important structures during surgery, it is nevertheless a legitimate concern. The evidence appears to indicate that even severing of the submandibular duct will not impede salivary flow. This subject is covered in greater detail later in this chapter.

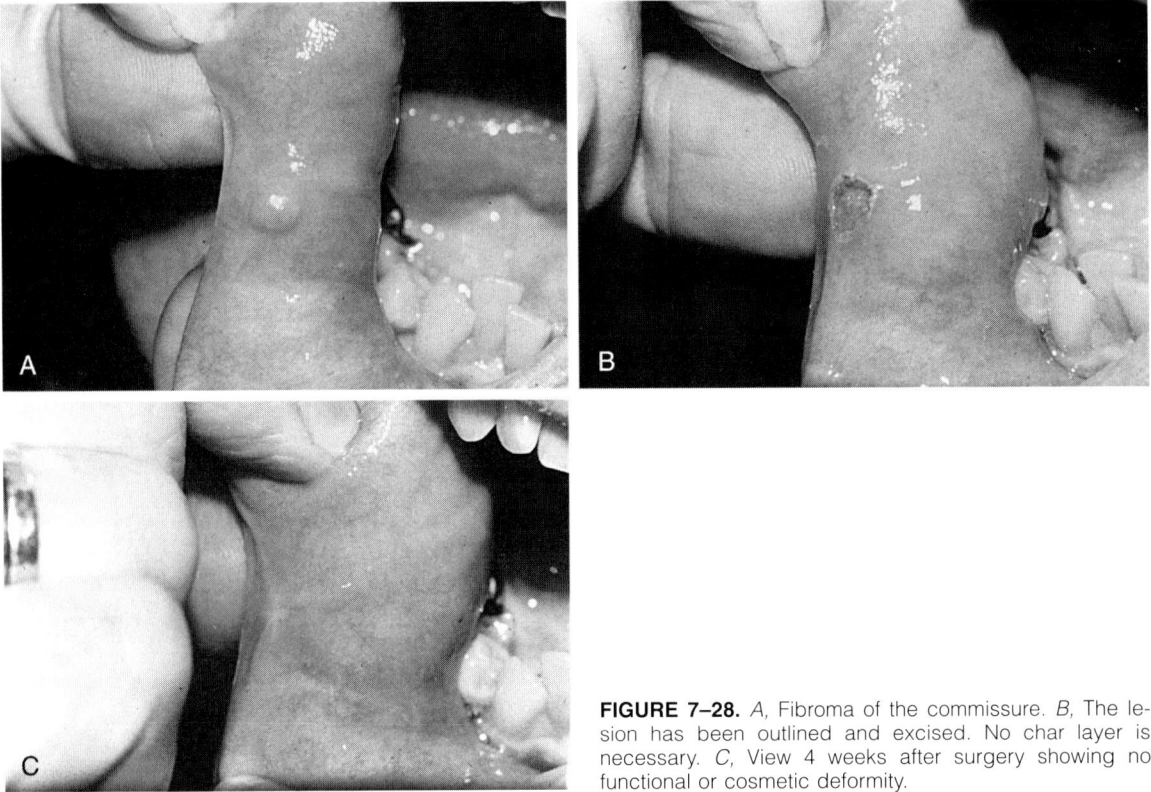

FIGURE 7–28. *A,* Fibroma of the commissure. *B,* The lesion has been outlined and excised. No char layer is necessary. *C,* View 4 weeks after surgery showing no functional or cosmetic deformity.

One major advantage of the use of the laser in the floor of the mouth is the diminished cicatrix formation seen postoperatively. Even large lesions may be effectively treated without restriction of mobility of the tongue. Mucosal or skin grafts to prevent cicatrix formation are unnecessary with use of the laser and are less likely to survive owing to the minimal imbibition possible from the lasered graft recipient site.

Some lesions treatable by laser include

- "Ranula" (mucous escape phenomenon)
- Salivary gland tumors
- Sialolithiasis
- Hemangioma
- Lymphangioma
- Dysplasia/leukoplakia
- Ankyloglossia

CASE HISTORIES

1. Figure 7–29: A 39-year-old woman with a 1 cm sialolith of Wharton's duct. The stone was not palpable in the floor of the mouth. The carbon dioxide laser was used at 4 watts in continuous fashion to make an incision over the duct. When the stone was reached, a small flash of light was seen, indicating the location of the sialolith. Brief lasering on either side of the sialolith enabled easy visualization and access to the stone, which was then removed with a forceps. No suturing was necessary, and healing was uneventful.

2. Figure 7–30: A 17-year-old boy with ankyloglossia. The carbon dioxide laser was used at 4 watts in slightly defocused mode to ablate the frenum. Depending on the surgeon's level of controllability, this may be performed either continuously or intermittently at 2 to 20 pulses per second, 20 to 200 milliseconds per pulse. Upward traction of the tongue is very useful in aiding dissection with the laser.

3. Figure 7–31: A Moderate-sized "ranula" in the floor of the mouth. The carbon dioxide laser may be used to marsupialize the lesion. The dome is grasped with forceps, and the laser is used to first outline the periphery of the lesion in continuous or intermittent fashion, then continuously at 4 to 8 watts to excise the dome. The base of the ranula is then lasered to obtain a hemostatic field. No suturing is necessary, and the wound heals without difficulty. Definitive treatment of the pseudocyst, if desired, involves excision of the offending sublingual salivary gland with or without the use of a laser modality.

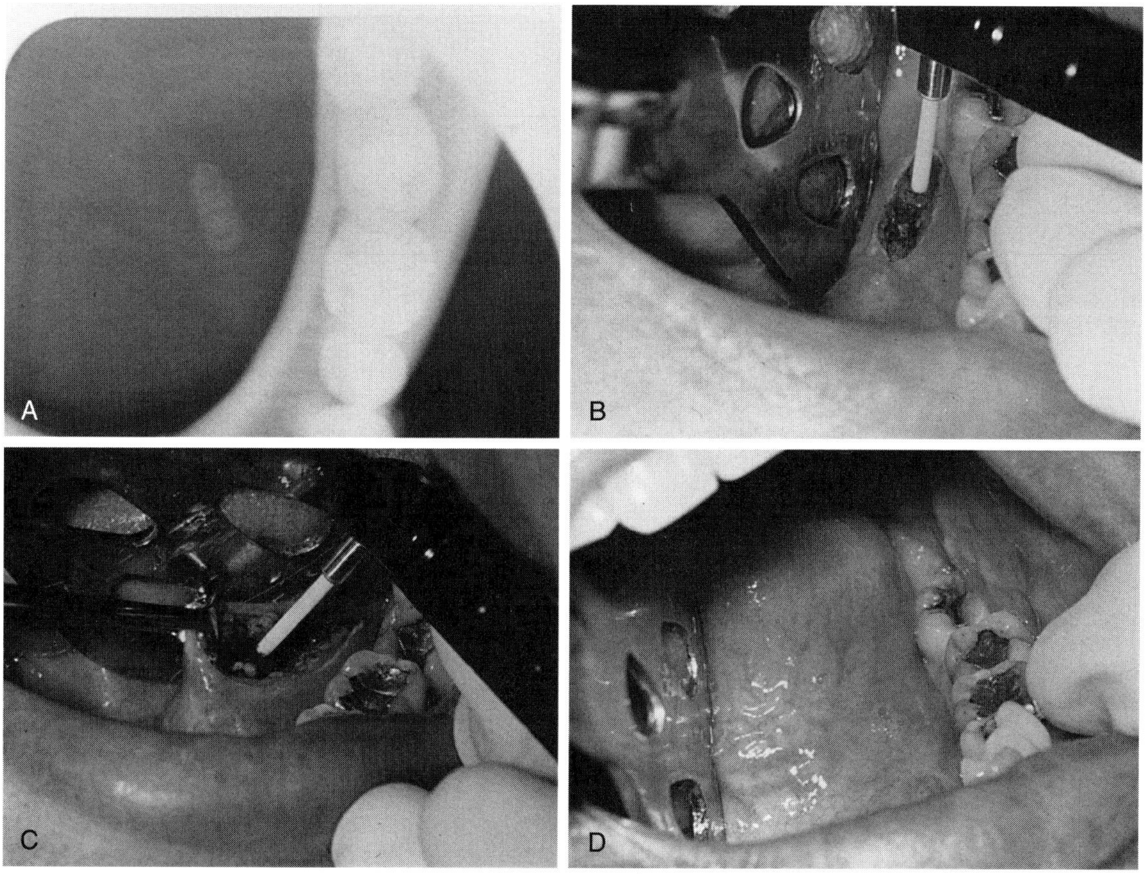

FIGURE 7–29. *A,* Radiograph of stone in Wharton's duct. *B,* Incision parallel to anticipated duct location. *C,* The stone is isolated by the flash of light seen when it is subjected to the laser. Minimal exposure to the laser on either side of the stone then delivers the sialolith; the wound is left unsutured. *D,* Four weeks after surgery, excellent healing is seen.

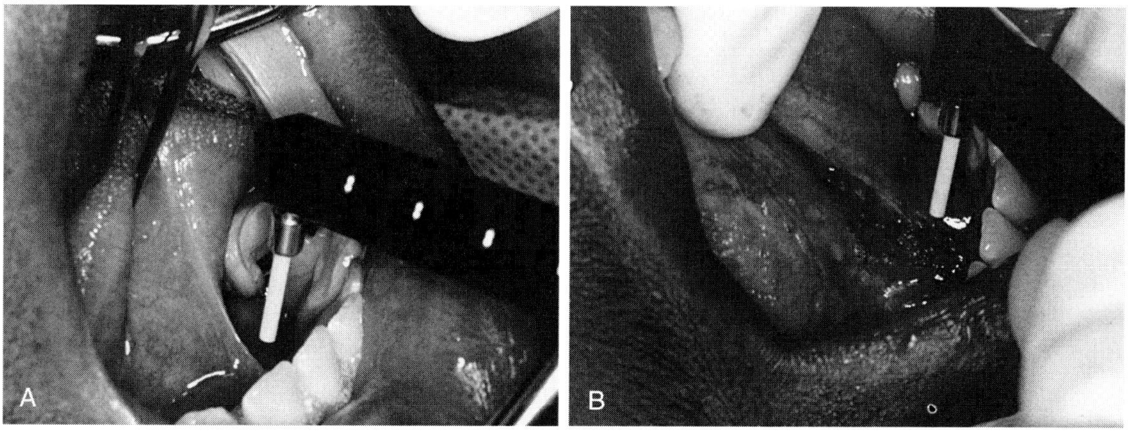

FIGURE 7–30. *A,* Ankylosis resulting from lingual frenum. The laser is slightly defocused while tension is placed on the tongue. *B,* Postoperative view.

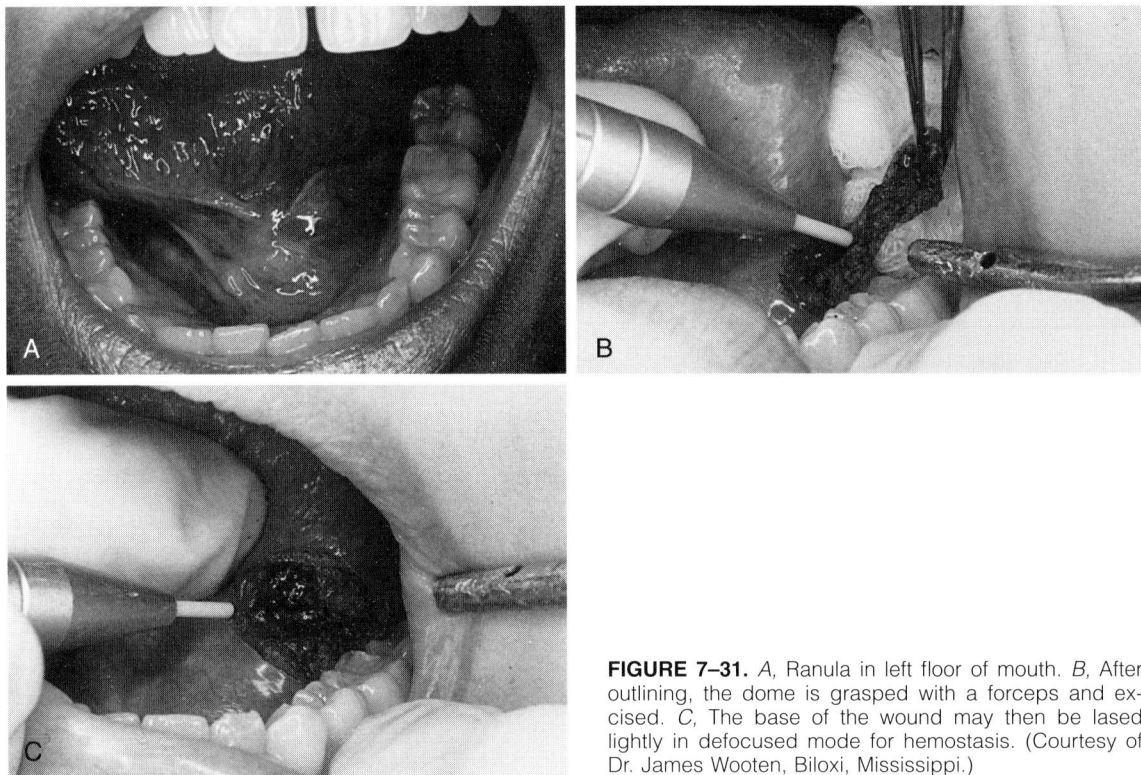

FIGURE 7–31. *A,* Ranula in left floor of mouth. *B,* After outlining, the dome is grasped with a forceps and excised. *C,* The base of the wound may then be lased lightly in defocused mode for hemostasis. (Courtesy of Dr. James Wooten, Biloxi, Mississippi.)

Gingiva

As with the hard palate, great care must be exercised when treating lesions of the gingiva owing to the proximity of the underlying bone. Failure to avoid bone exposure will lead to osseous necrosis and prolonged healing. Another danger posed by this region is the close relationship to the teeth. Carbon dioxide laser energy applied to teeth with energy densities greater than 1 joule (1 watt for 1 second using a 1-mm spot size) can lead to reversible enamel damage, and greater than 4 joules using a 1-mm spot size can lead to pulpal damage. This corresponds to an increase in pulpal temperature of 5°F (-2.35°C). Nd:YAG noncontact irradiation (with less absorption by hydroxylapatite) may not cause visible enamel damage but may lead to pulpal damage by direct penetration of the Nd:YAG wavelength through enamel and normal dentin to its likely chromophore, hemoglobin.

Owing to the differential effect of the laser on keratinized and nonkeratinized tissue, this factor must be taken into account when treating lesions that cross the mucogingival junction. Greater depth of effect will be seen on the nonkeratinized mucosa, and an uneven effect may be seen if equal power densities are applied to both nonkeratinized and keratinized tissues.

Because of these concerns and despite the kera-

tinized nature of the gingiva, modest power densities are recommended. Five to seven watts in focused mode (0.1- to 0.35-mm spot size) or slightly defocused mode (1 to 1.5 mm) will allow for reasonable efficiency and safety. Increasing the spot size slightly when crossing the mucogingival junction into mucosa, or lowering the power 1 to 2 watts, will alter the power density enough to provide a uniform effect across the lesion. In addition, to avoid osseous necrosis when removing full-thickness gingival lesions, it is recommended to use the laser down to the periosteum and then perform any subperiosteal curettage with a periosteal elevator or curette. Superficial lesions, of course, may be treated with the laser alone, and supraperiosteal dissection is actually greatly enhanced by the visibility afforded by the laser's hemostasis. Supraperiosteal dissection in the alveolar mucosa may be made even easier by applying tension to the lip or cheek while using the laser in focused mode for the procedure. This allows the tissue to be literally peeled off the periosteum. The use of the laser for drug-induced hyperplasia may prolong the case a few minutes, but it does provide excellent, long-lasting results.[16] When time is important, a combination of scalpel and laser surgery may be indicated (using the scalpel for rapid debulking and the laser for the finishing and fine aspects).

Gingival lesions amenable to laser surgery include

- Lichen planus
- Pyogenic granuloma
- Peripheral giant cell granuloma
- Fibroma
- Papilloma
- Drug-induced gingival hyperplasia
- Hyperplastic gingival tissue
- Verruca

CASE HISTORIES

1. Figure 7–32: A 28-year-old man with gingival hypertrophy secondary to calcium channel antagonist medication usage. The laser is used for its hemostasis, decreased postoperative discomfort, and minimal scarring. The procedure is performed by first using the laser at 4 to 8 watts in focused mode (i.e., with high-power density) to incise a new gingival margin. The underlying teeth must be well protected with a Freer elevator or metal matrix band. This tissue is then removed. The submarginal hypertrophic tissue is then ablated and sculpted to an appropriate level above the periosteum. This is usually performed with 6 to 10 watts continuously in defocused mode. In cases of massive hypertrophy, consideration should be given to performing a gross excision with a scalpel and then finishing the procedure with the laser for its beneficial effects. In addition, interproximal tissue tags should still be removed manually with a curette for safe and adequate débridement.

2. Figure 7–33: A 10-month-old child with pyogenic granuloma of the gingiva around the lower right deciduous central incisor. Despite the diagnosis, a previous attempt at scalpel surgery for excisional biopsy by another surgeon was met with profuse bleeding, requiring hospital admission. The patient was intubated in the outpatient clinic, and the lesion was outlined and excised using 4 watts of continuous carbon dioxide laser energy. No bleeding was encountered, the patient was discharged immediately, and the area went on to heal uneventfully.

3. Figure 7–34: A 48-year-old woman with an extremely large epulis covering the maxillary ridge. The laser hemostatic properties make the dissection bloodless and more easily visualized. The epulis is excised using 6 watts of continuous

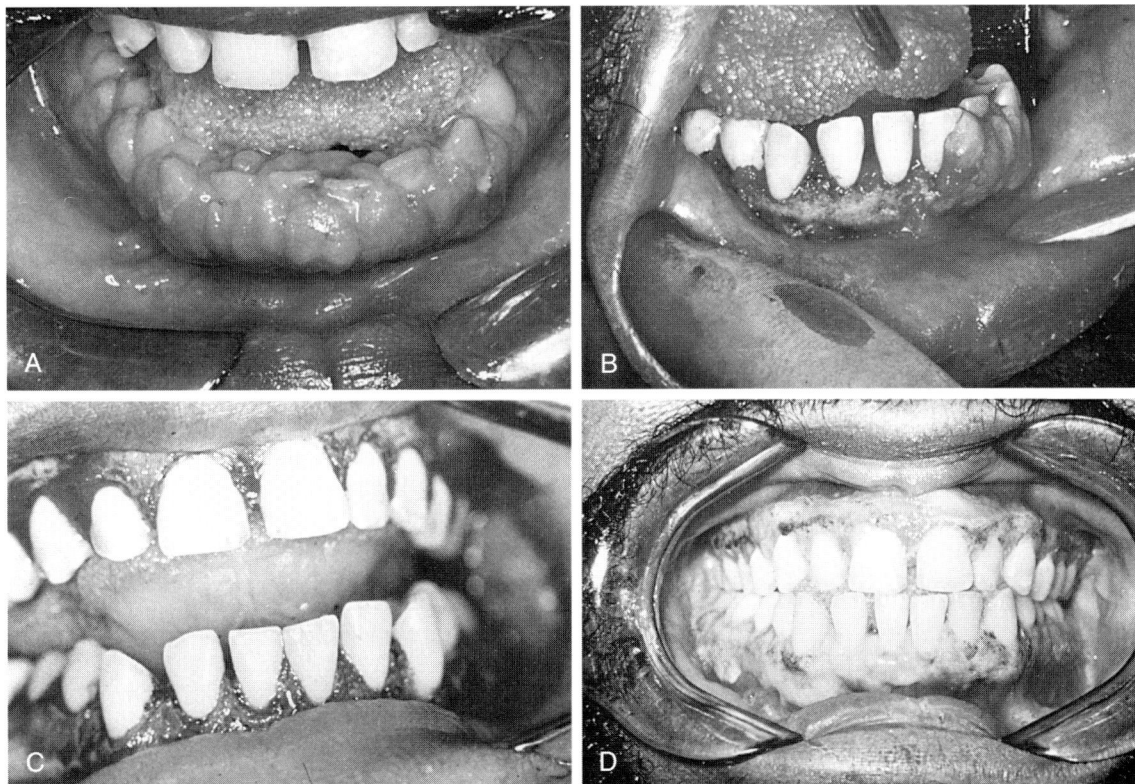

FIGURE 7–32. *A,* Drug-induced gingival hyperplasia. *B,* Gingival margin is contoured in focused mode, and inferior tissues are ablated in defocused mode up to the left lower central incisor. *C,* Immediately after laser gingivectomy. *D,* Two weeks after surgery.

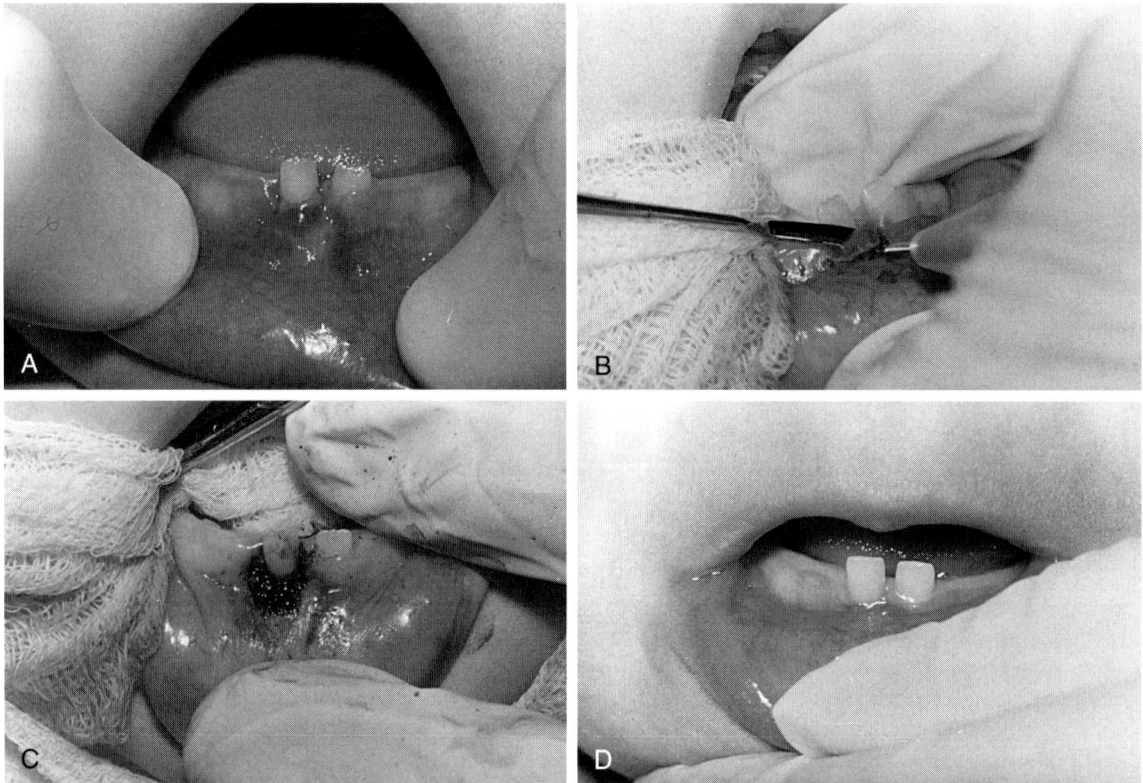

FIGURE 7–33. *A,* Pyogenic granuloma of the lower deciduous central incisor. *B,* Lesion excised in focused mode and sent to pathology. Note Freer elevator used for protection of tooth. *C,* Hemostasis is ensured by slight defocusing of the laser and by covering the surface of the wound. *D,* Wound 6 months postoperatively.

carbon dioxide laser energy in focused mode and may be sent for pathology, if desired. The muscle is then dissected superiorly using 4 watts in a continuous fashion. This margin can then be sutured or a splint may be placed. Healing is somewhat prolonged but is usually comfortable and excellent.

4. Figure 7–35: A 52-year-old man with verruca vulgaris of the left tuberosity, soft palate, and tonsillar pillar. This patient had undergone five previous attempts at surgical excision without success. The lesion was outlined at 6 watts, 10 pulses per second, and 10 milliseconds per pulse. The lesion was then ablated using 6 watts continuously in defocused mode. A relatively wide peripheral margin was used owing to the tendency of the lesion to recur if inadequately excised. The lesion healed without recurrence on follow-up at 1 year.

Soft Palate

The soft palate has traditionally represented one of the most complicated areas of the oral cavity to treat. Because of the distance from the oral stoma, access to the soft palate is limited with the use of a scalpel or electrosurgical unit. The functional importance of the soft palate in swallowing, phonation, and airway maintenance requires extremely diligent surgical planning and execution to prevent swift and potentially catastrophic complications. Both scalpel surgery and electrosurgery of the soft palate have been associated with significant airway edema, deglutition difficulties, and postoperative velopharyngeal incompetence.

Interestingly, exactly because of its anatomic location (line of site to the oral stoma), laser surgery of the soft palate is usually a relatively simple process. The minimal edema and postoperative scarring seen with the laser dramatically reduces the morbidity traditionally associated with surgery in this region. Certainly, that should not induce the surgeon to operate without concern in this vital area, but with appropriate planning and wound care, surgery in this region is safe, rapid, and effective.

Depending on the specific procedure to be performed, effective power densities may range from modest (4 to 6 watts at 1- to 2-mm spot size for surface ablation) to fairly high (14 to 15 watts at

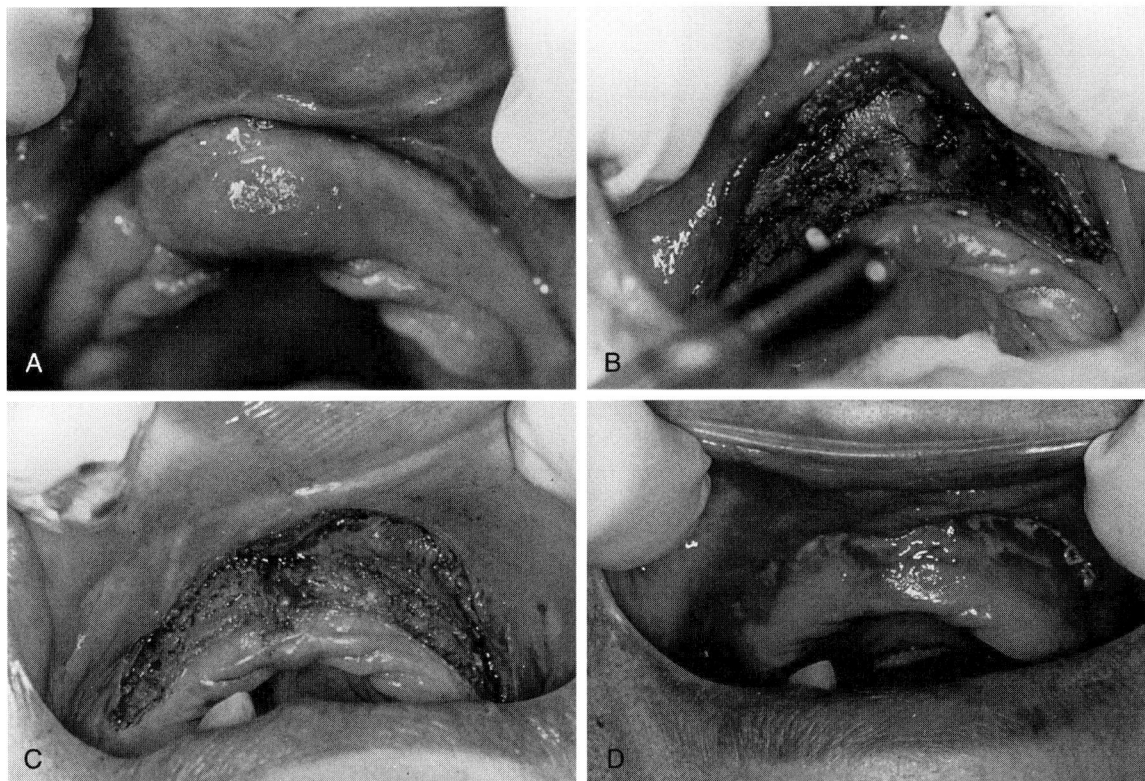

FIGURE 7–34. *A*, Epulis fissurata of maxillary ridge. *B*, Epulis has been excised with the laser in standard fashion, and muscle is being dissected superiorly with the laser. Applying tension to the upper lip makes dissection considerably easier. *C*, Finished supraperiosteal dissection. No splint was used in this case. *D*, Ten-day postoperative view.

0.8- to 2-mm spot size for laser-assisted uvulopalatostomy). Straight handpieces for both the articulated arm and hollow waveguide carbon dioxide lasers, as well as fiberoptic handpiece for the Nd:YAG, may be used for surgery in the soft palate. In addition, the straight line of site allows for articulated-arm lasers to be attached to a microscope and controlled by a micromanipulator for extremely precise surgery when necessary.

Lesions of the soft palate and uvula treated with laser include

- Salivary gland tumors
- Papilloma
- Verruca
- Pyogenic granuloma
- Hemangioma/lymphangioma
- Mucous retention phenomena
- Palatal/uvular hypertrophy

CASE HISTORIES

1. Figure 7–36: A 20-year-old man with papilloma of the uvula. The patient had noted some dysphagia from growth of the lesion. The lesion was excised with a carbon dioxide laser at 10 watts continuously in focused mode using a backstop handpiece to prevent inadvertent damage to the pharyngeal wall.

2. Figure 7–37: A 50-year-old man with significant nicotine stomatitis despite cessation of smoking. At the patient's request, the lesion was ablated at 6 watts in continuous mode. The procedure was performed under local anesthesia, and the patient was discharged to home immediately afterward. He tolerated food well but complained of a moderate burning sensation 2 to 4 days postoperatively. Swelling was minimal as was scarring.

One specific use of the laser in the soft palate and uvular region is for laser-assisted uvulopalatoplasty. Because of its recent introduction, this procedure is discussed later in greater detail.

Hard Palate

Because of its anatomic position, surgery of the hard palate is often difficult by any method. The ability of the many lasers to function in a hands-off

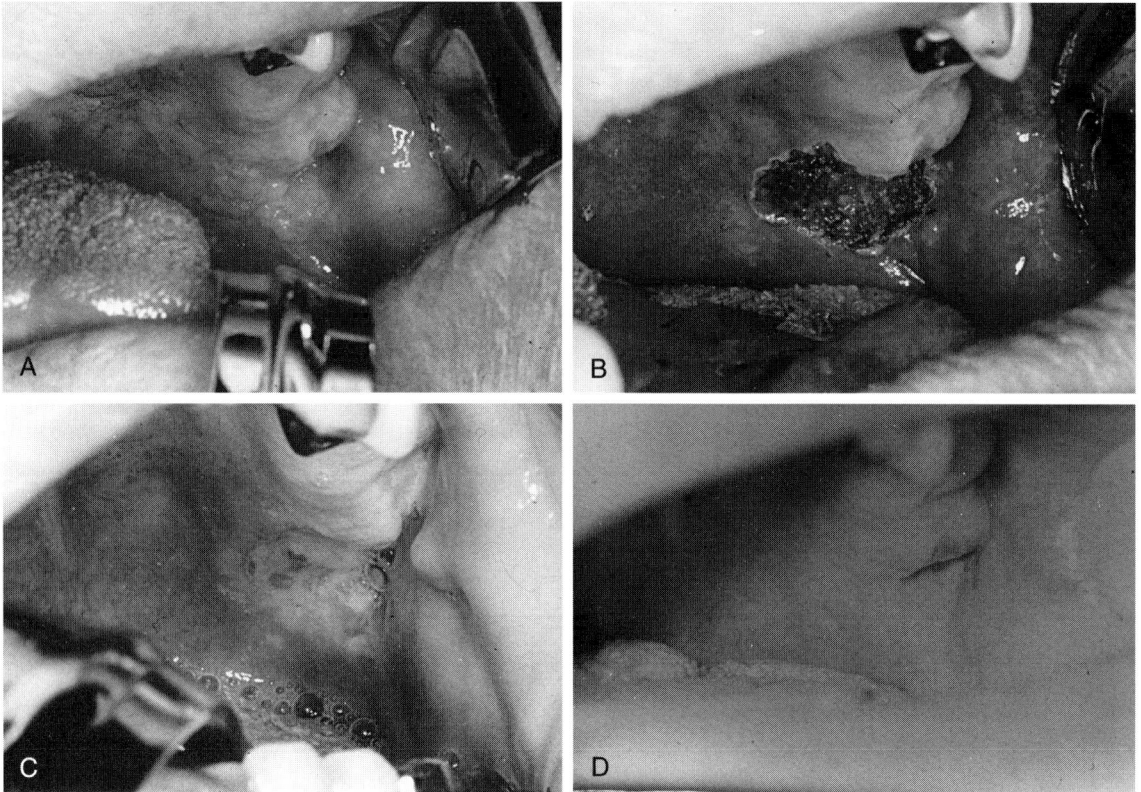

FIGURE 7–35. *A,* Area of verruca vulgaris of tuberosity, soft palate, and anterior tonsillar pillar. *B,* Area is ablated at 6 watts of continuous power with 3-mm margins. *C,* One-week postoperative view. *D,* One-year postoperative view showing no recurrence.

fashion and the availability of a variety of angled and curved fiberoptic and hollow waveguide handpieces, however, make access less problematic than in the past.

Another factor that must be considered is the attached, keratinized nature of the epithelium in this area. Because of the relatively decreased water content of the tissues, it is sometimes necessary to provide slightly higher power densities to achieve expected tissue effects when using the carbon dioxide laser. Incisions with the carbon dioxide laser are usually made at 8 to 10 watts in the focused mode (0.1- to 0.35-mm spot size), and vaporization may be effectively obtained with 8 watts at a spot size of 1.5 to 2.2 mm.

Unlike many other areas of the mouth, greater care must be exercised in the palate due to the proximity to the underlying bone. Failure to avoid the osseous tissue will result in osteonecrosis and prolonged or lack of healing. Although vaporization techniques are less likely to instigate this complication than are incisional or excisional techniques, these may be performed if the depth of the cut is carefully observed and controlled. As with gingival lesions, it is advisable to carry laser incisions down to periosteum and then use a periosteal elevator or

curette to perform any needed subperiosteal dissection. This will minimize the potential for damaging bone.

Lesions amenable to laser treatment include

- Pyogenic granuloma
- Papilloma/verruca (see Figure 7–34)
- Salivary gland tumors, without bony invasion
- Aphthous ulcers
- Gingival hyperplasia (See Figure 7–32)
- Papillary hyperplasia

Dermatologic Uses

The carbon dioxide laser has been used extensively for several years by dermatologists for the management of a variety of skin lesions. Although there are many other lasers that have specific indications for dermatologic use (e.g., copper vapor or tunable dye for port-wine stains), the carbon dioxide laser's excellent surface absorption and ability to be focused and defocused while sealing vessels 0.5 mm or smaller makes it the laser of choice for many discrete lesions. Nevertheless, nowhere is it more important for the surgeon to understand laser-

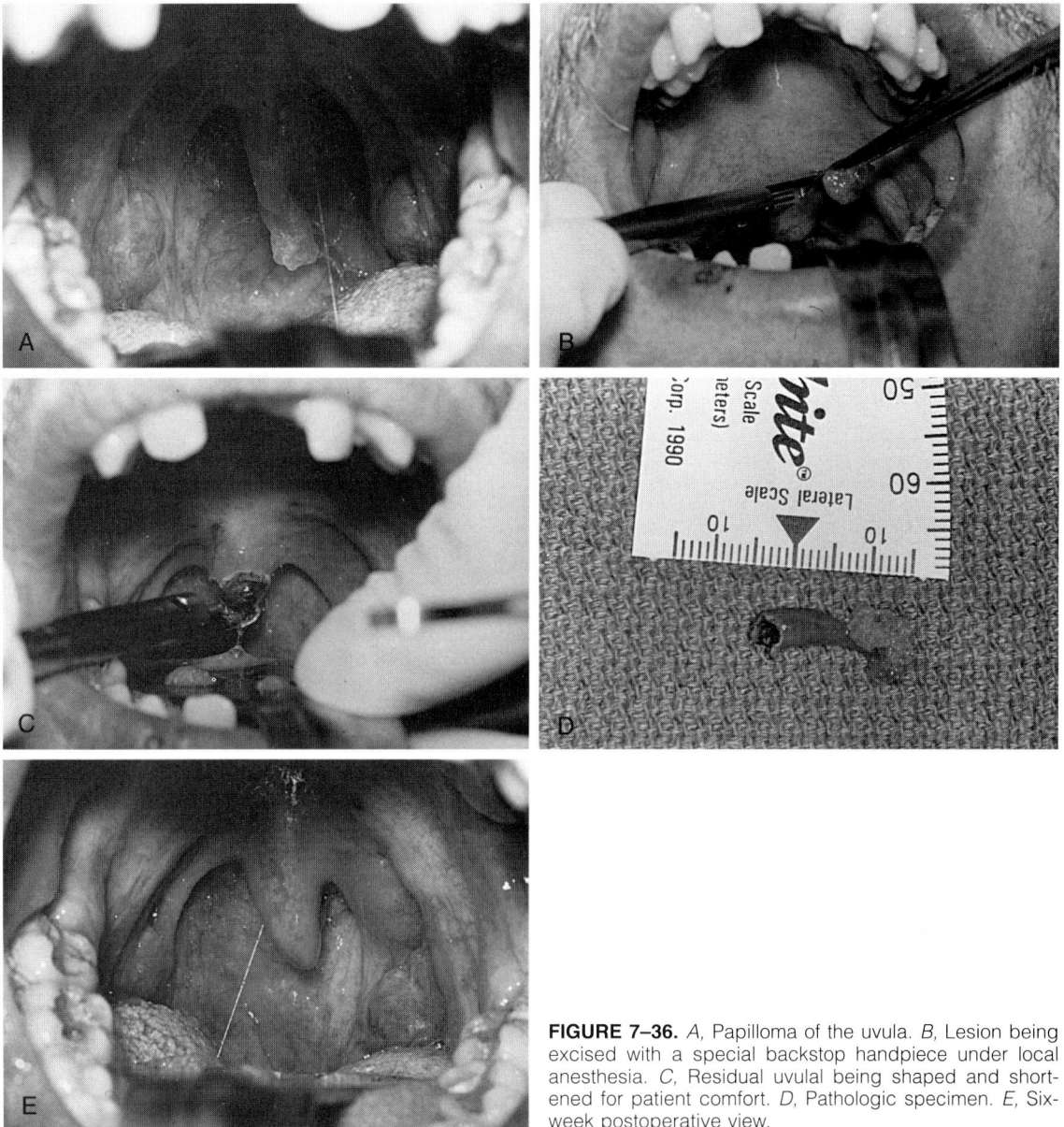

FIGURE 7–36. *A,* Papilloma of the uvula. *B,* Lesion being excised with a special backstop handpiece under local anesthesia. *C,* Residual uvular being shaped and shortened for patient comfort. *D,* Pathologic specimen. *E,* Six-week postoperative view.

tissue interaction and the indications for lasers of different wavelengths than it is for dermatologic facial lesions.

Although many surgeons prefer the scalpel for initial skin incisions owing to the precise lines produced and the tactile sensation its use renders, the laser has many advantages for use in the underlying tissues. In addition, the use of superpulsing, an electronic method of pulsing a continuous wave laser to produce high-peak powers for extremely short pulse durations, has been shown to dramatically improve the results of laser incisions in skin owing to the minimal zone of lateral thermal necrosis and damage. Superpulsing allows excellent incisional and excisional methods of treatment with

excellent cosmetic results. Many lesions are best treated not by excision, however, but by vaporization.[3] This method allows minimal destruction of normal tissue (by eliminating the need for elliptical incision) and precise control of the level of removal. This is especially important in areas where the precision of scalpel incisions is made difficult by access or tissue mobility, such as the eyelids. The lack of bruising and hematoma formation is also a significant benefit in areas such as these.

Healing following dermatologic surgery with the carbon dioxide laser is generally good. The lack of myofibroblasts in the wound, as discussed previously, limits the postsurgical contraction of the wound and amplifies the benefits produced by va-

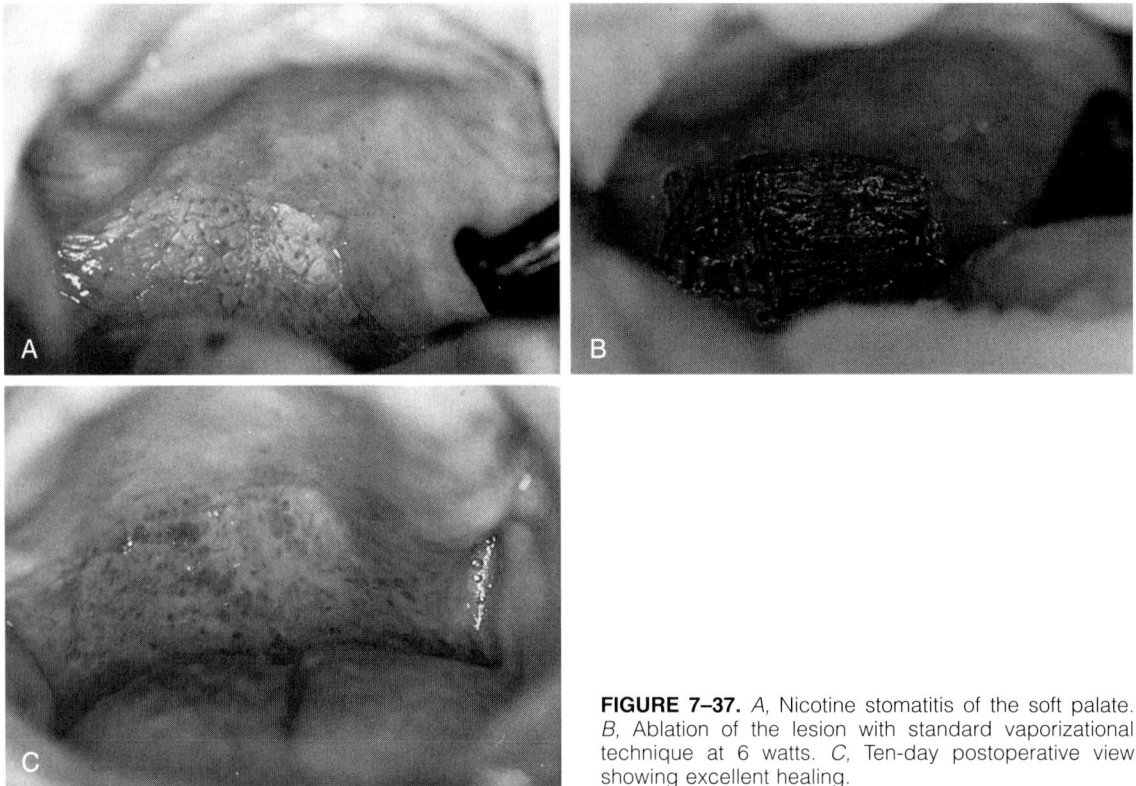

FIGURE 7–37. *A,* Nicotine stomatitis of the soft palate. *B,* Ablation of the lesion with standard vaporizational technique at 6 watts. *C,* Ten-day postoperative view showing excellent healing.

porization. When combined with the lack of bleeding (and subsequent lack of crusting), edema, inflammation, and pain, the laser provides an excellent modality for removal of selected lesions of the skin.[17] Of course, cosmetic results with the laser are not uniformly predictable and it is always advisable to perform a patch test in an inconspicuous area, when possible, if sensitive areas are to be operated on. Color and hypertrophic scarring changes should be looked for over the next 4 months. If the surgeon and patient are satisfied with the results, other areas should be considered for surgery.

When desired or indicated by cosmetic or functional reasons, the same variety of tissue closure options and suture materials exist for laser wounds as for scalpel wounds. The laser may even be used to quickly and efficiently undermine tissue, when necessary, for adequate tissue mobility. It must be remembered, however, that the tensile strength of laser wounds lags behind scalpel wounds for the next three weeks, after which the tensile strength of both wounds becomes comparable.[18, 19] Because of this temporary lack of tensile strength, sutures closing laser wounds should be left in place for a longer period of time than normal, even as long as twice the usual time period.[20] It should also be considered that any charring left on the wound edges during closure will remain for an extended period of time and cause unsightly darkening of the wound until

adequately removed by macrophages. This can easily be prevented by removing the charring on the wound edges with moist gauze prior to closure.

A large number of discrete dermatologic lesions are suited for laser removal, but some lesions are *ideally* treated with this modality. For example, the treatment of rhinophyma, an advanced form of acne rosacea, has been well described in the literature.[21–24] When treated at 10 to 15 watts in slightly defocused mode (1 to 2 mm), results are generally far superior to those achieved by conventional methods, and with little or no bleeding. By feathering the edges with lower power densities (4 to 6 watts and a spot size of 2 to 3 mm), the margins of the lesion can be well hidden.

The management of keloids has always been and remains difficult at best. Although the laser would seem to be an ideal tool for the management of keloids owing to its minimal scarring effect and surgical trauma and has been reported on extensively,[25, 26] this use has also been less than ideal in some cases.[17, 27] Techniques for the management of keloids include excision with primary closure, excision with healing by secondary intention (to eliminate any tension across the wound that might stimulate recurrent keloid formation), and creating numerous punctate holes in the keloid with the laser, which subsequently diminishes in size over time. It is apparent, however, that any of these modalities is best performed along with traditional ancillary therapy, including triamcinolone injections and pressure dressings.

Despite the lack of wavelength specificity for hemoglobin that is seen with some other dermatologic lasers, the carbon dioxide laser has been used effectively for the management of small telangiectasias.[27, 28] Without anesthesia, the small vessels are coagulated at 6 watts in gated mode for 10 to 15 milliseconds. Several pulses along the vessels may be needed for total obliteration, and some temporary depression of the skin may be seen postoperatively. Other vascular lesions of the face, such as port-wine stains, have been treated with the carbon dioxide laser, but this laser has been substantially replaced for this purpose by more wavelength-specific lasers (for pigment and hemoglobin chromophores), such as the tunable dye and copper vapor lasers. The Nd:YAG and KTP:YAG lasers have also been used for vascular and pigmented lesions, and although they are only moderately specific for these chromophores, may provide good results.

The easy control and small spot sizes associated with the carbon dioxide laser make it very useful for the removal of small facial lesions by slightly defocused ablation. Lesions such as benign nevi, tissue tags, and xanthelasma are rapidly and effectively treated in this manner. Powers of approximately 4 to 5 watts with a focal spot size of 1 to 1.5 mm are used in slow-gated mode (single-pulse or slow repeat mode at 1 to 2 pulses per second) in an overlapping fashion. The lesion is ablated down to normal tissue, removing only a minimal amount of adjacent tissue unless wider ablation is indicated by pathologic principles to prevent recurrence (e.g., in treating verrucae). Although larger lesions may also be treated in this fashion, it is advisable to perform test surgery as previously mentioned to determine if the final result will be cosmetically acceptable. When histopathology is desired on the lesions, this may be accomplished by standard incisional or excisional biopsy techniques, or by shave biopsy. This technique involves using a scalpel or razor blade to remove the superficial portion of the lesion (which is then submitted for histologic examination) and using the laser to vaporize the base of the lesion.

Lesions amenable to carbon dioxide laser surgery are listed in Table 7–1. Although this list is extensive, including many vascular lesions, the prudent surgeon should limit treatment to lesions that fall within his or her capability and level of experience. The important cosmetic effects of surgery in this area leave little room for error, despite the ease and effectiveness of laser surgery.

Finally, the use of superpulsing may dramatically improve the results of dermatologic carbon dioxide laser surgery for a wide variety of surgical proce-

TABLE 7–1. Indications for Dermatologic Uses of the Carbon Dioxide Laser

Actinic cheilitis	Lentigines
Angiofibroma	Neurofibroma
Basal cell carcinoma	Psoriasis
Bowen's disease	Pyogenic granuloma
Condyloma acuminata	Rhinophyma
Cylindroma	Scar revision
Epidermal nevus	Tattoo
Erythroplasia	Telangiectasia
Granuloma faciale	Verruca
Keloids	Xanthelasma

dures, including the recently developed cosmetic skin resurfacing procedure for small facial wrinkles.

CASE HISTORIES

1. **Figure 7–38:** A 58-year-old woman with a neurofibroma of the lip. The carbon dioxide laser was used owing to the difficulty in obtaining a cosmetic and functional incision line. The lesion was outlined at 4 watts in slow-intermittent mode (two pulses per second at 50 milliseconds per pulse) and was then excised in continuous fashion using 4 watts. The resultant char was removed, and the wound was dressed with antibiotic ointment and left unsutured. A superpulsed or ultrapulsed carbon dioxide laser would cause less charring and adjacent tissue damage than would a continuous-wave machine and would, therefore, probably result in an even better scar. These machines should be considered when performing dermatologic laser surgery.

2. **Figure 7–39:** A 30-year-old man with small telangiectasia of the lip. This lesion may be treated by a variety of lasers including the argon, Nd:YAG, KTP:YAG, or the carbon dioxide laser. The carbon dioxide laser was used in this case to gently vaporize the vessels involved and obtain hemostasis. This laser should be used only for small, superficial lesions. Larger lesions are best treated by hemoglobin-specific wavelengths. In this patient, 2 watts of power were used in very slow-intermittent mode (two pulses per second for 50 to 100 milliseconds per pulse). The lesion healed uneventfully over two weeks.

3. **Figure 7–40:** A 30-year-old man with two small pigmented nevi on his neck. Because these lesions were determined on history and physical examination to be benign, they were removed by the ablation technique. This is performed by using 2 to 4 watts in slow-intermittent mode (two pulses per second and 50 to 200 milliseconds per pulse) to vaporize the lesion down to adjacent skin level. Care should be taken to leave adnexal

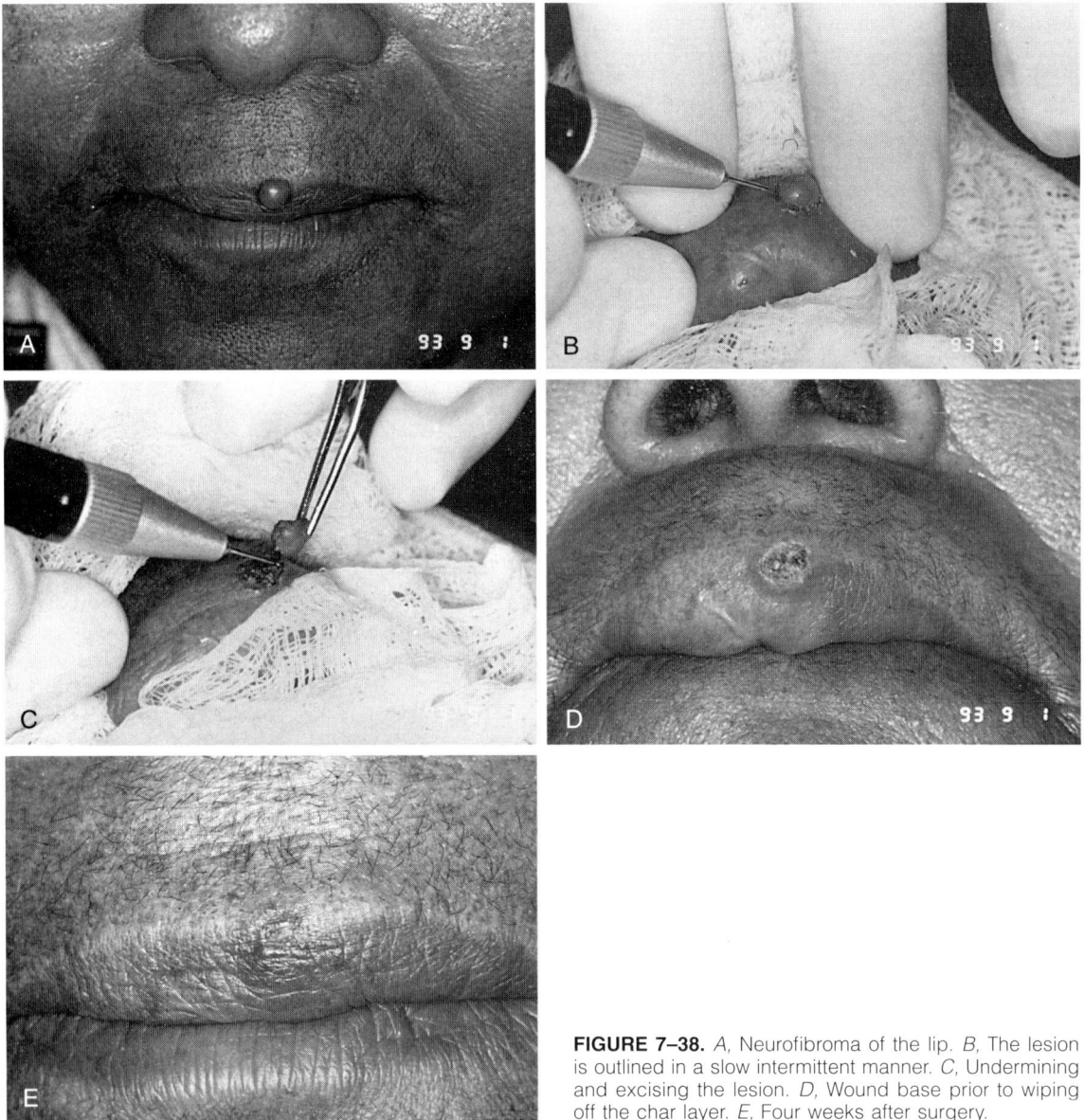

FIGURE 7–38. *A*, Neurofibroma of the lip. *B*, The lesion is outlined in a slow intermittent manner. *C*, Undermining and excising the lesion. *D*, Wound base prior to wiping off the char layer. *E*, Four weeks after surgery.

structures whenever possible because this provides epithelium for faster and better healing with less scarring.

4. Figure 7–41: A 29-year-old man with a pigmented lesion. Because the histology of this lesion was in question, an alternative to simple vaporization (which does not provide a pathologic specimen) is a shave biopsy. In this technique, the top of the lesion is sliced off using a scalpel or razor blade and sent for examination. The base of the lesion is then vaporized, as per normal procedure. This method provides a specimen for the pathologist but results in a similar postoperative appearance as does simple ablation. After removing the top of the lesion, hemostasis

is obtained by slightly defocusing the laser and covering the surface at 2 to 4 watts of power. The remainder of the procedure is the same as that used for simple vaporization.

LASER USE IN ANATOMICALLY DIFFICULT AREAS

Surgery in and around the oral cavity and face is complicated by the proximity to a number of vital structures. These include the submandibular and parotid ducts, the lingual nerve and artery, the vermilion border of the lip, the commissures of the mouth, and the airway space.

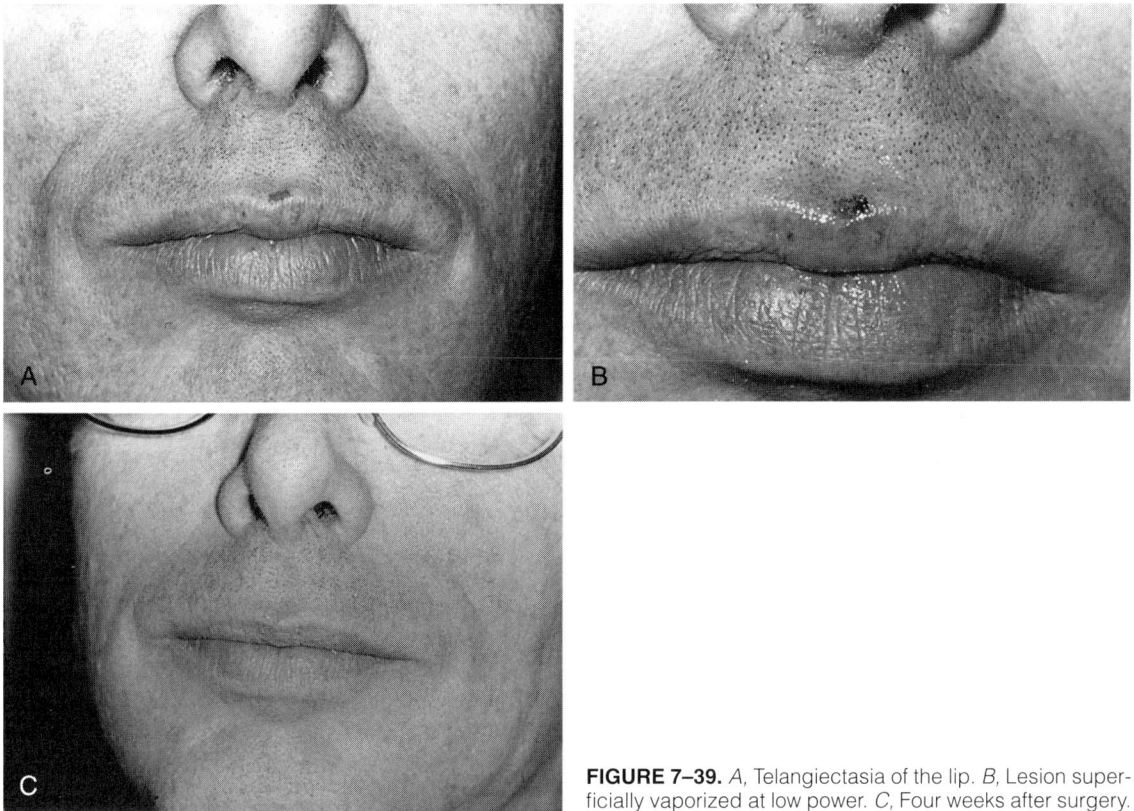

FIGURE 7–39. *A*, Telangiectasia of the lip. *B*, Lesion superficially vaporized at low power. *C*, Four weeks after surgery.

It has been the experience of many surgeons that carbon dioxide laser use near the submandibular and parotid ducts causes no long-term obstructive sequelae. Although a study by Mihail and associates[29] concluded that there was no difference in the incidence of stenosis between laser, scalpel, and electrosurgical transection of the submandibular duct, other studies have found no adverse effect on salivary flow following laser transection.[10] In this study, no histologic evidence of ductal stenosis or mucosal contraction around the ducts was found following healing. Another study involving a large number of patients showed that none had evidence of ductal constriction and salivary impairment.[30] It would appear that although consideration should always be given to possible postoperative ductal constriction, this should not preclude adequate surgical excision or vaporization; rather, long-term follow-up should be instituted to intercept possible problems early in their development.

Certainly, transection of the lingual nerve or artery will lead to serious morbidity. Although the use of the laser does not prevent these complications, the precise surgery possible and minimal lateral tissue damage seen with the laser minimizes the risks. In addition, the bloodless nature of the surgery in this highly vascular area also adds to the increased safety by allowing greater visibility of the surgical field.[31] Of course, the likelihood of neural or arterial damage is remote if controlled vaporizational techniques rather than excisional techniques are used. This ablative ability is a major advantage of laser surgery in the floor of the mouth, where the thin mucosa and superficial underlying structures make excisional techniques with a scalpel or a laser more likely to cause significant damage. The ability to vaporize tissues in successive layers in the floor of the mouth until the desired depth is reached (e.g., just the epithelium) rarely damages deeper structures if surgery is carefully performed.

Unlike conventional surgery and suture closure near the commissures, which can lead to wound contracture and deformity, laser surgery near this area appears to heal without this complication. The lack of myofibroblasts in the wound diminishes the ability of the wound to contract postoperatively following healing by secondary intention. It is recommended, therefore, that excisional or vaporizational techniques in this area may be performed without significant risk of deformity and should be carried out as necessary.

Surgery near the airway always involves a certain degree of risk. Even minimal swelling can result in ventilatory compromise. The minimal postoperative edema seen with laser surgery does, however, decrease the likelihood of airway compromise. Laser

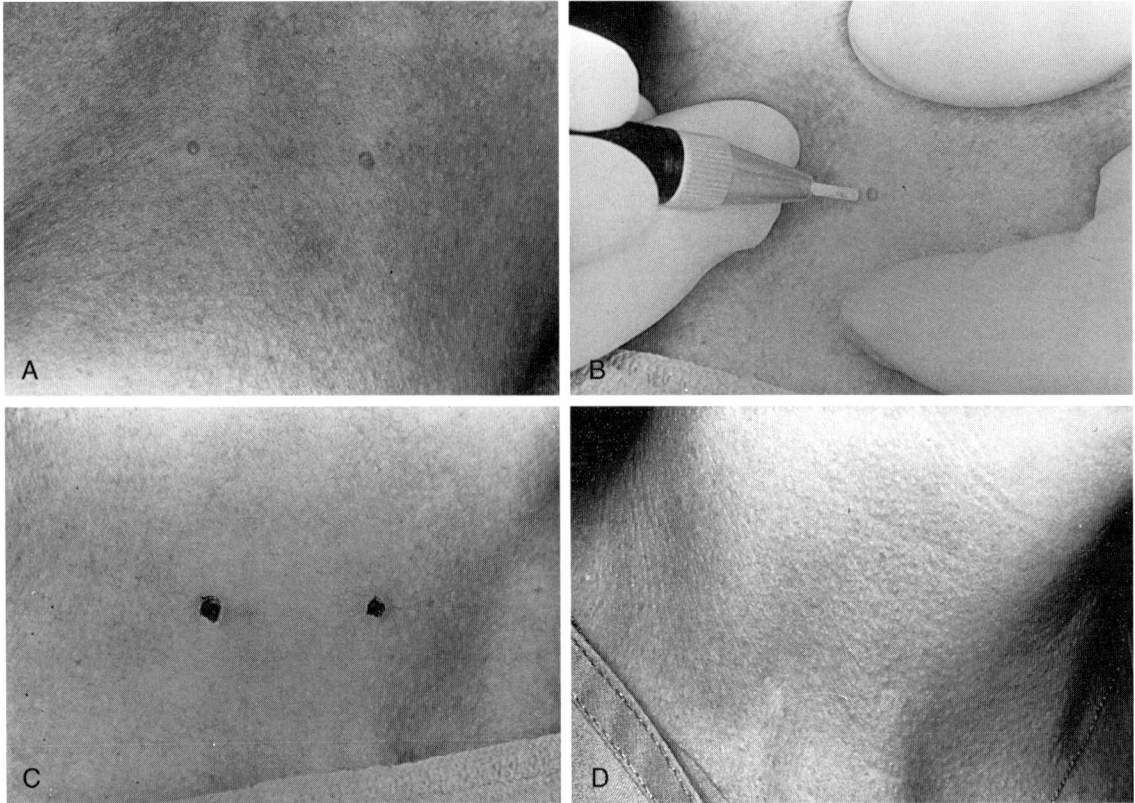

FIGURE 7–40. *A,* Two small pigmented nevi of the neck. *B,* Slightly defocused ablation at 2 to 4 watts. *C,* Immediately following surgery. *D,* Seven months after surgery. (Courtesy of Dr. James Wooten, Biloxi, Mississippi.)

procedures on the soft palate, uvula, and tonsillar pillars do not normally produce edema of the magnitude to cause airway problems, but the ensuing sore throat and the possibility of secondary bleeding must be explained to the patient, along with dietary instructions to prevent these problems. Because of the lack of postoperative airway complications seen with laser surgery, many procedures formerly performed under general anesthesia in the operating room are made possible under local anesthesia in an office setting with the use of the laser (a good example is the office-based laser-assisted uvulopalatoplasty versus a hospital-based uvulopalatopharyngoplasty [see Chapter 13]).

POSTOPERATIVE CARE

One of the main advantages of using the laser is the lack of postoperative problems and the minimal need for wound care. A thorough understanding of the effects of laser-tissue interaction is necessary, however, to be able to prevent postoperative sequelae and provide the patient with informed postoperative instructions.

Infection after laser surgery is rare, and the rou-

tine use of prophylactic systemic antibiotics is, in the opinion of this author, rarely indicated. This has been postulated to be a result of the sterilization of the operative site by the thermal effect on the bacterial flora. Several studies have demonstrated that the laser probably does not actually sterilize the site but possibly does disinfect it. In certain areas such as the periodontal ligament space, there is some evidence that recolonization by bacteria may be prolonged. It may also be that infection in the oral cavity is rare regardless of the surgical technique used. Some surgeons have advocated the use of chlorhexidine mouth rinse after surgery, and this certainly seems reasonable to aid in the local reduction of mouth flora. Further investigation in this area is warranted and will require large-scale studies to be accurate and clinically useful owing to the small incidence of infection that occurs under any circumstances.

Pain is an inevitable consequence of any tissue damage and certainly can, and often does, become manifest after laser surgery. Some laser surgeons have flatly stated that no postoperative pain occurs in their patients after laser incision or excision. Although this has been true in a minority of the author's cases, the majority of patients have fol-

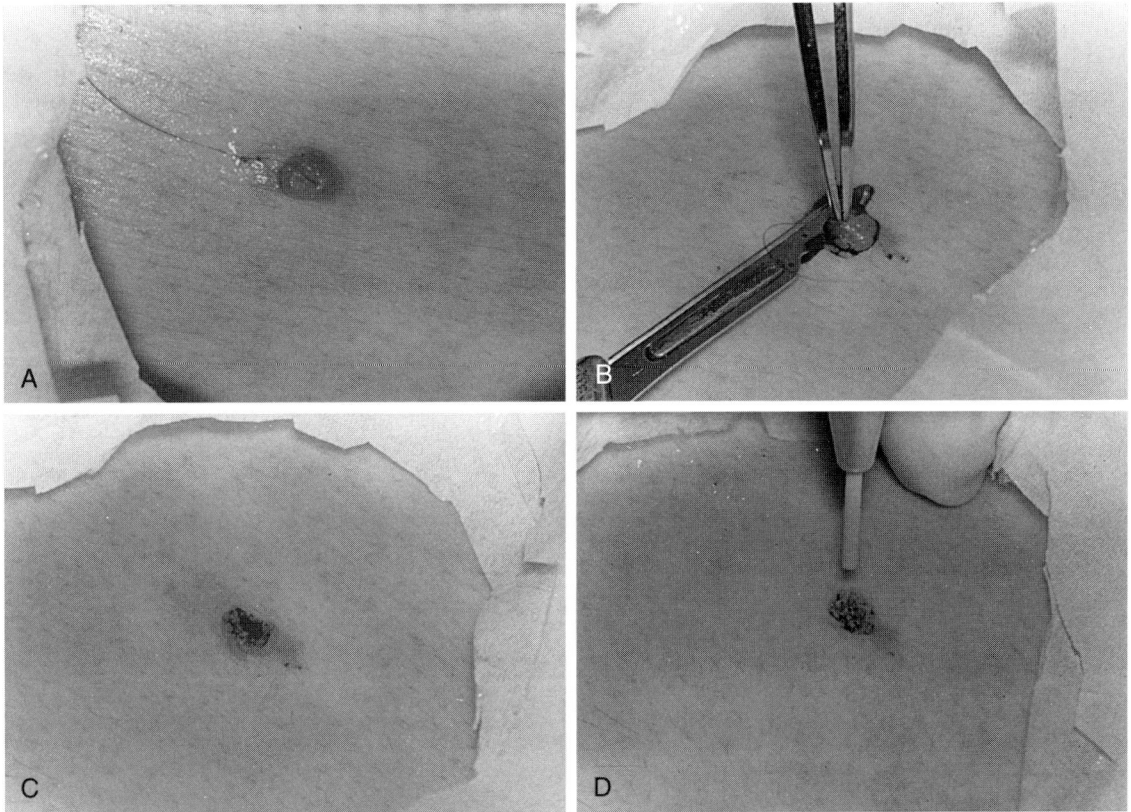

FIGURE 7–41. *A,* Raised melanotic nevus. *B,* Shave biopsy performed with a scalpel. *C,* Bleeding surface after shave procedure. *D,* The remainder of the lesion is vaporized to its base.

lowed a rather predictable and understandable postoperative course. As the laser incises through the tissues, it is thought that it is also essentially cauterizing, or sealing, the neural pathways. Although sealing is probably an inaccurate term,[31] this effect, in fact, often does limit the *immediate* postoperative discomfort felt by the patient. This effect is somewhat shortlived, however, because the nerves begin to regenerate 3 to 5 days after surgery. This is usually accompanied by a mild to moderate burning sensation and may be distressing to the patient, not so much by its intensity but rather by its timing. The uninformed patient will think that there is a postoperative complication when, after four days of no pain, the surgical site suddenly becomes painful. This problem is easily prevented by clearly informing the patient of this possibility and explaining the expected time course of any discomfort. In addition, even when pain does occur, it is commonly less problematic than with traditional methods of surgery. When pain begins immediately postoperatively, patients may dwell on the surgery and the discomfort. This only adds to the psychological trauma of the surgery. On the other hand, if and when discomfort begins 4 days postoperatively, the patient is usually back at work or school and

has resumed his or her normal lifestyle. This often minimizes the physical and emotional effects associated with the surgery. In terms of patient satisfaction after surgery, this can be a tremendous advantage for the use of lasers.

Postoperative edema is also a natural sequela to any surgery, and its extent, like the course of postoperative pain, can be explained on a physiologic basis and must be considered when performing laser surgery. Unlike postoperative pain, however, postsurgical edema in most cases is the exception rather than the rule. This has been studied extensively in the literature. The lack of edema undoubtedly is due to the fact that there is no efflux of mediators of inflammation into the wound via cut blood vessels as would normally be seen with scalpel or electrosurgical incisions.[32]

Postoperative scarring is an important issue for oral and maxillofacial surgeons to consider owing to its functional effects intraorally and its cosmetic effects extraorally. Scarring is considerably improved with the use of the laser for several reasons. The lack of myofibroblasts and collagen production in the wound with laser surgery compared with other modalities of treatment (e.g., scalpel surgery) limits postoperative contraction of the wound.[33] Hyaluronidase activity in the wound also appears to play an important part in wound healing, and it may be clearly distinguished in laser and scalpel wounds.[34] Finally, the relative resistance of intracellular matrix proteins to laser energy provides a scaffolding for tissue healing that may decrease surgical scarring.[35]

REFERENCES

1. Pogrel MA, McCracken KJ, Daniels TE: Histologic evaluation of the width of soft tissue necrosis adjacent to carbon dioxide laser incisions. Oral Surg Oral Med Oral Pathol 70:564–568, 1990.
2. Gáspár L, Szabó G: Removal of benign oral tumors and tumor-like lesions by CO_2 laser application. Laser Med Surg:33–36, 1989.
3. Bailin PL, Ratz JL, Wheeland RG: Laser therapy of the skin. Otolaryngol Clin North Am 23: 123–164, 1990.
4. Myers TD, Murphy DG, White JM, et al: Conservative soft tissue management with the low-powered pulsed Nd:YAG dental laser. Pract Periodontics Aesthet Dent 4(6):6–12, 1992.
5. Dederich DN: Laser/tissue interaction.: What happens to laser light when it strikes tissue? J Am Dent Assoc 124:57–61, 1993.
6. White JM, Goodis HE, Rose CL: Use of the pulsed Nd:YAG laser for intraoral soft tissue surgery. Lasers Surg Med 11:455–461, 1991.
7. Frame JW: Removal of oral soft tissue pathology with the CO_2 laser. J Oral Maxillofac Surg 43:850–855, 1985.
8. Pick RM, Colvard MD: Current status of lasers in soft tissue dental surgery. J Periodontal 64(7):589–602, 1993.
9. Hall RR: The healing of tissue incised by a CO_2 laser. Br J Surg 58: 222–225, 1971.
10. Fisher SE, Frame JW: The effect of the CO_2 surgical laser on oral tissues. Br J Oral Maxillofac Surg 22:414, 1984.
11. Frame JW, Das Gupta AR, Dalton GA, et al: Use of CO_2 laser in the management of premalignant lesions of the oral mucosa. J Laryngol Otol 98:1251, 1984.
12. Roodenburg JLN, Bosch JJ, Borsboom PCF: Measurement of the uniaxial elasticity of oral mucosa in vivo after CO_2–laser evaporation and surgical excision. Int J Oral Maxillofac Surg 19:181–183, 1990.
13. Colvard M, Kuo P: Managing aphthous ulcers: Laser treatment applied. J Am Dent Assoc 122:5153, 1991.
14. Stanley RJ, Roenigk RK: Actinic cheilitis: Treatment with the carbon dioxide laser. Mayo Clin Proc 63:230–235, 1988.
15. Horch HH, Gerlach KL, Schaefer HE: CO_2 laser surgery of oral premalignant lesions. Int J Oral Maxillofac Surg 15:19–24, 1986.
16. Pick RM, Pecaro BC, Silberman CJ: The laser gingivectomy. The use of the CO_2 laser for the removal of phenytoin hyperplasia. J Periodontol 56:492–496, 1985.
17. Olbricht SM, Arndt KA: Lasers in cutaneous surgery. In Fuller TA (ed): Surgical Lasers: A Clinical Guide. New York, Macmillan Publishing Co., 1987, pp 113–245.
18. Fry TL, Gerbe RW, Botros SB, et al: Effects of laser, scalpel, and electrosurgical excision on wound contracture and graft "take." Plast Reconstr Surg 65:729–730, 1980.
19. Hambley R, Hebada PA, Abell E, et al: Wound healing of skin incisions produced by ultrasonically vibrating knife, scalpel, electrosurgery, and carbon dioxide laser. J Dermatol Surg Oncol 14:1213–1217, 1988.
20. McBurney EI: Dermatologic laser surgery. Otolaryngol Clin North Am 23(1):77–97, 1990.
21. Bohigian RK, Shapshay SM, Hybels RL: Management of rhinophyma with carbon dioxide laser. Lahey Clinic experience. Laser Surg Med 8:397–401, 1988.
22. Shapshay SM, Strong MS, Anastasi GW, et al: Removal of rhinophyma with the carbon dioxide laser. Arch Otolaryngol Head Neck Surg 106:257–259, 1980.
23. Simpson GT, Shapshay SM, Vaughn CW, et al: Rhinologic laser surgery. Otolaryngol Clin North Am 16(4):829–837, 1983.
24. Simpson GT, Shapshay SM, Vaughn CW, et al: Rhinologic surgery with the carbon dioxide laser. Laryngoscope 92:412–415, 1982.
25. Bailin PL: Use of the CO_2 laser for non-pws cutaneous lesions. In Arndt KA, Noe JM, Rosen S (eds): Cutaneous Laser Therapy and Methods. New York, John Wiley and Sons, 1983, pp 187–199.
26. Carney JM, Kamat BR, Stern RS, et al: Cutaneous tissue repair after focused CO_2 laser irradiation. Lasers Surg Med 5:180–181, 1985.
27. Bailin PL, Ratz JL, Wheeland RG: Laser therapy of the skin: A review of principles and applications. Dermatol Clin 5:259–285, 1987.
28. Goldman MP, Bennet RG: Treatment of telangiectasia: A review. J Am Acad Dermatol 17:167–182, 1987.
29. Mihail R, Zajtchuk JT, Davis RK: Incidence of Wharton's duct stenosis in floor of the mouth cancers excised with scalpel or cautery versus CO_2 laser. Head Neck Surg 9:241–243, 1987.
30. Gaspar L, Szabo G: Manifestations of the advantages and disadvantages of using the CO_2 laser in oral surgery. J Clin Laser Med Surg 8(10):39–43, 1990.
31. Basu MK, Frame JW, Rhys Evans PH: Wound healing following partial glossectomy using the CO_2 laser, diathermy and scalpel: A histological study in rats. J Laryngol Otol 102:322–327, 1988.
32. Klein DR: The use of CO_2 lasers in plastic surgery. South Med J 70:429–431, 1977.
33. Fisher SE, Frame JW, Brownie RM: A comparative histologic study of wound healing following CO_2 laser and conventional surgical excision of canine buccal mucosa. Arch Oral Biol 28: 287–291, 1983.
34. Pogrel MA, Pham HD: Profile of hyaluronidase activity distinguishes CO_2 laser from scalpel wound healing. Ann Surg 217(2):196–200, 1993.
35. Luomanen M, Meurman JH, Lehto VP: Extracellular matrix in healing CO_2 laser incision wound. J Oral Pathol 16:322–331, 1987.

CHAPTER 8

Laser Management of Malignant Lesions of the Head and Neck

M. ANTHONY POGREL, MB, ChB, BDS, FRCS

Many of the inherent properties of lasers used for performing soft tissue surgery are advantageous in the surgical management of malignant disease of the oral cavity and related structures. The ability of the laser to perform hemostatic surgery by sealing blood vessels of a smaller diameter than the laser beam[1] is advantageous, because it means that more precise surgery can be carried out in a bloodless field, and sealing the vessels may decrease the seeding of malignant cells at the time of surgery.[2, 3] Similarly, the ability of the laser to seal the lymphatics at the time of surgery is advantageous in decreasing the swelling and edema associated with the surgery.[1] This, in turn, may decrease the need for a tracheostomy to be performed in the management of facial edema and may decrease the need for steroids to be administered postoperatively.[4] Sealing of the lymphatics may also decrease the possibility of seeding malignant cells into the lymphatics at the time of surgery.[2, 3] Also, the ability to seal nerve endings is advantageous in decreasing postoperative discomfort.[5]

The ability of the laser to leave a clean, dry, sealed wound is the probable reason for the noted low infection rate following laser surgery.[6] This is also advantageous in the management of malignant diseases because it decreases the need for prophylactic and therapeutic antibiotics. The fact that laser wounds heal with low levels of discomfort and relatively little scarring and wound contracture means that formal reconstruction by means of primary closure, skin grafting, or local flap procedures is not necessary because wounds can be left to heal by secondary intention, giving a good functional result with minimal scarring and lack of movement. It also can mean that some procedures previously performed in the hospital can now be performed on an outpatient basis using the laser.[7]

Some of these presumed advantages of laser soft tissue surgery have been questioned, but it does appear that there are genuine differences between laser ablation and excision and other modalities of tissue removal. Luomanen and coworkers have shown that extracellular matrix may be specifically protected from destruction by the carbon dioxide laser.[8] The pattern of hyaluronidase production differs in carbon dioxide laser versus scalpel wounds, with a bimodal pattern of hyaluronidase production in laser wounds.[9] Differences have also been shown in mast cell enzymes, with carbon dioxide laser wounds showing higher levels of lactate and succinate dehydrogenase than in scalpel wounds.[10] Laser wounds are generally believed to heal with little scarring and fibrosis, and this may be due to a relative absence of myofibroblasts in laser wounds.[11] More recently, however, myofibroblasts have been found in laser wounds, and scarring can occur and occasionally can be severe.[12, 13] The lack of fibrosis in laser wounds may simply be due to the decreased level of acute inflammatory cells and presumably inflammatory mediators.[14]

The use of the laser in and around the oral cavity is not, however, free of risks and complications. There are increased costs associated with the purchase and use of lasers in surgery, and additional measures must be taken to protect both the staff and patient. These measures include protection of adjacent structures on the patient and also any areas that may be affected by accidentally reflected laser beams. The surgeon, staff, and patient are protected by wearing goggles of the appropriate color to absorb the particular laser energy beam employed, and high filtration masks are worn in an attempt to eliminate inhalation of the laser plume, which may contain foreign protein and even infective agents.[15–18] High-volume suction must also be used close to the surgical site in order to evacuate the plume. Some lasers, particularly free-beam lasers, may have problems in gaining access to certain areas of the oral cavity. This can occur whether the beam is being directed free hand or via an operating microscope and joystick. Sometimes, the use of a front-reflecting mirror can enable access to previously difficult sites, such as behind the maxillary tuberosity and behind the lower incisor teeth. In some cases, front-reflecting mirrors are provided as an integral part of the laser guidance system, but in other cases, a free hand front-reflecting mirror can be used.

TYPE OF LASER AND MODE OF ACTIVITY

Conceptually, lasers fall into two groups: (1) those used as a free beam, such as the carbon dioxide laser, and (2) those most commonly used in a contact-tip mode, such as the neodymium:yttrium-aluminum-garnet (Nd:YAG) laser. Both of these systems are used for the management of oral and related malignancies. A free-beam laser can be focused or defocused. In focused mode with a narrow beam (in some systems, the beam can be as narrow as 0.1 mm), the laser acts as a surgical knife for carrying out surgical excision. However, by using a very narrow beam, some of the hemostatic and lymphostatic properties may be lost. By using a wider focused beam or a nonfocused beam of around 2 to 3 mm in spot size, the laser can be used to vaporize tissues. This is not a recommended treatment for invasive malignant disease because the surgical specimen is lost, but it is an appropriate means of treating dysplastic and premalignant mucosa, which often accompanies intraoral malignancy. In many cases, there is a field change present, possibly owing to risk factors such as smoking or alcohol intake, although in many cases the etiologic agent is unknown.

A contact tip laser such as Nd:YAG can be used as a surgical knife but lacks the precision and speed of a free-beam carbon dioxide laser. The beam of a contact tip laser is virtually always wider and more penetrating, causing more lateral damage. Access is, however, often easier in the contact tip mode

because the beam is fed through a fiber optic cable, which is usually flexible. When the contact tip is withdrawn slightly from the tissues, the beam rapidly increases in width and can then be used in vaporization mode. A free-beam laser such as the carbon dioxide laser can cause damage if it contacts teeth or bone because these structures will absorb laser energy but are not vaporized because they do not have a high enough water content and are generally raised to a higher temperature and charred.[19–21] At the present time, a laser system is not available that provides effective vaporization and cutting of hard tissues including teeth and bone, although excimer lasers operating in the ultraviolet wavelengths offer some promise of being able to cut bone and without unacceptable increases in temperature.[22–24] The contact tip laser causes less damage to teeth and bone because its energy is rapidly dissipated if the structure being vaporized is more than a millimeter or two away from the tip. A contact tip laser may, therefore, be safer when treatment is being performed around teeth.

THE MANAGEMENT OF SPECIFIC LESIONS

Premalignant or Dysplastic Lesions

Lesions falling into this category include many leukoplakias and most cases of erythroplakia and some cases of erosive lichen planus. In all cases, preoperative biopsy is mandatory and can be carried out with a scalpel or with the laser utilizing a narrow beam as a surgical knife. Biopsy must always be taken from the most dysplastic or premalignant area. The best evaluated means of identifying this area is by the use of toluidine blue staining.[25, 26] The most frequently used technique involves preoperative removal of mucus by means of a 1% acetic acid solution. After irrigating and drying, 1% toluidine blue is applied to the dysplastic area. Decolorization can then be carried out gradually by sending the patient away for 45 minutes to an hour with instructions to have a drink or a snack, or the area can be rapidly decolorized by reapplying 1% acetic acid. The acetic acid must be used judiciously because overaggressive use of acetic acid decolorizes all areas. Areas that preferentially retain the dye should be biopsied because these are areas with nuclei near the cell membrane and are therefore cells undergoing division, which are more likely to be the most dysplastic and may even show true malignancy. Whenever an incisional biopsy or definitive specimen that has been excised by laser is sent to the pathology laboratory, the pathologist must be informed of the mode of excision. This is because the laser denatures a thin rim of tissue around the edge of the specimen that may otherwise confuse the pathologist. The width of this zone of denatured tissue varies with the type of laser employed and the type of tissue incised. However, for the carbon dioxide laser, it varies between approximately 41 microns in salivary tissue to 86 microns in epithelium and muscle.[27]

Once an area of leukoplakia or erythroplakia has been biopsied under toluidine blue control, one has the choice of excising the area to the appropriate depth with a narrow beam laser used as a scalpel or vaporizing the area to the appropriate depth with a defocused wider beam, usually using a free-beam carbon dioxide laser. Vaporization usually is more rapid but does not leave a specimen for histopathologic examination. The excised or vaporized tissue bed is left to epithelialize secondarily and undergoes little scarring or contraction. Prior to excision, the area to be treated is normally outlined by making laser marks every few millimeters by using the laser in a slow, pulsed mode.

Sublingual keratosis, with its known malignant transformation rate of up to 25%,[28] is particularly amenable to vaporization or excisional biopsy with a laser and responds well to treatment with the free-beam carbon dioxide laser in particular[29] (Fig. 8–1). Behind the lower incisors, the beam may have to be reflected through a front surface reflecting mirror. The proximity of Wharton's ducts need not be of concern because they can be resected and left to open more proximally. The diameter of the ducts in relation to the diameter of the laser beam ensures that the duct orifices remain patent, and the relative absence of swelling with carbon dioxide laser treatment means that the ducts should not be narrowed by edema, causing submandibular swelling. The extent of the area to be treated by vaporization or excision can be outlined with the laser set on

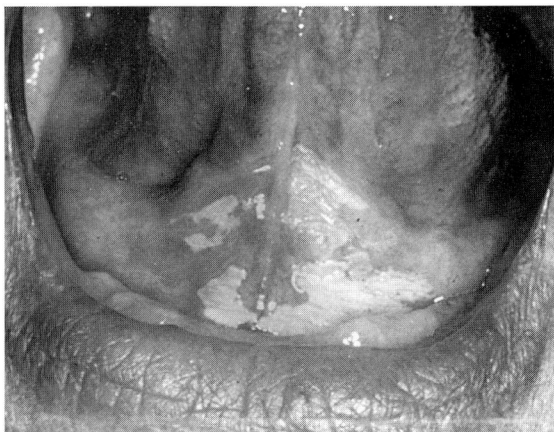

FIGURE 8–1. Sublingual keratosis, a lesion with a high potential for malignant transformation that responds well to laser vaporization.

intermediate or pulsed mode, as previously described for leukoplakia.

Carcinoma of the Tongue

Carcinoma of the lateral and ventral surfaces of the tongue is one of the more common lesions, representing over 29% of intraoral carcinomas and carrying a gloomy prognosis.[30] The 5-year survival rate for patients with carcinoma of the tongue is 67% for those diagnosed with localized disease only and 30% for those with spread at initial diagnosis.[31] This is probably related to the fact that metastatic spread to the regional lymph nodes occurs early, probably owing to an effect whereby malignant cells pass between the muscle bundles and are milked toward the posterior of the tongue by the constant movement of the tongue. For this reason, many specialists have advocated that tongue resections for carcinoma should be carried out as composite resections to include regional lymph nodes and should be incontinuity resections to encompass sound cancer principles of not cutting across malignant tissue. Treatment often included a mandibular resection or mandibulotomy for access, and the specimen was removed from the superior end to avoid unnecessary contamination of the neck tissues. Indeed, before 1970, transoral removal of carcinomatous lesions was criticized.[32] It has, however, been shown that strictly intraoral resection of the tongue carcinoma, coupled with a separate radical neck dissection when necessary, does not have an adverse effect on cure rate and prognosis and that when the laser is used for the intraoral resection, this is even more so.[32] The ability to carry out an intraoral laser resection for malignant tumors of the tongue brings a significant improvement in cosmesis and function because mandibular resection and mandibulotomy, as well as tracheostomy, can be avoided in many cases. Most papers have described the use of a free-beam carbon dioxide laser with a narrow beam as a cutting instrument for this lesion, but more recently, reports of contact tip Nd:YAG laser use have also appeared.[33] Because many cases of carcinoma of the tongue have surrounding areas of leukoplakia or erythroplakia, it is necessary either to include these in the dissection or to have biopsy evidence under toluidine blue control that the leukoplakia is nonmalignant, in which case it can be vaporized at the same time. As previously described, the outlines of the resection are marked with the laser set in a slow-pulse mode. For T_1 and T_2 lesions, a total resection is normally carried out with no primary repair. Normal cancer margins are preserved (1.5 to 2 cm beyond any visible or palpable tumor). Healing is often slow but is painless, and the final result leaves

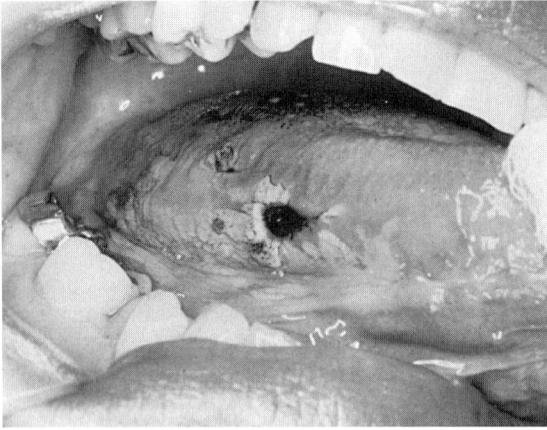

FIGURE 8–2. A biopsy-proven, toluidine blue–stained carcinoma of the left lateral tongue with a surrounding area of leukoplakia.

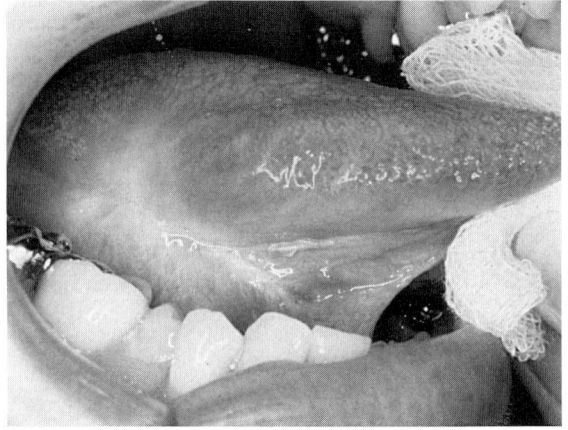

FIGURE 8–4. Appearance of tongue in Figure 8–2 when healing is complete. Note mobile tongue with minimal scarring.

relatively little scarring with a mobile functioning tongue (Figs. 8–2 to 8–4). Speech is rarely affected, and the tongue usually is mobile enough to cleanse the buccal sulci. Postoperative radiation therapy can be given once epithelialization is complete, normally between 4 and 6 weeks postoperatively. For T_3 and T_4 tumors, the same general principles of resection are followed, although in these cases, a larger tongue resection is necessary and reconstruction may well be required. Skin grafts normally do not take well on lasered surfaces because the lymphatics and blood vessels are sealed by the laser process. However, rubbing with wet gauze can remove the surface coagulation and cause pinpoint capillary bleeding, and then a skin graft or flap will take satisfactorily if indicated. These lesions also are more likely to require a concurrent radical neck resection and almost certainly necessitate combined

therapy, normally with postoperative radiation therapy. On occasion, a tracheostomy may still be required. However, in general terms, laser resection is still preferable because it avoids a mandibular resection or mandibulotomy and often avoids a tracheostomy. The overall prognosis and cure rate are at least as good as with conventional treatment[4, 7, 34–36] and may even be superior owing to the sealing of lymphatics and blood vessels at the time of resection, which may lessen the seeding of malignant cells and possible metastatic spread. This latter finding has been shown in animal studies[2, 3] and a small number of clinical studies,[35–37] although other studies have failed to confirm these findings.[38]

Lesions of the Tonsils and Oropharynx

In many cases, these lesions may be regarded as extensions of lesions of the posterior tongue and are treated similarly. The same indication for localized laser resection exists, although with surgery in this area, it is more likely that a concomitant tracheostomy may be required. Reconstruction of larger lesions is again by means of split-thickness skin grafts or a local or distant flap procedure, depending on which is most appropriate.

Lesions of the Palate

Malignant palatal lesions include squamous cell carcinomas and also malignant salivary gland tumors. Most squamous cell carcinomas and high-grade salivary gland tumors require a wide resection, which involves bone removal as either an inferior maxillectomy or total maxillectomy, depending on the size and histologic characteristics of

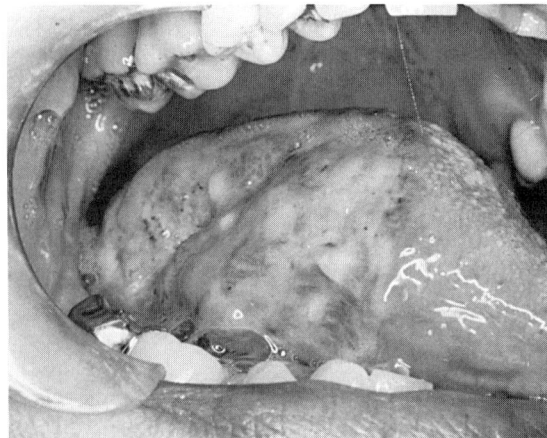

FIGURE 8–3. Appearance of tongue following laser excision of the lesion in Figure 8–2. No reconstruction was carried out.

the lesion. Because the present generation of lasers are inappropriate for bone cutting and bone removal,[19] the laser plays no part in these more extensive resections except as a means of outlining the lesion and making the superficial incision down to the periosteum. However, with low-grade lesions such as polymorphous low-grade adenocarcinoma, which has now been recognized to occur more frequently intraorally than was suspected,[39–41] and the low-grade mucoepidermoid carcinoma, if CT scans and other imaging techniques fail to reveal any bone involvement, then a localized laser resection can be performed. The surgical carbon dioxide laser is used in a narrow beam as a knife to carry out an excisional removal of the lesion, or a contact tip Nd:YAG laser can be used if preferred. Resection can be carried out in a bloodless field with great precision. However, care must be taken not to unnecessarily involve and char the palatal bone because this action may cause sequestration to occur. With the carbon dioxide laser, one knows when bone has been struck because the bright white reflected light is seen as the bone chars. Reconstruction of the palate is rarely necessary, and secondary epithelialization occurs uneventfully.

A similar technique can be used for severely dysplastic and early squamous cell carcinoma of the mucosa. Figure 8–5 shows a biopsy-proven, microinvasive carcinoma of the anterior palatal mucosa, which may have been aggravated by an ill-fitting upper removable partial denture. The malignant areas are stained with toluidine blue. In this case, conventional treatment would have consisted of an anterior palatal resection, including the loss of teeth and the necessity to wear an obturator. After discussion with the patient, laser vaporization of the area was carried out using a carbon dioxide laser with a nonfocused beam to vaporize down to

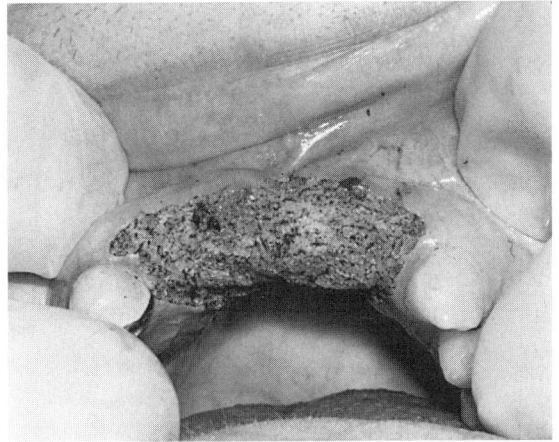

FIGURE 8–6. Mucosa vaporized down to the palatal bone with CO_2 laser. The area was left to epithelialize secondarily.

the palatal periosteum, avoiding the underlying bone (Fig. 8–6). The anterior palate reepithelialized satisfactorily with no scarring, and the patient went on to get a fixed bridge constructed. The final appearance approximately 8 years later is shown in Figure 8–7. Two biopsies were carried out over the intervening years, and both showed perfectly normal mucosa. This would appear to be an instance in which the use of a laser for vaporization for an early malignant lesion has saved the patient from a wider surgical procedure.

Lesions of the Lips

Exophytic lesions on the vermilion border or cutaneous surface of the lip can be excised with a surgical laser, and it also has been used in the management of actinic keratosis of the lower lip, which is known to have a premalignant disposition. On the mucosal aspect of the lips, both squamous cell carcinoma and salivary gland tumors can occur. Squamous cell carcinoma may lend itself to laser excision in the same manner as that described for such lesions of the tongue. Low-grade salivary gland carcinomas, such as the polymorphous low-grade adenocarcinoma or a low-grade mucoepidermoid carcinoma, particularly lend themselves to laser excision. Figure 8–8 shows a polymorphous low-grade adenocarcinoma of the left upper lip in a patient who was referred for laser treatment following incomplete scalpel excision of the lesion. Using local anesthesia, with the lip adequately retracted, a wide local excision with clear margins was carried out under direct vision. The resulting defect was left open to epithelialize secondarily, leaving an excellent result with only minimal scarring and contracture and no residual deformity of the upper lip

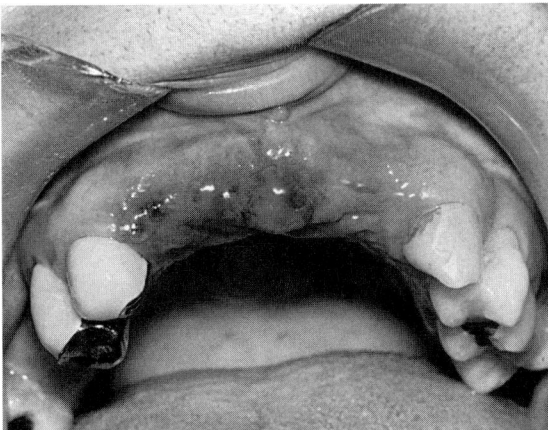

FIGURE 8–5. A biopsy-proven microinvasive carcinoma of the anterior palate stained with toluidine blue. Conventional surgery would involve an anterior palatal resection.

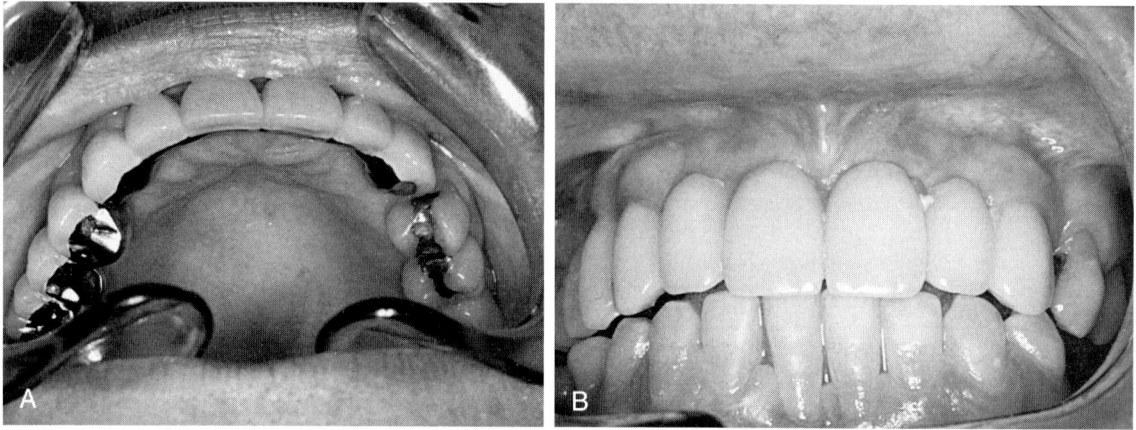

FIGURE 8–7. Appearance 8 years after laser vaporization, with normal-appearing mucosa and no recurrent or metastatic disease. Dental reconstruction was with a fixed bridge. *A*, Palatal view. *B*, Buccal view.

as can be seen in Figures 8–9, 8–10, and 8–11. This patient remains disease free after 6 years.

Verrucous Carcinoma

Verrucous carcinoma is a proliferative, superficial, noninvasive, and late-metastasizing form of squamous cell carcinoma.[42] It responds well to wide local excision, which is the treatment of choice. Radiation therapy has been contraindicated because it has been noted that the lesion can degenerate into a high-grade squamous cell carcinoma with radiation therapy. However, more recent evidence has disputed this finding, and radiation therapy may be effective for these lesions.[43] However, they are very effectively treated by means of the surgical carbon dioxide laser used in cutting mode to totally excise the lesion. Figure 8–12 shows an extensive verrucous carcinoma of the undersurface of the left

lateral tongue that was excised with a carbon dioxide laser, with the result shown in Figures 8–13 and 8–14. Healing was by secondary intention, and a mobile well-functioning tongue resulted. Follow-up in this patient for 7 years postoperatively has shown no evidence of recurrence or metastasis (Fig. 8–15). Verrucous carcinoma is often the end result of undertreatment of a proliferative verrucous hyperplasia, which shows an invariable progression to carcinoma.[44] When in the hyperplastic stage, it is adequately removed by means of a laser used either in an excision mode or in a vaporization mode. This is best carried out under toluidine blue control.

DEBULKING OF LESIONS

In inoperable head and neck malignancy, the laser may have a part to play in debulking lesions, either in vaporization or in excisional mode.[31] A major

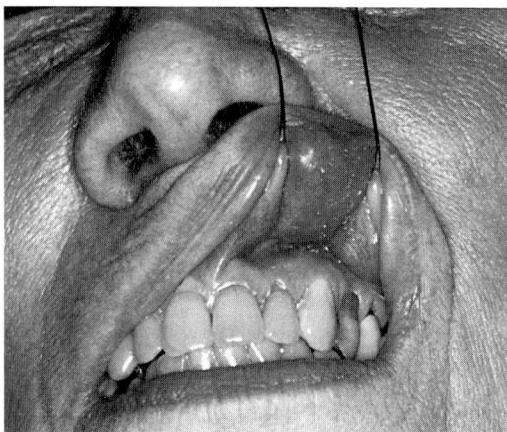

FIGURE 8–8. A polymorphous low-grade adenocarcinoma of the left upper lip suitable for laser excision.

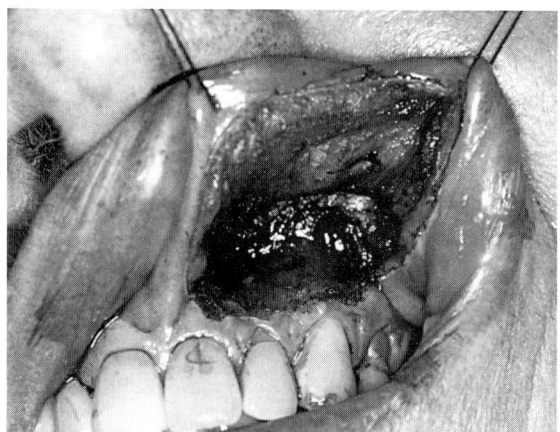

FIGURE 8–9. Patient in Figure 8–8 following laser excision. Note the defect is left to epithelialize secondarily.

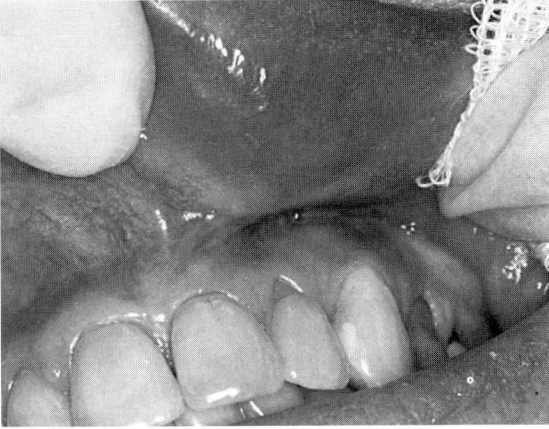

FIGURE 8–10. Patient in Figure 8–8 approximately 4 weeks after laser excision showing excellent reepithelialization and healing. There has been no recurrence or metastasis 6 years after the procedure.

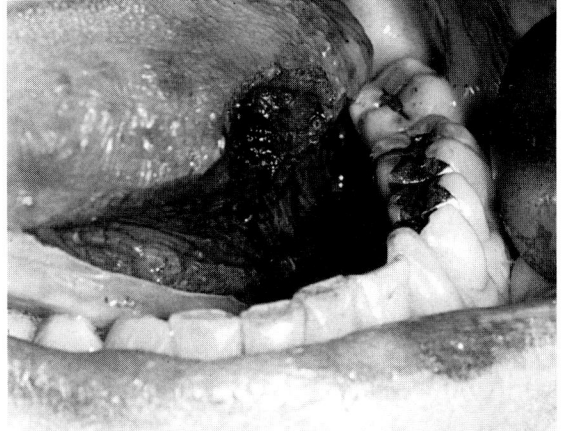

FIGURE 8–13. Appearance of tongue following laser excision. Wound was left to heal by secondary epithelialization.

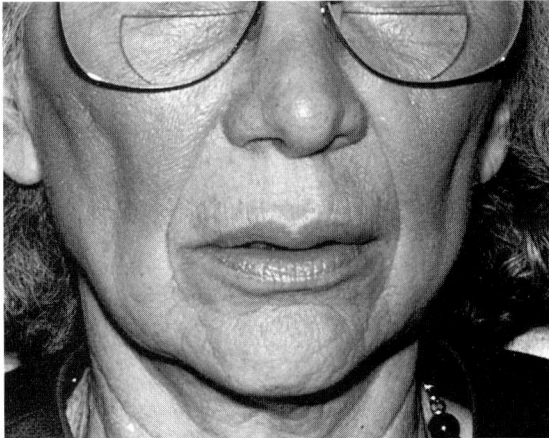

FIGURE 8–11. Final appearance of upper lip showing no residual deformity.

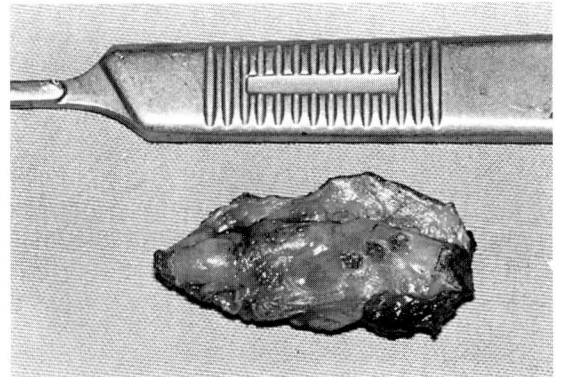

FIGURE 8–14. Laser-excised specimen from lesion in Figure 8–12.

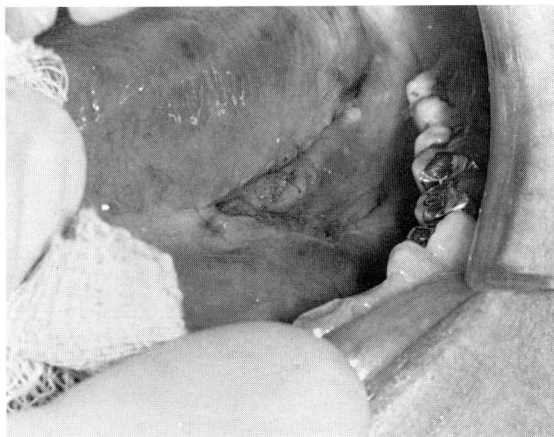

FIGURE 8–12. A verrucous carcinoma of the left lateral tongue stained with toluidine blue.

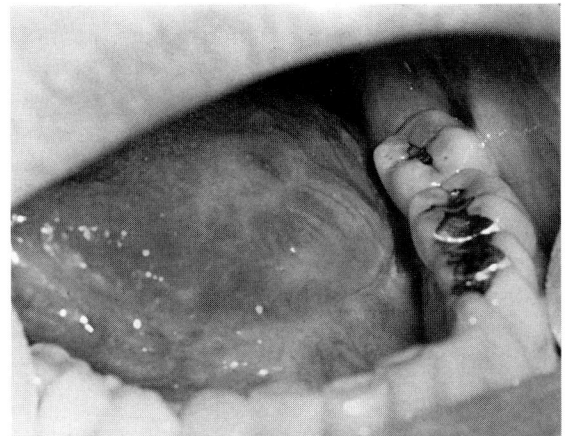

FIGURE 8–15. Appearance of the tongue from Figure 8–11 approximately 7 years postoperatively. The tongue is mobile and sensate, with no evidence of recurrence or metastasis.

advantage of the laser is the lack of bleeding and its ability to seal lymphatic and blood vessels so that reconstruction is simplified. Lesions can be debulked in order to clear the airway or gastrointestinal tract or, with large intraoral lesions, to enable mastication to continue. Debulking may also render a lesion more susceptible to radiation therapy or chemotherapeutic protocols. When debulking lesions of the airway or gastrointestinal tract, the contact tip mode of excisional vaporization is often preferred in the oropharynx and laryngeal regions because of access problems with the free-beam carbon dioxide laser.

HISTOLOGIC PATTERNS AMENABLE TO LASER TREATMENT

At the present time, laser ablation is possible with only solid tumors. The majority of malignant lesions of the oral cavity are squamous cell carcinomas; as has already been noted, not only are these suitable for laser surgery, but for many reasons, laser surgery may well be the treatment of choice. A variant of squamous cell carcinoma of the lips called keratoacanthoma is also amenable to localized laser excision. This is generally held to be a self-healing carcinoma, which undergoes spontaneous involution. Malignant salivary gland tumors may also be amenable to laser excision. The polymorphous low-grade adenocarcinoma and low-grade mucoepidermoid carcinoma, in particular, are amenable to wide local excision with the laser. High-grade mucoepidermoid carcinomas and adenocystic carcinoma require more radical excision, but when they are wholly within soft tissue such as on the tongue, lips, or cheeks, they may still be ideally excised with the laser. Localized palatal lesions can be excised with the laser, but more infiltrative lesions require a combination of laser, scalpel, and saws or drills because bone cuts also need to be made as part of a maxillectomy or one of its variants.

Mesenchymal malignant tumors such as the malignant fibrous histiocytoma and fibrosarcoma can be treated by radical excision using a laser, followed with radiation therapy when appropriate. Osteosarcomas require more conventional surgical techniques because bone is involved, but again the laser can be used as part of the soft tissue approach to the lesion.

THE LASER AS A SURGICAL KNIFE

In addition to the use of the laser for the removal of malignant lesions, the laser can also be used as a knife to assist in gaining access to a lesion for resection and also to aid in subsequent reconstruction. For instance, the laser can be used for such procedures as raising the cheek flap via a Weber-Ferguson incision in order to gain access to the maxilla or as part of a submandibular approach with or without the addition of a lip-splitting incision to gain access to the mandible for resection with or without simultaneous neck dissection. In these cases, the initial skin incision is still made with a scalpel, but all underlying incisions can be made with a surgical carbon dioxide laser with a narrow beam as a surgical knife. The inherent properties of the laser to minimize blood loss, seal lymphatics and nerve endings, and possibly minimize seeding of cells make underlying incisions an indication for laser surgery.

Similarly, the laser can be used to aid in raising soft tissue flaps for subsequent reconstruction following the excision of malignant lesions. Extraorally, it can be used to aid in the raising of such distant pedicle flaps as the deltopectoral flap and the pectoralis major myocutaneous flap, as well as variations of the trapezius and nape flap, which can be rotated for intraoral and extraoral reconstruction. It can also be used for raising the temporalis muscle flap, which can be turned down into the oral cavity once the zygomatic arch is sectioned.[45] It can also be used to raise nasolabial flaps based either superiorly or inferiorly for reconstruction of the floor of the mouth or other intraoral regions following scalpel skin incisions.[46] Intraorally, lasers can be used very effectively to raise a palatal island flap for reconstruction of the palate following excision of a salivary gland tumor or squamous cell carcinoma.[47]

PHOTODYNAMIC THERAPY

Photodynamic therapy involves the activation of a normally inert substance by means of light energy, converting it into an active substance. As such, the technique, in which plant extracts containing psoralens were applied to the skin of patients with vitiligo, which then darkened on exposure to sunlight, has been known for over 3000 years. More recent studies since the 1970s, however, have involved the intravenous injection of a chemosensitizing agent that is preferentially absorbed by malignant tissue or reticuloendothelial tissue.[48] When these tissues are then exposed to light energy, a photochemical reaction is catalyzed, releasing the toxic agents responsible for cellular death and tumor necrosis. The light energy usually is delivered by means of either a tunable dye laser or argon laser, if the tissues are deep to the surface, or a low-energy red laser beam for surface lesions. The most commonly used chemosensitizing agents are porphyrins and, more specifically, hematoporphyrin derivatives. Among the criteria that are included for application of a photosensitizer for the diagnosis and treatment of malignant tissue are the absence of permanent or severe systemic toxicity, photoactivation by a light wavelength transmitted by tissues, and the selective concentration of the drug in malignant tissues for enhancement of therapeutic ratio without destruction of normal tissues. Hematoporphyrin derivatives are preferentially concentrated in tumor tissue, liver, spleen, kidney, lung, muscle, and skin. This concentration in the skin is responsible for the temporary and generalized photosensitivity that often lasts approximately 30 days following drug administration. This property is a major disadvantage of current photosensitizing agents. Nevertheless, the technique has been used in preliminary studies of the management of head and neck cancer with promising results, and one study showed 11 of 12 metastatic deposits following photodynamic therapy.[49]

In order to get around the complication of photosensitivity, a search has been made for alternative photosensitizers. 5-Aminolevulinic acid is a naturally occurring precursor of heme whose production is controlled by negative feedback inhibition by heme. However, if excessive exogenous 5-aminolevulinic acid is given, the feedback control is bypassed, leading to a build-up of protoporphyrin IX. Because protoporphyrin IX is an effective photosensitizer, this mechanism makes it possible to sensitize cells capable of heme synthesis with photosensitization that lasts for only a few hours. Topical application of 5-aminolevulinic acid has been described for sensitization of cutaneous basal cell carcinomas,[50] and another study describes the oral use of 5-aminolevulinic acid in the treatment of oral squamous cell carcinomas.[51] In this case, protoporphyrin IX peaked after 4 to 6 hours, and subsequent irradiation with a nonthermal red laser light at 630 nm caused tumor necrosis in three of four patients. Photodynamic therapy may come to play a significant role in the primary treatment of intraoral malignant lesions and in the management of regional metastasis of head and neck carcinomas.

REFERENCES

1. Hall RP, Hill DW, Beach WD: Carbon dioxide surgical laser. Ann R Coll Surg Engl 48:181–188, 1971.
2. Lanzafame RJ, Rogers DW, Naim JO, et al: The effect of CO$_2$ laser excision on local tumor recurrence. Lasers Surg Med 6:103–105, 1986.
3. Lanzafame RJ, Rogers DW, Naim JO, et al: Reduction of local tumor recurrence by excision with the CO$_2$ laser. Lasers Surg Med 6:439–441, 1986.
4. Carruth JAS: Resection of the tongue with the carbon dioxide laser: 100 cases. J Laryngol Otol 99:887–889, 1985.
5. Tuffin JR, Carruth JAS: The surgical carbon dioxide laser. Br Dent J 149:255–258, 1980.
6. Kaminer R, Liebow C, Margarone JL, Zambow JJ: Bacteremia following laser and conventional surgery in hamsters. J Oral Maxillofac Surg 48:45–48, 1990.
7. Tradati N, Zurrida S, Bartoli C, et al: Outpatient surgical treatment with CO$_2$ laser in oral surgery: Immediate and long-term results. Tumori 77:239–242, 1991.
8. Loumanen M, Meurman JH, Lehto VP: Extracellular matrix in healing CO$_2$ laser incision wound. J Oral Pathol Med 16:322–331, 1978.
9. Pogrel MA, Pham HD, Guntenhoener M, Stern R: Profile of hyaluronidase activity distinguishes carbon dioxide laser from scalpel wound healing. Ann Surg 217:196–200, 1993.
10. Pinheiro ACR, Browne RM, Frame JW, Matthews JB: Assessment of thermal damage in precooled CO$_2$ laser wounds using biological markers. Br J Oral Maxillofac Surg 31:239–243, 1993.
11. Fisher SE, Frame JW, Browne RM, Tranter RMD: A comparative histological study of wound healing following CO$_2$ laser and conventional surgical excision of canine buccal mucosa. Arch Oral Biol 28:287–291, 1983.
12. Basu MK, Frame JW, Rhys-Evans PH: Wound healing following partial glossectomy using the CO$_2$ laser, diathermy and scalpel: A histological study in rats. J Laryngol Otol 102:322–327, 1988.
13. Schuller DE: Use of the laser in the oral cavity. Otolaryngol Clin North Am 23:31–42, 1990.
14. Pogrel MA, Yen CK, Hansen LS: A comparison of carbon dioxide laser, liquid nitrogen and scalpel wounds in healing. Oral Surg 69:269–273, 1990.
15. Sawchuk WS, Weber PJ, Lowy DR, Dzubow LM: Infectious papillomavirus in the vapor of warts treated with carbon dioxide laser or electrocoagulation: Detection and prevention. J Am Acad Dermatol 21:41–49, 1989.
16. Matchette LS, Farland RW, Royston DD, Ediger MN: In vitro production of viable bacteriophage in carbon dioxide and argon laser plumes. Lasers Surg Med 11:380–384, 1991.
17. Baggish MS, Poeisz BJ, Joret D, et al: Presence of human immunodeficiency virus DNA in laser smoke. Lasers Surg Med 11:197–203, 1991.
18. Wenig BC, Stenson KM, Weng BM, Tracey D: Effects of plume produced by the Nd:YAG laser and electrocautery on the respiratory system. Lasers Surg Med 13:242–245, 1993.
19. Small IA, Osborn TP, Fuller T, et al: Observations of the carbon dioxide laser in bone osteotomy of the rabbit tibia. J Oral Surg 37:159–166, 1979.
20. Pogrel MA, Muff DF, Marshall GW: Structural changes in dental enamel induced by high energy continuous wave carbon dioxide laser. Lasers Surg Med 13:89–96, 1993.
21. Leighty S, Pogrel MA, Goodis H, White J: Thermal effects of the carbon dioxide laser on teeth. Lasers Life Sci 4:93–102, 1991.
22. Dressel M, Jahn R, Neu W, Jungluth KH: Studies in fiber guided excimer laser surgery for cutting and drilling bone and meniscus. Lasers Surg Med 11:569–579, 1991.
23. Neev J, Liaw LL, Raney DV, et al: Selectivity, efficiency and surface characteristics of hard dental tissues ablated with ArF pulsed excimer lasers. Lasers Surg Med 11:499–510, 1991.
24. Lustmann J, Ulmansky M, Fuxbrunner A, Lewis A: 193 nm excimer laser ablation of bone. Lasers Surg Med 11:51–57, 1991.
25. Niebel HH, Chomet B: In vivo staining test for delineation of oral intraepithelial neoplastic change. J Am Dent Assoc 68:801–806, 1964.
26. Mashberg A: Tolonium (toluidine blue) rinse—a screening method for recognition of squamous carcinoma. J Am Med Assoc 245:2408–2410, 1981.
27. Pogrel MA, McCracken KT, Daniels TE: Histologic evaluation of the width of soft tissue necrosis adjacent to carbon dioxide laser incisions. Oral Surg 70:564–568, 1990.

28. Pogrel MA: Sublingual keratosis and malignant transformation. J Oral Pathol 8:176–178, 1979.

29. Frame JW: Treatment of sublingual keratoses with the CO_2 laser. Br Dent J 156:243–246, 1984.

30. National Cancer Institute: Cancer statistics review 1973–1987. Bethesda, MD, U.S. Department of Health and Human Services, 1990.

31. National Cancer Institute: Surveillance, Epidemiology and End Results program (SEER) 1973–1984. Bethesda, MD, U.S. Department of Health and Human Services, 1990.

32. Panje WR, Scher N, Karnell M: Transoral CO_2 laser ablation for cancer, tumors and other diseases. Arch Otolaryngol Head Neck Surg 115:681–688, 1989.

33. Shapshay SM: Laser technology in the diagnosis and treatment of head and neck cancer. Semin Surg Oncol 5:61–66, 1989.

34. Guerry TL, Silverman S, Dedo HH: Carbon dioxide laser resection of superficial oral carcinoma: Indications, technique and results. Ann Otol Rhinol Laryngol 95:547–555, 1986.

35. Nagorsky MJ, Sessions DG: Laser resection for early oral cavity cancer: Results and complications. Ann Otol Rhinol Laryngol 96:556–560, 1987.

36. Duncovage JA, Ossoff RH: Use of the CO_2 laser for malignant disease of the oral cavity. Lasers Surg Med 6:442–444, 1986.

37. Adams EL, Price NM: Treatment of basal cell carcinomas with a carbon dioxide laser. J Dermatol Surg Oncol 5:803–806, 1979.

38. Rhys-Williams S, Carruth JAS: The role of the carbon dioxide laser in treatment of carcinoma of the tongue. J Laryngol Otol 102:1122–1123, 1988.

39. Aberle AM, Abrams AM, Bowe R, et al: Lobular (polymorphous low grade) carcinoma of minor salivary glands. Oral Surg 60:387–395, 1985.

40. Evans HL, Batsakis JG: Polymorphous low grade adenocarcinoma of minor salivary glands. Cancer 53:935–942, 1984.

41. Freedman PD, Lumerman H: Lobular carcinoma of intraoral minor salivary gland origin. Oral Surg 56:157–165, 1983.

42. Kamath VV, Varma RR, Gadewar DR, Muralidhar M: Oral verrucous carcinoma. An analysis of 37 cases. J Craniomaxillofac Surg 17:309–314, 1989.

43. Vidyasager MS, Fernandes DJ, Kasturi P, et al: Radiotherapy and verrucous carcinoma of the oral cavity. A study of 107 cases. Acta Oncol 31:43–47, 1992.

44. Hansen LS, Olson JA, Silverman S Jr: Proliferative verrucous leukoplakia. A long-term study of 30 patients. Oral Surg 60:205–298, 1985.

45. Pogrel MA, Kaban LB: The role of temporalis fascia and muscle flap in temporomandibular joint surgery. J Oral Maxillofac Surg 48:14–19, 1990.

46. Worthington P: The management of the palatal pleomorphic adenoma. Br J Oral Surg 12:132–140, 1974.

47. Stell PM, Maran AGD: Head and Neck Surgery. London, Heinemann, 1978, p 347.

48. Davis RK: Photodynamic therapy in otolaryngology—head and neck surgery. Otolaryngol Clin North Am 23:107–119, 1990.

49. Schweitzer VG: Photodynamic therapy for treatment of head and neck cancer. Otol Head Neck Surg 102:225–232, 1990.

50. Kennedy JC, Polter RH: Endogenous proporphyrin IX, a clinically useful photosensitizer for photodynamic therapy. J Photochem Photobiol B 14:275–292, 1992.

51. Grant WE, Hopper C, MacRobert AJ, et al: Photodynamic therapy of oral cancer photosensitization with systemic aminolevulinic acid. Lancet 342:147–148, 1993.

Laser Management of Vascular and Pigmented Lesions

JOHN SEXTON, DMD, MSD

The selective absorption of different wavelengths of light by tissue chromophores makes the treatment of vascular or pigmented lesions via laser possible. In contrast to the carbon dioxide laser, whose tissue chromophore is water, lasers such as the argon, neodymium:yttrium-aluminum-garnet (Nd:YAG), dye, ruby, and KTP lasers emit wavelengths that can be differentially absorbed by endogenous or exogenous tissue pigments. The clinical efficacy of such lasers is due to their ability to photocoagulate, or photothermolyse, rather than excise. Variable but high absorption coefficients allow precise tissue destruction with minimal effect on surrounding tissues. In most cases, operative bleeding is eliminated. The following discussion briefly outlines the classification of vascular malformations found in the head and neck region, the components of the vascular lesion diagnostic work-up, and the usefulness of laser in the treatment of selected vascular or pigmented lesions.

CLASSIFICATION

Congenital vascular lesions can be generally categorized into two groups—hemangiomas and malformations. Acquired lesions may be traumatic or idiopathic in origin. Some lesions, such as venous lakes and varicosities, are part of the normal aging process.

The congenital anomalies may be further subdivided according to vessel type. Capillary, venous, and lymphomatous malformations are low-flow le-

sions, whereas arterial or arteriovenous (A-V) lesions are high flow. A-V malformations involve bone in many cases and may persist into adulthood. The hemangiomatous lesions are evident postnatally, are confined to soft tissue, and usually involute in early childhood. Almost all vascular lesions encountered in adults are malformations, especially when such lesions are found in bone.[1, 2]

Malformations may be seen in a number of different syndromes involving the oral cavity as well as the head and neck. Rendu-Osler-Weber syndrome is inherited as an autosomal dominant trait and manifests as multiple telangiectasias involving the skin as well as the mucous membranes of the gastrointestinal tract, nose, and oral cavity. The patient with Sturge-Weber syndrome demonstrates craniofacial angiomatosis, as well as meningeal hemangioma and cerebral calcification. The port-wine stain or capillary malformation seen in this syndrome tends to follow the first and second divisions of the trigeminal nerve. There may be pyogenic granulomas associated with gingival vascular ectasia.

Ataxia-telangiectasia is also an inherited disease that includes, in addition to neurologic and immunologic deficits, cutaneous and vascular telangiectasias.

Bleeding from angiodysplastic lesions may also be seen in Maffucci's syndrome, blue rubber bleb nevus, and hereditary hemorrhagic telangiectasia.[3]

In addition to the congenital or acquired vascular malformations, there are certain cutaneous diseases that have a small vessel component treatable via laser. Examples of such conditions are postrhinoplasty or post-traumatic red nose, the red nose of rosacea, and poikiloderma of Civatte.

Pigmented lesions that may be encountered in the oral or perioral regions and that may be amenable to laser treatment generally take two forms—(1) lesions attributable to melanin and (2) those due to exogenous pigment (i.e., tattoos). Melanotic pigmentation may be due to increased melanin production, as seen in freckles or melanotic macules, or it may be due to a developmental malformation, exemplified by the nevi.

Tattoos are classified into amateur tattoos, professional tattoos, and traumatic tattoos, each made up respectively of India ink, organometallic dyes, or traumatically implanted foreign material.

PHYSICS AND RATIONALE FOR TREATMENT

As briefly mentioned previously, the treatment of specific types of vascular and pigmented lesions is made possible by the ability of certain lasers to lyse precisely, via thermal injury, pigment-containing cells. This so-called selective photothermolysis targets hemoglobin, melanin, or exogenous pigment.[4] By using pulsed lasers in the treatment of these conditions, skin not containing the specific tissue chromophore is spared. The laser pulse width in conjunction with the specific wavelengths is calculated and delivered such that the thermal relaxation time of the target cell or organelle is not exceeded (thermal relaxation time being the time required for conductive cooling of the treated chromophore). Not only is the thermal damage very specific, but adjacent tissue structures are minimally affected by heat conduction. As an example, in the case of melanin-pigmented lesions, it is possible to target the melanosome and selectively explode it, leading to the disruption of melanocytes, nevus cells, or keratinocytes.[5]

Although pulsing the laser allows for much higher peak power and more selective tissue damage, continuous-wave lasers with either high or low tissue specificity also can be used to treat vascular or pigmented lesions. The occasional drawback to such lasers is a more diffuse tissue effect and thus less predictability with regard to tissue damage and ultimate healing.

TYPES OF LASERS

There are several types of lasers available for the treatment of vascular or pigmented lesions. The continuous-wave argon laser emits light in the blue-green portion of the electromagnetic spectrum, with two wavelength peaks at 488 and 514 nm, respec-

tively. This particular wavelength has excellent absorption by hemoglobin and natural skin pigments. In contrast to the carbon dioxide laser, which has a very high coefficient of tissue absorption and thus very little scatter, the argon laser scatters within the lesion, producing thermally induced coagulation.[6] The penetration of the beam is of the order of 1.0 to 1.5 mm beneath the epidermis.

The Nd:YAG laser has enjoyed most of its usefulness as a continuous-wave laser. Excited neodymium ions embedded in the YAG crystalline lattice are responsible for the laser transition, and the laser is pumped by a krypton arc lamp. The wavelength, in the near-infrared portion of the electromagnetic spectrum, is 1.06 μ. The Nd:YAG laser does not have a high coefficient of absorption by water and instead is scattered and diffused in the tissue, thus leading to deep penetration. Its advantage lies in its ability to coagulate vessels of 2 to 3 mm in diameter and its penetration of 5 to 7 mm. There is predilection for hemoglobin or tissue with dark pigment.[7] The disadvantages of the Nd:YAG laser is its depth of penetration and the possibility of tissue necrosis when treated areas are overlapped. Contact synthetic sapphire tips have helped minimize this effect.

More recently, the Q-switched Nd:YAG laser has been introduced for the treatment of pigmented lesions. Q-switched lasers deliver extremely high power with a pulse duration that is very short (pulse duration 10 nanoseconds). The Q-switched Nd:YAG laser can produce two wavelengths, those being 1064 nm and 532 nm, respectively. At 1064 nm, there is selective absorption by melanin and exogenous pigment in the dermis and epidermis. The altered frequency of 532 nm is absorbed by both melanin and hemoglobin.

Q-switched lasers such as the Q-switched Nd:YAG deliver such high energy in such a small amount of time that they can produce shock waves at the laser-tissue interface and thus cause some tissue tearing.[8]

Dye lasers have organic molecules, which are pumped by an argon laser, as the lasing medium. These lasers may be tuned, that is, made to emit in multiple portions of the electromagnetic spectrum. Dye lasers may be pulsed or continuous.

The pulsed-dye laser ruptures melanosomes at a wavelength of 510 nm and a pulse duration of 300 nanoseconds. It does not penetrate well into deep dermis. At a wavelength of 575 or 585 nm, there is superselective absorption by vascular tissue and little effect on melanin. There is also deeper penetration than with the argon laser. This selectivity coupled with a short pulse duration of 450 microseconds results a relatively painless, effective treatment with minimal scarring. The vascular relaxation time of small blood vessels less than 0.1 mm in diameter is 5 milliseconds. Thus, damage to surrounding tissue is avoided when this laser is used.[9, 10]

With experience, the dye laser can be used in a continuous mode, which is especially useful in tracing long or tortuous telangiectasias.

The Q-switched ruby laser is another of the more recently introduced lasers. The active medium is a ruby crystal doped with chromium ions, and the laser is pumped via a helical flash lamp. This laser produces 25 to 40 nanoseconds pulses and can generate 1,000,000 watts/cm^2 per pulse. The emitted wavelength of 694 nm is strongly absorbed by melanin and only weakly absorbed by hemoglobin. This makes the ruby laser a very effective tool for treating certain pigmentary disorders such as solar lentigines and nevus of Ota and also such unwanted skin blemishes as amateur tattoos.[11, 12]

Other lasers used in the treatment of vascular or pigmentary disorders include the copper vapor laser (578-nm wavelength, for vascular lesions), the KTP laser (532 nm, for vascular lesions), and the alexandrite laser (755 nm, for melanosomes).

TECHNIQUES

Argon Laser

The argon laser was one of the first lasers to be used in the treatment of vascular lesions. It was invented in 1964 and used initially to treat retinal detachment. Treatment of skin lesions gained popularity during the 1970s.

Use of the argon laser to treat oral mucosal vascular malformations usually involves using a continuous-mode setting and power outputs of 0.5 to 1.5 watts. The laser is delivered through a fiber optic cable to a hand piece. The spot size normally used is 0.1 cm, and the beam is defocused. Prior to treatment, local anesthesia must be used, generally avoiding vasoconstrictors to allow dilatation of the target vessels.

When commencing treatment, the lesion is stabilized by an assistant and the affected area is slowly but continuously ablated using either a to-and-fro painting motion or a circular technique, starting in the center of the lesion and working gradually outward. Superficial vessels may be simply traced. The end point for the treatment of mucosal or submucosal lesions is collapse of the lesion with whitening of the surface mucosa. Deep venous lakes of the lip may be more effectively treated by the glass slide technique. In this technique, a clear glass slide is pressed onto the venous lake in order to flatten the lesion and bring its deeper aspect closer to the surface. It is important, especially when using a continuous-wave laser, to keep the beam moving,

albeit slowly, to avoid excessive penetration and thus postoperative scarring.

Postoperatively the treated area ulcerates in 4 to 7 days following sloughing of the overlying mucosa. There may be swelling of the treated area, especially the lips, and the patient is advised to use ice immediately following treatment. The patient is also advised to avoid aspirin-containing medicine for a week, to avoid hot or spicy food, to refrain from using straws, and if the lesion is on the vermilion border, to apply antibiotic ointment 3 to 4 times daily. Pain medication usually is not required.[13]

In the treatment of skin lesions using the argon laser, lower power settings may be used in order to avoid excessive dermal scarring. Treatment of small areas may be undertaken at one visit, whereas larger lesions, such as port-wine stains, require multiple sessions. Again, local anesthesia is required. Following treatment, a transudate develops, lasting 1 to 3 weeks. There may be scab formation, and eventually the skin turns bright red. This is followed by gradual lightening over the course of about 4 months.

In the treatment of skin, the argon laser frequently is used in a gated mode. In order to avoid overlap and thus overtreatment, robotized devices are available (Hexascan) that are of help in this regard. Small vessel ectasia may be treated in a continuous mode, slowly tracing out the vessel. In this case, small power outputs, usually under 1 watt, are used. When using the argon laser, protective goggles must be worn that selectively eliminate or screen the two major wavelength bands (488 nm and 514 nm). Inadvertent shining of the beam into the eyes of operator, assistant, or patient could damage the retina.

Complications related to argon laser treatment generally are related to scarring. Although a successful outcome stems from a controlled dermal scar, excessive exposure can result in unacceptable scarring. This is especially true in children, and for this reason the argon laser is seldom used in children. Other potential complications include granuloma formation, bleeding, or nonresolution of the lesion.[14]

Nd:YAG Laser

Two types of Nd:YAG lasers are discussed. The continuous-wave Nd:YAG laser emits light in the near-infrared portion of the electromagnetic spectrum and thus also can be delivered through a quartz fiber optic cable. In the noncontact mode, the Nd:YAG laser has limited value in the oral cavity because of deep penetration and scatter. Superficial lesions, therefore, are better treated with argon or dye lasers. Thicker, deeply situated lesions, however, may be treated with the continuous-wave Nd:YAG laser, usually of the order of 20 to 30 watts. The clinical end point is visible shrinking of the malformation. Care must be taken not to overtreat by using too high a power. Overtreatment can lead to excessive scarring or coagulation necrosis with subsequent postoperative bleeding. For intraoral lesions, patients are advised to follow the same protocol as for treatment with the argon laser.

Newer continuous-wave Nd:YAG lasers fitted with sapphire tips have overcome many of the drawbacks of using this laser in the oral cavity. There is more of a sense of tactile control, depth of penetration and scattering are greatly reduced, and probes of different sizes or shapes can be chosen to incise, ablate, or coagulate. In spite of these advantages, however, tissue destruction is still dependent on the experience of the surgeon regarding appropriate laser power and speed of operation[15] (see Figs. 9–1 to 9–9; see also Color Plates 2 to 4).

CASE HISTORIES

The following nine cases (Figs. 9–1 to 9–9) represent vascular lesions amenable to treatment with the Coherent Lambda Plus argon dye laser. All patients were treated with the laser using a 1-mm spot size and a power setting of 0.5 to 2.0 watts. During treatment in some cases, the power setting was changed to a higher wattage if the tissue response was judged to be inadequate at the lower setting. All treatment was performed using local anesthesia on an outpatient basis. There were no complications.

Pulsed-Dye Laser*

The continuous- or pulsed-dye laser has become an excellent modality for the treatment of superficial vascular lesions such as telangiectasias, hemangiomas, angiomas, port-wine stain, red nose, and poikiloderma of Civatte. Intraorally, it may be used to treat venous lakes or ectasias. Because of its excellent selective absorption by hemoglobin with little or no effect on surrounding tissue, the dye laser, especially pulsed-dye, has found usefulness in the treatment of children, in whom postoperative scarring is minimal.

Treatment with the pulsed-dye laser may require local anesthesia without a vasoconstrictor, especially in children. The patient senses slight discomfort, like that from an elastic band being snapped

*Cynosure Incorporated, Bedford, MA.

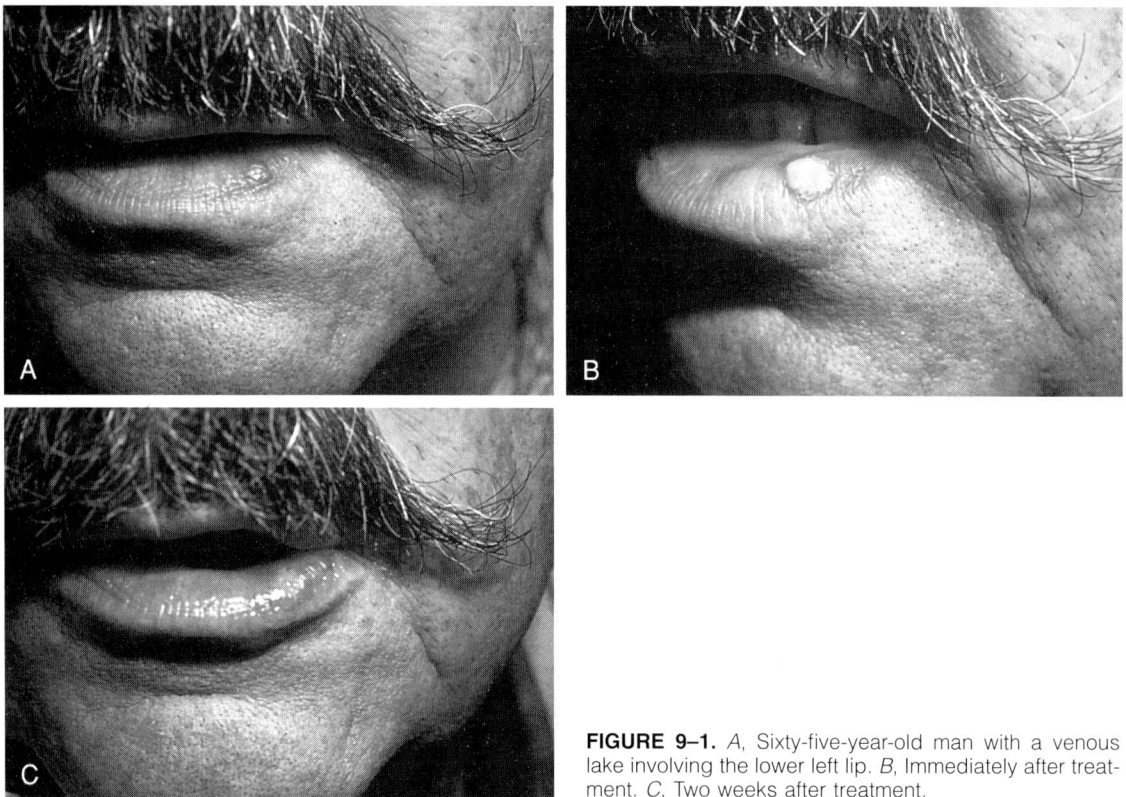

FIGURE 9–1. *A*, Sixty-five-year-old man with a venous lake involving the lower left lip. *B*, Immediately after treatment. *C*, Two weeks after treatment.

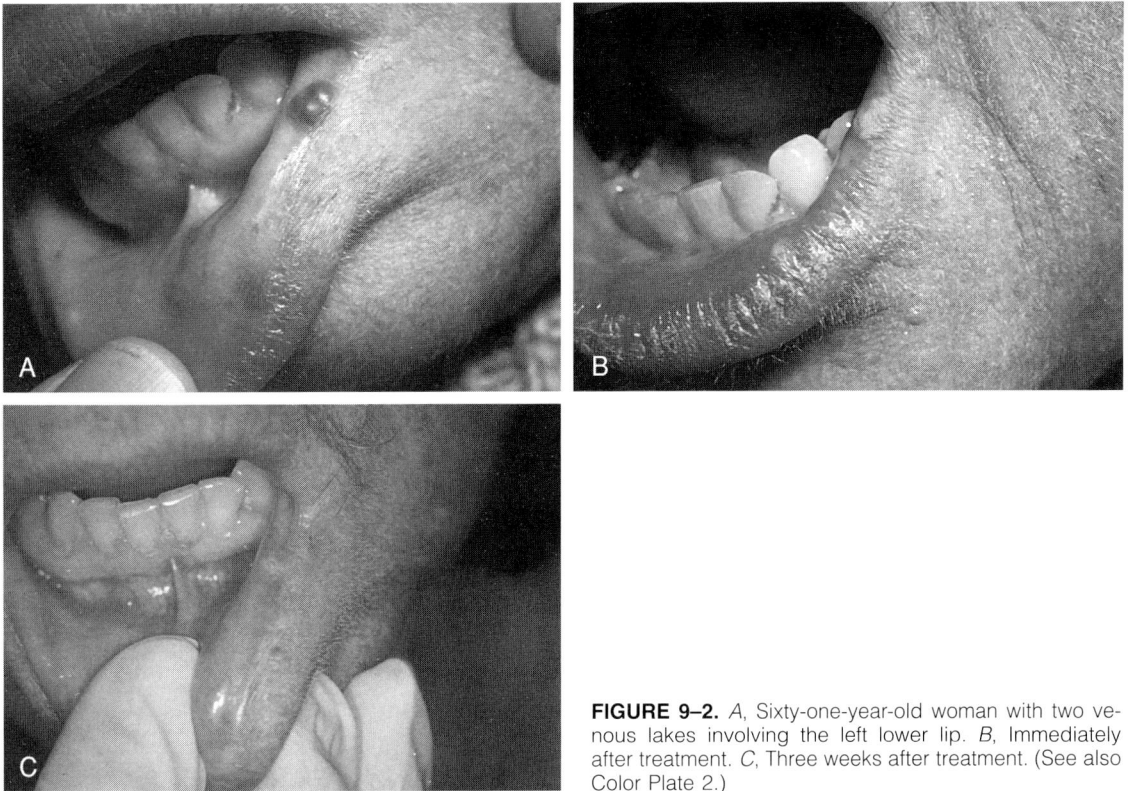

FIGURE 9–2. *A*, Sixty-one-year-old woman with two venous lakes involving the left lower lip. *B*, Immediately after treatment. *C*, Three weeks after treatment. (See also Color Plate 2.)

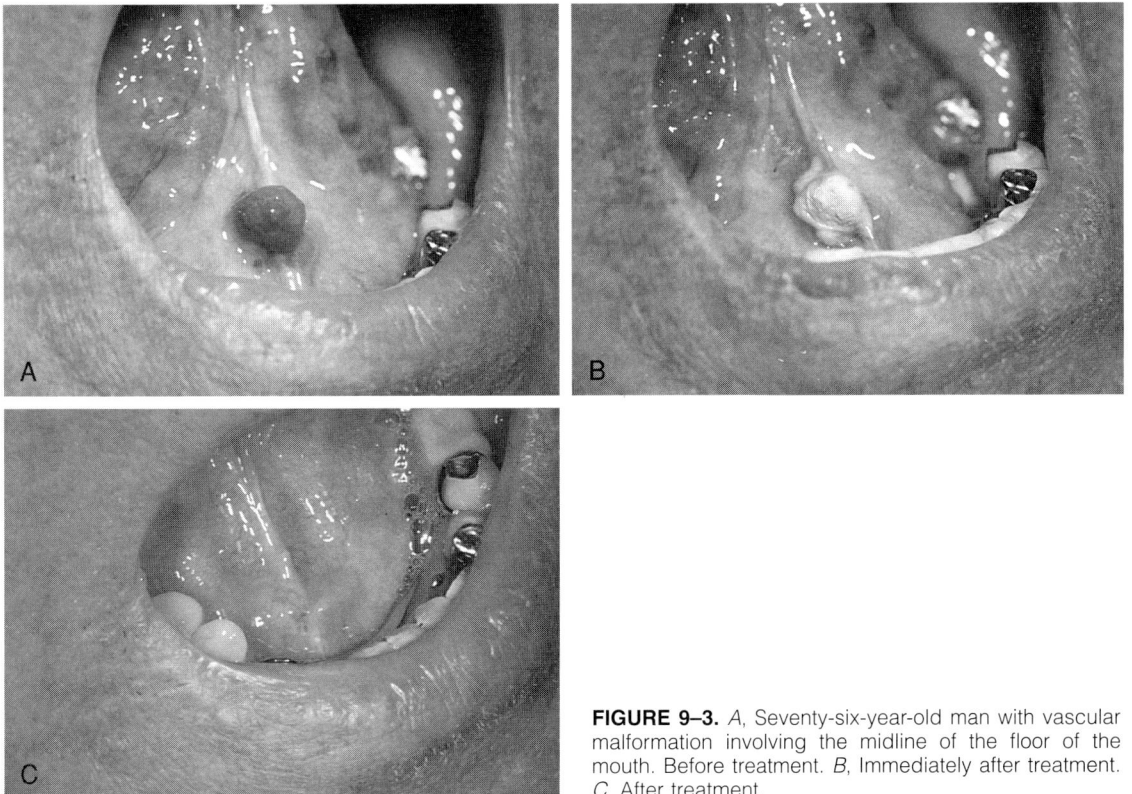

FIGURE 9–3. *A*, Seventy-six-year-old man with vascular malformation involving the midline of the floor of the mouth. Before treatment. *B*, Immediately after treatment. *C*, After treatment.

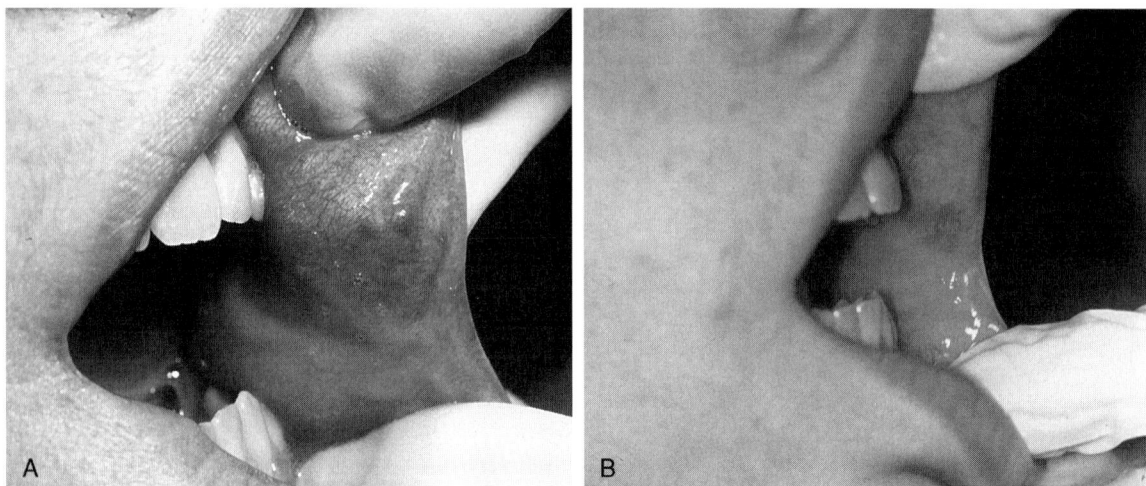

FIGURE 9–4. *A*, Twenty-nine-year-old with a hemangioma involving the left upper lip and oral commissure. Before treatment. *B*, Two months after treatment.

against the skin. The spot size used is 5 mm, and the energy required ranges from 6 to 8 joules/cm^2, with lower energy used for supervascular ectasias and higher energy used for darker, larger ectasias or malformations. After treatment, the treated area assumes a purple hue, which is bothersome to some patients and for which they should be prepared. This discoloration may take several weeks to clear.

During treatment, the lesion is simply followed with the laser, tracing out the telangiectasia or sequentially ablating larger lesions. Spots are overlapped by about 10%.

Postoperatively, again patients have little discomfort. Bacitracin and Vigilon are applied daily until the skin lightens. Postoperative complications from pulsed- or continuous-mode dye laser surgery in-

clude granuloma formation, hypopigmentation, and in inexperienced hands, scarring or a polka-dot effect.[16, 17]

As with all lasers, use of the dye lasers mandates the wearing of protective eyewear that selectively screens damaging wavelengths. All personnel in the laser suite must wear goggles (see Figs. 9–10 to 9–14; see also Color Plate 5).

CASE HISTORIES

The following cases illustrate the use of the pulsed-dye laser in the treatment of cutaneous vascular lesions (Figs. 9–10 to 9–14). Power settings were of the order of 6 to 7 joules/cm^2.

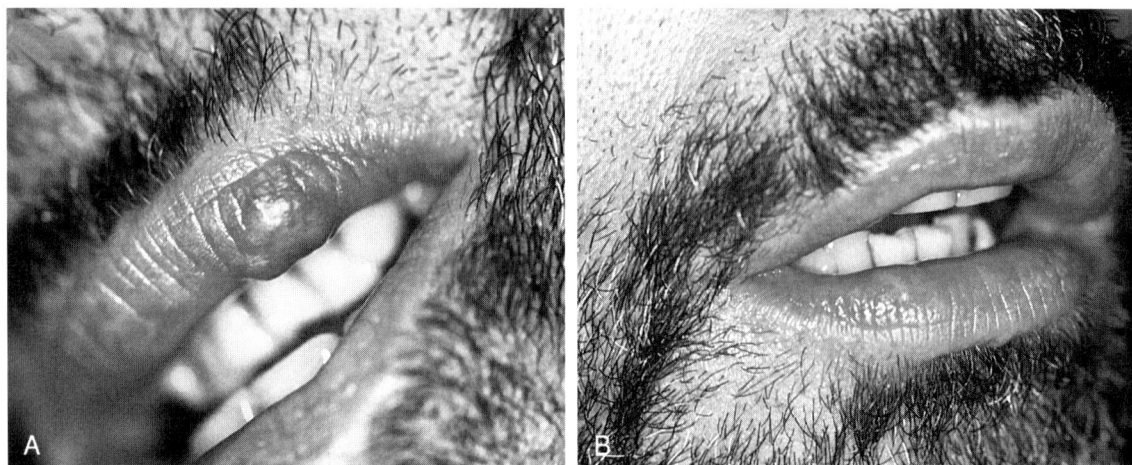

FIGURE 9–5. *A*, Forty-five-year-old man with large venous malformation involving right lower lip. *B*, After treatment.

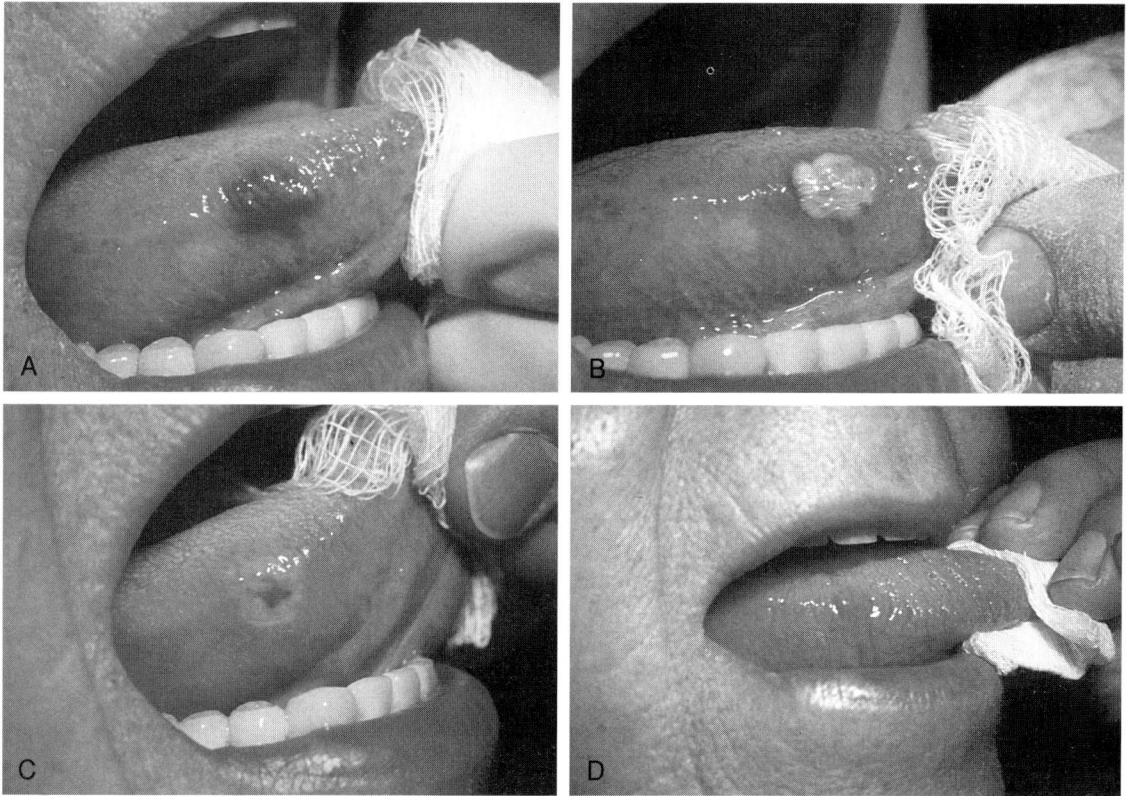

FIGURE 9–6. *A,* Seventy-two-year-old female with a hemangioma involving the right posterolateral border of the tongue. *B,* Immediately after treatment. *C,* One week after treatment. *D,* After treatment. (See also Color Plate 3.)

Q-Switched Nd:YAG Laser*

The Q-switched Nd:YAG laser represents a more recently introduced laser technology that delivers the laser light at very high peak energies. It has found great usefulness in the treatment of tattoos as well as certain pigmented lesions such as lentigines.

---
*Continuum Biomedical, Wantagh, NY.

Some lesions, such as cafe-au-lait spots, respond but in a less predictable manner. As of 1992, the Q-switched Nd:YAG laser has full FDA approval for tattoos only.[8]

In the treatment of intraoral tattoos, predominantly the amalgam tattoo, this author has found the Q-switched Nd:YAG laser very useful. Local anesthesia is used, and the laser hand piece is fitted with a shield because of tissue or blood splatter

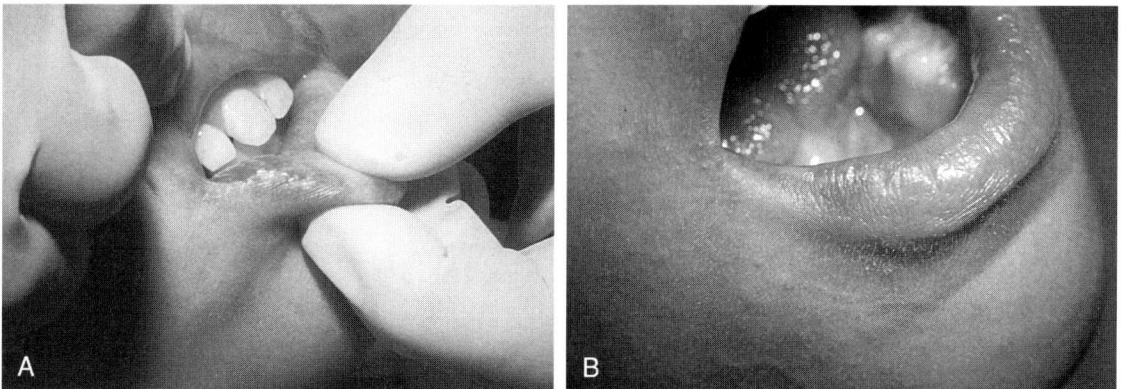

FIGURE 9–7. *A,* Twelve-year-old boy with hemangioma involving the right lower lip, commissure, and buccal mucosa. Before treatment. *B,* After treatment.

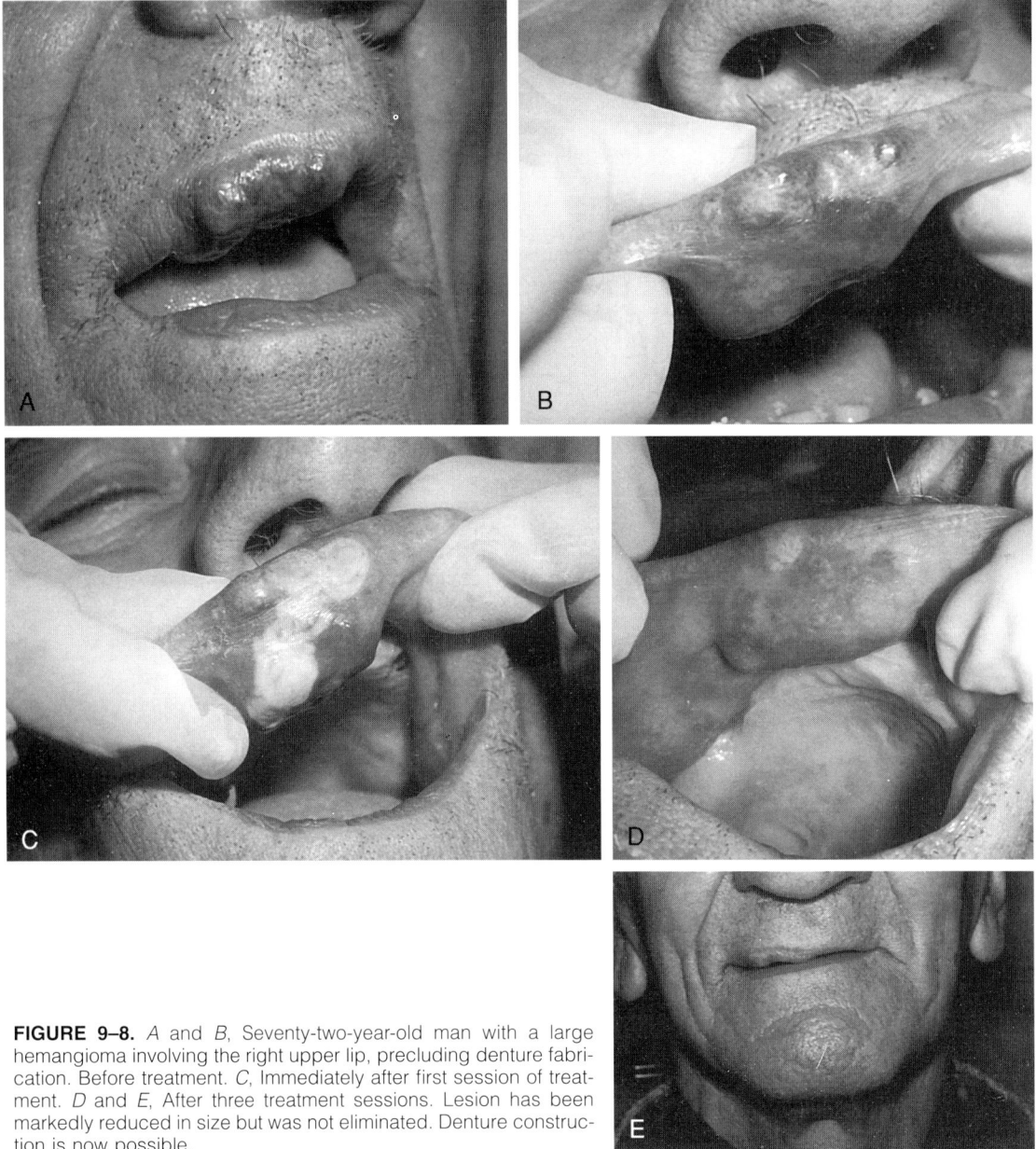

FIGURE 9–8. *A* and *B*, Seventy-two-year-old man with a large hemangioma involving the right upper lip, precluding denture fabrication. Before treatment. *C*, Immediately after first session of treatment. *D* and *E*, After three treatment sessions. Lesion has been markedly reduced in size but was not eliminated. Denture construction is now possible.

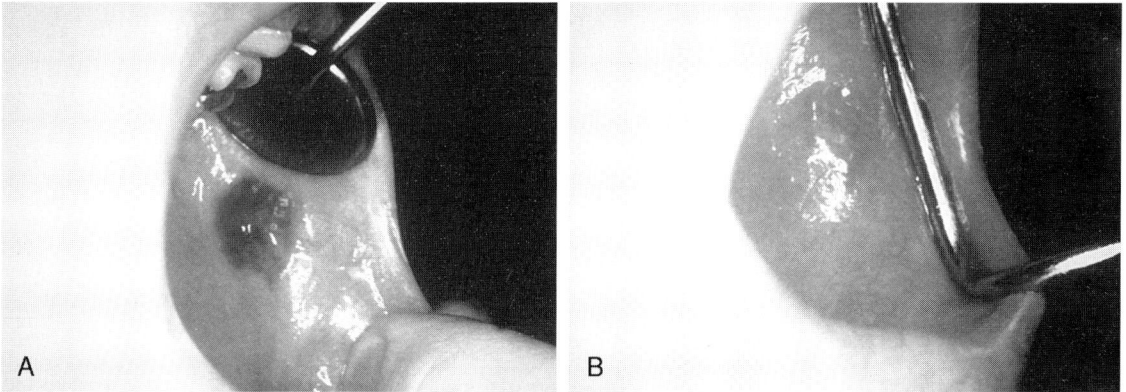

FIGURE 9–9. *A*, Forty-nine-year-old female with hemangioma involving the left buccal mucosa. Before treatment. *B*, After treatment.

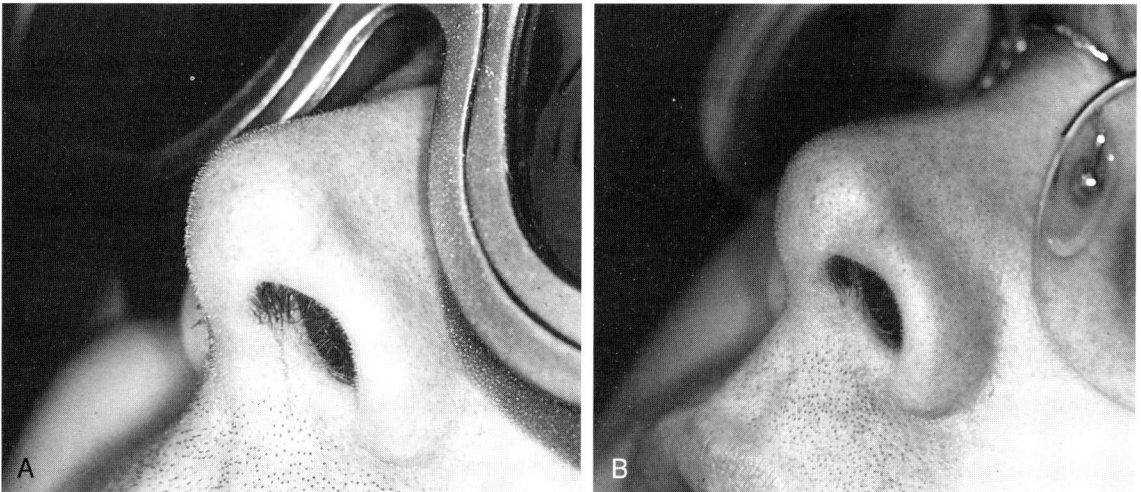

FIGURE 9–10. Pulsed-dye laser. Telangiectasia. *A*, Preoperative appearance. *B*, Postoperative appearance. (See also Color Plate 4.)

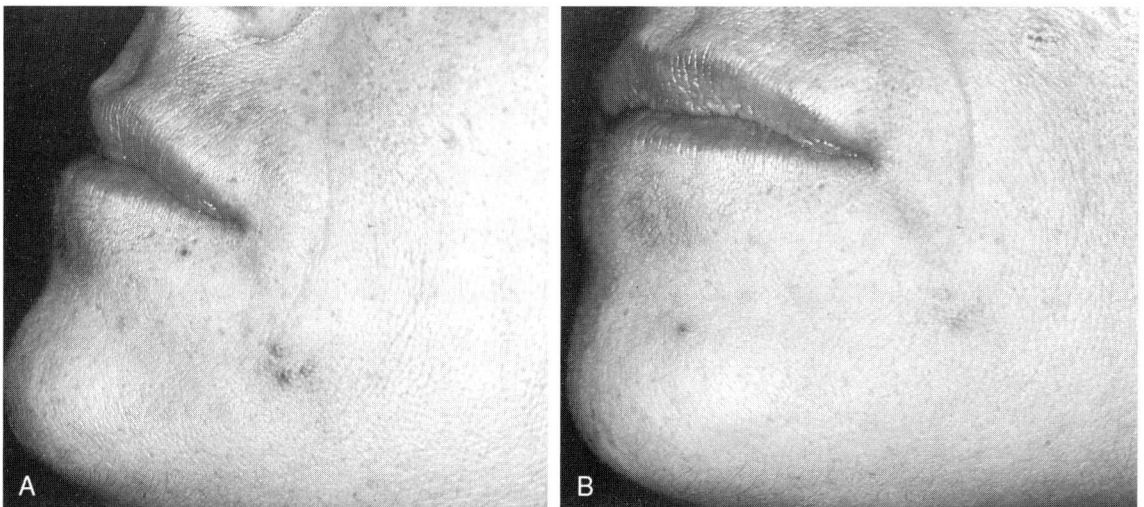

FIGURE 9–11. Pulsed-dye laser. Telangiectasia. *A*, Preoperative appearance. *B*, Postoperative appearance.

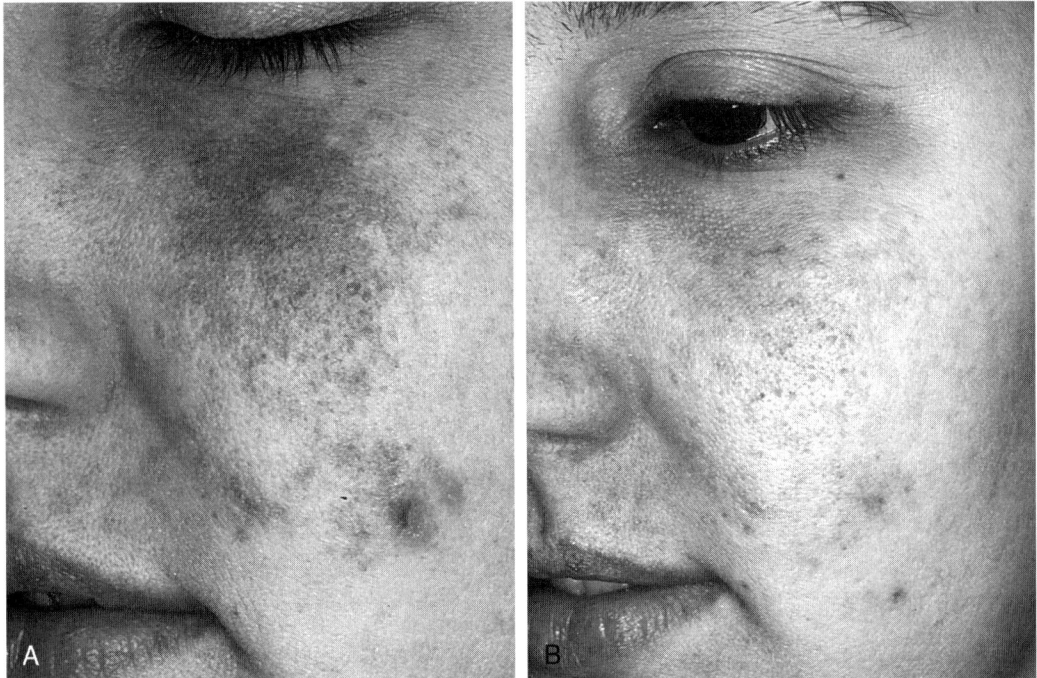

FIGURE 9–12. Pulsed-dye laser. Port-wine stain. *A*, Preoperative appearance. *B*, Postoperative appearance. (Courtesy of Dr. Kenneth Arndt.)

seen on occasion, which is due to tissue shock. The laser is set at 8 to 10 joules/cm^2, with the clinical treatment end point being whitening of the surface mucosa. The laser makes a snapping sound as the pulses are delivered.

Postoperatively, patients experience a little discomfort, and postoperative care is the same as that for argon laser treatment.

In the treatment of skin tattoos, amateur tattoos or tattoos that are a combination of black and red respond best to Q-switched Nd:YAG lasers. Green tattoos respond poorly. Multiple treatment sessions may be required, usually spaced at 4- to 8-week intervals. Postoperative wound care consists of bacitracin and, if indicated, a dressing. Postoperative scarring is very uncommon, and this factor is an advantage to this technique. An occasional unwanted postoperative sequela is hyperpigmentation or hypopigmentation (see Figs. 9–15 to 9–17; see also Color Plate 6).

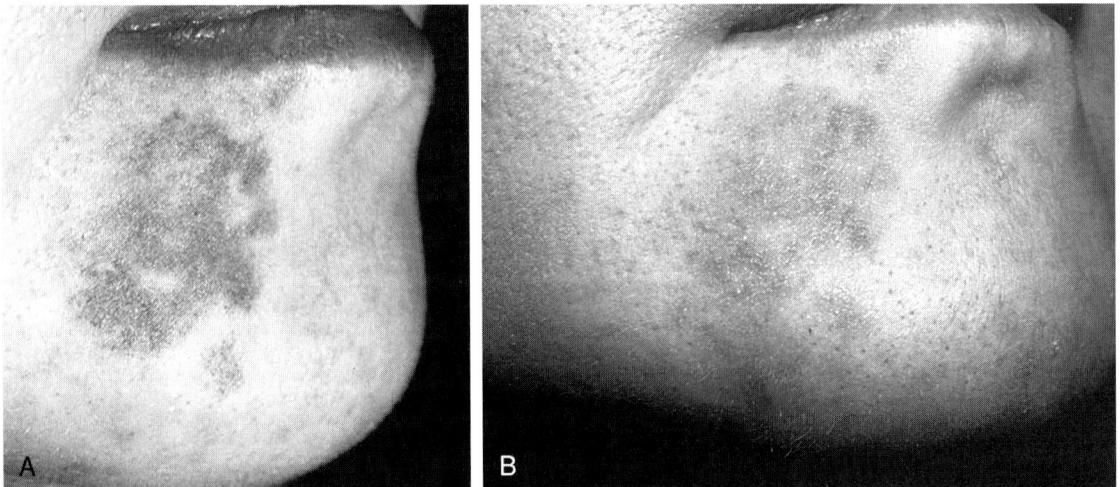

FIGURE 9–13. Pulsed-dye laser. Port-wine stain. *A*, Preoperative appearance. *B*, Postoperative appearance. (Courtesy of Dr. Kenneth Arndt.)

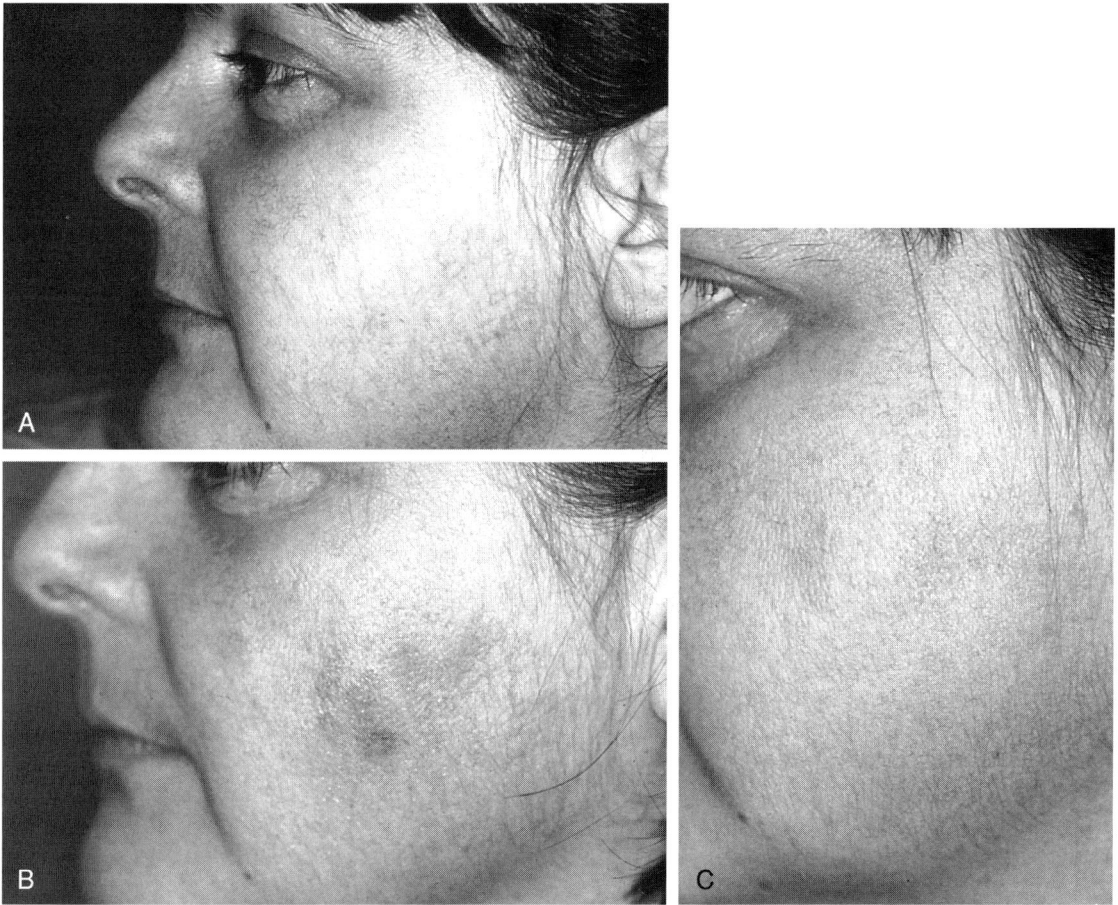

FIGURE 9–14. Pulsed-dye laser. Small vessel ectasias of the face. *A*, Preoperative appearance. *B*, Postoperative appearance (1 to 2 weeks). *C*, Postoperative clearing. (See also Color Plate 5.)

CASE HISTORIES

The following cases indicate use of the Q-switched Nd:YAG laser for the treatment of pigmented lesions (Figs. 9–15 to 9–17; see also Color Plate 6). Power settings were on the order of 0.7 to 1 joules/cm^2.

Q-Switched Ruby Laser

The Q-switched ruby laser is ideally suited for the treatment of pigmented lesions, including tattoos, nevi of Ota, melanotic macules, lentigines, and cafe-au-lait spots. Melasma and postinflammatory hyperpigmentation respond less favorably. Preoperative local anesthesia may or may not be required for treatment with this laser.

Again, the patient senses only slight, fleeting discomfort during the pulses. Power settings for the Q-switched ruby laser varies depending on the lesion. Lower power settings are used for lentigines (4 to 5 joules/cm^2) and higher settings for tattoos

(5 to 9 joules/cm^2). Healing takes place in 1 to 2 weeks, and there may be some crusting. Antibiotic ointment is applied daily after washing. Incidence of scarring with the Q-switched ruby laser is very low. Hypopigmentation may occur in some patients, but this condition is usually transient. Hyperpigmentation occurs in a small percentage of patients.[11, 12, 18]

SUMMARY

The principle of selective photothermolysis as effected with many of the aforementioned lasers has made possible simplified treatment of many vascular and pigmented superficial lesions. Selective photocoagulation of thicker and deeper vascular anomalies is facilitated by continuous-wave lasers such as the argon and Nd:YAG lasers.

Although the selective destruction of endogenous or exogenous tissue pigment via laser is well established, the mechanism for clearing is still undefined. In spite of this factor, however, long-term clinical

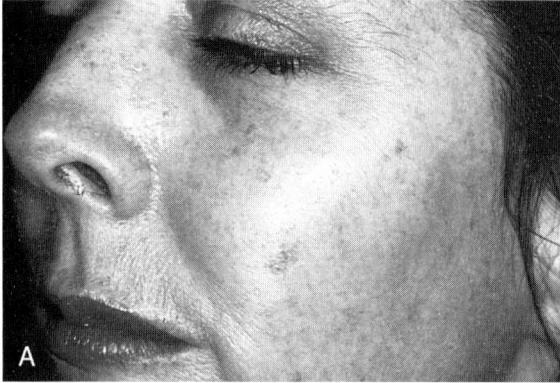

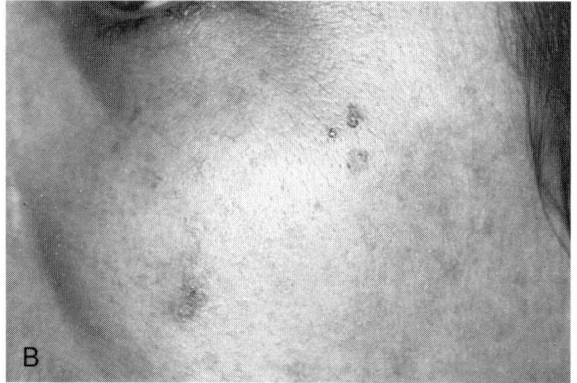

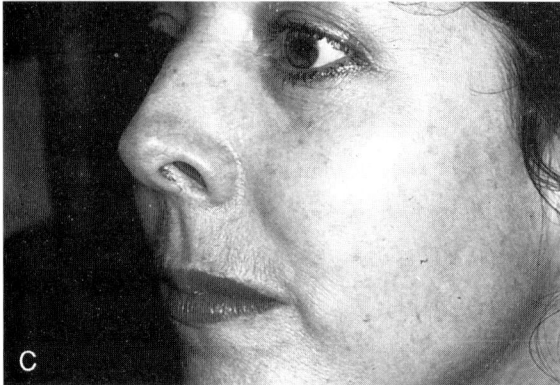

FIGURE 9–15. Q-switched Nd:YAG. Melasma. *A*, Preoperative appearance. *B*, Immediately after surgery. *C*, After treatment.

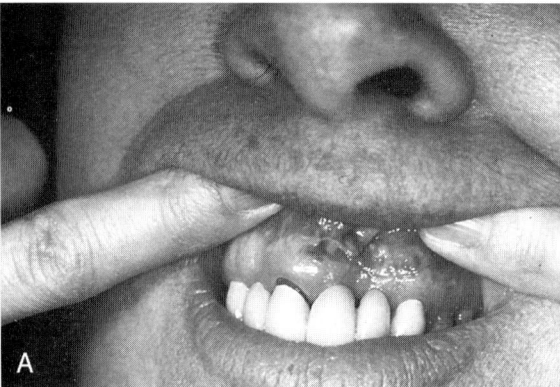

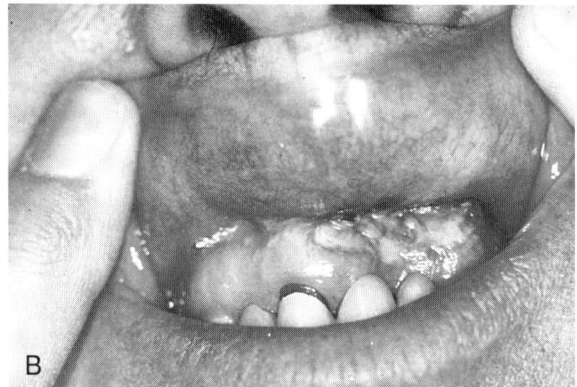

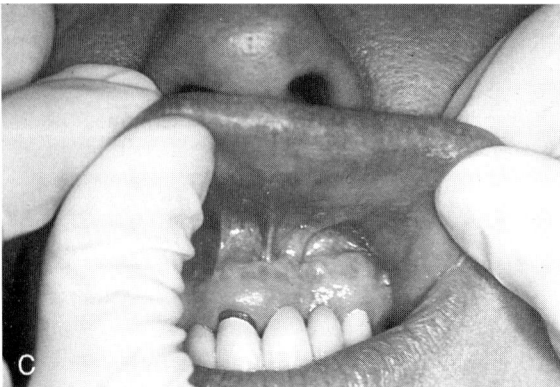

FIGURE 9–16. Q-switched Nd:YAG. Amalgam tattoo. *A*, Preoperative appearance. *B*, Immediately after surgery. *C*, Postoperative appearance. (See also Color Plate 6.)

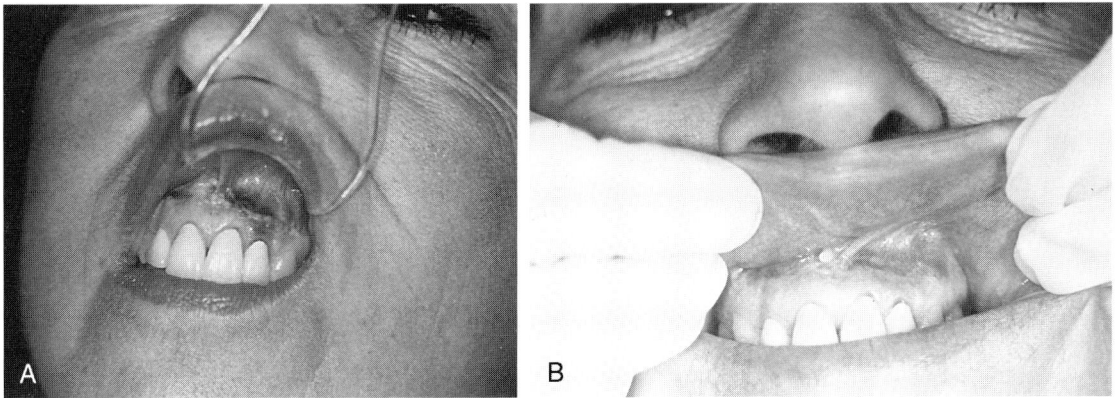

FIGURE 9–17. Amalgam tattoo treated first with carbon dioxide laser, then with Q-switched Nd:YAG. *A,* Preoperative appearance. *B,* After treatment.

use has demonstrated remarkable success in targeting and eliminating unwanted pigment while preserving normal tissue structure.

REFERENCES

1. Kaban LB, Mulliken JB: Vascular anomalies of the maxillofacial region. J Oral Maxillofac Surg 44:203, 1986.
2. Mulliken JB, Glowacki J: Hemangiomas and vascular malformations in infants and children: A classification based on endothelial characteristics. Plast Reconstr Surg 69:412, 1982.
3. Gorlin RJ, Pindborg JJ: Syndromes of the Head and Neck. New York, McGraw-Hill, Inc., 1964.
4. Anderson RR, Parrish JA: Selective photothermolysis: Precise microsurgery by selective absorption of pulsed irradiation.
5. Polla LL, Margolis RF, Dover JS, et al: Melanosomes are a primary target of Q-switched ruby irradiation in guinea pig skin. J Invest Dermatol 89:281–286, 1987.
6. Olbricht S, Arndt K: Lasers in cutaneous surgery. In Fuller TA (ed): Surgical Lasers: A Clinical Guide. New York, Macmillan, 1987, pp 113–145.
7. Shapshay SM, David LM, Zeitels S: Neodymium-YAG laser photocoagulation of hemangiomas of the head and neck. Laryngoscope 97:323–330, 1987.
8. Hruza GJ, Margolis RJ, Watanabe S, et al: Selective photothermolysis of pigmented cells by Q-switched Nd-YAG laser pulses at 1064, 532 and 355 nm wavelengths. J Invest Dermatol 88:495, 1987.
9. Anderson RR, Parrish JA: Microvasculature can be selectively damaged using dye laser: A basic theory and experimental evidence in human skin. Lasers Surg Med 1:263–276, 1981.
10. Gonzalez E, Gange RW, Momtaz KT: Treatment of telangiectasias and other benign vascular lesions with the 577 nm pulsed dye laser. J Am Acad Dermatol 27:220–226, 1992.
11. Taylor CR, Gange RW, Dover JS, et al: Treatment of tattoos by Q-switched ruby laser: A dose response study. Arch Dermatol 126:893–899, 1990.
12. Reid WH, McLeon PJ, Ritchie A, Ferguson-Pell M: Q-switched ruby laser treatment of black tattoos. Br J Plast Surg 36:455–463, 1983.
13. Sexton J, O'Hare D: Simplified treatment of vascular lesions using the argon laser. J Oral Maxillofac Surg 51:12–16, 1993.
14. Noe JM: Laser therapy of port-wine stains. In Mulliken JB, Young AE (eds): Vascular Birthmarks: Hemangiomas and Malformations. Philadelphia, W.B. Saunders Company, 1988, pp 91–102.
15. Catone GA: Lasers in dentoalveolar surgery. Oral Maxillofac Surg Clin North Am 5:48–49, 1993.
16. Reyes BA, Geronemus RG: Treatment of port-wine stains during childhood with the flashlamp-pumped pulsed dye laser. J Am Acad Dermatol 23:1142–1148, 1990.
17. Ashinoff R, Geronemus RG: Capillary hemangiomas and treatment with the flash-lamp pumped pulsed dye laser. Arch Dermatol 127:202–205, 1991.
18. Geronemus RG, Ashinoff R: Use of the Q-switched ruby laser to treat tattoos and benign pigmented lesions. Lasers Surg Med 11 (Suppl 3):64–65, 1991.

CHAPTER 10

Lasers in Periodontal Surgery

GUY A. CATONE, DMD

Periodontal disease is endemic in human populations, and the term refers to a host of interrelated conditions that have their origin within the supporting structures of the dentition. Although it can affect persons of all ages, it is well referenced in the medical and surgical literature as the singular cause of loss of teeth in a vast cohort of patients over age 40 years. An enormous effort has been expended to determine the cause of periodontal disease, and the reader is referred to any standard textbook on periodontology. A cursory evaluation of the literature demonstrates that the disease can be managed by conventional methods of prevention and diagnosis and by nonsurgical and surgical means. Surgical treatment has focused on the control of osseous defects and the eradication of diseased soft tissue. This has been accomplished successfully with manual instrumentation by scaling, curettage, débridement, and osseous recontouring.[1]

INITIATION OF LASERS FOR PERIODONTAL CONDITIONS

Laser technology has an adjunctive role in the field of periodontal surgery. However, a position paper has been issued opposing unsupported therapies using the laser and advocating further scientific inquiry into the potential salubrious applications of laser technology in periodontal treatments.[2]

LASER APPLICATIONS FOR GINGIVAL ENLARGEMENT

One of the earliest uses of laser devices was the use of the carbon dioxide laser initially to treat specific conditions of the periodontium.[3–5] The vast majority of cases to which laser technology has been applied in periodontal surgery have been classic periodontitis, although it has not gained wide acceptance. It has been used in gingival hyperplasias, where acceptance has been more widespread (Fig. 10–1). These latter conditions include the gingival hyperplasias caused by phenytoin sodium, which has been associated with gingival problems in approximately 50% of patients receiving it and, more recently, with drugs used to control the immune response to transplanted organs such as cyclosporine (Fig. 10–2). The cardiac drugs nifedipine and diltiazem have also been implicated in

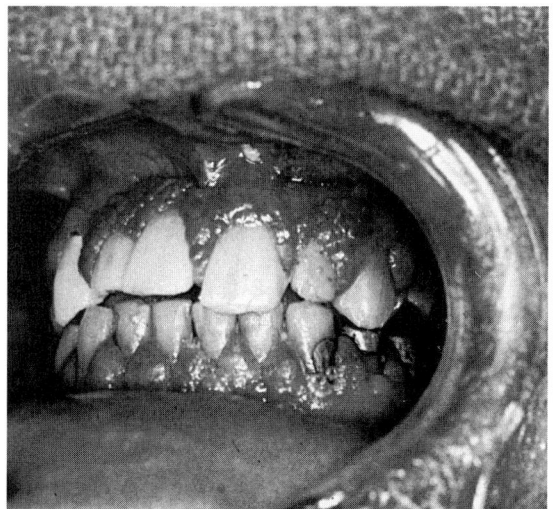

FIGURE 10–1. Typical gingival enlargement caused or associated with drug use (see text). In this case phenytoin was used to control seizure activity.

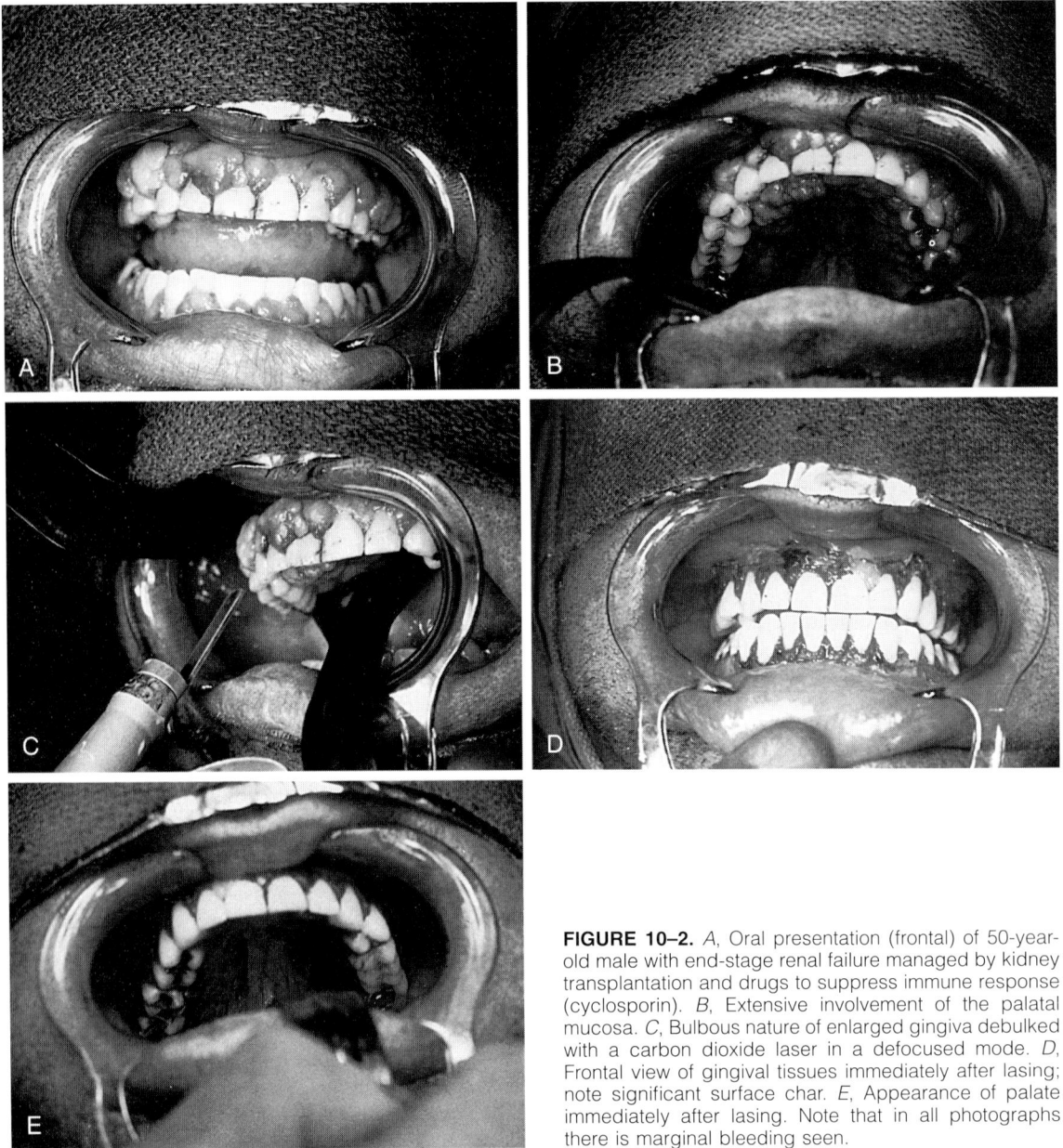

FIGURE 10–2. *A*, Oral presentation (frontal) of 50-year-old male with end-stage renal failure managed by kidney transplantation and drugs to suppress immune response (cyclosporin). *B*, Extensive involvement of the palatal mucosa. *C*, Bulbous nature of enlarged gingiva debulked with a carbon dioxide laser in a defocused mode. *D*, Frontal view of gingival tissues immediately after lasing; note significant surface char. *E*, Appearance of palate immediately after lasing. Note that in all photographs there is marginal bleeding seen.

gingival overgrowth. The laser has demonstrated practical applications in patients who exhibit gingival hyperplasia associated with a systemic hemorragic disorder and classic periodontitis concurrent with similar coagulopathies.[6]

The obvious major problem with the use of lasers in the oral cavity is the dental hard tissues (i.e., the teeth that are literally contiguous to the soft tissue that requires treatment). It is well known that teeth tolerate thermal or traumatic injury very poorly. Therefore, it is incumbent on the laser surgeon to protect the teeth, as noted below. The reader is referred to Chapter 2 and to the work of Luomanen

and colleagues on the effect of carbon dioxide laser energy on soft tissue.[7–11]

DIFFERENCES IN PERIODONTAL TISSUE RESPONSE TO LASERS AND CONVENTIONAL THERAPY

Luomanen and colleagues studied the cellular and extracellular components of healing and repair of the overlying epithelium and the subjacent connective tissue following incisions by the carbon dioxide laser in rat mucosa, and they compared

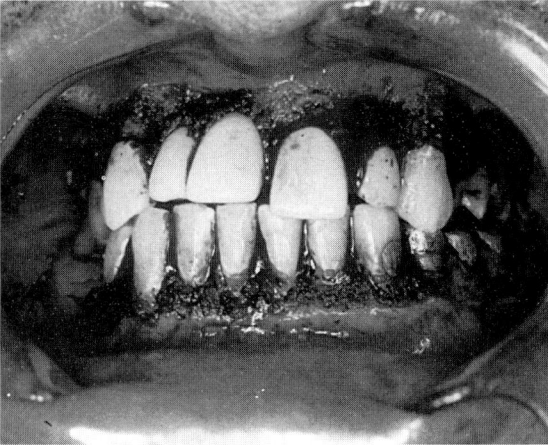

FIGURE 10–3. Appearance of gingival tissues in patient in Figure 10–1 after vaporization by a carbon dioxide laser. Note that the carbonaceous layer is thought by some investigators to offer protection during healing by secondary intention; others believe that the char layer acts as a foreign body and can cause inflammation and granuloma formation.

these with conventional scalpel incisions. From this research, it was clear that there were differences in the response of tissue when either conventional instruments or laser modalities were used to make incisions. These authors conclude that the differences seen clinically (for example, slower healing and decreased scar formation) when the carbon dioxide laser is used are related to the specific properties of the laser. Moreover, the character of laser ablation of tissue and specific thermal effects produced are products of the control exerted by the

laser surgeon by using the optimal spectrum of optical properties of the laser when irradiating tissue with either the continuous-wave or the pulsed carbon dioxide laser.[12–14]

The early observations of Goldman and colleagues in 1968 seemed to promote caution in the use of the carbon dioxide laser near bone tissue, as would be the case in the management of periodontal disease.[15] These concerns were countered by the investigations of Clayman and coworkers, who demonstrated that the carbon dioxide laser causes marginal injury to the subjacent bone residing near treated periodontal tissues. They found that the gingival tissues healed without incident but over a longer time period.[16]

Most initial reports that suggested the efficacy of the laser (usually carbon dioxide) for periodontal problems were limited to the laser gingivectomy and consisted mainly of reports of the management of gingival hyperplasias caused by drugs or congenital lesions (Fig. 10–3).[4, 17, 18] Pecaro and Garehime reported on the use of the free-beam carbon dioxide laser to perform a variety of procedures in the treatment of oral lesions ranging from epulis fissuratum to carcinoma in situ[3] (Fig. 10–4). Forty patients were cared for within a 2-year period using the Sharplan 743 laser unit (Sharplan, Tel Aviv, Israel) set, in most cases, at 20 W in a continuous mode. Patients were hospitalized for 2 days or less and examined on postoperative day 7 and again 1 month later. In the variegated group studied, there were no complications or significant blood loss (usually less than 10 ml). There were no reported postoperative hemorrhage, airway compromise, injury to contiguous hard or soft tissues, aspiration,

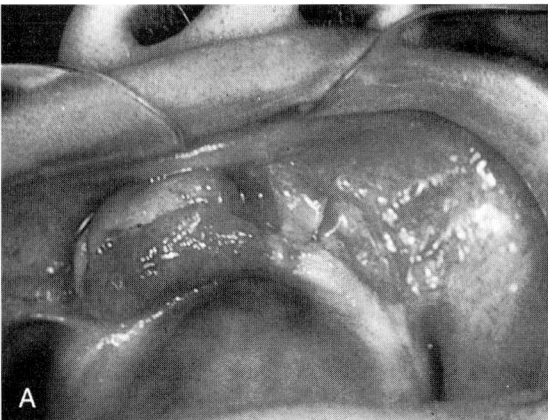

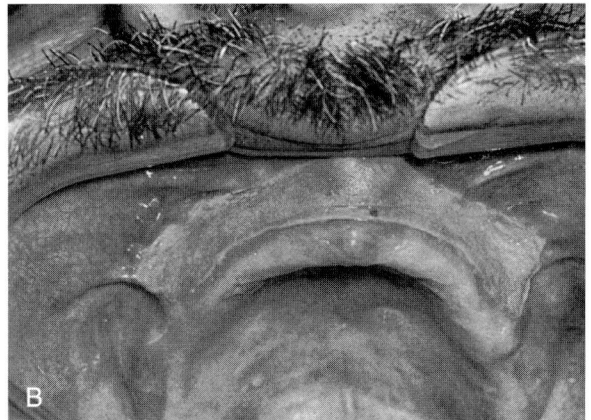

FIGURE 10–4. *A,* Example of large granuloma fissuratum easily managed by the vaporization and debulking properties of the carbon dioxide laser. *B,* Skin graft site after earlier vaporization of hyperplastic tissue with a carbon dioxide laser using UltraPulse (Coherent Laser, Palo Alto, California) in a defocused mode. This pulsing characteristic significantly reduces the formation of a char and, therefore, eliminates at least one barrier against acceptance of the skin graft. Wiping the lased surface with moistened gauze after each successive use of the beam not only removes most of the char but also presumably inhibits the sealing effects of the laser, thus enabling plasmapheresis or imbibition to nourish the grafted tissue. Although mucosa is ideal for grafting, especially in the maxilla, skin is useful when implants are contemplated.

or unusual pain that could not be managed by oral analgesics. The authors noted the decreased postoperative pain that would become apparent 4 to 7 days postoperatively, raising a concern in patients that a complication had occurred. They also noted a delay in healing, as compared with conventional scalpel surgery. It was postulated that the delay was related to the extensive coagulation of the remaining tissue layer that was evident after lasing. Such a coagulated base retarded epithelialization. Although no biometric analyses were performed, the authors noted complete healing after carbon dioxide lasing at 17 to 21 days, versus 10 to 14 days for healing from scalpel wounds. The focus of this article was not periodontal disease, but it did review the advantages of the carbon dioxide laser (see Chapter 5), and a case is highlighted of gingival hyperplasia associated with spontaneous bleeding in a patient with idiopathic thrombocytopenia who was also receiving phenytoin. The hyperplasia was removed with the carbon dioxide laser, with blood loss of less than 200 ml, despite a platelet count that was never more than 15,000.

A more focused article on laser gingivectomy for removal of phenytoin hyperplasia using the carbon dioxide laser was reported by Pick and colleagues, in which 12 cases of phenytoin hyperplasia were managed by laser ablation.[4] Importantly, before surgery all patients were prepared with instruction in proper flossing and were taught a modified Bass brushing technique. Patients were also scaled ultrasonically to remove gross debris and large calculus deposits. Periodontal scaling and root planing were also performed. Laser power settings varied much, but the range of power output was 5 to 20 W, with an unfocused laser spot and using a continuous-wave mode. These latter continuous-wave and pulsed modes were used for enhanced operator control and around tooth structures to decrease the chance of tooth injury. Pulsating laser application reduces laser time on target tissue, thus decreasing total radiant energy per unit time and per volume of tissue (energy density). The authors also used adaptors with mirrors of 45 and 90 degrees attached to the distal end of the laser handpiece to gain access to difficult anatomic areas. A No. 7 wax spatula was placed between the tooth surface and the enlarged gingival tissue during lasing. There were no recorded instances of injury to contiguous dental structures. The investigators also noted that all areas were lased until normal parabolic gingival architecture was the result. To deal with the interproximal tissue, curettage was performed and the tooth root planed to avoid laser pitting of enamel or root surfaces. No complications were reported, and re-epithelialization occurred within 10 to 11 days. The authors argue against the use of conventional periodontal surgical methods because the tissue of phenytoin hyperplasia is usually of uneven

bulk and the papillae are bulbous and often freely movable, thus encumbering classic gingivectomy. They conclude that all the advantages of the laser, such as reduced bleeding, decreased operative time, and the ability of the laser to coagulate, vaporize, or cut by varying the power and time of application, sterilization of the operative site, and decreased postoperative pain, are reasons to select the laser as the instrument of choice for this kind of lesion.[19]

As part of a series of oral soft tissue lesions addressed by the laser and reported by Pick and Pecaro,[6] the authors used a carbon dioxide laser—both the focused and defocused beam—at power settings of 5 to 20 W. A focal spot of 0.2 mm with a focal distance of 2.5 cm was used. Usually, a continuous mode was used, but they changed to a pulsed mode when working near hard dental tissue. A wide range of lesions were managed, such as papillomas, fibromas, pyogenic granulomas, hemangiomas, and premalignant, malignant, and preprosthetic lesions, in a total of 250 patients. Most of the lesions were treated with power settings of 8 to 15 W and vaporized or painted away, layer by layer; the carbonization was wiped away to permit visualization and to judge whether further lasing was necessary until unlased connective tissue was exposed. The authors left the layer of carbonized tissue to act as a bandage and permit a traumatic healing beneath (see Fig. 10–3). They included a group of gingival hyperplastic lesions (they reported no specific numbers but provided a description of the nature of the hyperplasias and their management). These hyperplasias included idiopathic gingival fibromatosis (Fig. 10–5), phenytoin hyperplasia, and irritation from orthodontic appliances in patients whose home care is poor. These patients were managed as reported earlier by Pick

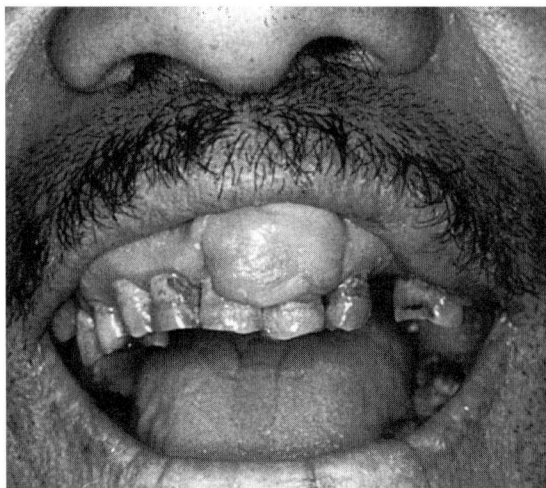

FIGURE 10–5. Presentation of idiopathic gingivofibromatosis managed by the laser, as in all gingival hyperplasias and hypertrophies.

and colleagues, with similar results.[4] Patients with coexisting hemorrhagic or coagulation disorders were also managed with the laser and incurred minimal loss of blood; the diagnoses of the patients included hemophilia, Sturge-Weber syndrome (encephalotrigeminal angiomatosis) with multiple intraoral growths resembling pyogenic granulomas, and idiopathic thrombocytopenia.

For patients with Sturge-Weber syndrome the laser is especially indicated. This rare congenital disorder has been attributed to aberrant embryonic development of ectoderm and mesoderm. Angiomatous lesions of the leptomeninges extending over the cerebral cortex lead to degeneration, resulting in convulsions, contralateral hemiplegia, and mental retardation.[5] Hylton notes that there are oral manifestations in approximately 38% of cases, and these include various angiodysplasias occurring in the mouth. Because convulsive disorders are seen in 80% of these patients, many take sodium diphenylhydantoin. An important decision is the management of the consequences of the anticonvulsant and the concomitant presence of an angiomatous lesion involving the gingival tissues. It should be understood, therefore, that, owing to the overarching syndrome, laser gingivectomy could be complicated by more hemorrhage than would be expected from gingival hyperplasia alone. In these cases, the author recommends the availability of either whole blood or other blood products. Assiduous attention to oral hygiene control is recommended to decrease the chronic inflammation promoted by the presence of dental plaque. It should be recognized that a major feature of the carbon dioxide laser is its ability to debulk excessive tissue, provided the appropriate laser parameters are used.

Several authors have noted the response of the gingival tissues to the use of nifedipine for its cardiovascular effects (at times complicated by the use of an anticoagulant).[18, 20–23] In a patient reported by Barak and Kaplan, the patient, whose status was post–myocardial infarction, was taking nifedipine as well as warfarin sodium.[18] Intraoral examination revealed entensive gingival hyperplasia of a nodular type on the buccal and lingual surfaces of the mandibular dentition and on the buccal surfaces of the maxillary dentition. Following a common protocol of ultrasonic scaling followed by periodontal scaling and root planing, the patient was scheduled for laser surgery using the Sharplan 1040 carbon dioxide laser (Sharplan, Tel Aviv, Israel). It was decided not to withdraw anticoagulation therapy after determining the prothrombin value to be 28%. Laser gingivectomy was performed under intravenous sedation and local anesthesia with the carbon dioxide laser, using both the continuous and pulsed modes. The contiguous dentition was protected during lasing by the use of silver paper. They noted that the

patient experienced marginal postoperative discomfort and pain. Three weeks after the laser surgery they observed complete healing, and 1 year later, no recurrence of the gingival hyperplasia upon discontinuation of the nifedipine.

When oral health is compromised by the presence of gingival hyperplasia, fibromatosis, or common periodontitis, the laser can excise or vaporize diseased tissue after appropriate preparation of the oral tissues; the preparation includes instruction in proper brushing and flossing, ultrasonic scaling, periodontal scaling, root planing, chlorhexidene mouth rinsing, and an appropriate antibiotic if an acute or chronic infection exists. Diseased, enlarged, or hyperplastic gingiva can be managed with the carbon dioxide laser set at a slightly defocused position and using a continuous wave at 5 to 10 W of power. After target tissue has been lased away, the interproximal tissue tags can be removed by curettage. Gingival tissues can be sculpted to an external bevel consistent with accepted conventional scalpel techniques. Although several prescribed drugs can cause gingival hyperplasia, such overgrowth occurs in about 50% of patients receiving sodium phenytoin.[24, 25] Apparently, the overgrowth of gingiva occurs in 67% to 95% of patients who are also mentally retarded.[26] Brunsvold and colleagues note that surgical intervention is required for approximately 30% of such patients.[27] For surgeons dealing with this intraoral lesion, aside from cosmetic defects, altered phonation, malocclusion, and effects on mastication, significant problems may be associated with compromise of the upper airway associated with gingival hyperplasia.

Bolger and colleagues reported a case of retrograde displacement of the tongue secondary to gingival hyperplasia.[28] An 11-year-old patient with a constellation of physical and mental problems presented with symptoms of respiratory distress, mild cyanosis, and stertorous breathing. Nasopharyngoscopy revealed posterior displacement of the tongue against the pharyngeal wall, causing vibratory stertor and partial airway obstruction. After an appropriate work-up and consultation with the parents, it was decided to use an operating microscope (see Chapter 8) with a 400 × magnification to permit a midline V wedge resection of the base of the tongue using a carbon dioxide laser, pulsed initially at 20 to 30 W and 0.1 second, then increased to 40 to 60 W. The resection was begun just behind the circumvallate papillae and carried down to the vallecula. A second procedure to revise the first one debulked the tongue sufficiently to allow an unobstructed airway when followed up at 9 months. The importance of this case lies in the fact that patients who present with gingival hyperplasia even after discontinuation of phenytoin, which may result in gingival fibromatosis that is resistant to regression despite drug withdrawal, is the possible association with an obstruction of the airway; that is, gingival hyperplasia may progress to a gingival fibromatosis after withdrawal of phenytoin. A nasopharyngoscopic examination and sleep studies to rule out sleep apnea as an associated phenomenon may be indicated for patients who present with unusual gingival enlargement.

An important use of the laser is in the clinical setting of phenytoin-induced gingival hyperplasia coexisting in a patient with mental retardation. In view of the potential for noncompliance in a mentally retarded patient, the carbon dioxide laser can be used to provide postoperative hemostasis; therefore, the risk that the retarded patient might either aspirate or remove a periodontal dressing is avoided, and the fibrin coagulum caused by the action of the laser is an effective dressing. Roed-Petersen used a standard free-beam carbon dioxide laser at 10 W with a focal spot of 0.2 mm and a defocused spot diameter of 0.4 mm; the exposure time was 0.1 second in narrow areas and continuous in larger areas of mucous membrane.[29] O'Neil and Figures noted the efficacy of 0.2% chlorhexidene gluconate rinse and Drew and coworkers demonstrated that patients with phenytoin hyperplasia experienced a significant reduction in gingival hyperplasia using a topical folate rinse (1 mg/ml), 5 ml per rinse for 2 minutes twice daily.[30, 31]

POTENTIAL USE OF LASERS TO CONTROL APICAL MIGRATION OF SULCULAR EPITHELIUM

A consistent observation after surgery around the dentition, as in routine periodontal procedures, is that the epithelium migrates faster than the healing connective tissue. The epithelium moves rapidly over the surface of the root, resulting in a deep pocket adjacent to the tooth. Repair is not possible because the epithelial and connective tissue cellular elements cannot generate a new attachment.[32] Bacteria and oral debris accumulate within these pockets and are not readily cleanable by routine home care. Accordingly, the detritus within the pocket continues the cycle of periodontal breakdown further, creating a poor postoperative prognosis.[33] It is the major thrust of periodontal therapy to restore or to regenerate the periodontal attachment that is destroyed by periodontitis. Control of the epithelial migration would seem to be a means of providing the existing progenitor elements in the periodontium an environment as well as time to reattach coronally. At least one attempt at managing the epithelium was presented in the initial investigations of Gottlow and coworkers using guided tissue regeneration techniques.[34, 35] Using several biologic barri-

ers, investigators have attempted to block and/or prevent apical migration of epithelial and gingival connective tissue cellular elements into the wound sites created by traditional periodontal incisions. Some of these barrier membranes have included GoreTex, Teflon, expanded polytetrafluoroethylene, Millipore filter, collagen, oxidized cellulose, and polyglactin 910.[36–49]

A series of clinical and laboratory investigations also used the technology of guided tissue regeneration in the management of furcation lesions.[50–55] Although other sites have been selected to regenerate the periodontal epithelial attachment—for example, in the region of integrated endosseous implants[56]—these studies have been isolated reports and were not characterized by statistically accepted methods of controlled cohorts and prospective analysis. Enhancements with the use of barrier techniques have included fibrin, fibronectin, and citric acid as biochemical reagents designed to enhance the generation of a viable periodontal attachment.[57, 58] With the advent of resorbable materials in guided tissue regeneration and the use of highly osteogenic cancellous bone harvested from extraoral sites in combination with demineralized lyophilized human cortical particulate bone, many of the disadvantages of the use of a barrier system are less compelling[59] (Fig. 10–6A and B).

The Nd:YAG laser used in the continuous and pulsed modes has been demonstrated to be an efficient instrument for managing a variety of dentoalveolar problems.[60] This was reported earlier by others in the management of dental and head and neck neoplasms.[61, 62] This laser has also been used to affect curettage of sulcular epithelium.[63] Meyers presented several uses of the Nd:YAG laser in other dentoalveolar procedures but focused on periodontal adjunctive procedures, including crown lengthening, removal of subgingival mineral deposits, and reduction of periodontal pocket depth by a minimum of 2 to 4 mm by using a technique of laser curettage.[64, 65] Meyers notes that indicated candidates for laser curettage are patients with periodontal pockets of 3 to 7 mm. In this procedure, the author uses a 320-micron fiber inserted to the depth of the pocket and lases the sulcus in a crisscross manner while the fiber is withdrawn slowly from the pocket. The fiber is parallel to the root contours toward the diseased epithelium, resulting in vaporization. Another application of laser energy demonstrated by Meyers is the lasing of exposed dentinal tubules, which results in closure of the tubules. The author notes that lased dentin is harder than non-lased dentin. The effects produced by the laser can explain the observation that patients suffering from dentinal hypersensitivity can be treated successfully by lasing the dentinal surfaces with the Nd:YAG laser. Meyers points to the studies by White and

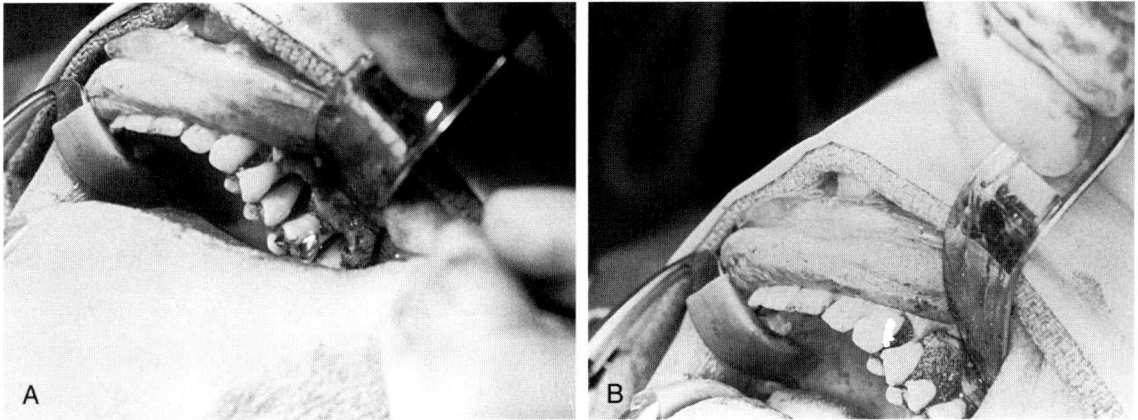

FIGURE 10–6. *A,* Deep infrabony defects are débrided with a combination of laser energy and curettage. *B,* Bone graft of cancellous bone from the proximal tibial metaphysis packed into all bony defects, followed by placement of resorbable guided tissue regeneration membrane.

associates, which demonstrated dentinal tubule closure by scanning electron microscopy as well as a change in hydraulic conductance or the rate of fluid flow through the dentinal tubules and a morphologic change in the odontoblasts.[66] Patients usually report lack of symptoms for up to 2 years after a single treatment, followed by recurrence, which presumably was due to the vulnerability of exposed dentin, which can be retreated if necessary.

To deal with vertical pockets associated with severe bone loss, most surgeons using the laser would combine it with traditional instrumentation. Usually, the defect is débrided with conventional flap surgery, followed by laser de-epithelialization weekly for several weeks. After flap surgery the defect is débrided and root planing is performed. The wound is next treated with a pulsed Nd:YAG laser for closure and healing. The root surfaces and alveolar bone are treated with the laser set at 1.8 W and 15 pulses per second (pps) and the soft tissues with energy of 3.0 W and 20 pps. The specific use of the laser was to de-epithelialize the tissues and to provide for other properties recognized as advantages of laser energy (e.g., hemostasis and disinfection). After initial débridement and lasing the periodontal defect is de-epithelialized weekly for 10 weeks. The quartz fiber of the laser is placed apical to the periodontal ligament attachment and the epithelium, and gingival connective tissue is removed coronally. After lasing, the defect is débrided and root planing is performed.[67] The authors report partial reattachment of the periodontal ligament with decreases in pocket depth and reduction in tooth mobility. This preliminary report suggested the use of the laser to interrupt apical migration of the epithelium so that elements within the remaining periodontal ligament could generate a new attachment.

LASERS AND CLASSIC PERIODONTITIS

Controversy surrounds the efficacy of lasers in the management of classic periodontitis; this is in sharp contrast to its usefulness for treating various forms of hyperplasias. Rossman and coworkers studied the effectiveness of the carbon dioxide laser in the retardation of epithelial migration in experimentally produced periodontal defects in monkeys.[68] The maxilla was chosen as the experimental site, one side serving as a control. Simultaneous treatment of both sides was performed using an inverse bevel incision 1.0 mm below the free gingival margin to remove the crevicular epithelium. Mucoperiosteal flaps were raised on the palatal and buccal surfaces; the intraosseous defects were débrided; and the root surfaces were lightly planed. On the experimental side the outer surface of the flaps was irradiated with the carbon dioxide laser beam held perpendicular to the surface and using a 2-mm spot size with a 400-mm focal length lens. The laser parameters were power densities of 10 W with impacts of 0.5-second durations. After lasing, the tissue flaps were securely adapted to the teeth and coapted over the intraosseous defects, as on the nonlased but débrided control sides. The animals studied at 7 and 14 days following laser radiation revealed delayed epithelial downgrowth along the root surface. It appeared that epithelialization was retarded by at least 7 days as compared with the control sides. Epithelial migration was roughly equal by 28 days. Significantly, connective tissue on the irradiated side did not reveal delayed healing. The authors speculated on the results of possible experiments with the Nd:YAG and the argon laser, as these beams literally pass through epithelium and are absorbed by tissue chromophores lying deeper within the tissues. Although no hypothesis testing of the data was performed, it was clear that the carbon dioxide laser did delay reepithelialization of the tissue flap and thus retarded downgrowth of epithelium in this animal model. Further, the authors reported no evidence of root resorption using the carbon dioxide laser as is seen in the use of other laser devices.[69, 70] Moreover, the authors speculate that the carbon dioxide laser is better able to de-epithelialize only and not damage the underlying connective tissue.

Investigations by Gold and Vilardi have examined the effects of the pulsed Nd:YAG laser in the removal of pocket lining epithelium in humans with moderate periodontitis.[71] This laser used at 20 Hz with a pulse duration of 150 micoseconds and using a quartz silica contact tip of 320 microns in diameter débrided the inner soft tissue wall of the pocket. The energy levels were set at 1.25 and 1.75 W, which delivered 62.5 and 87.5 millijoules per pulse at 1.25 and 1.75 W, respectively. Pockets were treated for 2 to 3 minutes. After lasing, a standard palatal flap was reflected and any remaining marginal tissue was resected with the border of the normal tissue left attached for orientation. The authors believed that laser curettage is a less invasive and a more controlled procedure than manual instrumentation. With the laser energy parameters used in this study, the sulcate epithelium was removed without damaging underlying connective tissue.

Because it has been shown that the simultaneous use of carbon dioxide and Nd:YAG laser beams in tissue (rather than using them separately) resulted in reproducible benefits, a study was designed by Arcoria and colleagues to compare soft tissue reattachment to the bony portions of posterior roots treated by conventional periodontal surgery with that of tissue exposed to two levels of laser irradiation using a coaxial carbon dioxide/Nd:YAG laser in the canine model.[72] The combined laser energy was used to ablate the bony portions of root surfaces to increase reattachment of soft tissue in experimentally produced periodontal defects. Two coaxial laser radiation energies were examined, a defocused, continuous-wave laser beam with a power density of 42.46 W/cm^2 and an energy density of 424.63 pulses per square centimeter and a coaxial beam at double the energy at a power density of 84.93 W/cm^2 with an energy density of 849.3 joules per square centimeter; these were compared with traditional flap periodontal surgery and an untreated control. The authors hypothesized that the use of the coaxial laser system could supplant conventional periodontal surgical techniques. Moreover, the fact that other studies had demonstrated enhancement of tissue results secondary to the use of a combination or coaxial method as compared with independent use of each laser device, they

expected that the use of a lower energy density would be beneficial in generating positive effects on wound healing rates in soft tissue. The overall conclusion of these investigators was that the use of the carbon dioxide/Nd:YAG coaxial laser as it was used in their study with continuous-wave output resulting in energy densities in excess of 100 joules per square centimeter was not indicated, despite the potential rationale of beneficial effects. Reduction of the power density parameters to 6W CO_2/6W Nd:YAG did not produce the beginning osteonecrosis and associated tissue degradation seen with ablations at 12W CO_2/ 12W Nd:YAG and did not compare favorably with conventional periodontal surgical sites. The authors were optimistic that the coaxial system demonstrated potential benefits, but a model device must be developed to reduce thermal production and transmission to calcified tissue.

ROOT PREPARATION AND CONTROL OF SULCULAR MICROFLORA

Root preparation using the pulsed Nd:YAG laser, alone or in combination with manual curettage, was studied by Cobb and coworkers.[73] This study involved topographic examination of root surfaces via scanning electron microscopy and DNA probe sampling to access the effects of laser application in advanced periodontal pockets of microbial populations as well. At energy levels of 3.0 W at 20 pps, 2.25 W and 20 pps, and 1.75 W and 20 pps with changes in time of application from 1 to 3 minutes, with pre- and postlasing manual curettage, the authors found changes in the topography of the root surfaces with a significant residuum of plaque and calculus deposits in all specimens. Moreover, although there was a significant reduction of populations of putative microorganisms mainly consisting of *Actinobacillus actinomycetemcomitans, Porphyromonas gingivalis,* and *Prevotella intermedia* in the period immediately after lasing, there was a gradual repopulation of these species. The earlier studies on the laser effects of subgingival flora support more recent reports; namely, that the Nd:YAG wavelength is absorbed well by melanin-producing bacteria such as *P. gingivalis* and *P. intermedia.* Pale organisms such as *A. actinomycetemcomitans* can be destroyed by the introduction of a dark laser–enhancing medium into the target sulcate areas to act as a photosensitizer for the laser beam.[74–77] Indeed, the altered topography of the root surface seems to lend itself to enhancement of reestablishment of contamination, and changes in the root surface, along with altered calculus deposits, apparently could serve as a nidus for further deposition of unwanted new plaque and calculus. Neither the physiochemical nature of the process the authors described as meltdown and resolidification of the root surface nor the makeup of the end products was fully elucidated, owing to the design of the study, which was strictly topographic in presentation.

In contrast, earlier studies by Melcer used the laser to manage periodontal pockets and root surfaces and contiguous bone.[78] He detoxified root surfaces with the laser without manual instrumentation, and he also used a technique of laser furcation plasty to gain access to the interradicular space. Melcer used a 5-W focus carbon dioxide beam with a pulse duration of 0.1 second, and the root surface was detoxified by a 3-W beam using a defocused beam of pulses of 0.05 second. He also described osteoplasty with the carbon dioxide laser with a continuous-wave beam set at 5 W; the resultant osseous reaction was not presented in detail. Although Cobb and coworkers and Melcer's studies cannot be compared to judge whether a salutary effect was produced as a result of the use of the laser, especially because two different lasers and contact versus free-beam modes were used, the thermal effect on dental hard tissues is an important outcome. Melcer postulated that the conversion of mineralized tissue to an altered crystalline matrix decreased its vulnerability to acid dissolution or to resorption by osteoclasts.

Since the introduction of laser technology for periodontal surgery, there has been a paucity of scientific studies—or indeed clinical experiences—offered in refereed journals. The major application of the laser for periodontal problems has been for the management of lesions of the gingiva such as granuloma gravidarum or the enlargements or hyperplasias associated with the use of various drugs. Laser applications for moderate to advanced periodontitis have received less attention in the literature, even though there is a reduction of blood loss associated with the resection of vascular gingival tissues. There is also a notable reduction in postoperative pain with laser resection of hyperplastic gingiva. This may be the consequence of (1) the carbonaceous surface produced by the laser, under which a fibrinous coagulum forms to act as a bandage during the healing process or (2) the sealing of peripheral afferent nerve endings.[60] There are also conflicting data on the healing of laser wounds versus conventional scalpel incisions. Some studies propose that lased tissue heals more rapidly and with less cicatrix formation than tissue subjected to traditional sharp dissection.[79, 80] These studies are opposed by investigations that purport to demonstrate that in certain animal models laser wounds exhibit delayed healing and that laser wounds have less tensile strength, especially in the period early

after wounding.[81–83] A delay in re-epithelialization of the sulcular epithelium would be useful in delaying downgrowth of the lining of a periodontal pocket and enable time for the reattachment of the fibrous connective tissue component of the sulcus. Rossmann and Israel have demonstrated a technique using the carbon dioxide laser to de-epithelialize the connective tissue contiguous to the involved tooth.[84, 85] There was a demonstrable delay in epithelial ingrowth around the tooth. It appears that the carbon dioxide laser has the ability to vaporize a thin layer of sulcular epithelium, which is characterized by "controlled wounding," thus decreasing collateral tissue damage.

Perhaps the ultimate advantage of the laser for periodontal surgery lies in the hemostasis that enhances visibility and in the rapid advances being made to enhance access to the diseased tissue. In most patients one can produce a reverse bevel laser incision and expose 2 to 3 mm of marginal alveolar bone. Access is thus gained to any inflammatory tissue surrounding the neck of the tooth or within bony pockets. This tissue is easily vaporized by the laser and the root surface detoxified by methods described earlier. One can then use the laser to de-epithelialize the sulcate tissues, followed by suturing in the usual fashion. Recognizing that, even with a combination of root planing followed by lasing, there is still residual diseased tissue, it may be prudent to stage periodontal procedures, because full-mouth treatments require much time. During periodontal laser surgery it is a given that teeth must be protected; sophisticated studies have been conducted that have demonstrated that radiant exposure of the enamel surface is followed by melting and recrystallization of the matrix, causing alterations in its physical properties. In enamel, there is an increase in mineral content and crystal growth, and dentin undergoes molecular changes to mimic the crystalline structure of enamel. These crystalline and molecular alterations decrease the vulnerability of enamel and dentin to acid destruction.[86–90]

PERI-IMPLANT CARE WITH THE LASER

Lasers, originally used in oral and maxillofacial surgery, have assumed an expanded role, beyond their traditional usefulness in dealing with the peri-implant tissues, and now are used. Indeed, in most phases of implantology various lasers have been found invaluable in the preparation of the oral tissues to receive dental implants.

It is of considerable practical use for the oral and maxillofacial surgeon to understand the interactions of laser radiant energy with the materials with which implants are fabricated. It is commonplace that certain welding techniques used in dentistry use the wavelength of the Nd:YAG laser, essentially for welding and soldering gold and chrome-cobalt alloys. It has been demonstrated that the Nd:YAG laser has properties suitable for welding titanium and, further, that such use of this laser welding ability produces superior results as compared with other techniques such as plasma welding or soldering. Owing to such welding properties the Nd:YAG device derives further importance in its role in the welding of implant-supported superstructures. This affinity of the wavelength of the Nd:YAG laser for unalloyed titanium is an advantage as well as a potential hazard. Block and coworkers have demonstrated melting and surface alterations on titanium implants after use of a dental Nd:YAG laser.[91] It has become clear that the use of the Nd:YAG laser for treatment of peri-implantitis, hyperplasia of surrounding gingival tissues, and exposure of an implant during the second stage before prosthodontic rehabilitation is contraindicated, owing not only to the gross thermal effect on the implant but also to the observations that Nd:YAG laser radiation can result in the dissolution of the surface layer from plasma-sprayed titanium implants. Unnecessary thermal injury to the contiguous peri-implant tissues and to supporting bone could occur when laser energy is used near endosseous implants. This has been borne out by the considerable documentation in the literature of the negative effects of excessive thermal energy on bone during implantation and, ultimately on the life of the implant. The surgeon is cautioned not to select electrosurgical methods for dealing with implant problems. All metallic implants have registered high temperatures—in some instances greater than 125°C—when inadvertently exposed to electrosurgical energy.

As is discussed in Chapter 5, one of the major advantages of the wavelength of the carbon dioxide laser is its ability to be reflected from polished metallic surfaces or mirrors. This occurs in reaching a critical population inversion within the laser cavity as well as being directed through the articulated arm of the laser in which strategically placed metallic mirrors direct the beam. The obvious disadvantage lies in specular reflection from nontarget metals or metallic instruments that may divert the beam with hazardous consequences. In implantology the highly polished metallic surface reflects the carbon dioxide beam, and therefore, there is significantly less time for unwanted thermal energy to develop within the implant. The carbon dioxide laser can, therefore, be used in gingival tissue contouring near implants and during the exposure of implants in second-stage procedures.

Inadvertent exposure of the surfaces of hydroxyapatite-coated titanium implants by the radiant energy of infrared lasers (i.e., Nd:YAG, carbon dioxide, and erbium:YAG) could result in the exposure of the metallic core of the implant and is not recommended. However, the use of such lasers for routine tissue recontouring about implants can be accomplished provided the implant surface is protected by a suitable barrier such as a No. 7 spatula or a segment of flat plastic sheeting.

Most lasers cannot be used to manage bone during implant procedures. Standard implant drills are advocated because the level of thermal energy transfer to the bone during drilling or bone recontouring can be controlled somewhat by water cooling. In contrast, bone necrosis is common when a laser such as the Nd:YAG is applied to osseous tissue.[92] Similarly, in separate studies, Clayman and Small and their respective coworkers demonstrated the effects on bone of attempted osteotomy incisions; the properties of the carbon dioxide laser, with its limited absorption in water-deficient tissue, required high wattages and longer applications of the beam, which delayed healing owing to undesirable thermal effects and carbonaceous particles.[16, 93]

Since the development and clinical application of endosseous implants, a common observation has been, that very similar to natural teeth, they react with (or are acted upon) by the oral ecosystem. Dental plaque forms on the surface of titanium implants and pocket formation similar to that in teeth involved with periodontitis is a common finding.[94–96] Lekholm and coworkers and Holt and associates have demonstrated that the supra- and subgingival microflora cultured from titanium endosseous implants are similar to organisms associated with natural teeth.[97, 98] In view of the response of implants, which react as do natural teeth to the oral ecosystem, a schedule for implant maintenance should be routine policy for every implant practice. Such a peri-implant maintenance service should be based on techniques established for the maintenance of natural teeth with due regard for findings from laser investigations.

An example of one such investigation is that of Fox and colleagues in which they noted unpredictable surface alterations occuring after débridement of titanium implants with metal instruments made of either stainless steel or titanium alloy.[99] It is known that the use of dissimilar metal instruments such as curettes could contaminate the surface of the noble titanium implants and change the oxide layer, rendering the implants vulnerable to corrosion. It was also noted that disruption of an epithelial seal during maintenance procedures could result in permanent detachment, owing to enhanced plaque adherence to the roughened surface caused by the disintegration of the oxide layer of the implant.

The core of this study was the use of a helium-neon laser to demonstrate the relationship between specular reflectance and surface roughness. The authors cited Whitley and colleagues, who demonstrated that reflectance (of laser light) was independent of alloy type or the finishing process and that the specular reflectance decreased as roughness increased.[100] The purpose of Fox and colleagues' study was to begin to qualify the optimal methods of maintaining dental implants with respect to the instrumentation that should be used. An unexpected finding was that titanium alloy curettes produced more surface roughness than similar stainless steel instruments. This was confirmed by scanning electron microscopy. The importance of the laser study using reflectance as a measure of surface topography is supported by studies demonstrating that epithelium can form hemidesmosomal attachments to titanium and that trauma to such an attachment by the improper instrument would result in failure of reattachment of a junctional epithelium and subsequent vulnerability of the implant.[101, 102] The result of Fox and coworkers' study suggested the use of plastic instruments for implant maintenance, although their efficacy has not been fully studied.

There has been some concern that manipulation of titanium implants during the commercial packaging process could negatively alter important properties of the fixtures and lead to decreased ability to osseointegrate.[103] This was noted by Block and colleagues, who suggested that the surfaces of endosseous implants be treated immediately before surgical implantation, in effect to enhance the sterile, high-energy, bioreactive surface that was believed to be crucial for implant success.[104] A variety of methods of enhancing surface properties of implants have been advocated. These have included radiofrequency glow discharge treatment (RGDT) and exposure to ultraviolet (UV) light. RGDT and UV exposure just before implantation appeared to have a positive effect at 5 weeks and an even better response at 3 months.[103] Singh and Schaaf demonstrated that RGDT and UV treatments produced high critical surface tension, high surface free energy, and cleanliness. Only UV exposure actually sterilized the implant.

Implant maintenance has included methods that mimic the care of the periodontium after periodontic manipulations or surgery. Both the use of ultrasonic scalers and metal curettes, as well as chemical treatments have produced alterations or damage to the surface of endosseous implants. These implants have included the titanium and the hydroxyapatite-coated titanium varieties. These observations gave impetus to the use of plastic instruments for scaling and root surface planing, simply because the plastic scaler appeared to create less surface damage, although the actual efficacy of this instrument to long-term survival of the implant has not been established.[99, 105–107] Teleologically it would appear

a priori that the surfaces of implants cannot be detoxified for the long term, especially the hydroxyapatite-coated implant, and methods should be developed to treat the acute peri-implantitis setting only, because most current attempts to cleanse and/or débride the implant surface are fraught with the worrisome result of disruption of the protective surface of the implant and ultimately lead to its disintegration. This is no less true in studies involving lasers.

With the objective in mind of avoiding deleterious alterations of the surface of implants during routine maintenance procedures or in the treatment of failing implants, the Nd:YAG laser was studied as a possible modality for detoxifying, débriding, and sterilizing the surfaces of hydroxyapatite-coated and titanium plasma–sprayed (TPS) implants. Using a dental Nd:YAG laser in the contact as well as the noncontact mode, the effects on the surfaces of titanium implants, hydroxyapatite and nonhydroxyapatite TPS types were evaluated, including the effects of the laser after contamination of the implant with spores of *Bacillus subtilis.* The use of the Nd:YAG laser at energy settings of 0.3, 2.0, and 3.0 W resulted in surface melting, loss of porosity, and other alterations, including physical changes in the crystalline structure of the hydroxyapatite coating. Moreover, in samples of implants contaminated by *B. subtilis* spores, total sterilization of the surface was not achieved. These studies in vitro must be compared with in vivo findings to determine whether or not Nd:YAG radiation and its effects on implant surface topography could affect the ability of an implant to osseointegrate or, indeed, could salvage a failing fixture.[104]

It has been determined that the carbon dioxide laser can be used for second-stage uncovering procedures in endosseous implants, sculpting tissue around existing implants, control of mucosal abnormalities, and the treatment of implant soft tissue complications.[108] The carbon dioxide laser is ideal for surgical manipulations around implants because carbon dioxide radiant energy is rapidly absorbed by the high water content of the mucosa so that the depth of tissue necrosis or vaporized tissue is minute (only 100 to 200 microns). The potentially harmful thermal energy is dissipated rapidly and does not reach the metal surface of the implant. Indeed, the specular reflection of the carbon dioxide wavelength is so rapid that if laser beam contact is made, there is not enough time for the energy to be transferred to the implant and to increase its temperature to a critical degree that causes damage. Ganz studied the effects of carbon dioxide laser energy on pure titanium endosseous implants, both uncoated and coated with hydroxyapatite.[109] Ganz used the concept that in placing an osseointegrated implant it is standard protocol to avoid an increase in temperature beyond 47°C (116.6°F).[110] Ganz concluded that it is safe to use the carbon dioxide laser around both hydroxyapatite-coated and titanium screws at power levels not exceeding 2 to 4 W in a continuous mode or 5 to 6 W with a mode-6 pulse. Ganz also believed that a pulsed laser beam was more appropriate for reducing the time the laser energy is actually in contact with the implant surface. One could begin with the continuous mode and, when in proximity to the implant as measured by a periodontal probe, switch to the pulsed mode.

The coaxial carbon dioxide–Nd:YAG laser, at equal continuous-wave settings of 6 and 12 W each, was used to determine whether or not such a combination was equal to or superior to the use of conventional periodontal surgical techniques in the canine model.[72] Soft tissue hyperplasia and osseous defects were replicated experimentally by using orthodontic wire and elastics, after which the coaxial laser was used as a treatment modality. The laser was directed at root surfaces and bony pockets using power densities from 42.46 to 84.93 W/cm² and energy densities from 424.63 to 849.3 joules/cm². Other quadrants were treated with conventional periodontal methods, and still others were left untreated, both serving as controls. Examination 2 weeks after lasing revealed no improvement of soft tissue attachments as compared with conventional therapy. Indeed, at higher energy densities significantly less tissue attachment and increased tissue necrosis was observed. Despite some observed potential benefits with the use of the coaxial device related to decreased time and ease of operation, the authors believed that the application of higher energy densities in a continuous-wave mode directed at soft tissue lesions close to vital calcified tissue was not indicated; however, it was noted that if a laser model could be developed to reduce the heat production and transmission to hard tissues, the coaxial device could not be used with energy densities over 100 joules per square centimeter. Further, they did not recommend the use of the infrared coaxial laser in preference to conventional means in the treatment of periodontal disease.

The Ho:YAG laser was studied by Leukauf and coworkers for its efficacy in experimental studies using the rat model in which the laser was directed to the sublingual tongue and periodontal tissue surfaces.[111] The pulsed Ho:YAG was compared with the pulsed excimer laser. It was noted that the excimer laser exhibited the most favorable damage profile as compared with the erbium:YAG or the Ho:YAG laser, but its application to macrosurgery was limited because its ablation rate and maximum energy output at the fiber tip were not sufficient for surgical manipulations. The tissue ablation caused by the Ho:YAG laser is a result of a rapid increase in pressure by the heating of intracellular contents causing a so-called microexplosion, followed by the demonstration of cellular elements being ejected as microscopic particles. They noted that photoablation was generated if there was an irradiance in the range of 0.1 to 10 joules per square centimeter at pulse durations of less than 3 microseconds, conditions attainable with both the excimer and the Ho:YAG lasers. Further, the authors noted excellent control of tissue ablation with the Ho:YAG laser at the slow repetition rate of 2 Hz. The Ho:YAG laser was observed to exhibit hemostasis coincidentally with tissue ablation, in contradistinction to the excimer laser, which required extensive thermocautery to achieve hemostasis despite atraumatic tissue ablation. Moreover, wound healing with the Ho:YAG laser was without complications after 3 weeks by primary re-epithelialization without scarring, so that the original ablation sites no longer were detectable. The excimer exhibited a much slower ablative process and poor tissue penetration. The authors' conclusion was that the Ho:YAG laser appeared to be well-suited for atraumatic ablation of oral lesions and for periodontal surgery.

Laser technology has been explored for use in determining the vascular perfusion of mucoperiosteal flaps used in guided tissue regeneration (GTR). Zanetta-Barbosa and colleagues conducted a pilot study using a canine model, which examined the prognosis of flaps as it related to the use of a biodegradable polylactic acid membrane placed over an area of the alveolar process where teeth were removed and the buccal cortex excised.[112] Following the removal of the buccal bone plate, titanium fixtures were placed, and the GTR membrane was placed between the mucoperiosteal flap and either bone or the fixtures. A laser Doppler flowmeter was used to determine the blood perfusion. Notable decreases in flowmetry values were noted on the alveolar surfaces, which contained GTR membranes destined to exhibit premature exposure as compared with the control sides. The pilot study suggested that there may be a positive prognosis related to reduced relative laser Doppler flowmetry and premature exposure of the GTR membrane to the oral environment.

Lasers can be used in the oral cavity to débride granulation tissue in relatively inaccessible areas, especially in furcation sites, circumferential defects, three-wall osseous defects, and intrabony defects where indolent tissue makes manual extirpation problematic. Care must be taken to avoid thermal injury to the crystalline structure of cementum or bone or the creation of an unwanted pulpal inflammatory reaction.

OTHER LASER-DIRECTED PERIODONTAL MANIPULATIONS

Most lasers can be used to release mucosal or mucomuscular frena, especially when the frenum is causing recession of the attached gingiva. This is observed in hypertrophic lingual frena, which can cause loss of one or more of the mandibular incisors. In this instance the tongue can be retracted superiorly and posteriorly by using a skin hook or retraction suture at its tip. An extraordinary carbon dioxide laser that has found broad application in oral and maxillofacial surgery, the Coherent carbon dioxide laser (Coherent Laser, Palo Alto, Calif.) is well-designed for frenectomy (Fig. 10–7). By setting the laser on ultrapulse (see Chapter 1) and using 10 W and 250 joules per square centimeter, the frenum can be incised in a focused mode and the underlying muscle resected, which contracts laterally, while lasing proceeds. The focused beam is kept posterior to the sublingual caruncle and in the midline to avoid any trauma to the submandibular gland ducts or the sublingual (ranine) veins. Submucosal bleeding is controlled either by the primary beam or by defocusing the spot and using a continuous mode.[6] An important application in children is concomitant use of the laser and ketamine anesthe-sia (Parke-Davis, Detroit, Mich.). One of the problems with this anesthetic is laryngospasm in an unintubated patient when fluids (saliva, blood) are able to flow from the oral cavity to the larynx. In this clinical setting, the laser, though it does not create a completely bloodless field, certainly provides significant hemostasis, so such a complication is less likely.

Pick and others have used the laser for crown-lengthening procedures to remove excessive soft tissue or a passive eruption problem.[113, 114] The procedure is greatly facilitated by the laser, especially when access is difficult. There is no need for reflection of a flap or suturing. The angled mirror adaptors for the carbon dioxide handpiece and the angled scalpel probe of the contact Nd:YAG laser are most suitable for this task. Lasers can also be used for sculpting procedures in distal wedge and tuberosity reductions.

Lasers, especially the Nd:YAG, have been considered for use in scaling, root planing and curettage, and pocket sterilization, and results have been

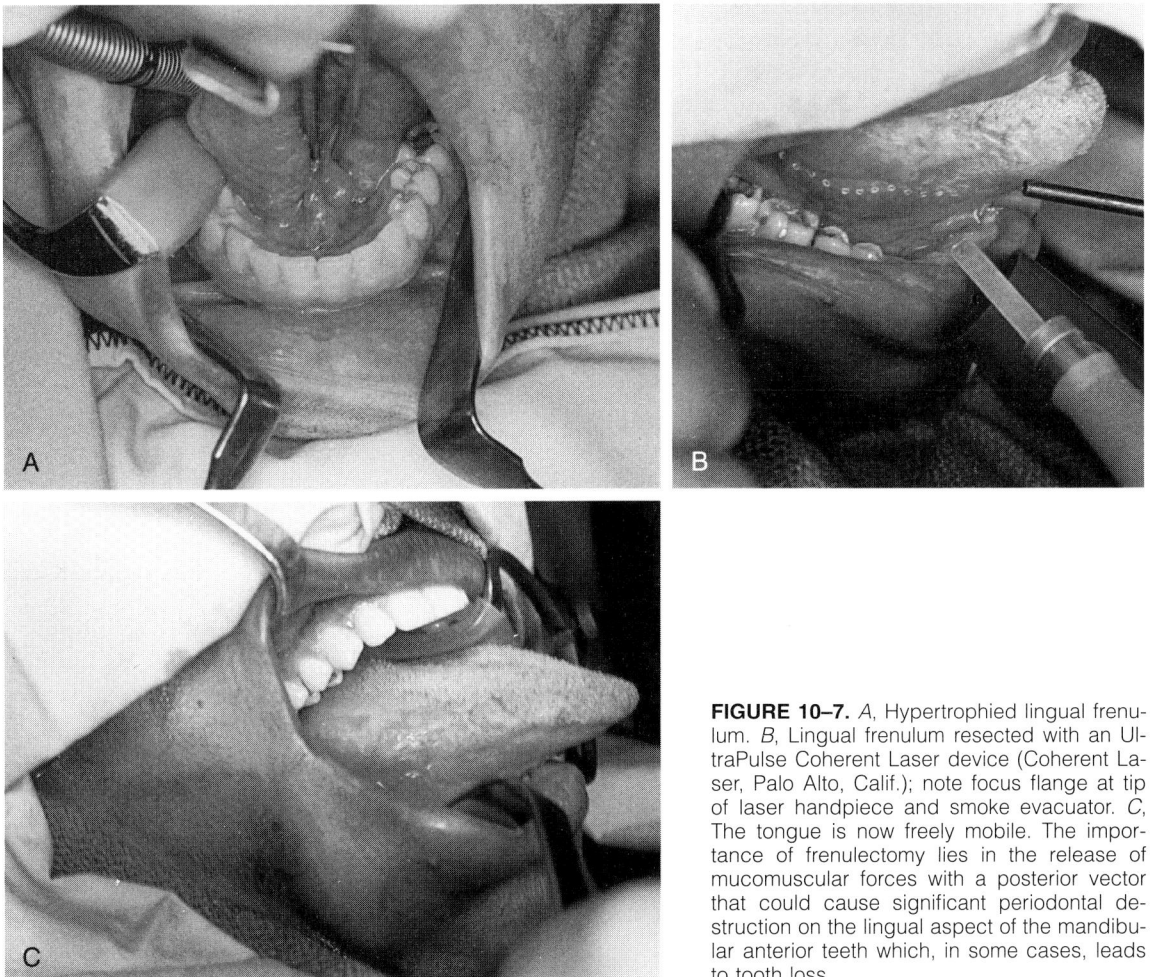

FIGURE 10–7. *A,* Hypertrophied lingual frenulum. *B,* Lingual frenulum resected with an UltraPulse Coherent Laser device (Coherent Laser, Palo Alto, Calif.); note focus flange at tip of laser handpiece and smoke evacuator. *C,* The tongue is now freely mobile. The importance of frenulectomy lies in the release of mucomuscular forces with a posterior vector that could cause significant periodontal destruction on the lingual aspect of the mandibular anterior teeth which, in some cases, leads to tooth loss.

compared with those of conventional hand instrumentation.[113, 115–119] Pick notes that only in recent publications have the effects of lasers on root surfaces, gingival attachments, and subjacent bone been explored to any extent using valid scientific and statistical controlled studies.[113] He notes that several investigators have shown that the use of raw Nd:YAG fibers in studies in vitro reveal tracking, charring, and poor fibroblastic attachment to root surfaces.[120–122] The Nd:YAG contact sapphire probe has been used in proximity to root surfaces and at less than 6 W power density produces an effect similar to that from manual instrumentation.[123] The newer contact probes that use the Wavelength Conversion Effect (Surgical Laser Technologies, Oaks, Pennsylvania) for more accurate power application have not been studied for these purposes (see Chapter 4).

SUMMARY

Advances in the use of laser devices in periodontal surgery will continue. It is true that specific safety precautions must be observed to shield not only nontarget tissue from laser damage but also operating room personnel or office staff from hazards. There is no direct evidence from prospective randomized double-blind studies in humans that lasers of free-beam or contact types have any significant value in the removal of detritus or accretions from the root surface, or, indeed, for any type of root débridement. There is promise in the area of subgingival curettage for the efficacy of lasers in the removal of the epithelial lining of the pocket but not for long-lasting bacterial decontamination. Clearly, there is no place for lasers in periodontal osteoplastic procedures; however, when used with the proper energy parameters their untoward effects on bone may be less dramatic than was previously surmised. Further laboratory and clinical experimentation may determine a significant place for lasers in periodontal surgery when power densities and energy densities have been tested and found to be as effective or more effective than conventional instrumentation.

REFERENCES

1. O'Leary TJ, Barrington EP, Gottsegen R: Periodontal therapy: A summary status report 1987–1988, J Periodontol 59:306, 1988.
2. The American Academy of Periodontology: Research in lasers in periodontics (position statement). Chicago, American Academy of Periodontology, 1992.
3. Pecaro BC, Garehime WJ: The CO_2 laser in oral and maxillofacial surgery. J Oral Maxillofac Surg 41:725, 1983.
4. Pick RM, Pecaro BC, Silberman CJ: The laser gingivectomy: The use of the laser for the removal of phenytoin hyperplasia. J Periodontol 56:492, 1985.
5. Hylton RP: Use of CO_2 laser for gingivectomy in a patient with Sturge-Weber disease complicated by dilantin hyperplasia. J Oral Maxillofac Surg 44:646, 1986.
6. Pick RM, Pecaro BC: Use of the CO_2 laser in soft tissue dental surgery. Lasers Surg Med 7:207, 1986.
7. Luomanen M, Virtanen I: Fibronectins in healing, incision, excision, and laser wounds. J Oral Pathol Med 20:133, 1991.
8. Luomanen M, Meurman JH, Letho V-P: Extracellular matrix in healing CO_2 laser incision wound. J Oral Pathol 16:322, 1987.
9. Luomanen M, Virtanen I: Healing of laser and scalpel incision wounds of rat tongue mucosa as studied with cytokeratin antibodies. J Oral Pathol 16:139, 1987.
10. Luomanen M: Oral focal epithelial hyperplasia removed with CO_2 laser. Int J Oral Maxillofac Surg 19:205, 1990.
11. Luomanen M: Experience with a carbon dioxide laser for removal of benign oral soft tissue lesions. Proc Finn Dent Soc 88:49, 1992.
12. Walsh JT, Flotte FJ, Anderson RR, et al: Pulsed CO_2 laser tissue ablation: Effect of tissue type and pulse duration on thermal damage. Lasers Surg Med 8:108, 1988.
13. Walsh JT, Deutsch TF: Pulsed CO_2 laser tissue ablation: Measurement and modeling of ablation rates. Lasers Surg Med 8:264, 1988.
14. Walsh JT, Deutsch TF: Pulsed CO_2 laser ablation of tissue: Effect of mechanical properties. IEEE Trans Biomed Eng 36:1195, 1989.
15. Goldman L, Shumrick DA, Rockwell RJ, et al: The laser in maxillofacial surgery. Arch Surg 96:397, 1968.
16. Clayman L, Fuller T, Beckman H: Healing of continuous-wave and rapid superpulsed, carbon dioxide laser–induced bone defects. J Oral Surg 36:932, 1978.
17. Rossman JA, Gottlieb S, Kondelka BM, et al: Effects of CO_2 laser irradiation on gingiva. J Periodontol 58:423, 1987.
18. Barak S, Kaplan I: The CO_2 laser in the excision of gingival hyperplasia caused by nifedipine. J Clin Periodontol 15:633, 1988.
19. Misenendino LJ, Nieburger EJ, Pick RM: Current status of lasers in dentistry. Ill Dent J 56:254, 1987.
20. Barak S, Engelbery IS, Hiss J: Gingival hyperplasia caused by nifedipine: Histopathologic findings. J Periodontol 58:639, 1987.
21. Ledermann D, Laumerman H, Reuben S, et al: Gingival hyperplasia associated with nifedipine therapy. Oral Surg, Oral Med, Oral Pathol 57:620, 1984.
22. Lucas RM, Howell LP, Wall BA: Nifedipine-induced gingival hyperplasia: A histochemical and ultrastructural study. J Periodontol 56:211, 1985.
23. Kaplan I, Giller S: CO_2 laser surgery, 1st ed. Berlin, Springer-Verlag, 1984.
24. Jones JE, Weddell JA, Mckown CG: Incidence and indications for surgical management of phenytoin-induced overgrowth in a cerebral palsy population. J Oral Maxillofac Surg 46:385, 1988.
25. Steinberg SC, Steinberg AD: Phenytoin-induced gingival overgrowth in severely retarded children. J Periodontol 53:429, 1982.
26. Kapur RN, Girgis S, Little TM, et al: Diphenylhydantoin-induced gingival hyperplasia: Its relationship to dose and serum level. Dev Med Child Neurol 15:483, 1973.
27. Brunsvold MB, Tomasovic J, Ruemping D: The measured effect of phenytoin withdrawal on gingival hyperplasia in children. ADSC J Dent Child 52:417, 1985.
28. Bolger WE, West CB Jr, Parsons DS: Upper airway obstruction due to massive gingival hyperplasia. A case report and description of a new surgical treatment. Int J Ped Otorhinolaryngol 19:63, 1990.
29. Roed-Petersen B: The potential use of CO_2-laser gingivectomy for phenytoin-induced gingival hyperplasia in mentally retarded patients. J Clin Periodontol 20:729, 1993.
30. O'Neil T, Figures K: The effects of chlorhexidine and

mechanical methods of plaque control on recurrence of gingival hyperplasia in young patients taking phenytoin. Br Dent J 152:130, 1982.

31. Drew H, Vogel R, Molofsky W, et al: Effect of folate on phenytoin hyperplasia. J Clin Periodontol 14:350, 1987.

32. Melcher AH: On the repair potential of periodontal tissues. J Periodontol 47:256, 1976.

33. Wigor HA, Walsh JT, Featherstone JDB, et al: Lasers in dentistry. Lasers Surg Med 16:103, 1995.

34. Gottlow J, Nyman S, Lindhe J, et al: New attachment following surgical treatment of human periodontal disease. J Clin Periodontol 13:604, 1986.

35. Gottlow J, Karring T, Nyman S: Guided tissue regeneration following the use of GoreTex. J Dent Res Abstr 1987.

36. Karring T, Nyman S, Lindhe J: Healing following implantation of periodontitis-affected roots into bone tissue. J Clin Periodontol 7:96, 1980.

37. Nyman S, Karring T, Lindhe J, Planten S: Healing following implantation of periodontitis-affected roots into gingival connective tissue. J Clin Periodontol 7:394, 1980.

38. Iglhallt J, Aukhil I, Simpson DM, et al: Progenitor cell kinetics during guided tissue regeneration in experimental periodontal wounds. J Periodont Res 23:107, 1988.

39. Gottlow J, Karring T, Nyman S: Guided tissue regeneration following treatment of recession type defects in the monkey. J Periodontol 11:685, 1990.

40. Salonen J, Perrson GR: Migration of epithelial cells on materials used in guided tissue regeneration. J Periodont Res 43:215, 1990.

41. Schallhorn RG, McClain PK: Combined osseous grafting, root conditioning, and guided tissue regeneration. Int J Periodont Restor Dent 4:8, 1988.

42. Caffese RC, Smith BA, Castelli WA, Nasjleti CE: New attachment achieved by guided tissue regeneration in beagle dogs. J Periodontol 9:589, 1988.

43. Dahlin C, Linde A, Gottlow J, Nyman S: Healing of bone defects by guided tissue regeneration. Plast Reconstruct Surg 5:672, 1988.

44. Nyman S, Gottlow J, Lindhe J, et al: New attachment formation by guided tissue regeneration. J Periodont Res 3:252, 1987.

45. Selvig KA, Nilvens RE, Fitzmorris L, et al: Scanning electron microscope observation of cell population and bacterial contamination of membranes used for guided tissue periodontal regeneration in humans. J Periodontol 8:515, 1990.

46. Chung KM, Salkin LM, Stein MD, Freedman AL: Clinical evaluation of a biodegradable collagen membrane in guided tissue regeneration. J Periodontol 12:732, 1990.

47. Blumenthal NM: The use of collagen materials in bone-grafted defects to enhance guided tissue regeneration. Periodont Case Rep 1:16, 1987.

48. Aukhil I, Pettersson E, Suggs C: Guided tissue regeneration—an experimental procedure in beagle dogs. J Periodontol 12:727, 1986.

49. Golgut PN: Oxidized cellulose mesh used as a biodegradable barrier membrane in the technique of guided tissue regeneration. A case report. J Periodontol 12:766, 1990.

50. Pontoriero R, Nyman S, Lindhe J, et al: Guided tissue regeneration in the treatment of furcation defects in man. J Clin Periodontol 14:618, 1987.

51. Pontorerio R, Lindhe J, Nyham S, et al: Guided tissue regeneration in degree II furcation–involved mandibular molars. J Clin Periodontol 15:247, 1988.

52. Pontorerio R, Lindhe J, Nyham S, et al: Guided tissue regeneration in the treatment of furcation defects in mandibular molars. J Clin Periodontol 16:170, 1989.

53. Lekovic V, Kenney EB, Kovacevik K, Carranza FA Jr: Evaluation of guided tissue regeneration in Class II furcation defects. J Periodontol 60:694, 1989.

54. Caffese R, Dominguez L, Nasjleti CE, et al: Furcation defects in dogs treated by guided tissue regeneration. J Periodontol 61:45, 1990.

55. Caffese R, Smith B, Duff B, et al: Class II furcations treated by guided tissue regeneration in humans: Case reports. J Periodontol 61:510, 1990.

56. Nyman S, Lang N, Buser D, Braggar U: Bone regeneration adjacent to titanium dental implants using guided tissue regeneration. A report of two cases. Int J Oral Maxillofac Implants 5:9, 1990.

57. Prato G, Lortellini P, Clauser C: Fibrin and fibronectin sealing system in a guided tissue regeneration procedure. A case report. J Periodontol 59:679, 1988.

58. Pettersson EC, Aukhil L: Citric acid conditioning of root affects guided tissue regeneration in experimental periodontal wounds. J Periodont Res 21:543, 1986.

59. Catone GA, Reimer B, McNeir D, et al: The proximal tibial metaphysis: An alternative donor site for maxillofacial grafting. J Oral Maxillofac Surg 50:1258–1263, 1992.

60. Catone GA: Lasers in dentoalveolar surgery. Oral Maxillofac Surg Clin North Am 45–61, 1993.

61. Ohyama M, Katduda K, Nobori T, et al: Treatment of head and neck tumors with contact Nd:YAG dental laser surgery. Auris Nasus Larynx 12:138, 1985.

62. Nagasawa A: Nd:YAG laser therapy in dental and oral surgery. In Joffe SN, Oguro Y (eds): Advances in Nd:YAG Laser Surgery. New York, Springer-Verlag, 1988.

63. Meyers TD: Lasers in Dentistry: Their Applications in Clinical Practice. JADA 122:46, 1991.

64. Meyers TD, Meyers WD: In vivo caries removal utilizing in YAG laser. Mich Dent Assn J 67:66, 1985.

65. Meyers TD, Meyers WD: The use of a laser for debridement of incipient caries. J Prosthe Dent 53:776, 1985.

66. White JMM, Goodis HE, Rose CM: Effect of Nd:YAG laser treatments on hydrolic conductance of dentin (Abstr 481). J Dent Res 69:169, 1990.

67. Kutsch VK, Ochs W, Arend J: Guided tissue regeneration by intermittent Nd:YAG laser de-epithelialization. J Calif Dent Assn 19:52, 1991.

68. Rossmann JA, McQuade MJ, Turunen DE: Retardation of epithelial migration in monkeys using a carbon dioxide laser: An animal study. J Periodontol 63:902, 1992.

69. Lindhe J, Nyman S, Karring T: Connective tissue attachment as related to presence or absence of alveolar bone. J Clin Periodontol 11:33, 1984.

70. Morris ML, Thompson RA: Healing of human periodontal tissue following surgical detachment. Periodontics 1:189, 1965.

71. Gold SI, Vilardi MA: Pulsed laser beam effects on gingiva. J Clin Periodontol 21:391, 1994.

72. Arcoria CJ, Steele RE, Vitasek BA, et al: Effects of coaxial CO_2/Nd:YAG irradiation on periodontal wound healing. Laser Surg Med 12:401, 1992.

73. Cobb CM, McCawley TK, Killoy WJ: A preliminary study on the effects of the Nd:YAG laser on root surfaces and subgingival microflora in vivo. J Periodontol 63:701, 1992.

74. Midda M: Nd:YAG subgingival curettage. In Proceedings 2nd Congress of the International Society for Lasers in Dentistry, 1990, p 105.

75. Tseng P, Gilkeson CF, Palmer J, et al: The bacteriocidal effect of a Nd:YAG laser in vitro. IADR Austr NZ (Abstr), 1990.

76. White JM, Goodis HE, Cohen JM: Bacterial reduction of contaminated dentin by Nd:YAG laser. IADR/AADR (Abstr), 1991.

77. Midda M: Lasers in periodontics. Periodont Clin Invest 14:14, 1992.

78. Melcer J: The use of CO_2 laser beam in periodontology. In Yamamoto H, Atsumi K, Kusakari H (eds): Lasers in Dentistry. Tokyo, Elsevier Science, 1989.

79. Carruth JAS: Resection of the tongue with the carbon dioxide laser. J Laryngol Otol 96:529, 1982.

80. Fisher SE, Frame JW, Browne RM: A comparative histological study of wound healing following CO_2 laser and conventional surgical excision of the buccal mucosa. Arch Oral Biol 28:287, 1983.

81. Buell BR, Schuller DE: Comparison of tensile strength in CO_2 and scalpel skin incisions. Arch Otolaryngol 109:465, 1983.

82. Pogrel MA, Yen CK, Hansen LS: A comparison of carbon dioxide laser, liquid nitrogen cryosurgery, and scalpel wounds in healing. Oral Surg Oral Med Oral Pathol 69:269, 1990.

83. Loumanen M: A comparative study of healing of laser and scalpel incision wounds in the rat oral mucosa. Scand J Dent Res 95:65, 1987.

84. Rossmann JA: Current research using the CO_2 laser in guided tissue regeneration: Animal studies. *In* Proceedings Second Annual Advanced Application Seminar, Luxar Corporation, 1993.

85. Israel M: Current research using the CO_2 laser in guided tissue regeneration: Clinical studies. *In* Proceedings Second Annual Advanced Application Seminar, Luxar Corporation, 1993.

86. Kantola S: Laser induced defects on the tooth structure. V, Electron probe microanalysis and polarized light microscopy on dental enamel. Acta Odontol Scand 30:475, 1972.

87. Kantola S: Laser induced effects on tooth structure. IV, A study of changes in the calcium and phosphorus contents in dentin by electron probe microanalysis. Acta Odontol Scand 30:463, 1972.

88. Kantola S: Laser induced effects on tooth structure. VII, X-ray diffraction study of dentin exposed to a CO_2 laser. Acta Odontol Scand 31:381, 1973.

89. Yamamoto H, Ohabe H, Ooya K, et al: Laser effects on vital oral tissues: A preliminary investigation. J Oral Pathol 1:256, 1972.

90. Ferreria JM, Phakey PP, et al: Effects of continuous wave CO_2 laser on the ultrastructure of human enamel. Arch Oral Biol 34:551, 1989.

91. Block CM, Mayo JA, Evans GH: In vitro analysis of the Nd:YAG laser on implant surfaces (Abstract). J Dent Res 70:530, 1991.

92. Bahcall J, Howard P, Miserendino L, Walia H: Preliminary investigation of the histological effects of laser endodontic treatment on the periradicular tissues in dogs. J Endodont 18:47, 1992.

93. Small I, Osborn TP, Fuller T, Hussein M, Kobernick S: Observations of the carbon dioxide laser and bone bur in the osteotomy of the rabbit tibia. J Oral Surg 37:159, 1979.

94. Adell R, Lekholm U, Rockler B, et al: Marginal tissue reactions in osseointegrated titanium fixtures. I, A 3-year longitudinal prospective study. Int J Oral Maxillofac Surg 15:39, 1986.

95. Ericsson I, Lekholm U, Branemark P-I, et al: A clinical evaluation of fixed-bridge restorations supported by the combination of teeth and osseointegrated titanium implants. J Clin Periodontol 13:307, 1986.

96. Lekholm U, Adell J, Lindhe J, et al: Marginal tissue reactions at osseointegrated titanium fixtures. II, A cross-sectional restrospective study. Int J Oral Maxillofac Surg 15:53, 1986.

97. Lekholm U, Ericsson I, Adell R, et al: The condition of the soft tissue at tooth and fixture abutments supporting fixed bridges. A microbiological and histological study. J Clin Periodontol 13:558, 1986.

98. Holt R, Newman M, Kratochvil F, et al: The clinical and microbial characterization of peri-implant environment. J Dent Res 65:257, 1986.

99. Fox S, Moriarty JD, Kusy RP: The effects of scaling a titanium implant surface with metal and plastic instruments: An in vitro study. J Periodontol 61:485–490, 1990.

100. Whitley JQ, Kusy RP, Mayhew MJ, et al: Surface roughness of stainless steel electro-formed nickel standards using a HeNe laser. Opt Laser Technol 19:189, 1987.

101. Schroeder A, van der Zypen E, Stich H, et al: The reactions of bone, connective tissue, and epithelium to endosteal implants with titanium-sprayed surfaces. J Maxillofac Surg 9:15, 1981.

102. Gould TRL, Brunette DM, Westhuray L: The attachment mechanism of epithelial cells to titanium in vitro. J Periodont Res 16:11, 1981.

103. Singh S, Schaaf NG: Dynamic sterilization of titanium implants with ultraviolet light. Int J Oral Maxillofac Implants 4:139, 1989.

104. Block CM, Mayo JA, Evans JA: Effects of the Nd:YAG dental laser on plasma-sprayed and hydroxyapatite-coated titanium dental implants: Surface alteration and attempted sterilization. Int J Oral Maxillofac Implants 7:441, 1992.

105. Newman MG, Fleming TF: Periodontal considerations of implants and implant-associated microbiota. J Dent Educ 52:737, 1988.

106. Thomson-Neal DM, Evans GH, Meffert RM: Effect of various prophylactic treatments on titanium, sapphire, and hydroxyapatite-coated implants: An SEM study. Int J Periodont Rest Dent 9:300, 1989.

107. Zablotsky M, Diedrich D, Meffery R, et al: The ability of various chemotherapeutic agents to detoxify and endotoxin infected HA-coated implant surface. Int J Oral Implantol 8:45, 1991.

108. Mason ML: Using the laser for implant maintenance. Dent Today 11:74, 1992.

109. Ganz CH: Evaluation of the safety of the carbon dioxide laser used in conjunction with root form implants: A pilot study. J Prosthet Dent 71:27, 1994.

110. Branemark P-I: Osseointegration and its experimental background. J Prosthet Dent 50:399, 1983.

111. Leukauf M, Trodham A, Kautsky M, et al: Infrared laser soft tissue ablation versus ultraviolet excimer laser, experimental introduction of the Ho:YAG laser in oral surgery. Oral Surg Oral Med Oral Pathol 76:425, 1993.

112. Zanetta-Barbosa D, Klinge B, Svensson H: Laser Doppler flowmetry of blood perfusion in mucoperiosteal flaps covering membranes in bone augmentation and implants. Implant Res 4:35–38, 1993.

113. Pick RM: Using laser in clinical dental practice. JADA 124:37, 1993.

114. Meyers TD, Murphy DG, White JM, et al: Conservative soft tissue management with the low-powered Nd:YAG dental laser. Pract Periodont Esthet Dent 4:6, 1992.

115. Midda M, Renton-Harper P: Lasers in dentistry. Br Dent J 170:343, 1991.

116. Gold SI: Applications of the Nd:YAG laser in periodontics. NY J Dent 60:23, 1993.

117. Tseng P, Liew V: The potential applications of a Nd:YAG laser in periodontal treatment. Periodontol (Aust) 11:20, 1990.

118. Tseng P, Gilkeson CE, Pearlman B, et al: The effect of Nd:YAG laser treatment on subgingival calculus in vitro (abstr 62). J Dent Res 70:657, 1991.

119. Cobb CM, McCawley TK, Killoy WJ: A preliminary study on the effects of the Nd:YAG laser on root surfaces and subgingival microflora in vivo. Periodontology 63:701, 1992.

120. Trylovich DJ, Cobb CM, Pipplon DJ, et al: The effects of the Nd:YAG laser on in vitro fibroblast attachment to endotoxin treated root surfaces. J Periodontol 63:626, 1992.

121. Spencer P, Trylovich DJ, Cobb CM: Chemical characterization of lased surfaces using Fourier transform infrared photoacoustic spectroscopy. J Periodontol 63:633, 1992.

122. Murlock BJ, Pippen DJ, Cobb CM, et al: The effect of Nd:YAG laser exposure on root surfaces when used as an adjunct to root planing: An in vitro study. J Periodontol 63:637, 1992.

123. Arcoria CJ, Vitaset-Arcoria BA: The effects of low-level energy dentistry Nd:YAG irradiation on calculus removal. J Clin Laser Med Surg 10:343, 1992.

CHAPTER 11

Laser Surgery of the Temporomandibular Joint

PART I *Use of the Holmium Laser in Temporomandibular Joint Surgery*

Michael G. Koslin, DMD   James H. Quinn, DDS   Guy A. Catone, DMD

HISTORY

The holmium: yttrium-aluminum-garnet (Ho:YAG) lasers are among the recently developed rare earth solid state lasers. This pulsed mid-infrared–wavelength laser is transmitted fiberoptically in a fluid environment, which makes it appropriate for use in arthroscopic joint surgery. The Ho:YAG laser was originally studied for use in angioplasty.[1, 2] In 1986, Fanton and Dillingham clinically developed the holmium laser for use in orthopedic arthroscopic surgery. They published the result of a clinical double-blind study in 1988[3] using 51 patients, 18 to 65 years of age, whom they randomized into laser treatment and nonlaser treatment groups for knee meniscectomies. They did a preoperative and postoperative evaluation for pain, swelling, wound tenderness, range of motion, and crepitation. Patients were evaluated at 2-week intervals, for up to 12 weeks postoperatively. At 6 weeks postoperatively, patients treated with the holmium laser had less inflammation, swelling, pain, iatrogenic trauma, scuffing, and intraoperative bleeding and had greater range of motion than the conventionally treated patients. The conclusion was that the holmium laser was safe and effective for cutting and abrading tissue. Primarily as the result of this study in February 1990, the FDA approved the 2.1-μm holmium laser for orthopedic use.

Trauner and colleagues[4] reported a bovine study in 1990 in which the holmium laser was used in the abrasion of articular cartilage and meniscal fi-brocartilage. They found that the holmium laser precisely and rapidly cut cartilaginous tissue with only moderate necrosis in saline. Their conclusion was that the holmium laser was a useful tool for precise arthroscopic removal of intraarticular tissue in orthopedic surgery.

In 1992, Lane and colleagues[5] conducted a clinical study of the holmium used in the arthroscopic débridement of knees. One hundred and fifty patients were divided into groups of 50 patients undergoing débridement by one of three modalities. In the group that received carbon dioxide laser treatment, all had subcutaneous emphysema. Sixteen patients (32%) treated with the carbon dioxide laser, eight patients (16%) treated with the holmium laser, and 11 patients (22%) in whom mechanical surgical techniques were used had postoperative effusions. However, Lane and associates agreed with Fanton and Dillingham that the Hol:YAG laser may prove to be helpful in arthroscopic surgical procedures.

Stein and coworkers[6] reported a study in which they created osteotomies in facial bones in sinuses of rabbits. Postoperative follow-up revealed a vigorous healing response. Their analysis found that the holmium laser's ability to ablate bone in soft tissue by energy transmitted through a flexible quartz fiber may prove to be useful in endoscopic sinus surgical procedures.

In 1990, Koslin was the first to use the holmium laser in the human temporomandibular joint (TMJ). He gave the first course in advanced TMJ arthroscopic surgery in the use of the holmium laser in

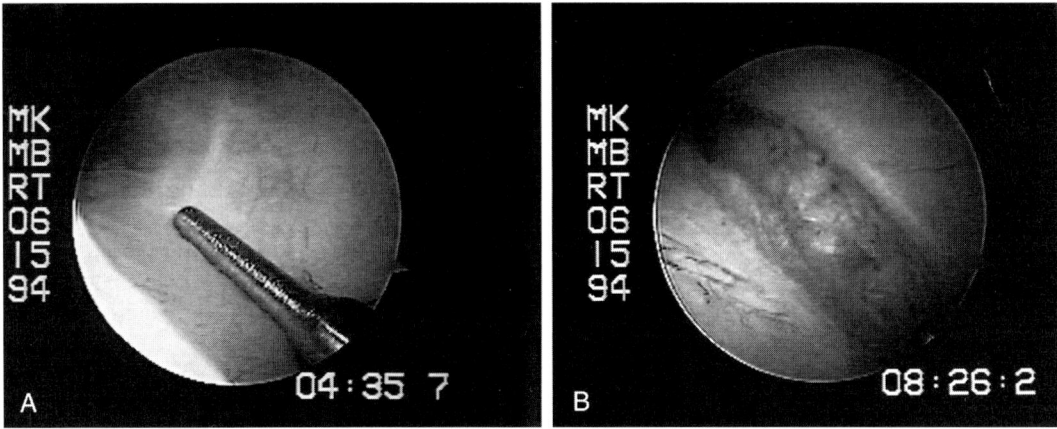

FIGURE 11–1. *A,* Right TMJ anterior articular disc dislocation, arthroscopic view, anterior recess, with a Ho:YAG laser surgical joint probe in position anterior to the disc margin to initiate releasing incision. *B,* The incision is made from medial as far laterally as possible, deepening it inferiorly to release attaching connective tissue to the fibers of the superior head of the lateral pterygoid muscle.

July, 1991. The preliminary experiences of the holmium laser in the TMJ in arthroscopic surgery were published by Koslin[7] and Hendler.[8]

Recently, the holmium laser was compared with an ultraviolet excimer laser in the ablation of oral tissues in animal model.[9]

HOLMIUM 2.1 μM YAG LASER—SURGICAL TECHNIQUES

The increased use of arthroscopic surgery for the treatment of TMJ problems has stimulated the search for new instruments to increase the surgeon's efficiency and safety. Cautery, mechanical, and suctioned-powered instruments have proved to be effective and safe for use within the TMJ. These instruments were sometimes not as efficient as we would desire, and multiple instruments were often needed for a single case because of the lack of multipurpose usage of each instrument. Cannula size had to be adjusted to accommodate different instruments, and heat was a consideration at times with the use of cautery instruments.

Laser technology related to TMJ surgery progressed rapidly. Early work with Nd:YAG on cadaveric specimens and dog models showed numerous problems with a few unique advantages. Nd:YAG contact surgery was awkward, with either ruby or ceramic tips being necessary for heat distribution. Unprotected quartz crystals were both dangerous and inefficient. Nd:YAG free-beam surgery had the major pitfall of beam penetration 3 to 5 mm deep to the intended surgical area.[10] The only major advantage of the Nd:YAG was its affinity for pigmented tissue, especially for the control of hemorrhage.

Early Studies

Cadaveric specimens were used to test the safety of the 2.1-μm holmium wavelength of the retrodiscal tissue laser wavelength. Advanced surgical procedures, such as anterior disc release, posterior scarification of the retrodiscal tissue, and débridement of degenerative joint fibrosis[11] were performed efficiently and safely. Temperature considerations were tested next, using the same techniques employed in studying electrocautery instruments.[12] The 2.1-μm Ho:YAG laser (Coherent Medical Palo Alto, CA) proved to perform surgical procedures with such an instantaneous release of heat because of the rapid pulsation that it was undetectable.[7]

Initial Surgical Techniques

At first, the energy was limited to less than 15 watts. This limitation provided a margin of safety.

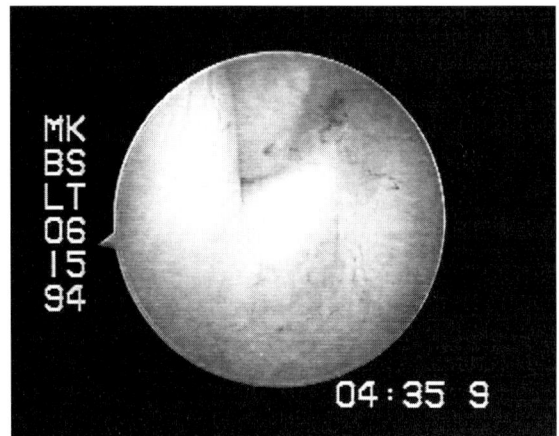

FIGURE 11–2. Retrodiscal scarification and synovectomy performed after disc release and reduction with Ho:YAG laser using reduced energy levels.

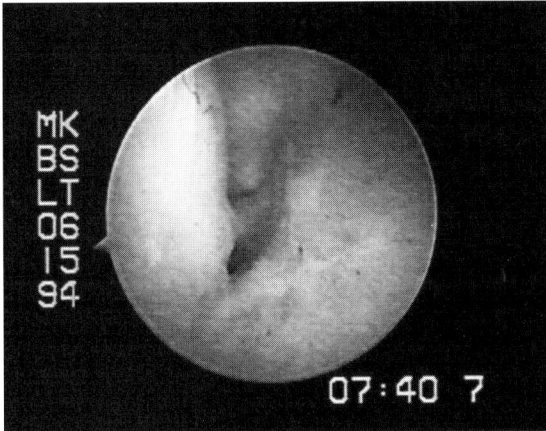

FIGURE 11–3. Tissue welding with Ho:YAG laser to produce fusion of the deeper retrodiscal connective tissues to control the reduced disc position.

TABLE 11–1. Surgical Follow-Up by Staging Classification Treated Arthroscopically

Stage (Wilkes)	Number Joints	Follow-up (Months)	Failures* (Joints)
II	31	26	4
III	69	22	3
IV	140	25	9
V	119	22	10

*(I) Painful joints requiring more than over-the-counter medications occasionally; (II) unable to obtain reasonable functional interincisal opening > 35 mm within one week of treatment; and (III) unable to return to a regular diet without pain.
Data from Koslin MG: Evaluation of temperature changes in the TMJ during arthroscopic surgery utilizing electrocautery instruments. New York, Second Annual Meeting of the International TMJ Study Club, Dec 10–12, 1988.

It has been demonstrated that without deliberate attempts, it is virtually impossible to penetrate the glenoid fossa at this energy level.[7] A down side to this energy was also observed—its fair to poor capability of stopping active bleeding. The effectiveness and efficiency of this surgery were proved daily through the ease of handling and the excellent patient results.

Current Surgical Techniques

The pioneering work of Dr. Joseph McCain[11] in the field of TMJ arthroscopic surgery has continued to be a standard throughout this decade. The application of laser instrumentation to our armamentarium requires minor adaptations of his well-recognized and published techniques. All TMJ laser surgery requires the use of double-puncture techniques with proficient skills in triangulation. Be-

cause many procedures are performed with a pulsed-beam technique, the correct placement of the cannulas is even more critical. Often, an additional portal is need to stabilize or manipulate tissue during laser surgery.

The anterior dislocated disc release is easily accomplished in a free-beam mode with settings of 1 joule of energy and 8 to 10 pulses per second (Fig. 11–1). This 8- to 10-watt setting allows for precise control while providing for efficient penetration with each pulsation.

The posterior retrodiscal scarification and synovectomy is a free-beam technique with settings of five pulses per second at 0.5 joules of energy which delivers a total energy of 2.5 watts. This energy level is easily controlled and restricts the ability of the laser energy to penetrate into deeper layers of tissue (Fig. 11–2). Tissue welding, a technique of decreasing posterior synovial tissue volume and fusion of the deeper retrodiscal tissue to control reduced disc position requires similar energy levels at a greater defocused distance (Fig. 11–3).

Débridement of fibrocartilage (Fig. 11–4) and

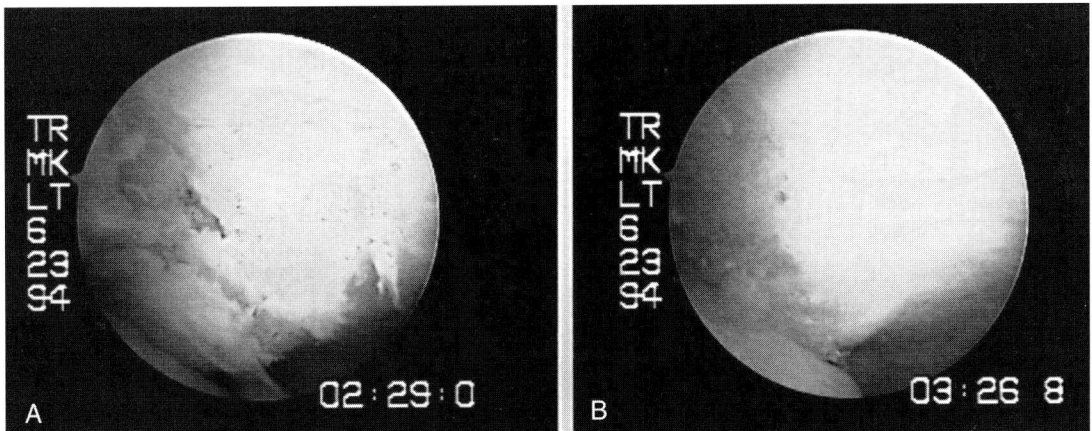

FIGURE 11–4. *A,* Left TMJ anterior recess arthrofibrosis. *B,* Débridement of arthrofibrosis adhesions; Ho:YAG laser vaporization.

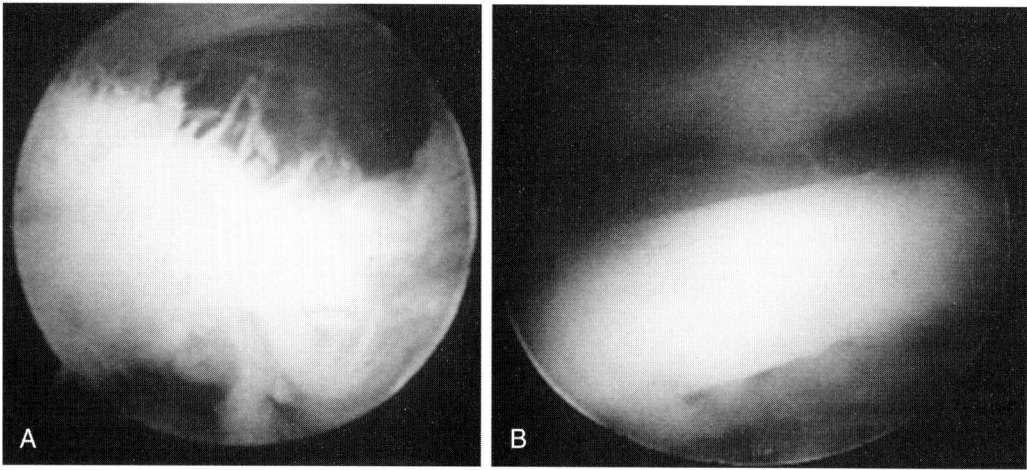

FIGURE 11–5. *A,* Articular disc perforation with marked fibrillation of the margin. *B,* Fibrillation vaporized and perforation margin smoothed by sculpting with the Ho:YAG laser to reduce joint friction during TMJ function.

TABLE 11–2. Results of Quinn's Study of Holmium Laser Arthroscopic Surgery of the Temporomandibular Joint

Patient Epidemiology

Number of Patients—83

Number of Joints—142

Bilateral—59 (71%)
Single—24 (28.9%)

Age Range—16 to 64 years (average age 36.2)
Females—75 (90.4%)
Males—8 (9.6%)

Preoperative Patient Evaluation

Pain

Minimal to none—6 (7.2%)
Moderate—41 (49.3%)
Severe—36 (43.3%)

Range-of-Motion—5 to 50 mm (50 mm in a hypermobility patient)
Average interincisal distance—27.8 mm

Eating Difficulty

None to minimal—47 (56.6%)
Moderate—28 (33.7%)
Severe—8 (9.6%)

Postoperative Results

Follow-up Range—6–29 months

Average—19 months

Pain (Joints)

Excellent—113 (79.5%)
Good—25 (17.6%)
Poor—4 (2.8%)
Excellent = minimal to no pain
Good = minimal pain
Poor = significant pain

Postoperative Results *(Continued)*

Patient Range of Motion

Interincisal (Distance)
Excellent—67 (80.7%)
Good—12 (14.4%)
Poor—4 (4.8%)
Excellent = vertical opening of 35–40 mm
Good = vertical opening of 30–35 mm
Poor = vertical opening < 30 mm

Patient's Diet

Excellent—60 (72.2%)
Good—19 (22.8%)
Poor—4 (4.8%)
Excellent, minimal dietary and functional restraints
Good, moderate dietary and functional restraints
Poor, significant dietary and functional restraints

Patient Satisfaction

Very satisfied—59 (71.0%)
Moderately satisfied—18 (21.6%)
Not satisfied—6 (7.2%)

Complications

Transient (3 days) neuropraxia frontal branch facial nerve—1

Eclipse Surgical Technology, Sunnyvale, CA

adhesions and the sculpting of perforated disc tissue (Fig. 11–5) require settings in the range of 12 to 14 pulses per second with an energy level of 1 to 1.2 joules. The increased number of pulsations allows for a smoother, more polished surface owing to the principles of tissue relaxation and elasticity (Tables 11–1 and 11–2).[7]

Results

Koslin's Study. To better understand the results of laser arthroscopic surgery, the joints were divided into groups according to the Wilkes-Bronstein-Merrill Classification of Internal Disc Disorders.[12, 13] All stages of disc disorders were treated with the Holmium 2.1 μm:YAG laser (Table 11–1).

Complications. Complications were very rare. One laser fiber broke and was retrieved in one Stage-III Joint and one stage-IV Joint. In one Stage-V joint, a laser fiber crumbled and was lavaged from the joint. A VIII TA nerve frontal branch weakness (which lasted 3 weeks) occurred in one stage-III joint.

Quinn's Study. The results of Quinn's study are found in Table 11-2.

REFERENCES

1. Furzikov NP: Different lasers for angioplasty: Thermoptical comparisons. IEEE J Quant Electron 23:1751–1755, 1987.
2. Brillhart AT: Arthroscopic laser surgery, holmium:YAG laser and its use. Am J Arthroscopy 3:7–11, 1991.
3. Fanton GS, Dillingham MF: Arthroscopic Meniscectomy Using the Holmium:YAG Laser: A Double-Blind Study. Presented at the Arthroscopic Association of North America Annual Meeting; Orlando, Florida, April 1990.
4. Trauner K, Nishioka N, Patel D: Pulse holmium:Yttrium-aluminum-garnet (Ho:YAG) laser ablation of fibrocartilage and articular cartilage. Am J Sports Med 18:316–320, 1990.
5. Lane GJ, Sherk HH, Mooar PA, et al: Holmium:YAG laser versus carbon dioxide laser versus mechanical arthroscopic debridement. SEM Orthop 7:95–101, 1992.
6. Stein E, Sedaleck T, Fabian RL, Nishioka NS: Acute chronic pain of bone ablation with a pulsed holmium laser. Lasers Surg Med 10:384–388, 1990.
7. Koslin MG, Martin JC: The use of the holmium laser for temporomandibular joint arthroscopic surgery. J Oral Maxillofac Surg 50:931–934, 1992.
8. Hendler BH, Gateno J, Mooar P, et al: Holmium:YAG laser arthroscopy of the temporomandibular joint. J Oral Maxillofac Surg 50:931–934, 1992.
9. Leukauf M, Trodhan A, Kautzky M, et al: Infrared laser soft tissue ablation versus ultraviolet excimer laser: Experimental introduction of the Ho:YAG laser in oral surgery. Oral Surg 76(4):425–432, 1993.
10. Bradrick JR, Eckhauser ML, Indresano AT: Early response of canine temporomandibular joint tissues to arthroscopically guided neodymium:YAG laser wounds. J Oral Maxillofac Surg 50:835–842, 1992.
11. McCain JP, De La Ruah, LeBlanc WG: Puncture technique and portals of entry for diagnostic and operative arthroscopy of the temporomandibular joint. Arthroscopy 7:221, 1991.
12. Koslin MG: Evaluation of temperature changes in the TMJ during arthroscopic surgery utilizing electrocautery instruments. Second Annual Meeting of the International TMJ Study Club, Dec 10–12, 1988.
13. Wilkes CH: Internal derangements of the temporomandibular joint. Arch Otolaryngol Head Neck Surg 115a:469–477, 1989.

PART II *Open Laser Temporomandibular Joint Arthroplasty*

Guy A. Catone, DMD

Prior to the widespread introduction of arthroscopy and then later laser-assisted arthroscopic surgery of the temporomandibular joint, laser modalities were used at Allegheny General Hospital, Pittsburgh PA to perform standard open arthroplasty of this articulation. Laser techniques can be used to perform the entire operative dissection or may be selected after an initial phase to gain access to the joint using conventional sharp dissection, followed by the use of a laser directed by a handpiece assisted by the operating microscope, or the laser could be used directly through a microscope once access is provided to the joint.

Temporomandibular joint surgery was introduced by Annadale in 1887,[1] who repaired a torn meniscus using a preauricular approach. Following this early articular surgery, Lanz in 1909[2] and Pringle in 1918[3] reported operative procedures for meniscectomy.

There followed multiple surgical approaches and techniques directed to the temporomandibular articulation and advocated by a host of authors. To address the problems associated with a painful dysfunctional and disabling TMJ, several major approaches have been described, such as laser and nonlaser arthroscopic surgery (laser techniques described within this chapter; nonlaser techniques are beyond the scope of this book and are found elsewhere in the maxillofacial literature); and open procedures including preauricular, postauricular, submandibular, and endaural techniques. Of these procedures, the preauricular appears to be more widely accepted, presumably because of its advantages in avoiding some of the complications reported in the other approaches, such as major facial nerve neuropathy and stenosis of the external auditory canal. Other approaches include the closed condylotomy, intraoral, and temporal flap, as well as other variations in design of the surgical flap, such as the use of a modified unicoronal or bicoronal flap technique (Fig. 11–6*A* and *B*)

In approaching the articulation while anticipating use of laser technology, we have found the preauricular approach to be satisfactory. However, the surgeon should select the approach he or she is most comfortable with based on his or her experience. Also, the extent of articular and extra-articular pathology may govern access and the properties of the laser energy, which will have unique and specific photobiologic effects on the soft tissue, bone, and most important, the hyaline cartilage of the external ear and fibrocartilage of the articular disc.

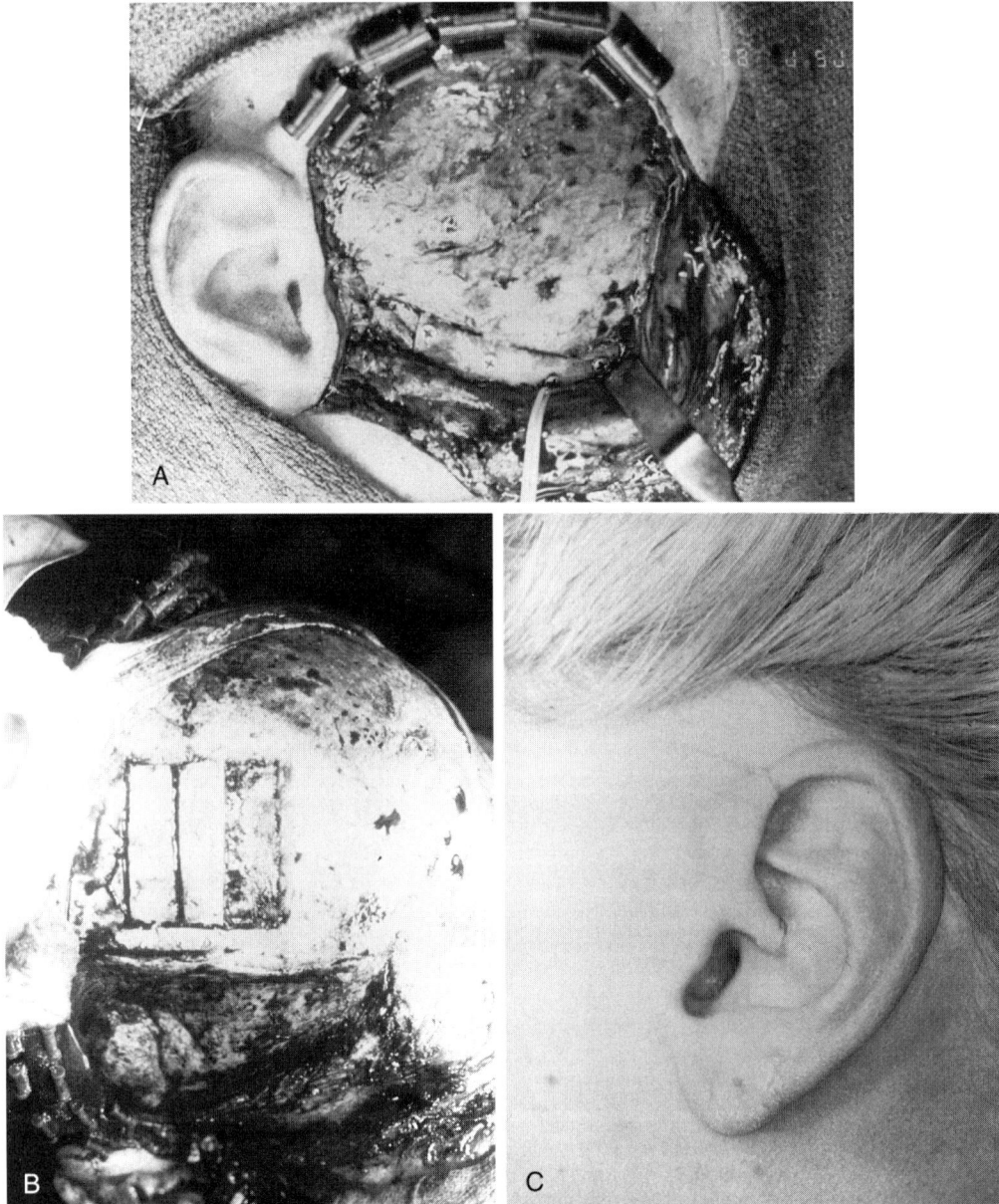

FIGURE 11–6. *A*, Modifications of the preauricular flap design—unicoronal scalp flap. *B*, Bicoronal flap for major reconstructive procedures, which may include calvarial bone harvest. *C*, Result of a modified preauricular incision involving dissection within the hair-bearing scalp, across the superior aspect of the helix, following the undersurface of the helix and following the crus helicis to the depth of the anterior skin of the concha, then inferiorly following the posterior aspect of the tragus to the incisura intertragica at its anterior aspect, then across the narrowest isthmus of the lobule to its most inferior attachment. (Method of Stark, Catone, and Kaltman.)

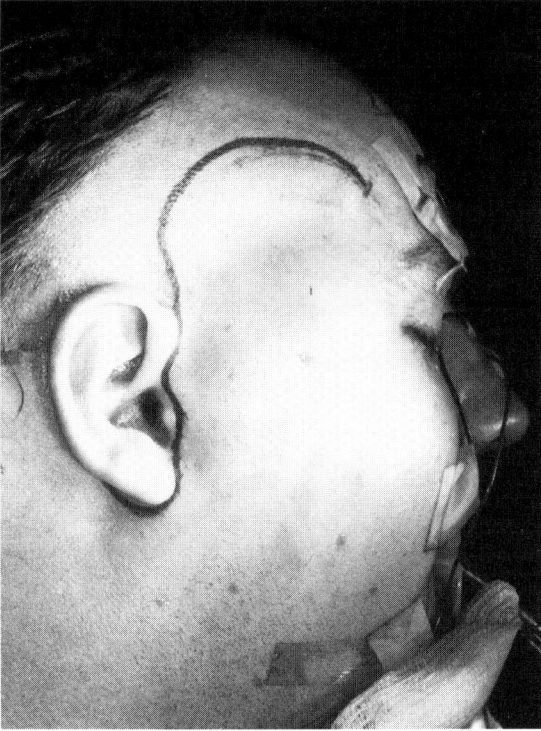

FIGURE 11–7. Question mark incision advocated by Al-Kayat and Bramley.

THE PREAURICULAR APPROACH

The preauricular approach has been described by numerous authors including Risdon,[4] Blair and Ivy,[5] Milch,[6] Henny and Baldridge,[7] McCann,[8] Rowe and Killey,[9] Giles,[10] Thoma,[11] Rowe,[12] and Poswillo.[13] The preauricular incision is placed anterior to the ear, with variable extensions into the skin of the temporal fossa. Variations in placement and design of the skin incision have been advanced to enhance access and visibility, decrease unacceptable aesthetic results, and reduce the probability of seventh nerve neuropathy. (Fig. 11–6*C*). By developing a more generous temporal fossa incision, access and visibility are gained. To this end, Rowe[12] advised that the superior aspect of the skin incision overlying the temporal fossa be inclined at a 45-degree angle to the zygomatic arch. It was also advocated by Middleton[14] to keep the operative dissection posterior to a line extending from the lobe of the ear to the lateral margin of the orbit. An additional modification of the skin incision to protect against nerve damage was advanced by Al-Kayat and Bramley,[15] who suggested the use of a "question mark" skin incision in the temporal fossa with its concavity turned anteriorly (Fig. 11–7). These authors performed meticulous cadaver dissections to locate the temporofacial branch of the facial nerve as it crossed the lateral aspect of the zygomatic arch and fused firmly in the confluence of these connective tissue layers, that is, the periosteum, superficial fascia, and superficial temporal fascia. (Fig. 11–8*A* and *B*). At our institution, the entire facial nerve arborization is continuously monitored during surgery by electromyography (Fig. 11–9).

Most authors describe the skin incision as ante-

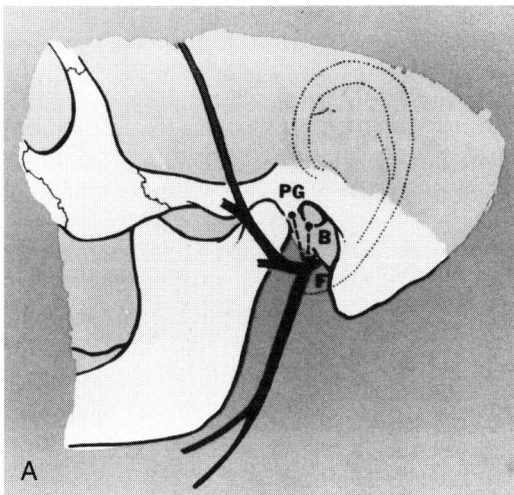

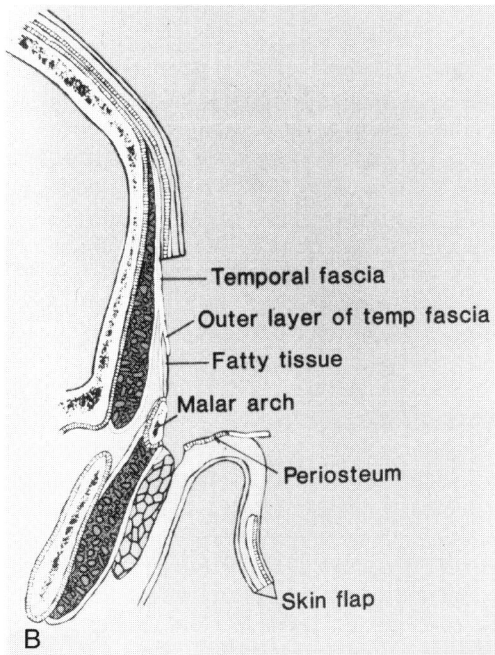

FIGURE 11–8. *A,* Average configuration and locus of the temporofrontal branch of the facial nerve, as determined by numerous cadaver dissections by Al-Kayat and Bramley. *B,* Coronal diagram of dissection for facial nerve branches and tissue planes.

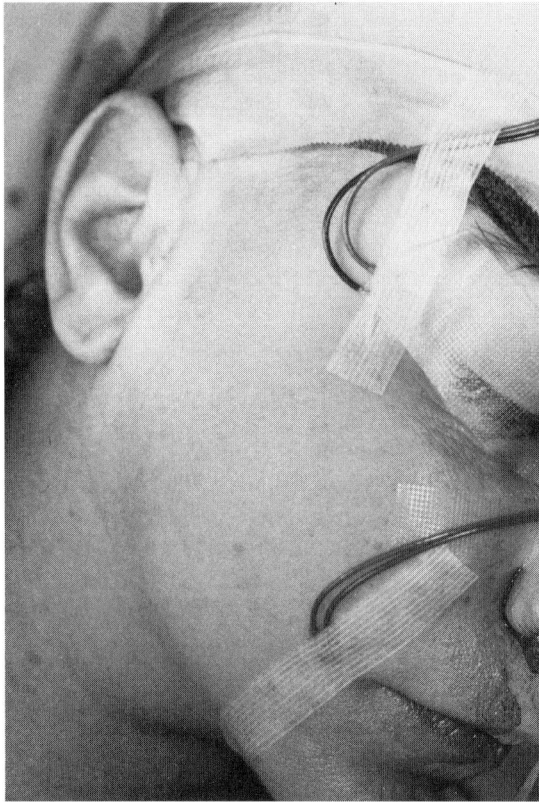

FIGURE 11–9. Use of electromyography to monitor the facial nerve during dissections involving the temporomandibular joint. This methodology has been extended to include all surgical approaches that may place the facial nerve branches at risk.

rior to the auricle beginning in the skin of the temporal region and closely adhering to the anterior margin of the helix and tragus and proceeding inferiorly to the attachment of the lobe of the ear. The skin incision then follows from the temporal component to the superior aspect of the groove at the superior attachment of the helix to the scalp and then extends inferiorly to the superior margin of the tragus. At this point, the incision may course straight inferiorly in front of the tragus or curve slightly posteriorly to the medial crest of the tragus. At the inferior margin of the tragus, the incision courses slightly anteriorly and inferiorly into a variable crease in the skin at the attachment of the lobule of the ear. The skin incision can be accomplished by a sharp scalpel, with the sharp dissection proceeding down to the level of the temporomandibular ligament as phase one of a two-stage sharp scalpel and laser technique as an alternative, the entire dissection can be performed using a laser in a free beam or contact mode. Care must be taken that excessive thermal energy is not directed to the cartilage of the external ear or cartilaginous canal because necrosis of part of these structures may

occur, leading of exposure to cartilage, delayed healing, and the necessity for additional reconstructive procedures.

Most surgeons advocate the development of a skin flap that is retracted anteriorly with stay sutures or skin staples. The dissection of the superficial skin flap and indeed the full open procedure can be accomplished with a carbon dioxide or contact Nd:YAG laser. Alternatively, a microscope can be located above the patient, establishing the appropriate focal distance, and the arm of the microscope containing the objective lens rotated out of the operative field and the first phase of the operation consisting of dissection to the temporomandibular ligament completed with sharp scalpel or laser handpiece (Fig. 11–10A and B). The second phase of the procedure could then involve the laser, which could be used to reshape the meniscus, release an adhesive capulitis, plicate the articular disc, or perform a meniscectomy.

During open dissection of the articulation, it is useful to dissect, clamp, and ligate the branches of the superficial temporal artery and vein in the most superior aspect of the wound prior to incising down to the temporal fascia. By sharp and blunt dissection, the incision is carried down to the superficial surface of the temporal fascia, beginning in the most superior aspect of the wound and proceeding inferiorly. The deep tissues just anterior to the cartilaginous aural canal are dissected free from the perichondrium, and by following the canal as it courses anteromedially and inferiorly, the root of the zygomatic arch is reached (zygomatic arch of the temporal bone). In most descriptions, the glenoid pole of the parotid gland is reflected anteriorly and inferiorly to gain access to the articulation. Dissection through the parenchyma of the glenoid pole of the parotid gland does not appear to offer significant advantages over an approach following the anterior margin of the cartilaginous aural canal.[16, 17]

Most variations of the preauricular approach have been attempts to preclude some of the disadvantages of this technique, namely, neuropathies of the facial nerve, especially the superior branches, development of salivary fistula or sialocele, neuropathy of the auriculotemporal nerve, auriculotemporal nerve syndrome (Frey's syndrome), hemorrhage, inadequate exposure of the articulation and infection. (Henny and Baldridge, 1957, Al-Kayat and Bramley, 1979).[7, 15, 18–23]

Once the posterior base of the zygomatic arch is reached, dissection proceeds through the periosteum of the bone and is carried subperiosteally anteriorly to avoid injury to the facial nerve branches. From this point on, surgical maneuvers vary depending on the nature of the articular pathology. In operations for internal derangements of the articulation,

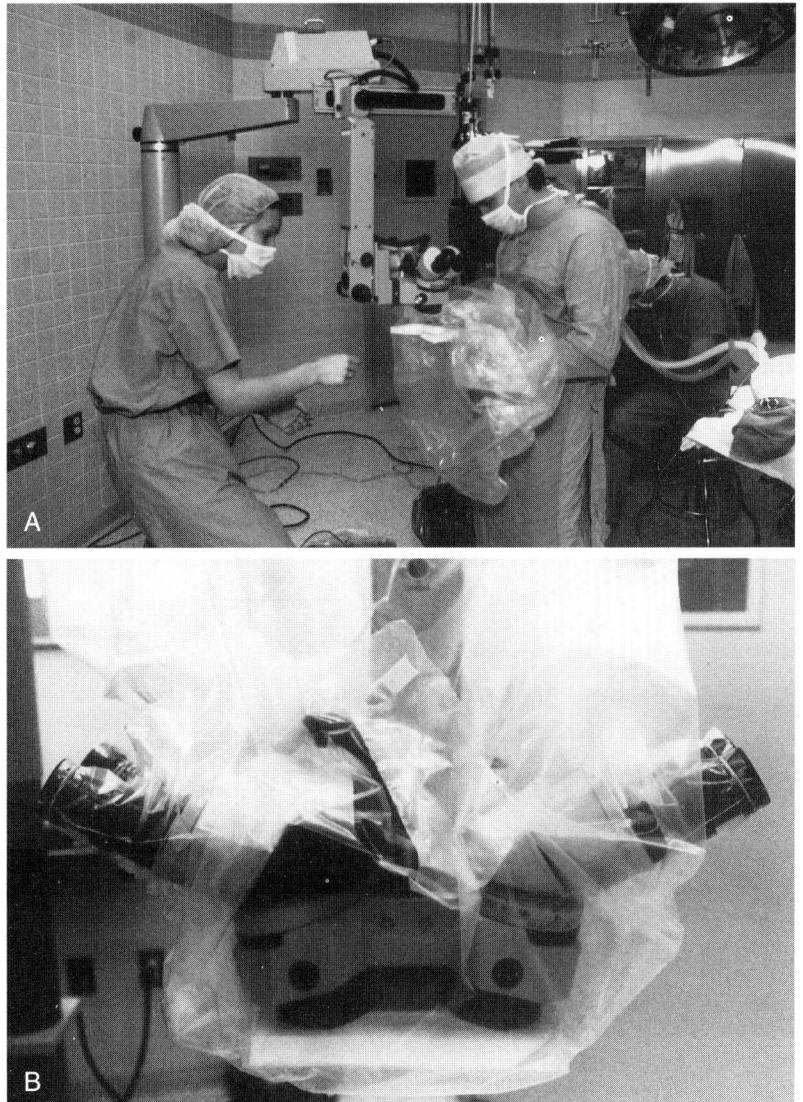

FIGURE 11–10. *A,* Example of operating microscope used for arthroplasty or "through-the-lens" laser microarthroplasty. *B,* Example of dual-head microscope, which was developed to allow the assistant surgeon to help the operating surgeon.

it is necessary to gain access to the joint spaces by appropriate incisions into the temporomandibular ligament and its underlying capsular ligament. These approaches to the internal structures of the articulation, as well as the operation designed to alter the individual articular components, have undergone changes in recent years.[20, 21, 24, 25] The major changes have been related to meniscoplasty and plication procedures of the articular disc, as described earlier by McCarty and Farrar.[16] A more detailed surgical description is described later with the use of the laser.

THE POSTAURICULAR APPROACH

The postauricular surgical design of the articulation was first developed by Bockenheimer,[26] and was later modified by Axhausen[27] and Hovell.[18] This approach is initiated behind the auricle, and the cartilaginous auditory canal is sectioned and reflected anteriorly with the auricle and parotid gland. Husted[28] and later Dolwick and Kretzschmar[29] have commented unfavorably on the use of this technique because it offers no major advantages over the preauricular approach. Indeed, Poswillo[13] observed that in proper hands the preauricular approach can yield good esthetic results and thus obviate some of the disadvantages of the postauricular approach. The postauricular approach can result in external auditory canal stenosis, otitis externa, infection of the cartilaginous aural structures, and neuropathy (paresthesia/anesthesia) and deformity of the auricle.[23] In contradistinction to previous reports by Eggleston,[23] there is a significant incidence of frontal nerve paresis.

The postauricular incision is made about 3 to 7 mm posterior to the auricular flexure. A variation of this approach is the perimeatal incision, which is a combination of the posterior and preauricular incisions.[29] The incision courses from a point 5 mm posterior to the most superior anterior attachment of the ear down to the mastoid process. Dissection is carried down to the mastoid fascia. This fascial layer is continuous with the temporal fascia so that dissection can proceed anteriorly along a common plane. The auditory cartilage is then divided and retracted forward. With the temporal fascia exposed overlying the root of the zygomatic arch, the technique of Al-Kayat and Bramley[24] is then used to prevent injury to the temporal branches of the facial nerve. With the facial and periosteal elements retracted anteriorly, the dissection is performed inferior to the zygomatic arch, and the capsule of the joint can be entered. Exploration of the joint can thus be carried out.[30] This approach has been used by Kreutziger[31] in a description of a microsurgical approach to the temporomandibular joint.

THE ENDAURAL APPROACH

The endaural approach was presented by Davidson in 1955.[32] In this approach, the incision is initiated just superior to the posterior aspect of the zygomatic arch and courses inferiorly and posteriorly in the intercartilaginous cleft between the tragus and helix. The incision continues medially on the roof of the auditory canal for approximately 1 cm and is extended in the sagittal plane around the anterior half circumference of the meatus at the junction of the cartilaginous tube and osseous meatus. At least two major modifications to the approach have been made by Rongetti[33] and Dias.[34] Rongetti noted that the incision should be extended anteroinferiorly in the incisura intertragica, resecting through the cartilage in that region. Dias suggested that previously reported endaural approaches were not truly endaural in view of the fact that they extended beyond the confines of the ear. He believed that they were preauricular versus endaural, and thus he described an approach that was restricted to the confines of the ear so that no visible external scar could be seen. He further indicated that there was no danger of meatal stenosis in this method, contrary to the observation of others.[35] In this procedure, the anterior meatal wall is reflected forward, thus affording the surgeon direct, although posterior, access to the articulation.

MICROLASERDISCOPLASTY/DISCECTOMY

An alternative to open, sharp scalpel procedures in arthroplasty of the craniomandibular joint and as a natural progression in failed attempts at noninvasive or arthoscopic nonlaser and laser techniques to treat temporomandibular joint disorders is the use of laser modalities, either by means of hand-held instruments or through an operating microscope. The procedure incorporating the operating microscope has been employed by one of the editors (GAC) since 1981, although its use has been highly selective. Use of laser technology for procedures involving the temporomandibular joint consists of two phases—the first phase involves dissecting down to the joint itself, which can be performed by sharp scalpel or usually a laser with a hand-held handpiece, following which the second phase is performed, which includes laser surgery with or without microscopic assistance to deal with the internal structures of the articulation. The operating microscope can vastly enhance the ability of the operating surgeon to visualize anatomic abnormalities and effectively and precisely apply laser energy.

The operating microscope has had a significant impact on modern surgical endeavors. Microsurgery, an entirely new surgical field, has evolved and has been used in most of the surgical specialties. This technology has just begun to find similar utility in the field of oral and maxillofacial surgery.

The use of microsurgical technology employing all of the accouterments of this field, such as operating microscopes, microinstrumentation, microsutures, microdrills, bipolar cautery, and coaxial through-the-lens radiant energy, has been rewarding in its application to the established procedure of arthroplasty of the temporomandibular joint. The introduction of diploscopes and triploscopes with fiberoptic lighting has permitted the surgeon and surgical assistants to view the same operative field. The advantages of this technology combined with laser energy are evident in the precision, accuracy, and decreased trauma of the procedure that follows as a consequence of enhanced visualization of the surgical field. What follows is offered to demonstrate microlasersurgery as an enhancement of an established operative procedure, that is, open arthroplasty of the temporomandibular joint via a preauricular approach. This surgical approach was chosen from the procedures described earlier as the best to use because the surgeon can avoid exposing structures to the harmful effects of the laser beam.

MICROSURGERY: BRIEF HISTORY

Microsurgery was initiated by Nylen in 1921, who used the microscope for surgical management of patients who had chronic otitis with labyrinthine fistulas. He used a monocular Brinell measuring microscope that had a magnification of 10 to 15 power.[36, 37] The advantages of microsurgical concepts were recognized by Holmgren,[38] who modified a Zeiss binocular slit lamp microscope, and others in the field of otolaryngology who developed new techniques, including stapedectomy, reconstruction of the middle ear, and resection of acoustic neuromas. The field of ophthalmology benefited by the introduction of the operating microscope by Perrit in 1946.[39] When Carl Zeiss, Inc., introduced a new operating microscope for mass production in 1953, the OpMi 1, which was devised by Dr. H. Littman essentially for aural surgery, a new phase of the development of this technology was initiated.[40] Ophthalmologists quickly improved their routine procedures and later began to devise innovative uses of this technology to be applied to the reconstruction of the anterior and posterior segments of the globe.[41] The development of the binocular microscope has been reviewed by O'Brien.[42]

Two major avenues of microsurgery progressed since the early 1960s—microneural surgery and microvascular surgery. Microneural surgery focused on primary fascicular nerve repair and interfascicular nerve grafts. This avenue of development was facilitated by research and clinical application in the grafting of long nerve transplants by the pioneering efforts of Smith,[43] Michon,[44] and Millesi.[45-47] Microvascular surgery was initiated by the early research of Jacobsen and Suarez.[48]

Microvascular surgery was given impetus by technical advances in microsutures, which enabled the successful anastomosis of human blood vessels of less than 0.5 mm in diameter.[49] The early clinical uses of microvascular surgery was related to the establishment of blood flow following severe injury.[50] With improvement in microsutures, the demonstration of the need for adequate venous drainage (two veins for each artery anastomosed), and the use of heparin, the initiation of widespread successful replantation procedures followed.[41] Komatsu and Tamai performed the first successful replantation of a thumb in 1956.[51] The first successful replantation of an upper limb was performed by Malt and McKhann in 1962.[52]

It was a natural evolutionary consequence that microvascular surgical technology and reimplantation procedures led to the concept of free transfer of tissues. This progress was facilitated by the concomitant indentification of skin areas supplied by a constant axial vascular network.[53] Multiple tissues, including intestines, glands, muscle, bone, joints, and nerves, have been transferred on a vascular pedicle.[54] Taylor, et al[55] reported the use of the free vascularized bone graft in defects of the tibia using the fibula, and Bunche[56] transferred rib with overlying skin. The first free vascularized nerve was used to repair a gap in the median nerve. Oktsuka and colleagues[57] reported composite tissue transfer in

which vessels, nerves, bone, and skin were anastomosed.

The application of microsurgical principles and techniques in maxillofacial surgery has followed closely the advances made in other surgical disciplines in this technology. Fugino[57a] demonstrated a microvascular deltopectoral dermal-fat flap transfer for facial reconstruction. In maxillofacial traumatology, mandibular defects have been repaired using a rib transfer based on its posterior vascular pedicle.[58] Harashina and associates[59] and Wells and Egerton[60] employed a free groin flap in the reconstruction of progressive facial hemiatrophy. Mandibular reconstruction using free osteocutaneous groin flaps and free rib transfers after facial oncologic surgery was presented by Daniel.[61] Similarly, David and Tan[62] reported the use of a de-epithelialized free groin flap for facial contour restoration. They later described the use of microvascular principles and techniques in cases after parotidectomy and mandibular ramus resection, hemifacial microsomia, hemifacial atrophy, and facial traumatology.[63] The biologic concept of the free tissue transfer greatly enhanced the practical evolution of the use of the operating microscope in maxillofacial surgery and provided fundamental principles that made the addition of coaxial laser energy that much easier. There is certainly significant controversy surrounding the use of free osteocutaneous tissue transfers to reconstruct the mandible to a functional organ. Most series indicate a limited volume of bone as a result and the inability of the maxillofacial prosthodontist to rehabilitate the patient from an oral prosthetic standpoint, especially because the marginal bone transferred can rarely support osseointegrated endosseous implants. The important spin off from such microsurgical procedures is the increased sophistication in the surgical specialties of the use of the microscope and the ever-increasing technical enhancement of the hardware and optics of the operating microscope to which the laser could be readily applied.

Microneural surgery was greatly advanced by the initial work in free autogenous nerve grafting by Smith,[43] Michon and Masse,[44] Millesi,[45-47] Berger and coworkers[64] and Samii.[65-70] In the field of oral and maxillofacial surgery, free autografts of sural nerves to replace defects of the inferior alveolar nerve have been reported to be successful by Hausamen and associates.[71] These authors[72, 73] later extended their work to include free transplants of the greater auricular and sural nerves to bridge defects in the facial, accessory, lingual, and inferior alveolar nerves. This research has been expanded by the work of Wessberg and Wolford and coworkers[74] and Wessberg and colleagues[75] in the reconstruction of the inferior alveolar nerve in cases of maxillofacial trauma and osteomyelitis. In certain cases, a transoral approach to the inferior alveolar nerve has been described that is claimed to enhance greatly the diagnosis, technique, and prognosis of microsurgical manipulations of this nerve. In the experience of one of the editors (GAC), microsurgical procedures are not facilitated by a transoral approach to the nerve but may be encumbered by the choice of this method.

MACRO/MICROLASER-ARTHROPLASTY OF THE TEMPOROMANDIBULAR JOINT

There is a rationale for reconstructive macro and microlaser-arthroplasty of the temporomandibular joint. Although there are a host of afflictions of this articulation that respond to surgical management,[76–78] we have found that laser technology for open joint procedures lends itself well in internal derangements[79, 80] of the articulation involving dysfunctional manifestations of reciprocal clicking, closed and open locking, and degenerative arthritis and fibrous ankylosis.[76, 77] These conditions may be associated with anterior dislocation of the articular disc with or without recapture, extreme thinning or rupture of the bilaminar zone, altered morphology of the articular disc and frank perforation of the disc, and rupture of one or more of its ligamentous attachments with anteromedial or anterolateral displacement of the disc. Altered morphology of the condyloid process, glenoid fossa, and articular eminence and the presence of osteophytosis are seen in degenerative arthritis of the joint and do not currently lend themselves to carbon dioxide on Nd:YAG laser surgery. However, the Holmium:YAG laser offers some promise.

Microsurgical exploration and microarthroplasty with adjunctive laser techniques are selected for patients with internal derangements involving intractable pain and dysfunction, and anterior displacement and perforation of the articular disc; severe degenerative arthritis, which has been verified by appropriate clinical findings, electromyography, and articular imaging; and in those in whom orthopedic occlusal therapy to reposition the condyle or articular disc, or both, is impractical or contraindicated; or when all noninvasive manipulations as well as marginal invasive therapies (e.g., arthroscopy) have been unsuccessful.

MICROSURGICAL PRINCIPLES

Although microsurgery is merely an extension of the surgeon's visual and manual capability, the application of such microtechniques on patients should come only after appropriate education in microsurgery principles and laboratory experiences. One of the observations that forms the foundation of microsurgery is the realization that the human hand can perform extraordinarily-precise manipulation at a microscopic level only if there is an appropriately magnified field from which the eye can send visual images to the brain to integrate and coordinate the necessary fine motor maneuvers.

The following presents a consistent, successful application of microsurgical technique for the repair of internal derangements and other arthropathies of the temporomandibular joint. The use of the hand-held contact laser is also included in this section for similar articular problems in the interest of brevity. Although the term microarthroplasty has been used to described the technique, it is merely a modification of the microsurgical techniques originated and elegantly described by Henny and Baldridge[7] and McCarty and Farrar.[16] Microarthroplasty is an attempt to increase the level of sophistication in the surgical care of temporomandibular arthropathies. The degree of magnification, illumination, and access to the microanatomy of the articulation provided by the microscope and microinstrumentation greatly enhances the skill of the surgeon in providing a successful result.

LOUPES VERSUS OPERATING MICROSCOPE

Operating loupes usually provide 2.5 power magnification. One can use 6-power loupes, but they are expensive and have several disadvantages. One of the chief drawbacks to loupes is that they must be worn on the surgeon's head. Because there is a single focal distance of 0.25 mm for 2-power magnification, the surgeon is forced to use telescopes. Loupes must necessarily move with movements of the head and cannot be held in a stationary position. At magnifications greater than 2.5 power, the head movements interfere with the concentration of the surgeon and thus with surgical manipulation. It is also evident in comparison with the operating microscope that loupes do not offer the same depth of focus at 6-power magnification as the microscope. Loupes must be worn in conjunction with a light source, and when loupes and a light are combined, it is an awkward arrangement. Moreover, the surgical assistant may or may not be wearing loupes or be viewing the same operating field, and therefore, surgical assistance suffers.

Although there are a variety of microscopes available, we use the Optosysteme (Newtown, Pennsylvania) Zeiss microscope, which is binocular and has a coaxial laser built in. This system consists of two optical and mechanical microsurgical systems with two independent (dual head) microscopes for the operating surgeon and the assistant surgeon. Thus, an advantage of this unit is that the surgical assistant can see almost exactly what the operating surgeon observes (Fig. 11–11). It is also equipped with a third part to allow for observation. This part is monocular with no stereopsis, and it cannot be used for surgical assistance. However, a 35-mm still camera can be mounted on it for still photographs or a video camera can be adapted by use of a C-mount standard 50/50 beam splitter. The operating team can thus view the microsurgery in real time or later via a standard video player.

Focus and zoom are motorized and operated by a footswitch device, thus freeing the surgeon's hands to concentrate on the operation. The two microscopic heads are mounted to permit 135 degrees of rotation and are preset to focus at the same point in the operative field. The distance from the objective lens to the surgical field is 200 mm (8 inches), which has been found to be comfortable in temporomandibular joint surgery. The eyepiece-to-field distance of 394 mm (15.75 inches) allows the surgeon to sit or stand while operating. In the microsurgical phase of temporomandibular joint surgery we prefer to sit to decrease unwanted hand movement and to ensure lower back comfort. There is a diopter register on each eyepiece to adjust the oculars to the individual surgeon's refractive error. By manually rotating the prism housing of the microscope, interpupillary adjustments are made. Each binocular microscope has an independently controlled zoom that is foot-operated. Depending on the eyepiece used, the magnification ranges from 3.5 to 36 power. We have largely used the 3.5 power (10 × eyepiece), and higher power was used only when we were engaged in nerve repair. The operative field is illuminated via a coaxial fiberoptic bundle that terminates in an illuminator lens housing located between the dual microscopes. At the powers from which we operate, this illumination is extremely intense and does not have an appreciable effect on the optics.

For temporomandibular joint microlasersurgery, the surgeons sit on either side of the operating table and use standard dental operatory operator and assistant chairs. There are special operating chairs available from manufacturers of operating microscopes that have control pedals to make individual adjustments. There is also a removable sterilizable and fully adjustable arm rest to attach to the chair. One can use motorized hydraulic chairs, but the cost-benefit ratio does not appear to be favorable for the microsurgery that is performed in the maxillofacial area. A simple maneuver to gain room for the surgeon's knees is to place the patient's head at the foot of the operating table because on most tables, the major controls are located at the head of the table and thus interfere with the positioning of the surgeon's knees.

MICROINSTRUMENTATION

Sutures

Laser surgery usually does not involve the use of multiple sutures, largely because of the nature of the surgical goals, such as ablation or vaporization of scar tissue or discal tissue within the temporomandibular joint. Moreover, the surgeon may require the use of the technique of tissue welding with low-power densities using the laser. After using many different kinds of sutures, a fine 7-0 to 9-0 monofilament suture has been selected. For

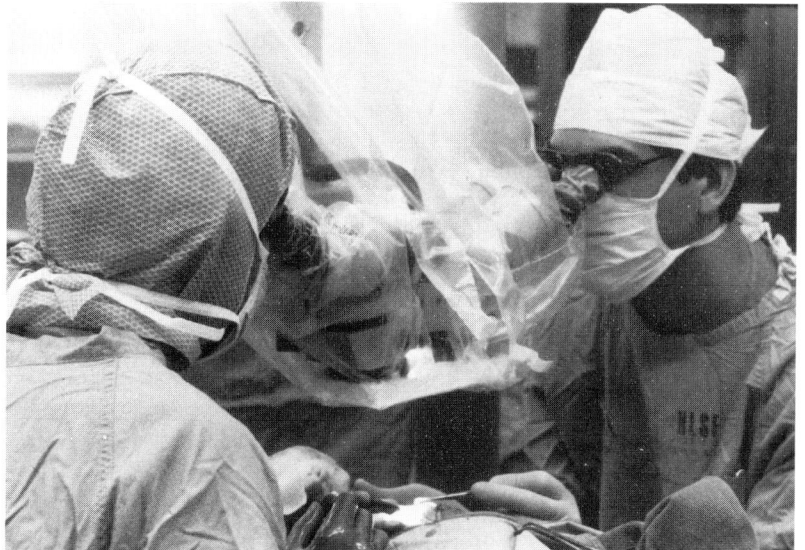

FIGURE 11–11. Surgeon and assistant surgeon viewing the operative field through the microscope.

example, if one is prepared to suture inadvertent nerve injury, the fine monofilament 9-0 is virtually nonreactive and can be passed through tissue with no appreciable friction or tearing of peri or epineurium. When suturing the bilaminar zone and articular disc, we originally began with 9-0 sutures but had to resort to larger gauges of 6-0 and 7-0. The major advantages of the fine gauge sutures are the size of the needle and the fact that numerous sutures could be placed in a small area for strength against the movement of the condyloid process. However, the needle was not strong enough to consistently penetrate the fibrocartilage of the disc, and we were also concerned about the ultimate strength of the sutures at fine gauges. Although the 6-0 or 7-0 suture is not extremely small gauge, the use of this suture with microinstruments, combined with the visibility provided by the operating microscope, makes suture placement easy. There has been no observable deleterious effect on the microneedle holder using these sutures but it is suspected that mechanical problems with these instruments will be traced to the use of the larger sutures and needles. One can use an 8-0 microsuture, which borders the small size of the 9-0 suture and shares some of its properties. The PC-3, 6-0 needle can be selected, which is I-beam shaped in cross-section, with the cutting edge in the inner surface of the curvature of the needle. It should be mentioned that microlaser welding to plicate the articular disc eliminates the need for sutures if only for security until the build-up of connective tissue reinforces the plication area.

Hand-Held Instruments

There are multiple hand-held instruments available for microlaser procedures, but only a few essential ones need to be used. The jeweler's forcep numbers 3C, 4, 5, or 7 can be used, but 3C and 5 are most useful in handling the articular ligamentous tissue, bilaminar tissues, and the articular disc. (Fig 11–12) All macroinstruments can be anodized for safety during laser use. When handling neural tissue, the number 5 forcep is useful because it is less traumatic to fragile neural tissues. These forceps are inexpensive, and if they are dropped and the tips bent, they should be discarded. Do not attempt to rebend barbed forcep points. They can also be labeled in large numbers with their size to facilitate their selection with the naked eye during surgery. It is important not to use the electrocautery with the forceps because the tips will be rapidly deformed. Use of a bipolar electrocautery with foot control is the preferred method of controlling larger bleeding vessels at the microlevel if they cannot be controlled with a defocused free-beam laser or use of a frosted contact laser tip with the Nd:YAG laser.

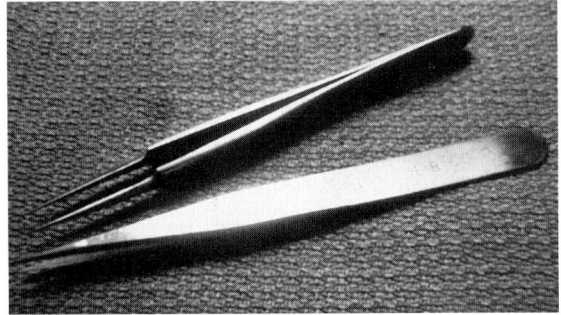

FIGURE 11–12. Examples of microforceps used during a microlaserdiscectomy or other intra-articular microsurgical maneuvers.

Needle holders may be of the nonlocking, spring-loaded type or the locking type, which disengage by gentle finger pressure. (Fig. 11–13). These needle holders are held in the hand as one would hold a pencil rather than a pair of scissors. One can rest the palm of the hand or hypothenar eminence on the patient while manipulating only the fingertips to pass the needle through tissue. The semilocking type of needle holder produces a jarring effect and may tear the delicate portion of the bilaminar tissue when the needle is disengaged. By applying firm but gentle pressure to the point that the needle disengages, no appreciable jarring will occur. Loading the needle on the needle holder is done by viewing them through the microscope and simply holding the needle with the forceps with one hand then taking up the needle with the holder in the other hand. A surgical knot tie under the microscope is the most important maneuver in microsurgery. The surgeon should practice with nerves and blood vessels in the small animal laboratory before at-

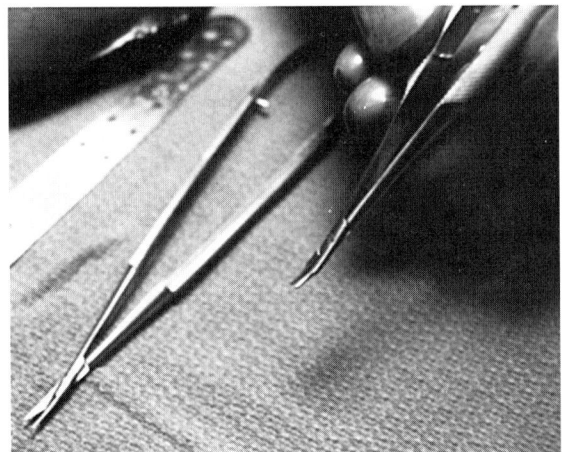

FIGURE 11–13. Microneedle holder with a nonlocking, spring-loaded socket that disengages with light finger pressure, thereby not creating significant vibration that could lacerate tissues.

tempting a surgical case involving the tying of multiple knots in humans.

Microscissors may be straight or slightly curved and many times may have a variset wheel in the handles. According to most manufacturers of such instruments, the rotation of this wheel displaces the handles laterally, which enhances the cutting action of the blades. With the wheel in the closed position, the scissors function as a standard spring scissors. The open position is only occasionally required to cut either very dense tissue or paradoxically very thin elastic tissue. The curved-tip scissors are used to dissect tissue in the region of the capsule and bilaminar zone. The straight-tip scissors are used to cut sutures. In laser microdiscectomy, the articular disc is sculpted and reshaped, and scar tissue is vaporized from its surface, as is done in the treatment of adhesive capulitis, with the laser beam directed through the microscope lens. A joystick and laser firing button mounted directly on the binocular housing on the surgeon's side can be operated by the thumb and index fingers to accomplish ordinary functions of the microscissors. Further, the laser firing mechanism can be used to vaporize remnants of the medial aspect of the articular disc in a very precise manner, avoiding the often encountered heavy bleeding from the depths of the wound usually arising from the medial vascular network.

The microinstruments can be kept in a small metal tray on the Mayo stand, or the tray holding the instruments can be clipped to the patient's chest drapes. This is done to avoid dropping them, which usually causes irreparable damage.

MICROSURGICAL LASER TECHNIQUE

When scheduling a microsurgical procedure in the operating suite, it is important to determine whether or not the microscope is functional and that the appropriate instruments are available. A laser-trained nurse must be present at all laser procedures. Because the microscope is a highly technical item of instrumentation, adjustments and repairs must be made periodically. To borrow an operating microscope from another surgical service may not be possible or desirable (one gets comfortable using one's own) on the day of surgery.

Before surgery, the anesthesiology team is advised to be positioned on the contralateral side of the patient opposite the side of surgery. Their position is slightly angled and at waist level to the patient. It is also requested that they produce a controlled hypotensive state of anesthesia so that the blood pressure is maintained at a mean arterial pressure of 80 to 90 mm Hg, depending on the cardiovascular status of the patient. Nasoendotracheal intubation is performed to permit manipulation of the mandible during the early phase of surgery to palpate the lateral pole of the condyloid process prior to skin incision and later to visually and manually evaluate the movements of the condyle and articular disc during function before and after the joint is entered. An anesthetic agent is used to permit the injection of epinephrine (2% Xylocaine with 1:100,000 epinephrine). A vaporized anesthetic agent is employed, and muscle relaxants are not ordered to enable continual monitoring of the facial nerve. An electromyograph is used throughout the operation after placement of strategic facial electrodes. All the laser safety procedures discussed in Chapter 3 are used to protect the patient and operating room personnel during the entire operation.

The patient is placed on the operating table with the head at the foot of the table. (Fig. 11–14). As mentioned earlier, this allows room for the surgeon's knees while sitting so that hyperflexion of

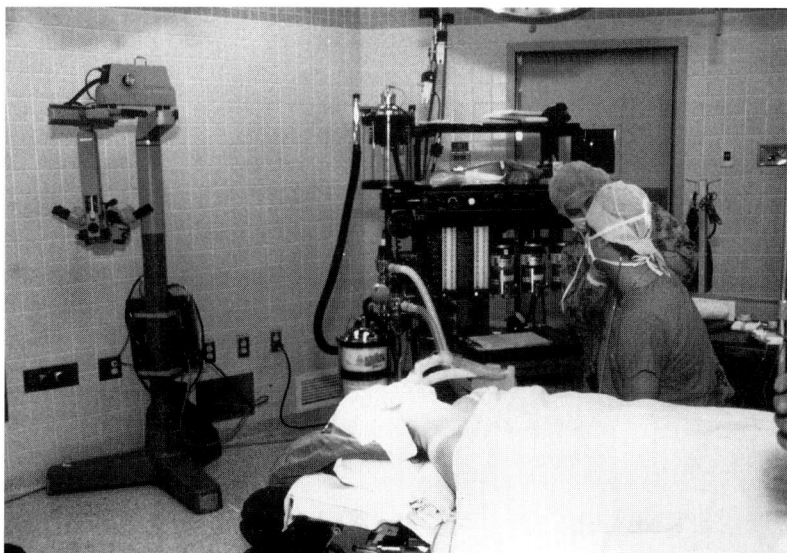

FIGURE 11–14. Positioning of patient on the operating table. Note that the patient is "reversed" so that the head of the patient is placed toward the foot of the table, thus enabling the surgeon and assistant to sit comfortably at the operative site.

the surgeon's neck is avoided because he or she can assume a position closer to the operative field. After induction of anesthesia, the head and neck of the patient is placed in the thyroid position, and the head is placed in a soft "horseshoe" or "doughnut" pillow and the head is rotated to the contralateral side, exposing the surgical site. At this point, the table may be rotated in the longitudinal axis of the patient to ensure that the surgical side is flat. This position assists in subsequent focus of the microscope. The patient may also be placed in the reverse Trendelenberg position to decrease venous congestion in the head and neck region. This, of course, depends on anesthetic considerations and if hypotensive agents have been used.

While the anesthesia team is gradually decreasing the blood pressure and establishing surgical anesthesia, the microscope is positioned over the operative site and the focal distance is adjusted with the operators in a seated position. The vertical support column of the microscope is then locked in position at that height. The horizontal microscope carrier arm is also locked with respect to the vertical column. The microscope arm supporting the binocular housing can be swung out of position but will return to the original focal length and location above the operative field. Adhesive tape, which is used in the microsurgical phase of the operation, is then placed on the floor corresponding to the location of the floor supports (legs) of the vertical column of the microscope. The rollers of the microscope are then unlocked, and the microscope is removed from its position near the operating table. This method saves time subsequently during the operation when the microscope is brought into position over the field of surgery. At this time, the microscope and other portals and attachments (camera) are covered with a sterile plastic, and the plastic drape is secured with sterile adhesive strips or rubber bands.

The patient's hair is shaved approximately 1.5 cm above the attachment of the helix to the temporal skin. The operative site is then prepared with an antiseptic solution, followed by gentle irrigation of the ear canal with saline. Ear drops containing a topical antibiotic mixed with a steroid are placed within the ear canal, and a small cotton pledget or cottonoid soaked in sterile mineral oil or antibiotic and steroid suspension is gently placed in the canal also. Antibiotic ointment or skin adhesive is used in the previously antiseptically prepared hair to keep the hair away from the operative field. Sterile towels are then stapled to the skin outlining the surgical site. The patient is then totally draped in the usual fashion.

There are at least two methods of using a laser to perform an open procedure or arthroplasty of the temporomandibular joint. In one approach, the surgeon can use laser energy delivered by a hand-piece with a contact tip, as in use of the Nd:YAG system, or a focused carbon dioxide laser using a handpiece with an attached waveguide. Thus, in these two approaches, the surgeon has tactile sense when dealing with surgical tissue. On the other hand, the surgeon can select use of a laser delivered through a microscope after reaching the temporomandibular ligament and employing a standard sharp scalpel technique, which has been well described in the surgical literature, or by the use of laser energy dissection delivered by a handpiece.

An outline of the skin incision in the preauricular region is made with a marking pen, as described earlier in the preauricular approach. Local anesthesia containing epinephrine is injected into the incision site and along the perichondrium of the anterior aspect of the aural canal. It is not advocated to inject a vasoconstricting agent into the joint space because the action of the vasoconstrictor will alter the character or extent of inflammatory reaction involving the intra-articular tissues. The incision may extend from the skin of the temporal fossa region, arching from the anterior attachment of the helix, with the concavity of the incision presenting forward. This superior extent of the incision only extends no more than 1 cm into the hair-bearing scalp. The incision then courses inferiorly along the anterior margin of the helix to the superior aspect of the tragus, then to the medial crest of the tragus. It is then carried inferiorly along the preauricular region just anterior to the tragus to the inferior attachment of the lobule of the ear to the skin of the neck. This initial incision is easily accomplished using the fine-tipped contact tip of the contact Nd:YAG laser (Surgical Laser Technologies, Oaks, Pennsylvania). It can also be accomplished by using a highly focused carbon dioxide laser (UltraPulse, Coherent Laser, Palo Alto, California) set on 5 to 15 watts. When using the Nd:YAG contact tip, it is important to use 10 to 15 watts and to move the tip of the contact scalpel lightly over the tissue, maintaining constant contact. If the contact tip is removed from the tissue bed, the laser should be placed on standby. Keeping the laser on while away from the tissues may result in burn up or deformation of the tip. As the contact tip is drawn across the tissues, the assistant should keep tension perpendicular to the incision line because this facilitates the cutting action of the contact laser energy. The incision is made through skin and subcutaneous fat, and a skin and fat flap is developed by undermining with the scalpel contact tip of the laser anteriorly to approximately 3 cm. Bleeding vessels are controlled with the dome-shaped contact tip of the Nd:YAG handpiece or by defocusing the carbon dioxide laser and applying its energy to the wall of the vessel if it is less than 0.5 to 1 mm in diameter. The skin flap thus created can be fixed to the skin of the face using skin staples.

At this junction, the author (GAC) prefers to develop an intermediate flap just above the superficial surface of the temporal fascia. This landmark is easily identified by using a Kitner (peanut) to push the tissue in the superior aspect of the wound to reveal the underlying glistening white surface of the temporal fascia. The tissues adhering to the temporal fascia are easily brushed away with the laser, and care should be taken not to stay in one spot for any appreciable time while the laser is active. Within this layer, the peripheral vessels of the superficial temporal artery and vein can be identified at the superior or temporal aspect of the wound, and these can be clamped to decrease intraluminal blood flow and the wall of the vessels "shrunk" and then divided by the laser. Indolent bleeding vessels are simply electrocoagulated or ligated, if necessary. There is a relatively constant plexus of veins anterior to the perichondrium at the root of the zygomatic arch, which are easily managed by the application of laser energy. It is important to leave a layer of perichondrial tissue on the cartilage of the auditory canal and to avoid the inadvertent contact of the laser with exposed cartilage, which could result in cartilaginous necrosis. The intermediate flap thus courses over temporal fascia in its superior extent and is superficial to the fat pad, underneath of which is located the variable presence of the frontotemporal branches of the facial nerve. The dissection can be carried anteriorly and inferiorly using the lateral aspect of the posterior zygomatic arch as a limit to the depth of the wound, the floor of which is made up of the lateral fibers of the temporomandibular ligament.

One of several techniques can be used to avoid injury to the branches of the facial nerve, whose distribution has been exhaustively studied by McCormack and colleagues[81] and Davis and associates,[82] who dissected hundreds of cadavers to outline the surgical anatomy of its superficial branches, and specifically the relations of the temporal ramus to the superficial fascia. Al-Kayat and Bramley[15] performed cadaver dissections of the facial nerve and used a modification of the preauricular approach to avoid injury to the facial nerve. It was noted that as the temporal fascia extends from the superior temporal line inferior to the zygomatic arch, it divides about 2 cm superior to the arch, thus defining a superficial plane and a deep plane attached to the lateral and medial periosteum of the zygomatic arch, respectively. This division of the temporal fascia thus forms a pocket containing a small quantity of fat, the zygomatic branch of the superficial temporal artery, and the zygomaticotemporal branch of the maxillary nerve. It has been demonstrated that the lateral periosteum of the arch

is firmly fused with two other connective tissue layers—the superficial fascia and the outer layer of the divided temporal fascia. The temporofacial branch of the facial nerve courses through the substance of the parotid gland and ascends anterolateral, crossing the zygomatic arch within the fusion of the above-mentioned connective tissue layers. The nerve can be found on average 2 cm from the anterior concavity of the external auditory canal with a range of 0.8 to 3.5 anteriorly. The intermediary flap is easily pushed by the tip of the laser contact probe along its entire anterior margin, the tissue falling away ahead of the tip.

By developing a thin skin flap, one can decrease injury to the temporofacial nerve branches that may lie in the loose superficial fascia. Dissection is carried anterior to the cartilaginous aural canal and superiorly to inferiorly along the temporal fascia, thus defining the intermediary flap, which is not to exceed 2 cm anterior to the concavity of the external auditory canal. It is preferable to reach the root of the zygomatic arch and not to stray beyond 1 cm anterior to the external auditory canal, but access and visibility can be limited by the thickness of the flap. This is especially true when skin is included in a full-thickness flap, which must be retracted firmly forward. Once the intermediary flap is fully developed, it can be stapled to the undersurface of the skin flap. A Wheatlander retractor can now be used to maintain the access gained by careful laser dissection.

The surgeon can easily palpate the curvature of the root of the zygomatic arch, the most posterior aspect of which can now be used as an starting point to develop a third flap. This flap will include the superficial layer of the temporal fascia and keep intact the underlying temporalis muscle fascia. One can make an incision with a sharp laser contact tip (scalpel probe) perpendicular to the posterior arch down to periosteum and then use a periosteal elevator to identify the underlying bone. Next, the temporal fascia is divided vertically, sparing the temporalis fascia, which prevents the temporalis muscle from extruding partially into the wound and proving to be an annoyance. This can be accomplished by bluntly dissecting beneath the temporal fascia with blunt scissors and then inserting a small anodized malleable retractor to protect the underlying temporalis fascia overlying the temporalis muscle. The surgeon can also release the superior aspect of the temporal fascia by angulating the incision in the fascia anteriorly. Further release can be gained inferiorly by incising through the posterior fibers of the temporomandibular ligament and, more inferiorly, the periosteum of the neck of the condyloid process. One can now use a blunt nasal freer or Woodson elevator to reflect the periosteum from the arch anteriorly to the articular eminentia. The temporal fascia flap can be quickly undermined with dissecting scissors and retracted from the field by retraction sutures or, if possible, the self-retaining retractor. The temporomandibular ligament can thus become part of the anteriorly retracted third flap, exposing the lateral capsular ligament. In the posterior dissection, it may be necessary to clamp and ligate the middle temporal artery, a branch of the superficial temporal artery that perforates the temporal fascia to supply the temporalis muscle.

At this juncture in the operation, the operator may choose to continue to use the laser handpiece with or without microscopic enhancement, or position the arm of the binocular apparatus to proceed using the laser through the lens of the microscope. When gross pathology exists, which may require meniscectomy, it may be expeditious to continue using the laser handpiece, although thorough resection, especially of the medial remnants of the disc, is greatly facilitated by the visual enhancement provided by the microscope. The Wheatlander retractor is repositioned exposing the zygomatic arch, articular eminence, lateral capsular ligament, and the neck of the condyloid process. The lateral capsular ligament can be entered by setting the power density of the laser to a cutting mode and, in the case of the carbon dioxide waveguide-mounted handpiece, drying the field to discourage absorption of the laser beam by water and incising through the ligament in a horizontal anterior to posterior movement. There are variations to this incision, especially if one uses the microscope in which highly focused but lesser required wattages are used to create, for example, a cruciate incision in which the flaps of the incision are retracted by fine sutures. At some point in the procedure in which the bone of the zygomatic arch and the neck of the condyloid process are exposed,

the operator can place the Wilkes joint spreader (Walter Lorenz, Florida). This apparatus, which is used in any standard open approach to the articulation, greatly facilitates access to the joint spaces (Fig. 11–15).

An assiduous attempt is made to control all bleeding. Anesthesia is checked to determine the blood pressure, which has been monitored with an arterial line at or just below 80 to 90 mm Hg in the healthy patient. An additional vasoconstrictor is not recommended at this time because it will obscure inflammatory conditions within the articulation.

If the operating microscope is chosen to be used, it is brought to the head of the operating table and located to its previously determined site by the markings on the floor. The horizontal arm is then rotated to a position above the operative site. The table is lowered to the original preoperative focal adjustment, and the surgeons can then sit opposite each other. The cruciate incision is then entered and is preferred as an alternative to the horizontal or inverted L–shaped capsular flap, which may force the surgeon to the large venous channels present in the posterior lateral aspect of the articulation. A periosteal elevator is used to outline the condyloid process to ascertain the presence of gross anatomic changes. Retractors designed by Dunn (Walter Lorenz, Florida) are used to expose further the condyloid process and protect the contiguous soft tissue, especially the highly vascular medial region. The condyloid process is inspected for deformation, osteophytosis, and loss of fibrocartilagenous. If possible, the surface of this structure is not violated because gross intervention may lead to further pathologic remodeling. Small osteophytes that can be observed to be interfering with joint function can be gently removed by using a diamond burr

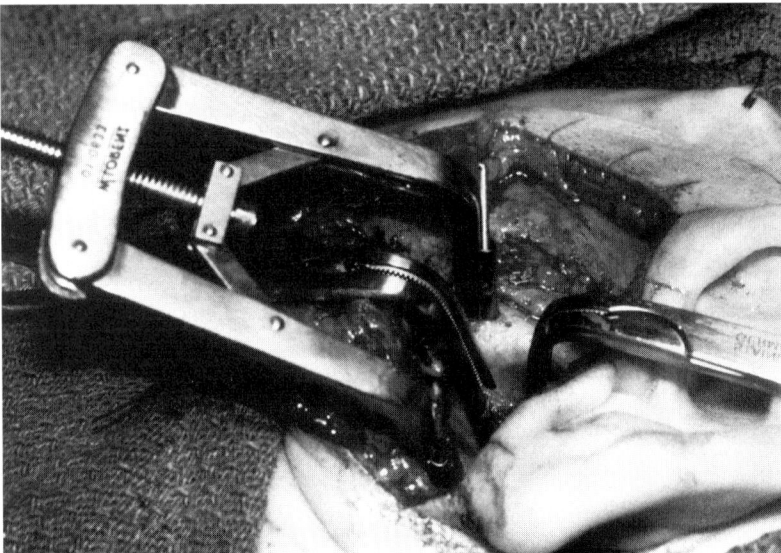

FIGURE 11–15. Good visual and manual access to the temporomandibular articulation is provided by the Wilke joint spreader.

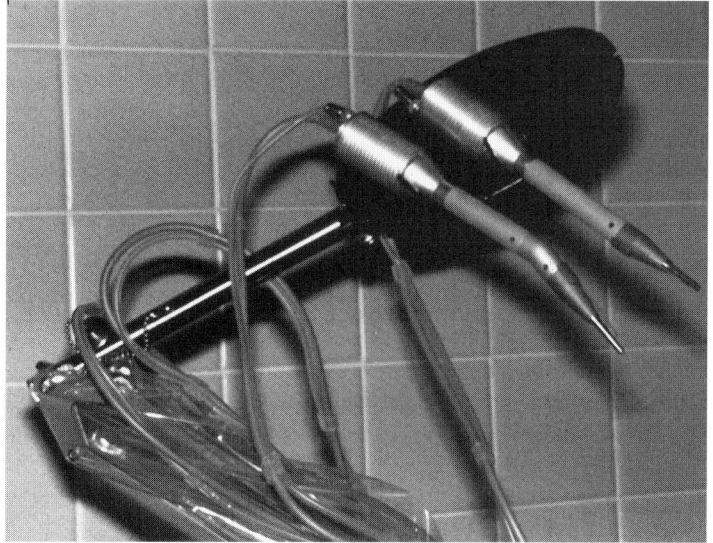

FIGURE 11–16. Xomed microsurgical handpieces. Note the angulated handpiece, which rests gently over the wrist of the surgeon.

in the angled Microcraft microsurgical handpiece (Xomed Corporation, Florida) (Fig. 11–16). Gross deformations and conditions such as bony ankylosis are probably best managed by alternative nonlaser methods.

With all retractors in place, the surgeon can insert moistened cottonoids around the entire articular space, thus protecting the bony surface of the glenoid fossa, the fibrocartilage of the condyloid process, the medial vascular tissues, and isolate the articular disc for the application of laser energy. If the metallic surfaces of the retractors within the operative field are not anodized, the cottonoids protect nontarget metal and tissue from inadvertent laser beam reflection. To temporarily control oozing from either the bilaminar zone or the lateral pterygoid muscle fibers in the anterior regions of the joint, DeBakey pediatric vascular clamps can be activated anteriorly and posteriorly.[83] (Fig. 11–17). Moreover, if a coaxial through-the-lens free-beam laser is used, it is kept away from the fiberoptic cord, which is taped to the joint spreader using

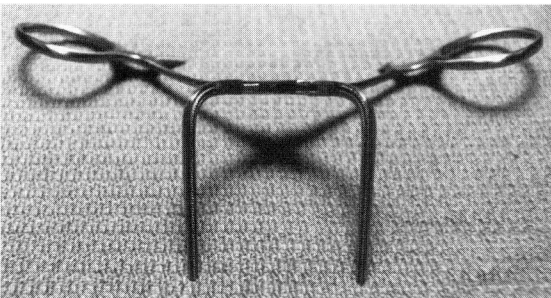

FIGURE 11–17. DeBakey clamps are used to enhance hemostasis and control of the articular disc and bilaminar zone.

sterile adhesive strips; the laser beam striking the end of the fiberoptic cord can destroy the light-transmitting fibers. The fiberoptic light cord is often used to supplement the light source, which is transmitted through the microscope, and also when the laser energy is applied using the handpiece or waveguide.

The focused free-beam carbon dioxide laser through the microscope can be used to perform a number of tasks by directing the coaxial helium: neon directional laser on the tissues to be incised, or it can be used in a defocused mode applied to tissue to cause vaporization, ablation, or hemostasis. With marginal power of 2.5 to 5 watts, the beam can be directed by using one hand (thumb and index finger) to control the directional joystick mounted between the ocular tubes and the firing of the laser controlled by a small button in the middle of the joystick lever. Anodized microinstruments can be used to grasp the soft tissues in order to direct the beam even more precisely. The hand-held laser (either carbon dioxide or the contact Nd:YAG laser) can be operated in a similar fashion using the operating microscope or loupes to enhance visibility. All of these lasers can execute a significantly varied range of surgical procedures with enhanced speed, more precise control of target tissue, and by limiting collateral tissue damage, less unwanted contiguous tissue injury than comparable equipment such as electrosurgical instruments, motorized shavers, and suction punch instruments.

All of these laser devices can be used to perform a host of intra-articular maneuvers, such as meniscectomy, lysing and ablation of adhesions and pseudowalls, excision of hypertrophic tissue, synovectomy, release of anterior band and muscle fibers, sculpting discoplasty, laser cauterization of the posterior attachment or oblique protuberance, removal of fibrillation of the articular fibrocartilage, hemostasis, increasing the width of the anterior or posterior recesses, and generalized débridement outlining the periphery of the articular disc. Moreover, in cases of perforation of the posterior attachment and when the need exists to debride diseased tissue and cicatrix formation in degenerative joint disease, laser devices have been used with beneficial results. In cases of perforation of the posterior attachment as well as débridement of diseased tissue and cicatrix formation in degenerative joint disease. Débridement with a laser device is especially interesting because it may be of value in eradicating most of the giant cell reactions seen after surgical placement of teflon and polymer temporomandibular implants. Advances in laser fusion of biologic tissues using computerized milliwatt laser parameters holds future promise in welding perforations in the articular disc or its bilaminar zone or other attachments.[84]

REFERENCES

1. Annadale T: On the displacement of the inter-articular cartilage of the lower jaw and its treatment by operation. Lancet 1:411–412, 1887.
2. Lanz A: Discitis mandibularis. Zentralbl Chir 9:289, 1909.
3. Pringle J: Displacement of the mandibular meniscus and its treatment. Br J Surg 6:385, 1918.
4. Risdon F: Ankylosis of the temporomandibular joint. J Am Dent Assoc 21:1933, 1934.
5. Blair VP, Ivy RH: Essentials of oral surgery. St. Louis, CV Mosby Co, 1936.
6. Milch H: Bayonet incision of temporo-mandibular arthrotomy. Am J Ortho Oral Surg 27:287, 1938.
7. Henny FA, Baldridge OL: Condylectomy for persistently painful temporomandibular joint. J Oral Surg 15:24, 1957.
8. McCann, CF: Bilateral subcondylar osteotomy. Report of a case. J Oral Surg 23:240, 1965.
9. Rowe, NL and Killey, HC: Fractures of the Facial Skeleton, 2nd ed. Baltimore, Williams & Wilkins, 1968.
10. Giles, HV: A useful incision to the parotid gland and fractures of the mandible. Intern Surg 51:76, 1969.
11. Thoma, KH: Oral Surgery, 5th ed., Vol I. St. Louis, CV Mosby Co, 1969.
12. Rowe, NL: Surgery of the temporomandibular joint. Proc R Soc Med 65:383, 1972.
13. Poswillo, D: Surgery of the temporomandibular joint. Oral Sci Rev 6:87, 1974.
14. Middleton, DS: Clinical approach to derangement of the mandibular joint. J Roy Coll Surg Edinb 17:287, 1972.
15. Al-Kayat A, Bramley P: A modified pre-auricular approach to the temporomandibular joint and malar arch. J Oral Surg 17:91–103, 1979.
16. Smith AE, Robinson M: Surgical correction of mandibular prognathism by sigmoid notch osteotomy with sliding condylotomy—a new technique. J Am Dent Assoc 49:46, 1956.
17. Stuteville OH: Surgical reconstruction of the temporomandibular joint. Am J Surg 90:940, 1954.
18. Hovell, JH: Condylar hyperplasia. Br J Oral Surg 1:105, 1963.
19. James P: The surgical treatment of mandibular joint disorders. Ann R Coll Surg Engl 49:310–328, 1971.
20. Eggedi P: Etiology of condylar hyperplasia. Aust Dent J 14:12, 1969.
21. Popowich L Crane RM: Modified preauricular access to the temporomandibular articulation. Oral Surg 54:257, 1982.
22. Alexander RW, James RB: Postauricular approach for surgery of the temporomandibular articulation. J Oral Surg 32:346, 1975.
23. Eggleston DJ: The perimeatal exposure of the condyle. J Oral Surg 36:369, 1976.
24. McCarty WL, Farrar WB: Surgery for internal derangements of the temporomandibular joint. J Prosthet Dent 42:191–196, 1979.
25. Dunn MJ, Bewza R, Moan D, Sanders J: Temporomandibular joint condylectomy: A technique and post operative follow-up. Oral Surg 51:363–374, 1981.
26. Bockenheimer P: Eine nerve methode zur freilegung der keifergelemky ohme sichtbare maubem unde ohme vevlezund des nervus facialis. Zemtralbl P Chir, 47:1560, 1920.
27. Axhausen G: De operative fueilegumg des kiefergelemks. Chirung 3:713, 1930.
28. Husted, E: Surgical management of temporomandibular joint disorders. Dent Clin N Am 601–607, 1966.
29. Dolwick MF, Kretzschmar DP: Morbidity associated with the preauricular and perimeatal approaches to the temporomandibular joint. J Oral Maxillofac Surg 40:699–700, 1980.
30. Walters P, Geist ET: Correction of temporomandibular joint internal derangements via the posterior auricular approach. J Oral Maxillofac Surg 41:616–618, 1983.
31. Kreutziger KL: Microsurgical approach to the temporomandibular joint. A new horizon. Arch Otolaryngol 108:422–428, 1982.
32. Davidson AS: Endaural Condylectomy. Br J Plast Surg 8:64–67, 1955.
33. Rongetti JR: Menisectomy. A new approach to the temporomandibular joint. Arch Otolaryngol 60:566–572, 1954.
34. Dias AD: A truly endaural approach to the temporomandibular joint. Br J Plast Surg 37:65–68, 1984.
35. Sarnat BG, Laskin DM (eds): The Temporomandibular Joint. Springfield, Massachusetts, Charles C Thomas, 1980.
36. Nylen CO: The microscope in aural surgery. Its first use and later development. Acta Otolaryngol 116 (suppl):226–240, 1954.
37. Dohlman CF: Carl Olof Nylem and the birth of the otomicroscope and microsurgery. Acta Otolaryngol 90:161, 1969.
38. Holmgren G: Some experiences in the surgery of otosclerosis. Acta Otolaryngol 5:460, 1923.
39. Perrit RA: Recent advances in corneal surgery. (Abstract.) Trans Am Acad Ophthalmol Otolaryngol 54:4238, 1949–1950.
40. Littman H: Ein Neves Operationsmikroskop. Klin Monatsbl Augenheilkd 124:473, 1954.
41. Silber SJ: Microsurgery, Baltimore, Williams & Wilkins Company, 1979.
42. O'Brien BM: Microvascular reconstructive surgery. Edinburgh, Churchill Livingston, 1977.
43. Smith JW: Microsurgery of peripheral nerves. Plast Reconstr Surg 33:317, 1964.
44. Michon J, Masse P: Le moment optimum de la suture nerveuse dans les plaies du membre superieur. Rev Chir Orthop 50:205, 1964.
45. Millesi H: Zum problem de uberbrucking von Defekten peripherer nerven. Wien Med Wochenschr 118:182, 1968.
46. Millesi H: Weiderherstellung durchtrennter peripherer nerven and nerventransplantation. Munch Med Wochenschr 111:2669, 1969.
47. Millesi H: Indikation and technik der autologen and interfazikularen nerventransplantation. Melsunder Med Mitteilungen 46:181, 1972.
48. Jacobsen JH, Suarez EL: Microsurgery in anastomosis of small vessels. Surg Forum 11:243, 1960.
49. Kubo T, Ikuta Y, Watari S, et al: The smallest digital replant yet? Br J Plas Surg 29:313, 1976.
50. Kleinert HE, Kasdan ML, Romero JL: Small blood vessel

anastomosis for salvage of severely injured upper extremity. J Bone Joint Surg, 45A:788, 1963.

51. Komatsu S, Tamai S: Successful reimplantation of a completely cut off thumb. J Plast Reconstr Surg 42:374, 1968.
52. Malt RA, McKhann C: Replantation of severed arms. JAMA 189:716, 1964.
53. Taylor GI, Daniel RK: The anatomy of several free flap donor sites. Plast Reconstr Surg 56:243, 1967.
54. Ostrup LT, Fredrickson JM: Microvascular surgery. Scand J Plast Reconstr Surg 10:18, 1976.
55. Taylor GI, Miller GDH, Ham FJ: The free vascularized bone graft. J Plast Reconstr Surg 5:533, 1975.
56. Bunche HJ, Furwas DW, Gordon L, et al: Free osteocutaneous flap from a rib to the tibia. J Plast Reconstr Surg 59:797, 1963.
57. Oktsuka H, Torigai K, Shioya N: Two toe-to-finger transplants in one hand. J Plast Reconstr Surg 60:561, 1977.
57a. Fugino T, Tanino R, Sugimuto C: Microvascular transfer of free deltopectoral dermal fat flap. Plast Reconstr Surg 55:428, 1975.
58. Tschopp HM: A Composite Living Bone and Muscle Graft for Reconstruction of the Mandible. Lettre d' information, No. 5, Groupe d'advancement Microchirurgie, 1976.
59. Harashina T, Nakajima T, Yoshimura Y: A free groin flap reconstruction for progressive facial hermiatrophy. Br J Plast Surg 30:14, 1977.
60. Wells JH, Egerton MT: Correlation of severe hemifacial atrophy with a free dermo-fat flap from the lower abdomen. Plast Reconstr Surg 59:223, 1977.
61. Daniel, RK: Mandibular reconstructive with free tissue transfers. Ann Plast Surg 1:346, 1978.
62. David DJ, Tan, E: A de-epitheliazied free groin flap from facial contour reconstruction. J Maxillofac Surg 6:249, 1978.
63. David DJ, Tan E: Microvascular surgery in maxillofacial reconstruction. Ann Acad Med Singapore 8(4):481–485, 1979.
64. Berger H, Meissl G, Sammi M: Experimentelle erfahrungen mit killagenfolien uber nahtlose nervanastomosen. Acta Neurochir (Wein) 23:141, 1970.
65. Samii M, Willebrand H: The technique and indication for autologus interfascicular nerve transplantation. Excerpta Med Interm Contr Ser 217:39, 1970.
66. Samii M, Schurmann K, Scheimpflung W, Wallenborn R: Experimental studied comparing grafting with autogenous and irradiation freeze-dried homologous nerves. Excerpta Med Intern Congr Ser 287:263, 1971.
67. Samii M: Die operative wiederherstellung verletzter nerven. Largebecks Arch Klin Chir 332:335, 1972a.
68. Samii M, Wallenborn R: Tierexperimentelle untersunchungen uber dem eimflu (b) der spanning anf den regenera-

tion ser folg nach nervennaht. Acta Neurochir (Wein) 27:87, 1972b.
69. Samii M: Interfaszikulare autologe nerventransplantation. Dtsch Arztebl 70:1257, 1975.
70. Samii M: Nerventransplantation. Bild der Wissenschaft 3:44, 1974.
71. Hausamen JR, Samii M, Schmidseder R: Repair of mandibular nerve by means of autologous nerve grafting after resecting of the lower jaw. J Maxillofac Surg 1:74–78, 1973.
72. Hausamen JE, Samii M, Schmidseder R: Indication and technique for the reconstruction of nerve defects in head and neck. J Maxillofac Surg 2:159–167, 1974.
73. Hausamen JE: Principles and clinical application of micronerve surgery and nerve transplantation in the maxillofacial area. Ann Plas Surg 7:(6)428–433, 1981.
74. Wessberg GA, Wolford LM: Bilateral microneurosurgical reconstruction of the inferior alveolar nerves view autogenous sural nerve transplantation. Oral Surg 52:465, 1981.
75. Wessberg GA, Wolford LM, Epker BN: Simultaneous inferior alveolar nerve graft and osseous reconstruction of the mandible. J Maxillofac Surg 40:384, 1982.
76. Kreutziger KL, Mahan PE: Temporomandibular degenerative joint disease: Part I. Anatomy, pathophysiology, and clinical description. Oral Surg 40:165–192, 1975.
77. Kreutziger KL, Mahan PE: Temporomandibular degenerative joint disease: Part II. Diagnostic procedure and comprehensive management. Oral Surg, 40:297–319, 1975.
78. Cherrick HM: Pathology. *In* Sarnat BG, Laskin DM (eds): The Temporomandibular Joint. Springfield, Massachusetts, Charles C Thomas, 1980, pp 180–204.
79. McCarty W: Diagnosis and Treatment of Internal Derangements of the Articular Disc and Mandibular Condyle. *In* Solberg, WK and Clark, GT (eds): Temporomandibular Joint Problems, Biologic Diagnosis and Treatment. Berlin, Quintessence Publishing Company, 1980, pp 145–164.
80. Katzberg RW, Keith DA, Guralnick WC, Manzione JD, et al: Internal derangement and arthritis of the temporomandibular joint. Radiology 146:107–112, 1983.
81. McCormack WL, Cauldwell EW, Anson BJ: The surgical anatomy of the facial nerve: with special reference to the parotid gland. Surg Gynec Obstet 80:620, 1954.
82. Davis RA, Anson BJ, Budinger JM, Kurth LRE: Surgical anatomy of the facial nerve and parotid gland upon a study of 350 cervicofacial halves. Surg Gynec Obstet 102:385, 1956.
83. Saunderson JR, Dolwick MF: Increased hemostasis in temporomandibular joint surgery by use of the DeBakey bulldog vascular clamp. J Oral Maxillofac Surg 41:271, 1983.
84. White JV, Leefmans E, Stewart G, et al: Laser fusion tissue repair with CO_2 laser. SPIE, 1066:35, 1989.

CHAPTER 12

Lasers for Use in Cosmetic Maxillofacial Surgery

JEFFREY MOSES, DDS

The use of lasers in conjunction with endoscopes in facial rejuvenation procedures has literally turned cosmetic surgery inside-out. Conventional surgical techniques, such as brow lifting, blepharoplasty, and rhytidectomy, have been adapted to incorporate these new technologies; they provide the desired aesthetic results and concomitantly offer the patient less postoperative discomfort and a more rapid recovery.

These revolutionary surgical techniques offer the surgeon a challenge to rethink traditional procedures and use the basic principles of orthodox surgery in a new métier: endolaser surgery replaces the bicoronal incision without the necessity of skin resection (therefore requiring minimal incisions), decreases bleeding, eliminates drains and problems with alopecia, and provides excellent visualization. Thus, in only the past 3 years, the paradigm has shifted away from fundamentals learned during formal education.

In this chapter, we discuss minimally invasive endoscopically assisted forehead surgery, blepharoscopy, and facial skin resurfacing using lasers with respect to established anatomic principles, traditional surgical techniques, and a new method of fixing the soft tissue to the cranium based on our experience with endolaser surgeries.

DEFORMITY PRIOR TO SURGICAL CORRECTION AND ITS CAUSES

Cosmetic facial surgery's goal is to correct the anatomic changes that occur in the aging face. As forehead wrinkles and horizontal skin lines form at the lateral canthus beginning approximately at the age of 40, the eyebrows steadily descend from a position well above the supraorbital rim to push infrabrow skin over eyelid folds. Patients with hyperactive corrugator muscles give the impression of anger or fatigue. The skin becomes lax and forms creases indicating the underlying muscles of facial expression.

Indications for endolaser brow lift are identical for patients who are candidates for the open technique, that is, ptotic brows, glabellar creases, and transverse forehead rhytids. This surgical technique is relatively contraindicated in patients who have previously undergone browplasty and those with an excessive amount of redundant or thick skin, or both.

Indications for upper and lower blepharoscopy include dermatochalasis (skin redundancy), blepharochatory eyebrow position, and blepharoptosis. The indication for removal of the anterior fat pads is determined preoperatively by palpation and pinching of the area of the superior lateral brow. Upper eyelid blepharoplasty is intended to eliminate excessive upper eyelid skin to provide a balanced vertical relation between the upper eyelid, the palpebral crease, and the brow, so that all are vertically equal. Lower eyelid blepharoplasty is directed at eliminating bulging or protruding fat and reducing excessive skin and fine rhytids. Elimination of wrinkles is accomplished with either chemical peel or laser resurfacing simultaneously with the transconjunctival removal of fat.

Indications for skin rejuvenation include photoaging effects such as rhytids in the periorbital and perioral areas, actinic keratosis, elastosis, and hyperpigmentation. Also, scars or disease states such as actinic cheilitis, rhinophymas, epidermal nevi, tumors, and superficial skin cancers prompt surgical intervention.

ANATOMY

Functional Anatomy of Forehead and Scalp

We present a thorough overview of the relevant facial anatomy from a surgical perspective and review the pertinent muscles, nerves, and vascular system to elucidate the surgical techniques discussed later in this chapter.

Figure 12–1 shows the four major muscles of concern for the facial rejuvenation procedure: the corrugator, the frontalis, the medial depressor fibers of the supercilli underlying the orbicularis oculi, and the procerus muscles.

The frontalis and corrugator muscles are the primary muscles of the forehead. The frontalis muscle extends transversely and inserts into the galea aponeurotica. It elevates the eyebrows and produces horizontal forehead creases. The corrugators arise from the medial orbital rim of the frontal bone near the superior orbit and insert into the frontalis muscle and the skin of the medial brow. The contraction of these paired muscles pulls the eyebrows together and causes glabellar frown lines. Although the contracture of the frontalis muscle opposes corrugator activity, the corrugator, the procerus, and the orbicularis oculi muscles act in concert to close the eyes and create facial expressions that produce transverse and oblique glabellar lines.

The superficial musculoaponeurotic system (SMAS) is a continuous fibromuscular layer interlinking the many muscles of facial expression. The SMAS divides the subcutaneous fat into two layers; it contains fibrous septa that extend through the fat and attach to the overlying dermis, acting as a network to distribute facial muscle contractions to the skin (Fig. 12–1A and B). In the upper face, the vessels and the sensory nerves are initially deep to the SMAS and small branches penetrate the SMAS to run within its superficial aspects or on its surface.

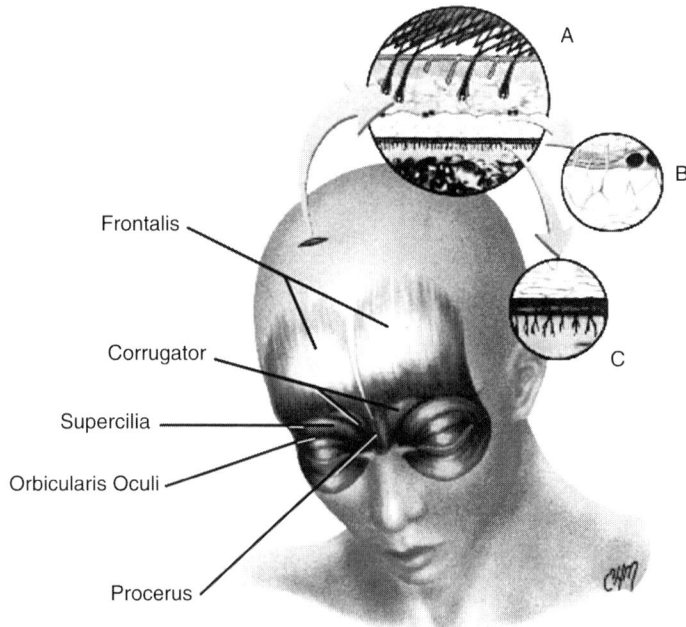

FIGURE 12–1. The four major muscles for facial rejuvenation: the corrugator and frontalis in the forehead, the medial depressor fibers of the supercilli underlying the orbicularis oculi, and the procerus muscles. These muscles move the skin of the face and scalp and are called the muscles of expression. A, The superficial musculoaponeurotic system (SMAS), a continuous fibromuscular layer composed of the epidermis, dermis, fibrous septum, vessels, fascia, muscle, and motor nerves. The SMAS splits to ensheath the frontalis, occipitalis, procerus, and some of the periauricular muscles. B, The SMAS divides the subcutaneous fat into two layers. In the upper face, vessels and nerves arise to penetrate the SMAS. C, Fibrous septa extending through the fat to the dermis create a network connecting the skin to the underlying muscles to distribute the muscle contractions throughout the system.

Above the zygoma, the SMAS is a more consistent layer that envelopes the frontalis muscle and then forms the galea aponeurotica. The temporal branch of the facial nerve courses within the SMAS in the temple and is particularly vulnerable over the zygoma, where it lies superficially just beneath the subcutaneous fat.

In the aging patient, the SMAS is useful as a deep layer to tighten; its surgical significance is that it acts as a guide to the level of important neurovascular structures. Undermining beneath the SMAS and above the periosteum is a safe, avascular plane during elevation of a forehead flap, allowing injury to the temporal branch of the facial nerve to be avoided. However, undermining at the subperiosteal plane releases the fixation at the supraorbital rims of the brows to give full release.

The galea aponeurotica, or epicranium, is composed of the frontalis, the galea, and the occipital muscles, and extends laterally into the SMAS. The frontalis muscle joins the orbicularis muscle at the orbital rim.

The temporalis muscle is covered by a dense, tough fascia, called the deep temporalis fascia, which is continuous with the periosteum of the skull. Some fibers of the temporalis arise from this fascia (Fig. 12–1C). A few centimeters above the zygomatic arch, at the temporal line of fusion, the deep temporalis fascia splits into its superficial and its deep layers, which then insert into the superficial and the deep aspects of the superior surface of the zygomatic arch.

Figure 12–2, a side view of the head, shows the subperiosteal dissection region, coronally to approximately 2.5 cm above the rim of the orbit; the subgaleal dissection region; and the conjoint ligament, which is defined as the location where the superficial temporal fascia joins in with the deep temporal fascia as it inserts to the galea at the level of insertion of the temporalis muscle on the parietal bone and frontal bone. The conjoint ligament connects the access of the temporal to parasagittal dissections.

The nuchal line, also known as the superior occipital line, is the place of attachment of the occipital, splenius, semispinus, and other muscles of the posterior superficial neck region at the nuchal ridge.

The SCALP mnemonic for its anatomy explains the five layers present:

S, Skin. The thickness of the epidermis and dermis of the scalp varies from 3 to 8 mm; it is thickest in the occiput and diminishes frontally and temporally.

C, Subcutaneous tissue. The second layer of the scalp is a dense layer composed of connective tissue and fat that binds the skin to the underlying galea. In its deepest half, the subcutaneous tissue contains

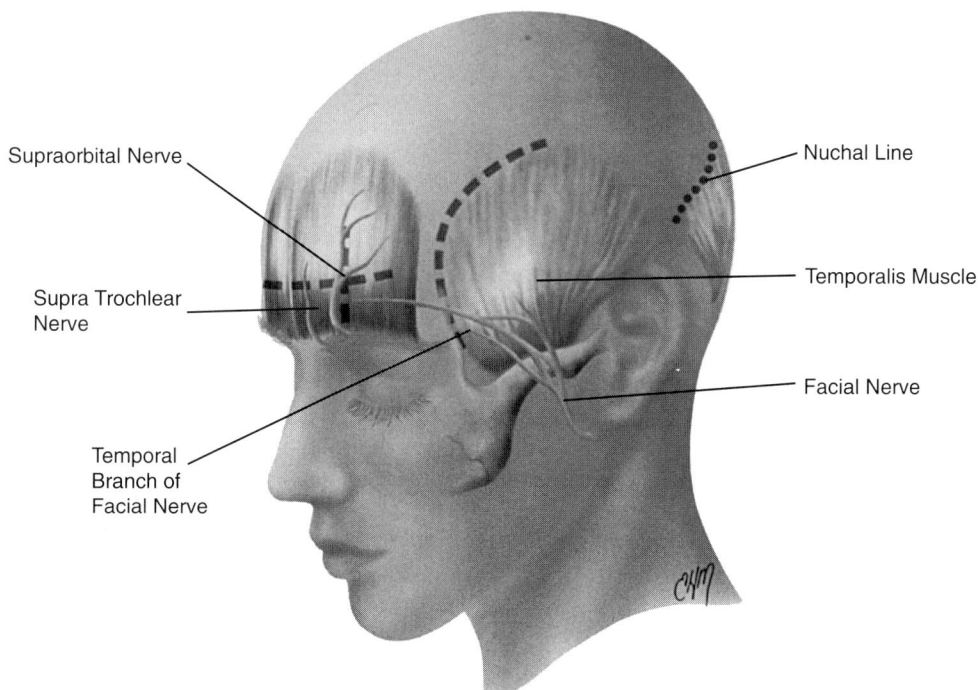

FIGURE 12–2. Subperiosteal dissection region and related anatomic structures. Motor nerves enter the deep surface of the muscles. Sensory nerves and vessels originate deep to the fascia, but their terminal branches run within or superficial to it.

adnexal tissue, nerves, lymphatics, and the principal arteries and veins of the scalp.

A, Galea aponeurotica, also known as the epicranium. The paired occipital and frontal muscles are connected over the vertex of the skull by the galea aponeurotica. The galea is the strongest layer of the scalp. It is a musculofascial layer supported by the areolar tissue of the subaponeurotic space. The attachment of the galea aponeurotica is extensive, stretching from the radix of the nose medially, along the supraorbital margins laterally, across the temporal area to the superior auriculocephalic angle, then posteriorly and slightly downward along the inferior nuchal line to the spinous process of the seventh cervical vertebra.

L, Loose areolar tissue. This connective tissue is loose, thin, and relatively avascular, situated between the galea and the periosteum. Its laxity provides the mobility of the scalp.

P, Pericranium. The innermost layer of the scalp adheres to the outer table of the skull, containing a rich vascular supply from underlying bone. In between the cranium tables, the diploë act as feeder vessels.

Figure 12–3 provides a view of the five layers of the scalp.

The zygomatic branch and the frontal branch of the facial nerve are two of the five major nerve branches most at risk of injury during brow lift. The frontal branch is also called the temporal nerve; both are terminal branches without anastomotic connections. These nerves are complex in terms of their horizontal branching patterns and in their relationship to fascial and muscular layers. The nerve rami exit the parotid, run within the SMAS over the zygomatic arch and the temple area, and enter the undersurface of the frontalis muscle. The nerve branches are superficial to both layers of the deep temporalis fascia. Therefore, to avoid injury when elevating flaps, the surgeon must undermine either in the immediate subcutaneous plane or deep to the SMAS on the temporalis fascia. Over the zygomatic arch, the nerve lies in the SMAS just beneath the subcutaneous fat and immediately overlies the bony prominence of the zygoma.

The scalp is extremely vascular, deriving its blood supply entirely from the external carotid system. In the preauricular region, the supratrochlear, supraorbital, and superficial temporal arteries are of significant importance. The superficial temporal artery is also the primary blood supply to the lateral aspect of the orbicularis oculi muscle.

The Anatomy of the Eyelids

The orbicularis oculi muscle is a thin, elliptic muscle that surrounds the eye and extends into both eyelids. It arises from the medial palpebral ligament and is arbitrarily divided into the orbital and palpebral portions. The palpebral portion is further divided into the preseptal and pretarsal portions, in which the pretarsal fibers are attached to the lateral orbital tubercle by the lateral canthal tendon and provide support for the lower lid margin.

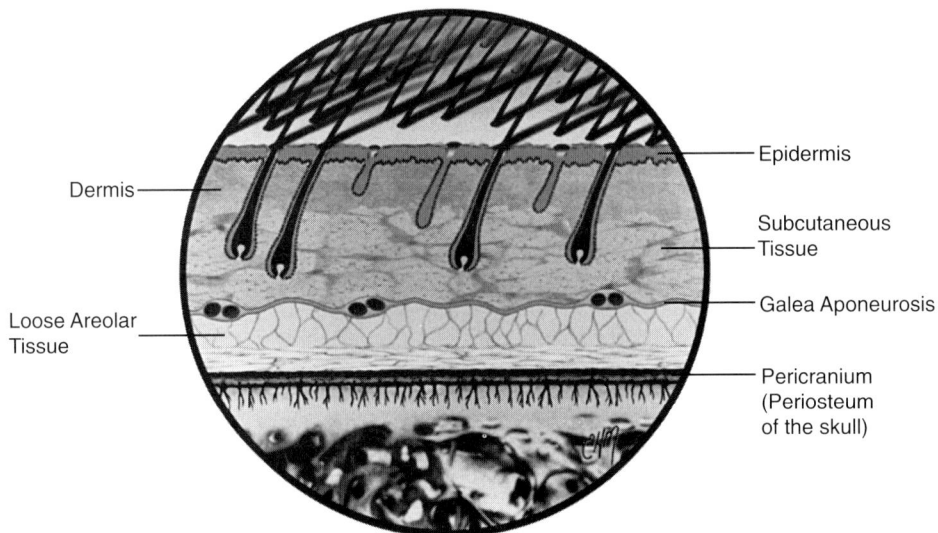

Dermis

Loose Areolar Tissue

Epidermis

Subcutaneous Tissue

Galea Aponeurosis

Pericranium (Periosteum of the skull)

FIGURE 12–3. The five layers of the scalp: the skin, the subcutaneous tissue, the galea aponeurotica (equal to the SMAS above the zygoma), the loose areolar tissue, and the pericranium. In reference to the structure of the skin, notice that the thin epidermis is composed of stratified squamous epithelium that overlies the more fibrous dermis. Collagen bundles of the superficial pupillary dermis are thinner and more randomly oriented than those of the deeper reticular dermis.

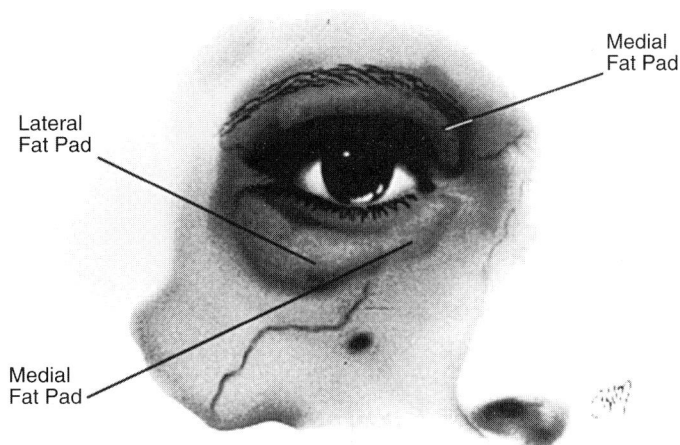

FIGURE 12–4. Fat pads surrounding the eyes; front view.

In the upper lid, the orbital portion extends over the corrugator, supercilli, and inferior portion of the frontalis muscle, whereas in the lower lid, the orbital segment may extend inferiorly into the cheek, overlying the nasalis muscle and lip levators. The orbital orbicular forms a continuous sphincter interrupted only at the medial canthus. The orbicularis oculi muscle is innervated by the facial nerve via the temporal branch.

In the upper lid, the levator aponeurotica attaches to the pretarsal muscle at the upper edge of the tarsus. It is covered by a distinct layer of fascia in the upper eyelid, which forms a pocket for the upper lateral fat pad.

The lower medial, lower central, and temporal fat pads are significant in blepharoscopy for the large blood vessels that transverse the fat. If the fat is not excised with extreme care, avoiding excessive tugging tension, these vessels can cause excessive bleeding and complications. Figures 12–4 (front view) and 12–5 (cross section) present the eye structures pertinent to this discussion.

The Anatomy of the Skin

The skin is divided into the thinner, more superficial epidermis and the more fibrous dermis. The epidermis varies in depth. It is thickest in the scalp and thinnest (0.04 mm) in the delicate skin of the eyelid. The dermis, composed of connective tissue, or collagen, contains nerves, blood vessels, muscles, lymphatics, and sweat glands. The more superficial and thinner dermis is termed the papillary dermis, which contains thin, randomly arranged collagen fibers and the superficial vascular plexus. The deeper and thicker dermis, called the reticular dermis, contains coarser bundles of collagen and the deep vascular plexus composed of larger vessels that surround skin appendages.

As previously discussed in the scalp anatomy, immediately beneath the epidermis and the dermis lies the firm, dense, and vascular subcutaneous tissue. Beneath the subcutaneous tissue lies the galea aponeurotica, a thick, tough, fibrous tissue that connects the frontalis muscle and the occipital epicra-

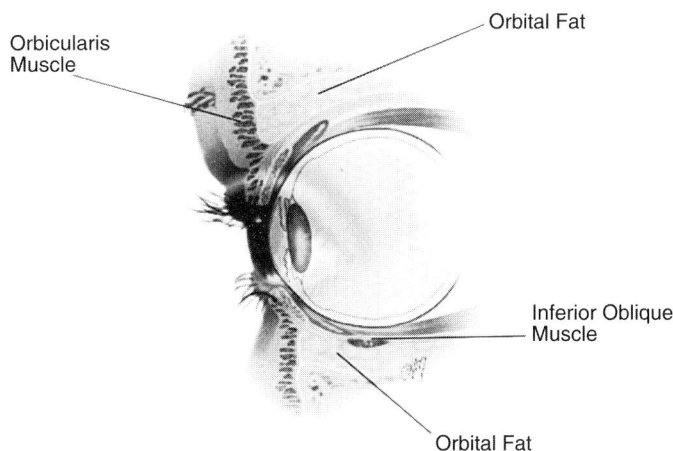

FIGURE 12–5. Cross-sectional view of eye structures analogous in upper and lower lids. The orbicularis oculi surrounds the orbit and extends into both eyelids.

nium, which inserts laterally into the temporalis. Beneath the galea is a plane of loose areolar tissue; next lies the pericranium or the periosteum of the skull. The deepest layer is the outer cortex of the skull.

Sharpy fibers are the ends of the collagen fibers embedded in the skull. They extend through periosteum to the bone (see Fig. 12–3).

The mechanical characteristics of skin are determined by the major connective tissues of the dermis, the elastic fibers, the collagen fibers, and the ground substance. Skin is anisotropic, meaning that skin tension and properties vary in different directions.

The hair follicle consists of the hair itself and the surrounding epithelial covering, which includes the sebaceous gland and the arrector pili muscle. The base of the hair follicle extends to the subcutaneous tissue deep to the dermis and can be damaged easily when elevating skin flaps. Because the direction and angle of hair growth vary over the scalp and the follicles are not perpendicular to the skin surface, incisions made in cosmetic maxillofacial surgery must follow the growth angle of the hair for the best aesthetic results. The surgeon must make an incision parallel to the growth angle of the follicles

to obtain future hair growth through a scalp incision. Figure 12–6 shows a hair follicle and its angle and direction of growth.

TRADITIONAL SURGICAL TECHNIQUE

The Surgical Armamentarium

The conventional surgical armamentarium, consisting of the surgical scalpel and electrosurgery, seems less accurate when compared with use of the laser for surgical incisions. Although fine surgical instruments offer precision to the half millimeter, separate cautery is required. The electrosurgical needle, loop, or probe can cause thermal necrosis, but the surgeon adept with a high-power laser controls not only the incision but cautery in one tissue-specific instrument.

The laser offers reproducible results in the depth it penetrates tissue and in focusing the beam to incision or ablative operating mode. Also, it permits a less invasive surgical approach when compared with conventional surgery. The differences are espe-

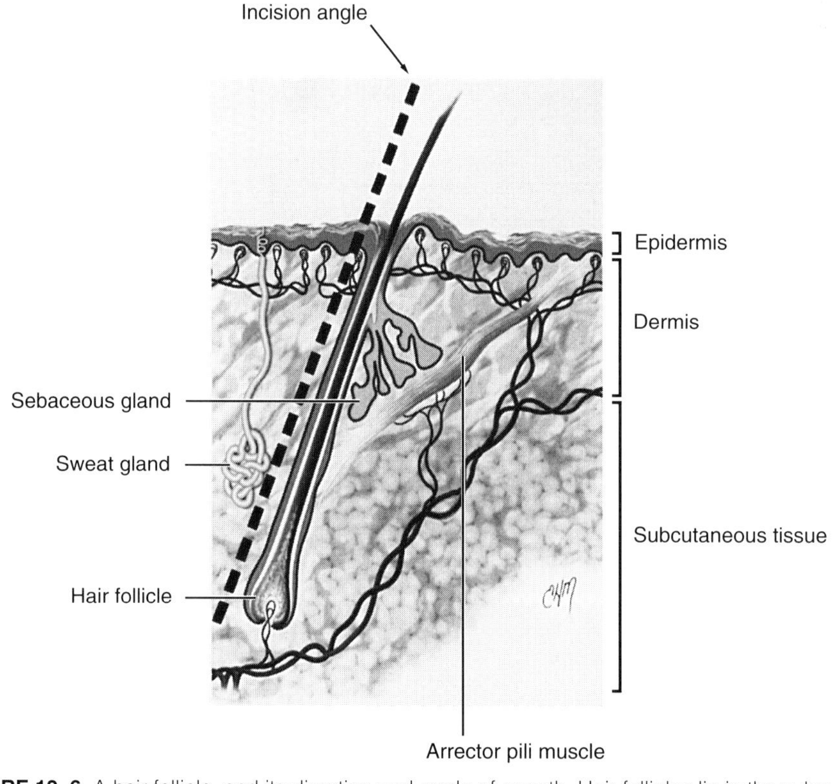

FIGURE 12–6. A hair follicle, and its direction and angle of growth. Hair follicles lie in the subcutaneous tissue deep to the dermis and are susceptible to damage when flaps are elevated. Surgical incisions should be beveled to include as many hair follicles as possible. These hair follicles will be in the suture line and will grow through the scar.

cially apparent after discussing the elements of traditional surgical techniques.

Forehead and Brow Lift

Surgeons who perform conventional lift procedures must concern themselves with the position of all incisions to minimize scarring. The forehead lift through a coronal incision posterior to the frontal and temporal hairline is a comprehensive operation; it allows elevation of the entire brow, direct attenuation of the action of the frontalis, corrugator, and procerus muscles, reduction of the transverse vertical creases, and scar camouflage in the scalp hair.

Local anesthesia requires infiltrations to block the supraorbital and supertrochlear nerves along the level of the eyebrows, augmented by infiltration along the intended line of incision using 1% lidocaine with 1:100,000 epinephrine. The extensive incision is marked within the hair, extending to or beyond the tragus of each ear.

Bleeding must be controlled, usually with pressure and bipolar cautery. The operation may proceed bloodlessly when the surgeon enters the subgaleal supraperiosteal plane using blunt dissection down to the supraorbital ridges. However, the surgeon may choose to use the subperiosteal plane instead.

With blunt dissection, the extent of the corrugator muscles is delineated and isolated from the bilateral supraorbital neurovascular bundles. Approximately 1 cm of muscle is excised after the corrugators are separated from their bony origin, and the section of muscle is cross-clamped. The procerus muscle is also partially removed; narrow transverse strips of galea, frontalis muscle, and subcutaneous tissue are excised, using cautery when required to control bleeding. After hemostasis is achieved, the forehead flap is advanced cephalically and redundant skin is excised in the hairline. (The scalp posterior to the coronal incision should be pushed forward to determine its elasticity, in turn, to determine the amount of skin excised from the forehead flap.)

Closure is accomplished with multiple buried galeal and dermal sutures to eliminate all tension; surgical staples supplement the closure in the hair-bearing scalp.

The patient is observed in recovery, then discharged on oral antibiotics and pain medication. Drains, if deemed necessary, are removed 1 day after surgery. Sutures may be removed between 1 and 2 weeks after surgery for incisions within the hairline.

Although the coronal approach to brow lift is a safe procedure, albeit extensive, complex, and time consuming, it offers the aesthetic results desired by the patient with the correct motivation. Healing requires rest for at least 6 days and elimination of vigorous activity for at least 4 weeks. Few complications are presented with this approach, but hematomas and infections can occur. The loss of hair along the incision and the loss of sensation in the scalp behind the incision are longer term events.

Blepharoplasty for Superior Eyelid Contour Improvement

The surgeon uses a marking pen to outline excessive upper eyelid skin by elevating the upper lid fold. The line begins where the lid creases, nasally above the upper punctum, and extends to the lateral canthus. It then slopes slightly upward in one of the lateral canthal creases, about 1.5 cm beyond the lateral canthus. The extent of excess skin is determined by grasping the skin at the central aspect of the marked line with a smooth forceps. The forceps pinches the skin to eliminate all excessive eyelid skin, everts the lashes, and minimally elevates the upper lid from its apposition to the lower lid. A mark is made at this superior site and also nasally and temporally to the midpoint; these three markings are connected.

Two percent lidocaine with 1:100,000 epinephrine is injected subcutaneously over the outlined upper eyelid and lateral canthus for anesthesia. A blade is used to incise along the upper eyelid marks, first over the lower line and then over the upper line. The skin is severed from the orbicularis muscle with scissors and then dissected. Any herniated fat is removed, as is the medial orbital fat pad. With slight pressure to the globe, the orbicularis muscle is picked up with forceps and severed with scissors, respecting the levator aponeurosis. Fat protrudes through the opening, and it is grasped with forceps, clamped with a hemostat, and severed. Cautery is required to achieve hemostasis.

The skin incisions are closed with continuous 6-0 Prolene suture in multiple close bites that are pulled snugly during closure. No dressings are used after surgery. The patient is instructed to apply ice cold saline compresses on the eyelids for the first 24 hours. To reduce edema, the head should be about 45 degrees higher than the rest of the body during bed rest. Patients must be watched closely for the first 3 to 4 hours after surgery for the development of hemorrhaging. The sutures are removed 4 days after the blepharoscopy. The incision may be supported with sterile tape applied over weak areas for an additional 3 days.

Transconjunctival Lipoplasty for Inferior Eyelid Contour Improvement

The traditional lower blepharoplasty incision may be transconjunctival or infraciliary, may be extended laterally to the lateral canthus, and may or may not include skin excision. Here, however, our discussion focuses on the transconjunctival technique.

A small vein retractor is used by the assistant to pull downward at the center of the lower lid while the surgeon holds the Jaeger retractor against the globe protector and the upper lid, allowing the surgeon to expose the inferior palpebral conjunctiva, where anesthetic is injected subconjunctivally. Two percent lidocaine with 1:100,000 epinephrine is injected with a 28- or 30-gauge needle into the fat pads and subconjunctival tissues. After the appropriate delay in time for hemostasis, the incision is made in the conjunctiva from the medial to temporal end of the eyelid. The surgeon grasps the inferior edge of the severed palpebral conjunctiva while the assistant grasps the adjacent more superior edge with another forceps. With the two forceps pulled apart, further dissection is carried out until fat is seen. Blunt dissection isolates the three orbital fat pads. The fat that prolapses with gentle pressure on the eye is clamped with a hemostat and cut along the hemostat blade. Then cotton-tipped applicators are placed underneath the hemostat as cautery is applied over the fat stump. The surgeon verifies that there is no residual bleeding prior to allowing the fat to slide back into the orbit. The other fat pads are removed in a similar manner. The conjunctiva is reapproximated with three 6-0 plain catgut buried sutures. Postoperative care, similar to that for the upper blepharoscopy procedure, is recommended for the next 24 hours.

Facial Skin Resurfacing

Responsive Wound Healing of Superficial Skin Damage and Applications to Cosmetic Treatments of Fine Facial Rhytids

Wound healing is a complex biologic event involving three phases. The initial phase is called the substrate or inflammatory phase, which lasts approximately 1 to 3 days. It is followed by a cellular proliferative phase, lasting 2 to 3 weeks, that is associated with increased fibroplasia in the wound. The maturation phase then develops, persists for 12 to 18 months, and is associated with collagen deposition and remodeling.

The healing sequence begins with initial wound edge bleeding that coagulates. Within 24 hours, a thin yellowish crust or scab forms. Reepithelialization occurs as migration from the wound margin and outer root sheaths of hair follicles, also occurring within 24 hours. Vascular dilation occurs, and the tiny vessels become filled with leukocytes.

Swelling in the wound develops as the cells and fluid escape the vascular channels. In cutaneous healing, during the regeneration of both epithelial and connective tissue components, the extracellular matrix, containing the collagens, acts as an adhesive substrate. Total resurfacing of the wound is completed in 7 days. As the wound matures, the rejuvenated collagen fibers of the dermis are realigned into the more parallel pattern of youthful skin. The auxiliary capillaries of healing regress. The wound softens, flattens, and becomes lighter in color.

Collagen develops in several different trimer configurations and constitutes approximately 98% of the skin's connective tissue. In uninjured skin, collagen fibers are unbranched and extremely long. When the skin is healing, collagen fibers have a haphazard orientation; during maturation, the randomly dispersed collagen fibers coalesce.

Lesions of the epidermis or connective tissue of the papillary dermis heal without scarring, whereas injury that extends into the reticular dermis always forms scar tissue.

Wound healing usually occurs more rapidly in covered wounds; the covering keeps the tissue fluid on the wound surface in a liquid state and crusting, a mechanical barrier to epidermal migration, is minimized.

Dermabrasion and Chemical Peel

Dermabrasion and chemical peeling are processes that affect both the epidermis and the superficial dermis, producing a smoothing of surface irregularities and altering skin pigmentation.

The face is anesthetized with 1% or 0.5% lidocaine containing 1:100,000 epinephrine. Regional blocks may be accomplished on the supraorbital, infraorbital, and mental nerves. In dermabrasion, the patient's skin is first cleaned, then frozen using freon and abraded using either a wire brush or a diamond fraise. A methodical procedure follows this order: preauricular and mandibular areas, then gradually continuing superiorly and anteriorly to the cheeks, chin, perioral area, forehead, and nose.

The quality of dermabrasion is related to the technique used in that the skin must be taut during abrasion. The wire brushes are motion dependent, and the appearance of white lines beneath the brush alerts the surgeon that he or she is planing in papillary or superficial reticular dermis. The surgeon must be concerned with maintaining the normal contour of the skin and altering it to a firm, solid state; the failure to dermabrade to an adequate depth in the papillary dermis gives inadequate results.

A biosynthetic dressing may be applied over topical antibiotic ointment onto the abraded surface. Crust formation is prevented by a thin application of petrolatum every 3 to 4 hours. Postoperatively, the patient experiences moderate to severe swelling, especially if the eyes and lips have been treated; the edema subsides on the fourth or fifth day.

In dermabrasion, regeneration of the injured collagen significantly augments the new collagen in enhancing skin contour. Wounds caused by dermabrasion heal by the same mechanism as unabraded wounds. For this reason, use of topical ointments following dermabrasion facilitates epithelialization.

Chemical peel, also known as chemexfoliation, produces favorable results in fine facial wrinkles, particularly in the perioral and periorbital regions. The process is the utilization of a controlled chemical injury to the skin resulting in limited exfoliation. The superficial effect allows for a regeneration of skin from the surrounding appendages and from the papillary layer of the dermis.

Phenol is the primary component of the chemical peel emulsion, although it may produce cardiac arrhythmias in the patient. To counteract the toxicity of phenol, the patient is hydrated with 500 ml of Ringer's lactate before applying the peel solution. Trichloroacetic acid can also be used in lighter peels with less skin bleaching than is experienced with phenol.

As in dermabrasion, the patient's face is cleaned to remove deep facial oils and the peel solution is systematically applied, allowing 10 to 15 minutes to elapse between facial region applications to reduce the likelihood of increased phenol blood levels. The emulsion is first applied to the forehead, then to the cheeks, then to the perioral regions, and finally to the eyelids. A thick, white frost indicates the areas where the peel solution is applied. Careful feathering of the solution into the hairline, around eyebrows, and in the mandibular area conceals the potential line of demarcation between the peeled and unpeeled areas. Extra care must be taken in the periorbital area to avoid any exposure to the eye.

The patient is monitored postoperatively for a minimum of 2 hours, and additional intravenous solution is administered. A moist dressing is applied.

The same complications result from both dermabrasion and chemexfoliation: Milia develop in approximately 50% of patients, usually 7 to 10 days after treatment. Acneform lesions may appear and clear spontaneously in 7 to 10 days. However, erythema may persist for 8 to 12 weeks, and pigmentary changes, of which hyperpigmentation is the most common, may take months to resolve. Scarring is possible when dermabrasion is carried to reticular dermal layers, especially over the zygomatic eminence and around the mandible. Rarely, hemorrhage, infection, and skin necrosis occur in overtreated areas.

Patients must limit the application of cosmetics that can cause dermatitis; sunscreens with sun protective factor (SPF) 15 should be used daily for 3 months after the dermabrasion procedure, and the patient should avoid unnecessary exposure to ultraviolet light during this time to avoid hyperpigmentation.

SURGICAL ADVANCES

An overview of the minimally invasive endoscopy and laser-assisted technique for brow lift is discussed in the section entitled Surgical Procedure. As with any new technology, the surgeon must invest his or her time and that of the staff in learning its application and the new surgical technique. Financial investment in the required equipment and auxiliary armamentarium is also necessary. However, during the review of the surgical procedure section, the surgeon should consider that this technology and approach offer several advantages to both the operator and the patient.

The laser enables the surgeon to work rapidly at a distance through smaller incisions and less dissection than conventional procedures to reach and modify target tissues, such as the corrugator, procerus, and orbicularis muscles. Surgery on muscle is simplified, and the laser approach is also useful for taking down the conjoint fascia. Incisions are cauterized by the laser, providing proactive control of bleeding, a bloodless working field, and therefore, better visibility in the surgical field. Smaller incisions and less dissection translate into less invasiveness and nerve preservation; fewer stitches are required, and in the case of hairline incisions, less tissue damage, skin necrosis, and alopecia result. A drain is not necessary when using a laser as the scalpel.

The patient enjoys a shorter postoperative recovery, and because the laser seals the lymphatics, it also produces less swelling, fewer stitches requiring removal, and better aesthetics realized from the smaller incisions and less resultant scarring and hair loss. The brow lift laser approach also diminishes forehead elevation possible for the patient with a naturally high forehead. Paresthesias are diminished, and ecchymosis in the immediate postoperative period is reduced.

This technique accomplishes the goals of reduction in forehead rhytids, elevation of the brows, and diminished lateral hooding and infrabrow skin overhang, and improves the upper face in approximately the same time of operation as traditional surgery.

Chemical peels and dermabrasion are time-tested procedures, but they are not without their respective shortcomings, especially in the ability to exfoliate facial zones selectively and precisely, without danger to nearby mucous membranes from peeling solutions and rotary hazards near the mouth and eyes.

When light or moderate peels are performed, circumoral rhytids are improved but usually remain. When heavy peels or deep dermabrasion is performed that effectively treats the wrinkles, hypopigmentation is an inevitable result.

Laser energy, if properly delivered, can also achieve layer-by-layer tissue ablation for skin rejuvenation. The high-energy pulsed beam accurately cuts with negligible char, coagulates, and delivers measured energy into the depths of the surgical field. Therefore, the surgeon has control over the incision depth during rhytidectomy. This new laser application offers less secondary tissue damage, reduced pain (as the nerves are sealed), less postoperative edema, cicatrix, and crusting, and therefore, a less traumatic and perhaps shorter recovery.

APPLICATIONS OF THE CARBON DIOXIDE LASER

Lasers are becoming an integral part of the surgical armamentarium; the surgeon must be able to assess the efficacy of this new technology and modify traditional surgical techniques in light of his or her applications.

A laser is composed of several structural elements. The most important is the active medium (lasant), for example, carbon dioxide, in a laser cavity, which is subjected to a specific externally applied energy. This results in optical resonance that, through focusing with mirrors or lenses, generates a beam of intense light (radiation) in a wavelength characteristic of the active medium. Variation in the active medium results in lasers of differing wavelength and power generation. For example, the neodymium:yttrium-aluminum-garnet (Nd:YAG) laser uses a solid active medium of Nd:YAG and emits energy at a wavelength of 1.06 microns. When it is focused to achieve a converging beam, the intensity is increased to form a focal spot. Past the focal spot, the beam diverges and its power decreases. Laser light is directional (nondivergent), which is termed coherent.

The ability of laser light to be focused to a very small focal spot allows the beam to destroy a defined volume of tissue by vaporization. The carbon dioxide laser is the first laser to produce a well-controlled, localized, precise thermal injury that can offer both incisional and ablative properties for surgical applications. The carbon dioxide laser emits radiation in the infrared portion of the electromagnetic spectrum, at wavelengths of 10.6 microns, and in the case of the Duolase 9.3 by Medical Optics,

Inc. (Carlsbad, California), 9.3 microns. The effect on soft tissue of any laser with a wavelength in the range of 9 to 10.6 microns or more is wavelength independent, because the constituent of soft tissue that dominates its absorption characteristics, known as the primary chromophore, is water. Therefore, the carbon dioxide laser's continuous high-power output is almost completely absorbed by the fluid present in most biologic tissues. The fluid (water) vaporizes, and the cells burst. Lasers do not cut tissue but disrupt individual cells in a layer that is one or two cells thick. For this reason, laser surgery is termed laser photocoagulation, photoablation, or photothermolysis.

The distance the energy transmits into the tissue is called the penetration depth. Coagulation depth is the deepest level where alterations in the tissue will occur owing to the laser's energy. The effect of this thermal energy on tissue is influenced by the time of exposure, type of tissue, laser wavelength, and skill of the practitioner.

Carbon dioxide lasers possess a unique design feature that offers the surgeon more choices in the resulting tissue effect: the ability to switch the laser instantly from an incision mode to one that can achieve ablation of large surface areas at low power levels. This capability has added an unprecedented degree of control to laser surgical procedures. This unique feature is due to the form of the carbon dioxide laser radiant energy: it can assume the shape of a continuous wave or emit in single or multiple pulses. Gated continuous-wave operation permits the low power of the continuous wave to be transmitted to tissue in discreet short bursts. In pulse operation mode, carbon dioxide lasers emit energy in short bursts and deliver higher peak powers during each pulse; but the average power, including the time between pulses, is comparable to that of continuous-wave mode. Operation in this mode decreases thermal conduction through nontarget tissue and allows time for tissue cooling between pulses, thus decreasing thermal tissue damage.

The histologic appearance of the epidermis and superficial dermis in human skin after laser treatment is shown in Figures 12–7 and 12–8. The healing time of laser-ablated tissue is probably not significantly different from that of wounds caused by a dermatome; however, lasers are technique dependent, which affects the overall clinical result.

Carbon dioxide lasers offer several advantages over the scalpel in surgical procedures and over chemicals in skin rejuvenation: Ablation is performed without char and bleeding, operating time is minimized, and the laser seals blood vessels during surgery with minimal thermal damage to surrounding tissues.

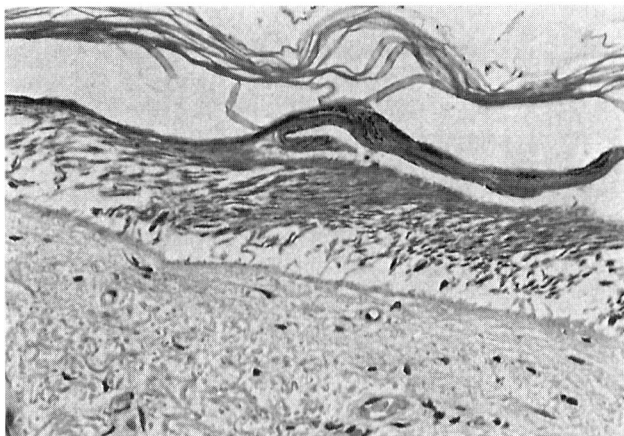

FIGURE 12–7. Histologic appearance of epidermis and superficial dermis after one 2-mm diameter laser impact with the Coherent Ambulase carbon dioxide laser at an SP1 setting 0.1 second pulse. The epidermis is focally detached with spindly alteration of the nuclei. The dermal necrosis is less than 0.1 mm in depth. (From Fitzpatrick RE, Ruiz-Esparza J, Goldman MP: The depth of thermal necrosis using the CO_2 laser: a comparison of the superpulse mode and conventional mode. J Dermatol Surg Oncol 17:340, 1991. Copyright 1991 by Elsevier Science Inc.)

THE LASER SURGICAL ENVIRONMENT

As new technologies become more commonplace for physicians, the operating room must be modified to accommodate the laser and endoscope. Consideration must be given for the comfort of the patient and surgical team, the ease of surgeon's access, and the correct equipment set-up for compliance with specific safety practices dictated by its use. A room that is dedicated to laser procedures is optimal, but it is not required if appropriate entrance signage is properly displayed with visitor access for laser-specific protective eyewear (Fig. 12–9).

The surgical suite must be designed with appropriate lighting and electrical service, and adequate ventilation and air conditioning for the comfort of the patient and surgical team, as well as to compensate for any heat generated by the instruments. Owing to tissue vaporization that releases particulate matter and gaseous products, lasers require smoke evacuation. A laser plume not evacuated from the room by a smoke evacuator should be evacuated to the outside through appropriately filtered conduits. The surgical suite should contain a minimal amount of flammable materials such as curtains, sheets, and towels, and reflective surfaces should be minimized. Special consideration should be given to light exiting the operating room because stray light could potentially harm an outsider during the procedure.

The surgeon should have a thorough understanding in laser biophysics, laser-tissue interactions, laser function, and safety precautions. Office personnel should also be familiar with the fundamentals of the endolaser procedure. The assistant should be prepared to make any adjustments in the laser's timing or power during the procedure. Although lasers are constructed with engineering safety controls, that is, enclosure of the beam, erection of shields and baffles, and door interlocks, in compliance with regulatory mandates, the surgical team must be familiar with emergency shut-down procedures.

Personal safety precautions must be taken for the patient and all members of the surgical team. The eyes are particularly susceptible to damage from the laser; therefore, suitable eye protection is required.

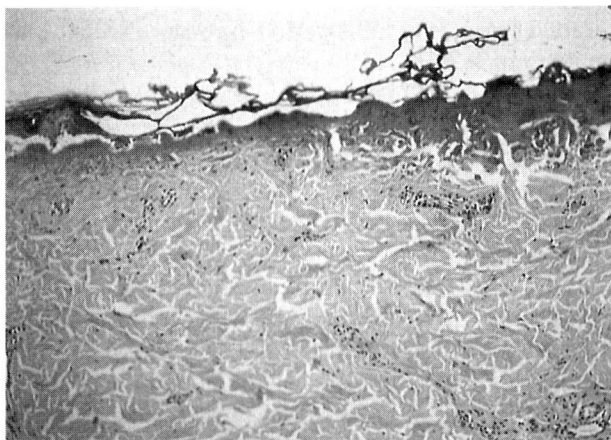

FIGURE 12–8. Histologic appearance immediately after laser impact with a 2-mm diameter spot from a carbon dioxide laser at a 13-watt, 0.2-second pulse. There is complete loss of the epidermis, with dermal necrosis exceeding 0.2 mm in depth. (From Fitzpatrick RE, Ruiz-Esparza J, Goldman MP: The depth of thermal necrosis using the CO_2 laser: a comparison of the superpulse mode and conventional mode. J Dermatol Surg Oncol 17:340, 1991. Copyright 1991 by Elsevier Science Inc.)

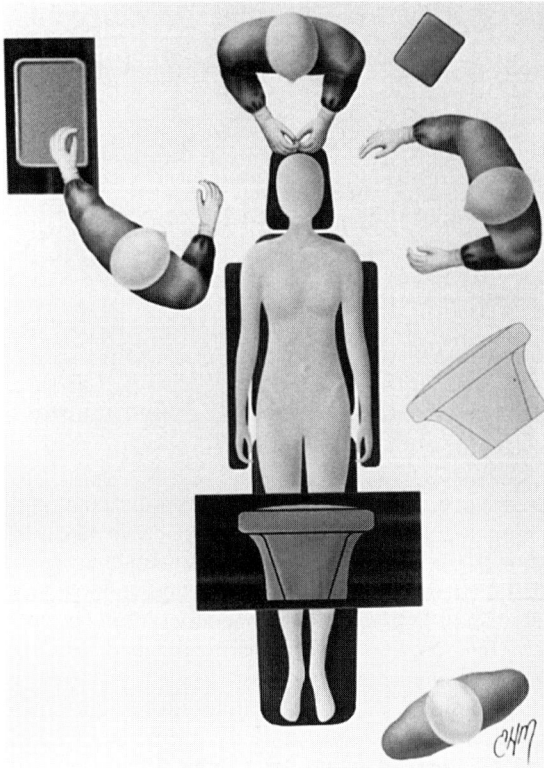

FIGURE 12–9. A bird's-eye view of the laser operatory: the surgeon is located at the patient's head, the anesthesiologist at the patient's feet, the nurse and surgical tray to the surgeon's right, and the assistant to the surgeon's left. The laser stand is located between surgeon and assistant, and monitors are positioned on a table above the patient.

Owing to the specific wavelength of energy emitted by commercially available medical carbon dioxide lasers, clear glasses with side protectors or goggles are sufficient. (Clear glasses allow the surgeon and the team to see tissue colors and textures as normally presented.) The skin must also be adequately protected from any potentially harmful laser effects. The patient may be protected with moistened drapes to protect exposed skin surfaces.

In addition to the dedicated endoscopic instruments mentioned below, the surgeon requires elevators, retractors, and other instruments on a standard face lift set-up.

The surgical suite should be equipped with a stand to hold the surgical equipment, anesthetic solutions, and other required instrumentation. The highly specialized instruments required to perform this procedure include an endoscope (4 to 5 mm in diameter and 170 mm long, 30-degree angle) carried on a duck bill sheath. Endoscopes require adequate optical filters for eye protection; if the surgeon is using a microscope, protective glasses are not necessary. A high-definition autofocus endoscopic microcamera, a color monitor, and an auto-

matically adjustable cold light source connected to the endoscope via an optical fiber are also essential. For the periosteum dissection, blunt and sharp instruments, such as special endoscopic scissors, forceps, and dissector probes for muscle identification and dissection and nerve isolation and protection are required. All metallic instruments to be used with the laser should be protected against glare (nonreflective). If the laser is not used for cautery, an endoscopically modified suction coagulation device is recommended. Laser access is usually accomplished by fiber-directed tips. Figure 12–10*A* and *B* shows the endoscopic armamentarium used in these procedures.

SURGICAL PROCEDURE

Minimally Invasive Endoscopic and Laser-Assisted Forehead and Brow Lift

State-of-the-art instrumentation is the first key to performing this surgery; the coupling of lasers with endoscopes provides a minimally invasive approach to the classic forehead and brow lift surgical procedure. Lasers can substitute for cold steel techniques and offer the surgeon more precise control of glabellar and frontal musculature, facile dissection of the conjoint fascia, and ease of cauterization. The endoscope provides a 30-degree magnified view angle, with irrigating portals to simplify the inside-out technique. Endolaser procedures employ smaller incisions and less dissection than conventional procedures to reach and modify target tissues.

The Duolase 9.3 (Fig. 12–11*A* and *B*) is a carbon dioxide laser that allows the clinician the opportunity to perform soft tissue procedures. The Duolase 9.3 has an UltraFlex flexible fiber delivery system that allows for easy access and precise control of each procedure.

The Ultrapulse carbon dioxide laser (Coherent Inc., Palo Alto, California) delivers high energy through a handpiece that collimates the beam. It employs a scanner for resurfacing applications but can also be used for incisions.

These lasers can be used in our surgical technique; the surgeon should notice that preoperative patient preparation involves the same planning, that is, anesthesia, markings, and consideration of the required incisions and dissection planes relevant to the traditional surgical approach.

The nerve blocks used are 1% lidocaine or 0.5% bupivacaine Marcaine with 1:100,000 epinephrine. Infiltration of the deep tissues consists of 2% lidocaine or 0.25% Marcaine with 1:200,000 epinephrine, administered as shown in Figure 12–12. Markings are also similar to the conventional approach as the patient is best marked while he or she is

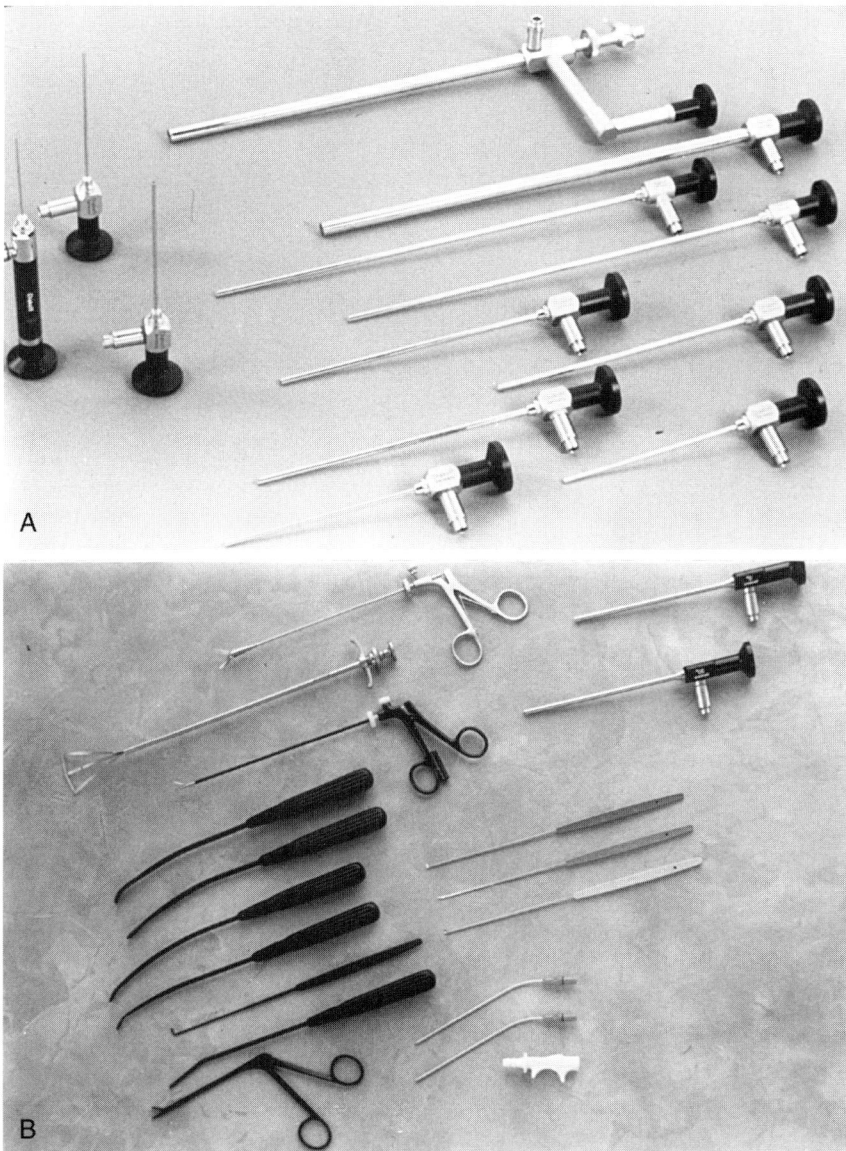

FIGURE 12–10. *A* and *B*, Endoscopic armamentarium. Notice the nonreflective surfaces.

awake and sitting facing the examiner for brow lift at the time of surgery. Occasionally, some surgeons delay marking the incision lines until after the patient is sedated.

First, the supraorbital nerve notch or foramen is marked; a vertical line is drawn upward from this point on both sides. If the supratrochlear foramen is palpable, it is also marked. All horizontal and vertical glabellar and forehead rhytids are marked, as is the lateral limbus. Brow position at rest, from the rim to the superior brow at the lateral limbus, is marked, and brow position when elevated to the desired position is measured (Fig. 12–13*A* to *C*). (This is the desired amount of brow elevation.) The incisions, as described below, are next marked.

Incisions

This endolaser technique requires the use of one midsagittal, two parasagittal, and two temporal incisions versus the extensive bicoronal excision of the open technique. Instruments are positioned through these incisions to employ our portal approach.

The midsagittal incision is a slightly curved horizontal incision of about 2 cm, which is placed about 2 to 4 cm behind the hairline. A vertical incision can also be justified for screw fixation of the central brow for cases involving male pattern baldness or where the hairline pattern will be greatly altered by a horizontal incision. This incision is carried through the frontalis muscle into the subgaleal

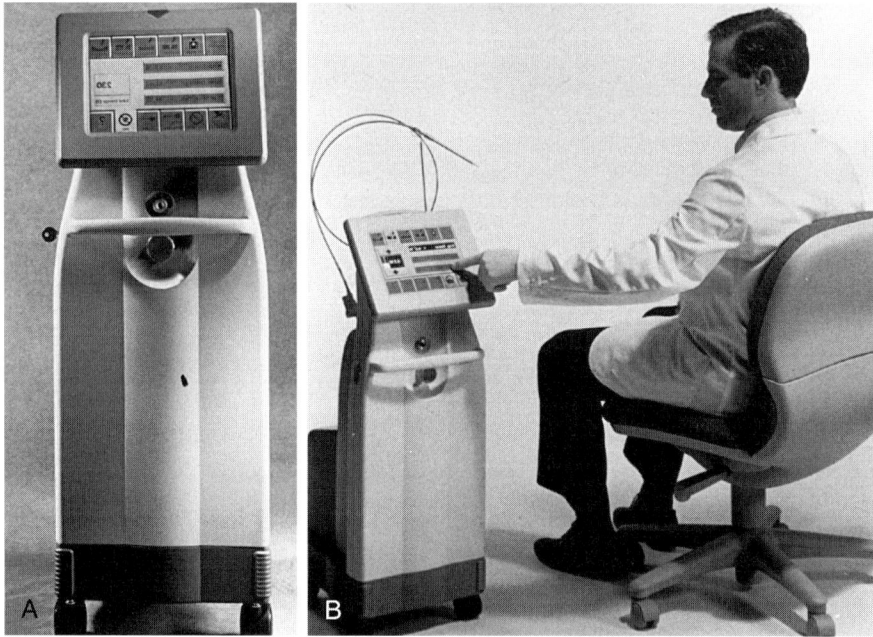

FIGURE 12–11. *A* and *B*, The Duolase 9.3 carbon dioxide laser from Medical Optics, Inc.

plane. This incision accepts the endoscope and can be extended, as long as it is limited to the supraorbital nerve corridor, with little influence on the ultimate aesthetic result.

The parasagittal incisions are 1- to 2-cm vertical incisions placed behind the hairline at the plane of the lateral canthus, depending on the direction of superior pull the surgeon desires when screw fixa-

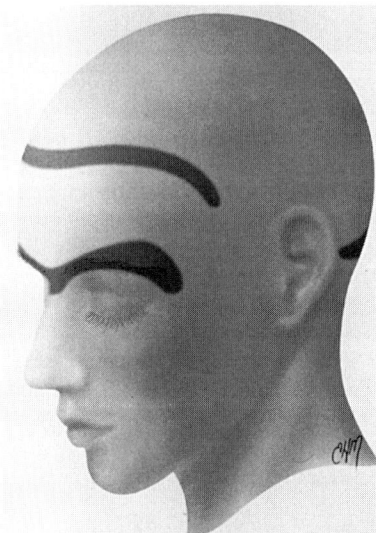

FIGURE 12–12. The administration of nerve blocks and areas of infiltration *(shaded)*. Local anesthesia with a vasoconstrictive agent (lidocaine with epinephrine) is the principal anesthesia used to diffuse the entire area. Deep anesthesia is unnecessary.

tion is used. These incisions should be marked on the bone with the high-output carbon dioxide laser, making a black mark on the bone, to establish each incision's original position once the scalp has been undermined.

The temporal incisions are positioned so that the midlines of these 2.5-cm horizontal or vertical incisions are at a point found by drawing a line at a 45-degree angle from the lateral canthus, approximately 2 to 5 cm posterior to the hairline. They follow the direction of a face lift incision used to undermine tissue over the temple. These incisions should extend to the deep temporalis fascia. Figure 12–14 depicts the endoscopic incision sites.

The best surgical technique focuses largely on the extent or plane of dissection. More extensive dissection entails greater risks of complications and longer recovery period. However, results are compromised with less dissection. This minimally invasive technique combines the subgaleal and subperiosteal dissection planes to realize the positive aspects of each dissection plane and to increase surgical exposure; it employs the location of the changing planes as the points of fixation. The subgaleal dissection extends both superiorly and inferiorly, and extends posteriorly as far as possible (Fig. 12–15). This is the same approach as that used for peeling through the conjoint ligament.

High-output carbon dioxide lasers dissect well in the subgaleal plane. A 0.1-mm spot laser handpiece is used to make the surgical incisions with the laser set to 250 to 300 millijoule at 5 to 10 watts. With its use, the corrugator and procerus muscles are

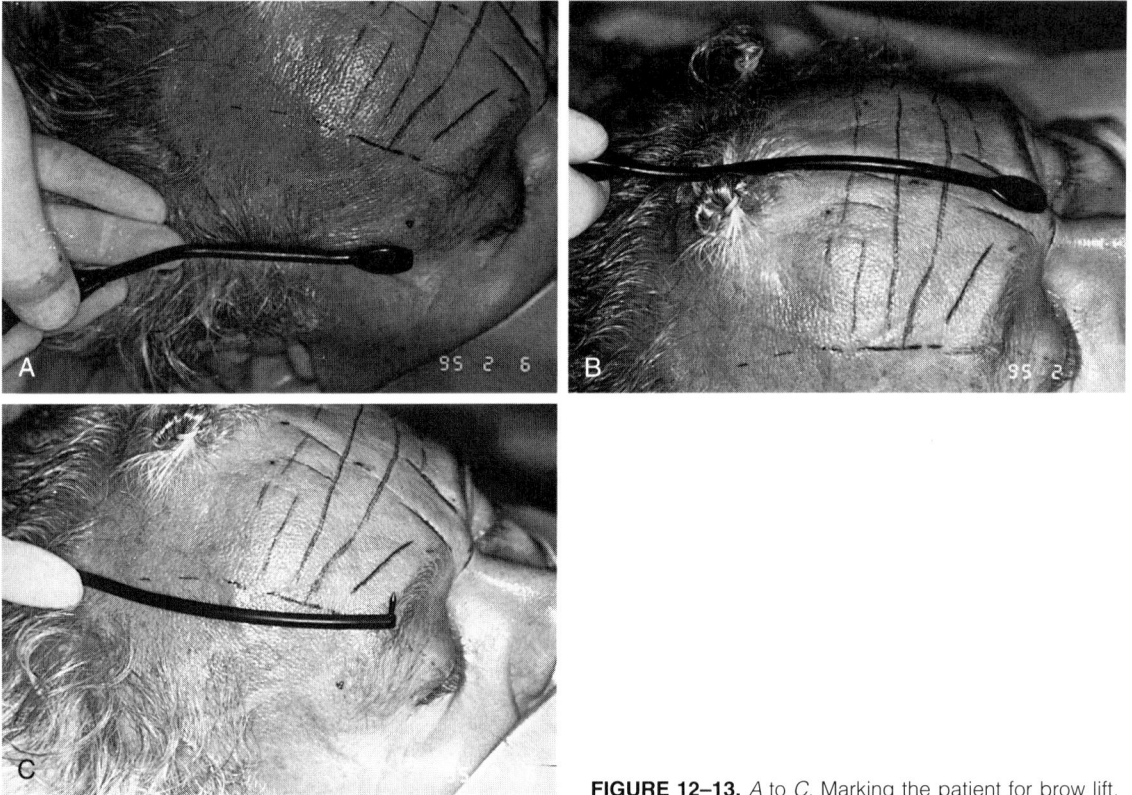

FIGURE 12–13. *A* to *C*, Marking the patient for brow lift.

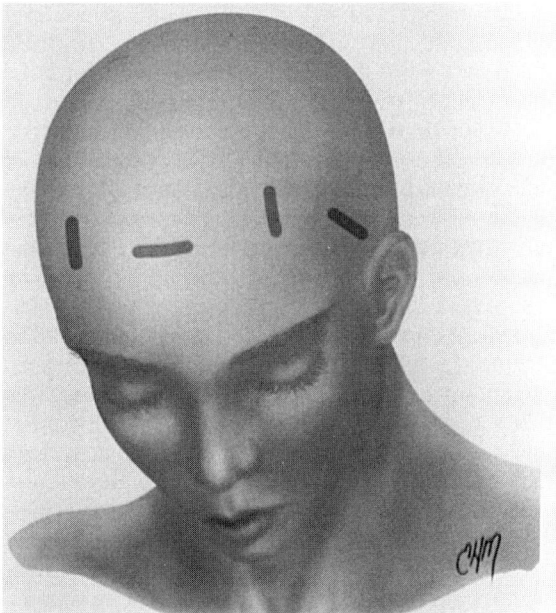

FIGURE 12–14. The location of the endoscopic incision sites: midsagittal, parasagittal, and temporal. The midline incision is vertically through the galeal periosteal layers (where there are no nerves) to allow easy introduction of the endoscope. Incisions in the temporal area are parallel to the direction of the superficial temporal vessels.

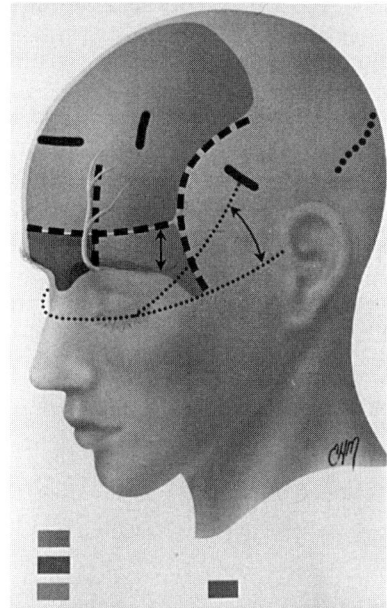

FIGURE 12–15. The laser-assisted forehead and brow lift planes of dissection combine the subperiosteal and subcutaneous approaches. Subperiosteal dissection allows better periorbital remodeling, whereas subcutaneous dissection preserves sensation posterior to the incision line. Notice the location of the supraorbital nerve, supraorbital wad, and conjoint ligament area.

easily released and easier to retract than with dissection in the subperiosteal pocket. It is more difficult to dissect in the subperiosteal plane and harder to retract outward than the subgaleal to obtain a good pocket for endoscopic visualization. However, the advantage of subperiosteal dissection is that it is the easiest endoscopic dissection to learn and provides good access to the midface, if needed.

Either the medial periosteum can be elevated or the subperiosteal and subgaleal planes can be joined. A point of fixation is created at the level of the cut edge of periosteum, which can be sutured to temporalis fascia.

The optic cavity is then created in the subgaleal supraperiosteal plane or the subperiosteal plane using the 4-mm 30-degree endoscope and the endoscopic brow lift elevators as shown in Figures 12–16 and 12–17.

Anteriorly dissect in the subperiosteal plane from the midsagittal and parasagittal incisions down to the subgaleal plane for muscle release using the temporal incision over the deep temporal fascia, through the conjoint ligament at the lateral orbital rim into the frontal dissection. Backcut along the conjoint ligament, with the endoscope placed in the frontal dissection and the surgical instruments in the temporal incision, releasing the conjoint ligament. Periosteal elevators are used to dissect the periosteum from the supraorbital rim in a subperiosteal plane lateral to the supraorbital nerve neurovascular bundle.

Centrally, attempts should be made to preserve the trochlear neurovascular bundle, which is possi-

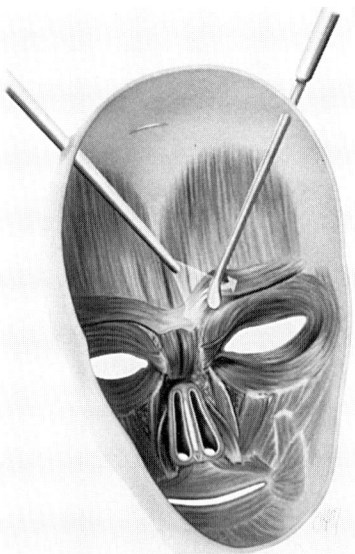

FIGURE 12–17. The subgaleal and subperiosteal dissection: view from the inside, using endoscope and laser. Endolaser techniques allow more accurate and controlled periorbital dissection and brow muscle modification.

ble through the subgaleal dissection. Thus, horizontal incisions and sections of the procerus, corrugator, and supracilli depressor muscles are made with a combination of dissectors, grasping forceps, and scissors or laser.

The flaps are easily elevated if the surgeon is in the correct dissection plane without spread of laser energy to the overlying skin. The surgical assistant provides traction and countertraction to facilitate the progress of skin flap elevation. In the SMAS zone, where the surgeon wishes to dissect more carefully, the laser is turned down to 5 to 8 watts.

By defocusing the carbon dioxide laser beam, or with the contact YAG laser, coagulation of bleeding points can be applied judiciously to provide hemostasis, using 250 millijoules at 10 to 20 watts. Alternatively, occasional brisk bleeding of larger vessel size may be managed with the endoscopically modified suction coagulation devices.

Frontalis release incisions can be made, if necessary, through fibers of the frontalis muscle at this time. It is helpful to make the muscle resections at the inferior portion of the pocket first and to work the next resections superiorly progressively to prevent pooling of blood inferiorly from superior incisions performed too early in the sequence.

Now the operator positions the blunt scalp dissector posteriorly through the incisions and carries subperiosteal dissection posteriorly to the nuchal line, indicated by the insertion of the occipital and the other superficial neck musculature (Fig. 12–18A and B). Over the temporalis muscle region, a more superficial plane is dissected over the temporalis

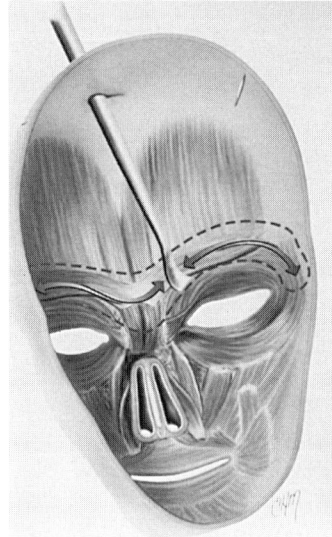

FIGURE 12–16. The endoscopic release of the supercilii: view from the inside, using endoscope and laser. Resection of the depressor supercilii muscle under endoscopic control and magnification.

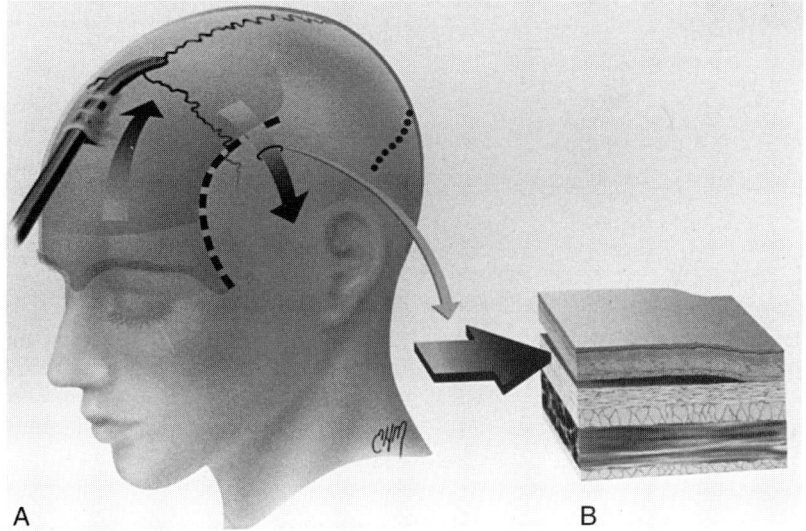

FIGURE 12–18. *A* and *B,* Laser-assisted forehead and brow lift dissection planes showing the layers of the scalp; the different shaded areas show the subgaleal and subperiosteal dissections and the location of conjoint ligament and nuchal line. Anterior dissection between the galea and the pericranium, with a change of plane to the subperiosteal plane approximately 2 to 3 cm above the orbital rim, protects the supraorbital and supratrochlear nerves.

A   B

fascia. Size 0 Gore-Tex sutures are then placed into the subgaleal aponeurotica layer at the appropriate position inferior to the incisions at the parasagittal and, occasionally, midsagittal regions and either tunneled posteriorly to a single screw fixation point, using a 1.5-mm (d) × 4-mm (l) titanium screw, or directed centrally to a curved seven-hole titanium plate with the marionette suspension technique, correction of developmental or acquired soft tissue asymmetries such as that with damage to cranial nerve VII from prior tumor pathology correction or surgical interventions such as those found with temporomandibular joint or cosmetic facial surgery.

If elevation of the midcentral brow is desired, or more than 1 cm of posterior displacement is required, the screw is placed 1.5 to 2 cm from the inferior edge of the incision, referencing the bone markings. A 0 Gore-Tex suture is placed in the galea in the inferior margin of the incision, and the suture is tied to the screw, pulling the forehead and midcentral brow upward.

Plate suspension employs three to six size 0 Gore-Tex sutures placed corresponding to the desired vector of upward pull. A separate incision is then made approximately 6 to 8 cm posterior to the midsagittal portal, where the microplate is fixed to the cranium. If needed, two separate microplates may be used and placed lateral to the midline. The Gore-Tex suspension sutures are then passed from the anterior portals under the intact but elevated scalp flap and secured to the horizontal bar of the T-plate. The patient may then be raised on the operating room table to a sitting position and the final brow height can be evaluated and adjustment made, if needed. The sutures are tied and cut. Myotomy incisions and suspension techniques are presented diagramatically in Figures 12–19 to 12–22.

Incisions are closed with either 4-0 or 5-0 nylon

suture and bandaged with a Barton skull pressure dressing covered with Spandex net. Usually, no drains are required. Theoretically, with appropriate immobilization of the scalp flap, periosteal reattachments occur with Sharpey fiber assistance and excess gathered scalp is accommodated posteriorly, thereby removing the requirement for scalp excision common to older techniques. This change in paradigm is based not only on satisfactory results and widespread experience of surgical colleagues but on the probable fact that scalp excision techniques closed with tension allow relapse through mechanical and biologic creep of the scalp tissues despite the surgeon's best intentions.

Postoperative care involves a 7-day regimen of

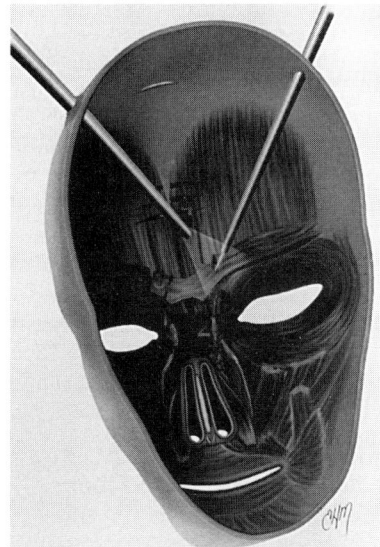

FIGURE 12–19. The myotomy incisions; view from interior, using endoscope and laser.

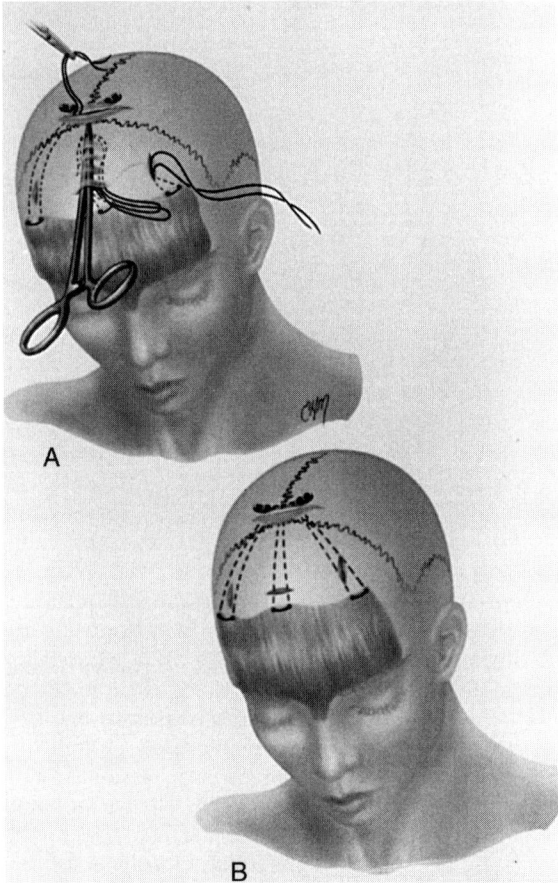

FIGURE 12–20. *A*, Midprocess of attaching sutures to the plate. Inclusion of the subperiosteal layer to the galea allows the use of this stronger structure for secure anchoring. *B*, One centrally placed plate with sutures attached to the plate.

pressure dressing application and regular dressing changes.

On the second postoperative day, the patient may wash his or her hair and wear a 3-inch Ace headband at home and at night for the subsequent 10 days. One week after surgery, the sutures are removed.

Complications of the minimally invasive brow lift approach include neurapraxia of the temporal division of the frontal nerve, forehead weakness, numbness, and hematoma, swelling, and exaggerated elevation of the corner of the eye, which is present for the first few weeks postoperatively. However, no skin necrosis has been found to date.

Technique of Contact KTP:YAG and Nd:YAG or Carbon Dioxide Fiber Laser–Assisted Brow Lift

Although blepharoscopy is an effective method of removing excess eyelid skin, it does not correct

coexisting brow ptosis. The brow lift procedure, discussed earlier, corrects brow ptosis; however, for patients desiring to avoid this procedure, the transblepharoplasty brow suspension can be performed concurrently with blepharoscopy.

The transblepharoplasty brow suspension is a relatively noninvasive method of stabilizing the brow through the blepharoplasty incision; the orbital portion of the orbicularis oculi muscle underlying the brow cilia is suspended to the periosteum of the frontal bone at a specified distance from the supraorbital rim. Because the muscle is sutured directly to periosteum, brow ascent during and after blepharoplasty is achieved.

This technique employs blepharoplasty anesthesia and markings as described in the following section, with the addition of two intrasurgical markings. Using a laser, a crescent of preseptal orbicularis muscle is excised. A muscle flap is elevated in the plane under the supraorbital fat pad, past the superior margin of the brow. Here, in the lateral portions of the dissection, the surgeon encounters branches of the superficial temporal artery and vein, which must be cauterized.

The anchoring suture must capture sufficient tissue remaining over the frontal bone and periosteum to be effective. At a vertical line drawn tangential to the lateral margin of the iris, a point is marked approximately 1 cm superior to the supraorbital rim. A marking suture is passed through the skin at the lower margin of the brow, and a point is marked where the suture intersects the orbicularis muscle on the underside of the flap. A 2-0 or 3-0 Gore-Tex suture is then passed through the periosteum at the

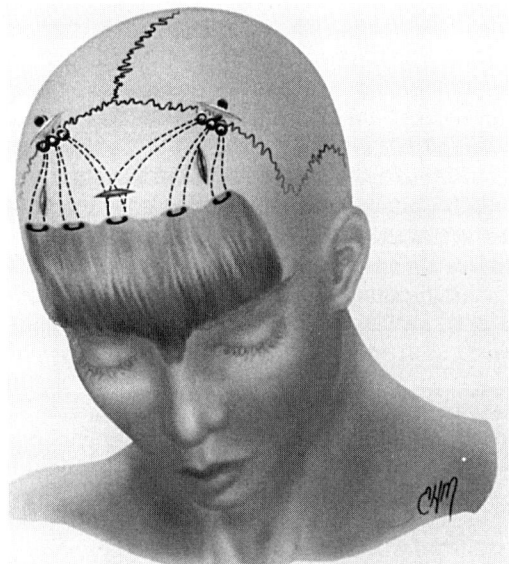

FIGURE 12–21. An alternate marionette suspension with two plates placed either side of center; sutures are attached to the plates.

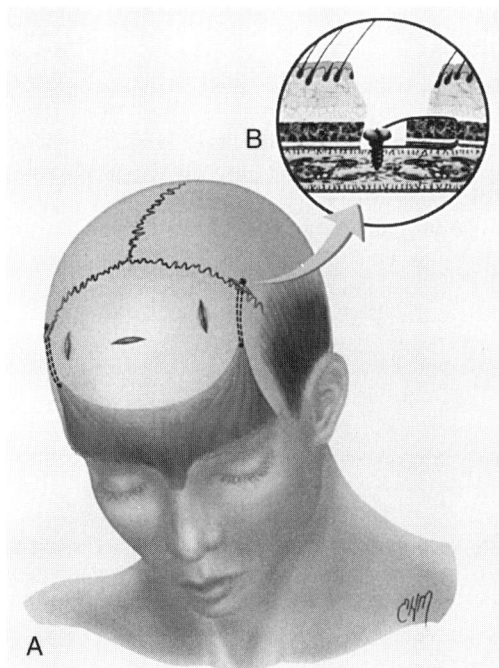

FIGURE 12–22. *A,* Two laterally placed single permanent screw sites with the elevation suture attached. Deep anchoring sutures allow a stable and reliable elevation of the brows and skin layer closure with minimal tension. *B,* Close-up view of the scalp and skull showing an alternate method of attaching a suture in the innermost scalp layers to the screw.

supraorbital rim marking, and through the orbicularis oculi muscle at the intersection of the marking suture at the underside of the flap, and the suture is tied. Two to four sutures are placed along this same horizontal plane to anchor the brow. It is important to suture only orbital orbicularis to prevent a pucker below the eyebrow. After these sutures are placed, brow stabilization is tested and the blepharoscopy incision is closed.

Short-term results are enhanced by the use of a laser, as noted previously, because intraoperative bleeding is reduced, and postoperative bleeding and ecchymosis are diminished.

Technique of Carbon Dioxide Laser–Assisted Transcutaneous Blepharoplasty for Superior Eyelid Contour Improvement

A blepharoscopy may easily be performed in conjunction with the endoscopic brow lift. A corneal shield, manufactured by Byron Medical Company (Tucson, Arizona), is placed in the patient's eyes after the markings are complete and before local anesthesia is injected to protect the patient's eyes from laser radiation and mechanical tissue

trauma. Customarily, tetracaine, a topical anesthetic, is administered and Lacri-Lube (Allergan Pharmaceuticals, Irvine, California) may be necessary for ease of insertion.

Accurate skin marking is essential. As in the conventional procedure, skin markings are made with the patient in the sitting position to determine the degree of gravity's effect on the redundant skin. The surgeon elevates the upper eyelid with a finger and marks the inferior incision where the natural supratarsal lid crease exists, at a distance of about 8 to 9 mm above the lid margin. This becomes the level of the supratarsal fold. Medially, this marking ends above the punctum, and the surgeon extends it laterally 1 to 1.5 cm to the lateral canthus with a slight upward slope. The superior incision line is marked to create a slight (1-mm) lagophthalmos while pinching the excess eyelid skin. First, a mark is made above the free margin of the lid at the midpupillary point. Once the central point is located, it is extended medially and, finally, the lateral lid tissue is marked to indicate the extent of skin excision in these areas. At the lateral canthus, the line angles upward approximately 3 to 4 mm, preferably in a normal skin crease. The upper line should parallel the lower line.

A syringe with a 30-gauge needle and 1% lidocaine with 1:100,000 epinephrine is injected; the anesthetic is infiltrated in the superior lid and rolled with a gloved finger, spreading the anesthetic throughout the lid tissue.

A David Baker retractor (Fig. 12–23) is inserted with the frosted shield underneath the upper eyelid and the frosted surface facing the conjunctiva. The small retractor prongs are placed superior to the tarsal plate and slid inferiorly, and the screw is tightened on the slotted arm to provide tension on the superior lid skin (Fig. 12–24).

The laser incises with one pass through the full thickness of the eyelid skin; the lower incision is

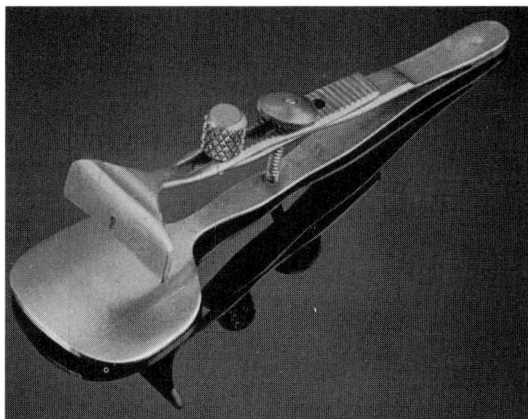

FIGURE 12–23. David Baker retractor.

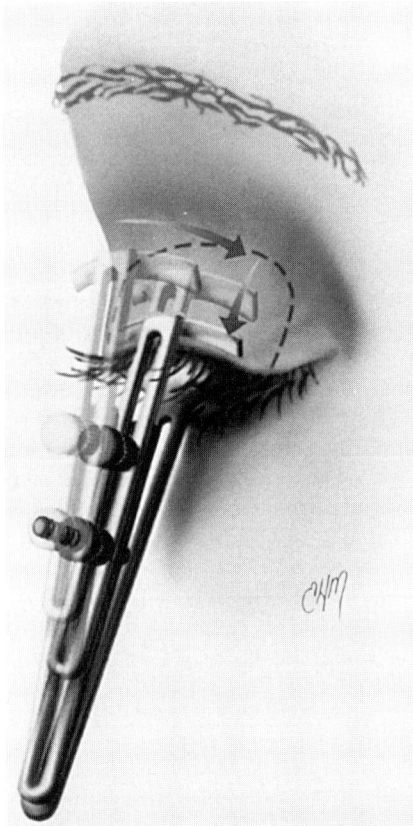

FIGURE 12–24. David Baker retractor in use.

beveled, and simultaneous hemostasis is achieved. At this level, the fibers of the orbicularis oculi muscle are visible and there is no subcutaneous fat separating the skin and muscle. Because the skin and muscle are attenuated, they have stretched together and have equal excess. Therefore, equal excision is indicated; muscle excision is begun just superior to the tarsal plate region and extends the length of the skin excision, first laterally, then undermined medially, separating it from the underlying septum orbitale. The laser scalpel requires two passes to excise the muscle completely. If preseptal muscle is left under the skin excision, there will be muscle over muscle when the final closure is performed. This redundancy can cause a heavier, fuller lid postoperatively.

A small artery is present under the orbicularis that should be controlled. The septum orbitale is opened to expose the underlying fat pads. It may be necessary to extend the dissection in the lateral half of the superior incision just beneath the orbicularis oculi muscle to remove the lateral fat pad. The lateral fat is removed, with the excision extending from about the midorbit to the level of the periosteum. With digital pressure on the globe and retraction laterally and inferiorly while the incisions are

made, the middle fat pad will present itself. After this is teased out, it is first clamped at its base and then removed with one pass of the laser. Consideration is given to the miniature vessels that require cauterization with the defocused laser. It is helpful to do this just before the laser cutting pass.

Before closure, the surgeon checks for hemostasis. The orbital septum is never sutured. Three tack sutures are created using 6-0 fast-absorbing gut suture, or depending on the surgeon's preference, none may be employed. Tissue glue, similar to Isodent (Ellman International Inc., Jersey City, New Jersey), is also used.

Figure 12–25 reveals a surgical series, whereas Figure 12–26 shows the presurgical patient and healing stages.

An antibiotic ointment should coat the incision lines, and the patient is advised to apply ice or cold compresses and sleep with head elevation. The patient should also avoid sun exposure.

Technique of Carbon Dioxide Laser–Assisted Transconjunctival Lipoplasty for Inferior Eyelid Contour Improvement

Lower eyelid laxity is determined by a preoperative pinch test. A few drops of topical tetracaine hydrochloride 0.5% ophthalmic solution are used to anesthetize the conjunctiva and cornea. Two percent lidocaine with epinephrine is deposited transcutaneously beneath the orbicularis oculi muscle over the entire lower eyelid for each eye. Additional anesthetic is injected subconjunctivally over the inferior palpebral conjunctiva along the planned line of incision. The corneal shield placed to protect the globe from laser energy is also important to protect the globe from mechanical tissue trauma (Fig. 12–27).

Of the three basic surgical techniques for lower lid blepharoscopy, we will employ the transconjunctival approach, which is excellent for the patient who exhibits primarily herniated orbital fat and fine rhytids. The herniated orbital fat is removed, and simultaneous skin resurfacing will tighten the skin and eliminate fine rhytids.

A vein retractor is placed to retract the lower lid toward the infraorbital rim. The conjunctiva is grasped with forceps beneath the inferior tarsal border about 4 mm beneath the lower lid, and with one pass of the laser, an opening is made through it into the orbital fat compartment. The tissue plane between the muscle and orbital septum is undermined to the level of the orbital rim, and then the conjunctiva is incised medially and laterally for almost the entire length of the lower lid.

The superior margin of the incised conjunctiva is held with a 6-0 gut suture on a clamp draped

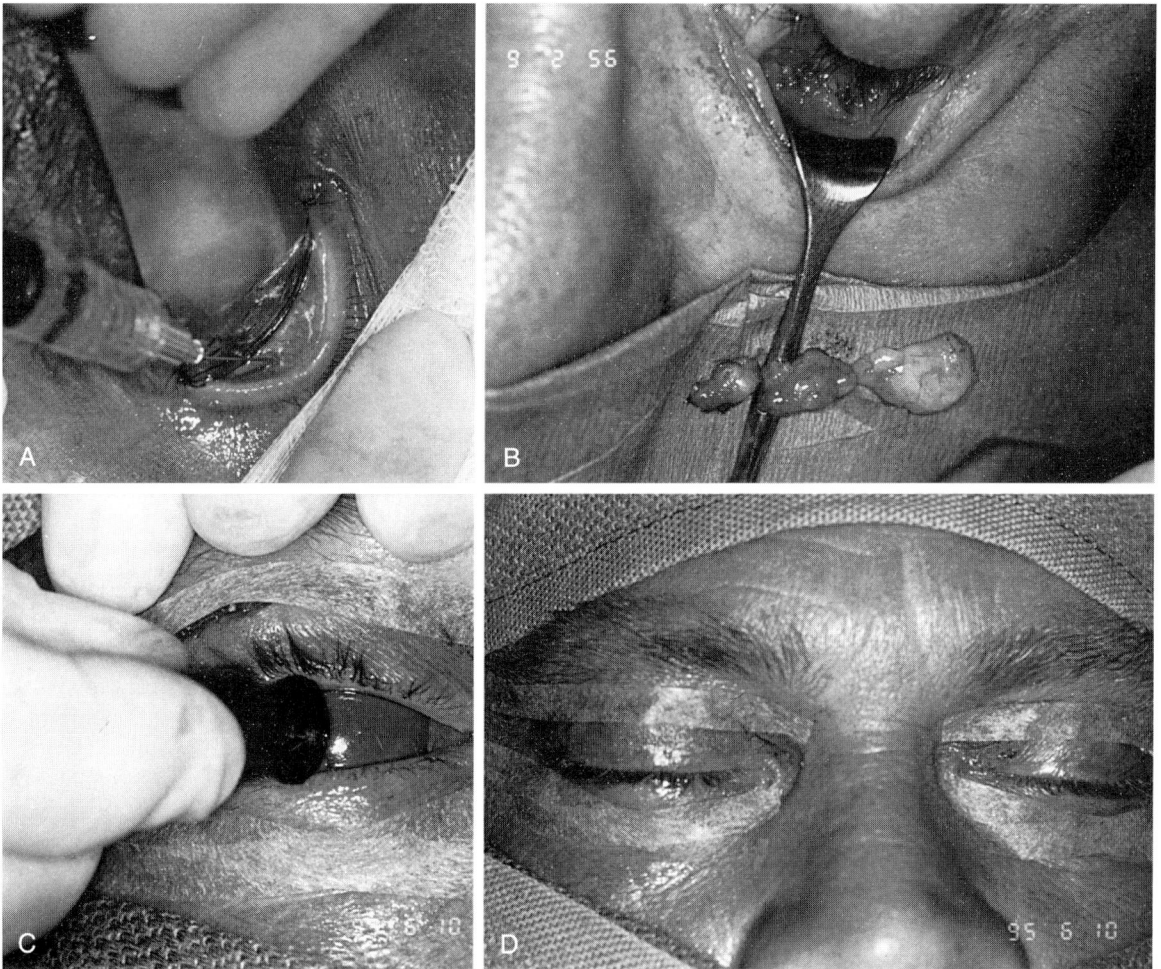

FIGURE 12–25. Surgical series of upper and lower blepharoscopy procedures. *A,* Anesthesia; *B,* removal of the lower fat pads; *C,* removal of the coronal shield; and *D,* after surgery.

superiorly while a frosted (modified for use with a laser) Jaeger-style metal protector is on top of the corneal shield and conjunctiva. A vein retractor holds down the inferior margin of the incised conjunctiva. Dissection separates the fat from the septum orbitale, and as this is done, the fat bulges into the field. The inferior oblique muscle delineates the central and medial fat compartments. Pressure applied to the eye through the upper eyelid will help prolapse the orbital fat into the field after the fascia is incised. The individual fat pads are held with a pickup and vein retractor managed by the assistant. As the fat is grasped with forceps (Fig. 12–28), it is positioned over the moistened sterile cotton roll and is incised with one pass of the laser. All fat pads are removed in this manner. Often, no sutures are placed in the conjunctiva; however, the author's preference is to place one resorbable tack of 6-0 fast-absorbing suture (Fig. 12–29).

Postoperative care includes the application of cold compresses for the first 48 hours, use of oph-

thalmic antibiotic ointment for 3 to 5 days, and head elevation during bed rest.

Similar to the traditional approach, upper and lower lid blepharoscopy complications are rare; however, the most serious complication, retrobulbar hemorrhage, requires mandatory consultation and management with lateral canthal release. Other complications include dry eye syndrome (conjunctivitis sicca), rare cases of surgical infection, hematoma, and ectropion or intropion.

Laser-Assisted Facial Skin Resurfacing

Advances in carbon dioxide laser technology have produced an extremely high energy pulsed laser beam that cuts with negligible char and excellent coagulation. The resulting depth of penetration of the injury will extend past the basement membrane of the epidermis and into the underlying papillary dermis. A setting of 250-millijoule pulses

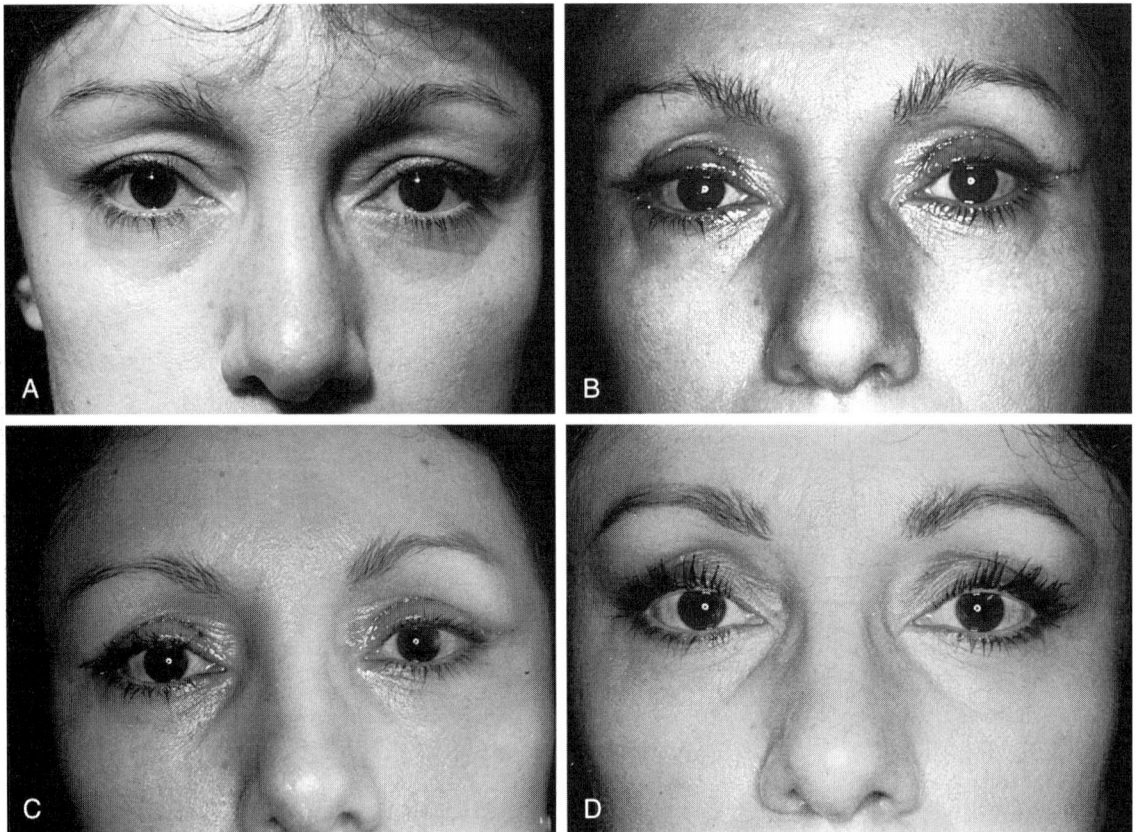

FIGURE 12–26. *A,* Patient presentation before upper blepharoscopy; *B,* 1 hour after surgery; *C,* 6 days after surgery; and *D,* 10 days after surgery. (Courtesy of Dr. Larry David.)

produces damage that preserves the basal layer of skin. Pulses of 300 millijoules produce damage into the upper papillary dermis; therefore, a laser can be used for resurfacing to the same depth as a chemical peel.

Skin resurfacing using carbon dioxide laser ablation can be administered around the eyes, cheeks, and lips, areas sensitive to traditional dermabrasion and chemical peel. In addition to smoothing rhytids, laser ablation is indicated for removal of excess skin around eyes after blepharoscopy. The controlled thermal injury to cells depends on the combination of lasing time and the resultant cells' temperature. During selective photothermolysis, extreme temperatures are present in target sites of the skin for very short durations. As a critical temperature is reached, ablation occurs.

Laser facial skin resurfacing is performed in the office under local anesthesia (lidocaine, as in the traditional approach, but epinephrine is not necessary) with a focused carbon dioxide laser operating in a pulsed mode. Seven watts of power is sufficient to vaporize variable-sized (2 to 4 mm diameter) craters in the epidermis, with no thermal injury to the underlying papillary dermis. (Depth of injury increases with increased power and pulse duration, but the depth decreases as focal size increases.) The technique involves lasing each shoulder of the rhytid, which is usually accomplished with two passes of the laser. After the shoulders of the wrinkle have been ablated, bursts of energy are directed down the center of the wrinkle, creating an area of overlap. This technique reduces the shoulders of the wrinkle and achieves general shrinkage of collagen underneath the area ablated. With healing, new collagen formation will raise the lower central points. Residual necrotized tissue above the papillary dermis is wiped off with saline-moisturized gauze.

A white skin endpoint is seen with each laser pulse. The collimated handpiece keeps the laser defocused properly, so that the procedure is uniform and laser dependent rather than technique dependent.

A 35% trichloroacetic acid solution can be used at the edge of the demarcation line of laser treatment to feather the result into adjacent skin. The vermillion border is approached, but the lips are not included in the feathering. The dermal layer is protected and moisturized with dressings, similar to the traditional procedural method.

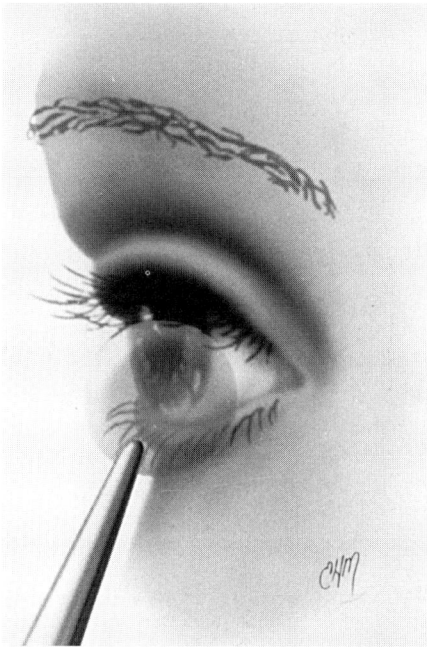

FIGURE 12–27. Placement of the corneal shield, which is used to protect the globe and cornea. Local anesthesia is injected through the conjunctiva and behind the orbital rim to numb the fat pockets.

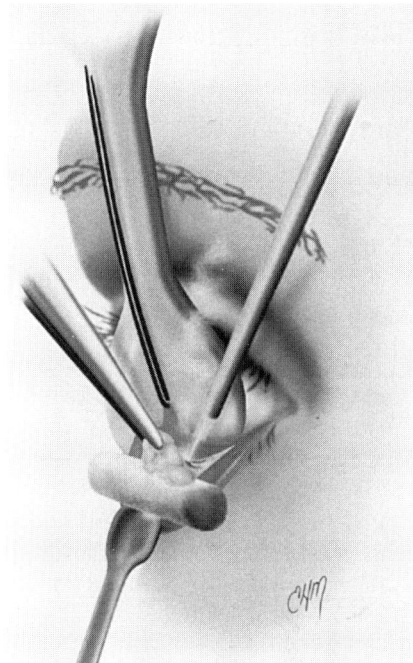

FIGURE 12–28. The laser incision, performed while employing a Jaeger retractor placed over the cornea to hold the lid away. The incision extends medially and laterally for almost the length of the lower lid; the curve of the lid is carefully followed, so fat is immediately visible. Fat over the moist cotton is excised using one pass of the laser.

A healing period of 4 to 5 days is required in which mild to significant edema is present. Erythema may be present but usually resolves spontaneously within the next month. After the initial healing process, the patient must wear sunblock and minimize exposure to ultraviolet radiation.

One treatment is usually sufficient, but a touch-up procedure may be necessary. Postoperative follow-up consistently shows excellent cosmetic results. Complications, such as scarring and hypopigmentation, are uncommon. Ecchymosis in the immediate postoperative period is reduced or nonexistent. Diminution of wrinkles is achieved with complete resolution in many patients (Fig. 12–30).

Lasers are a reliable way to eliminate problem wrinkles without the incidence of complications such as hypopigmentation and skin texture changes seen with deep chemical peels and dermabrasions. Laser energy provides excellent ablation depth control to the millimeter level; however, the precise selection of the power level (approximately 7 watts) depends on skin thickness and color. The recuperation time of 4 to 6 days is approximately half the time of a standard deep chemical peel or dermabrasion.

SUMMARY

The use of lasers in conjunction with video-assisted endoscopy is one of the most recent advances in facial rejuvenation surgical technique. These new technologies replace the bicoronal incision and its required skin resection in the conventional forehead and brow lift. In this chapter, we

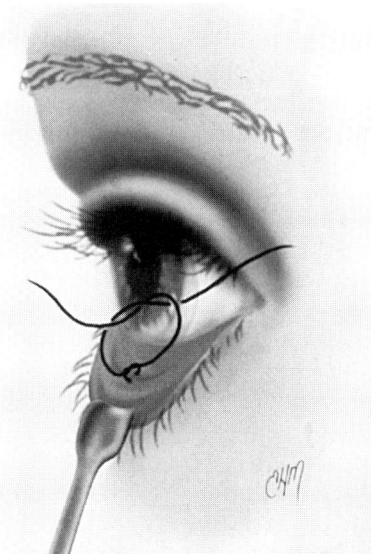

FIGURE 12–29. Placement of single resorbable suture to close the incision partially. The conjunctiva does not need closure.

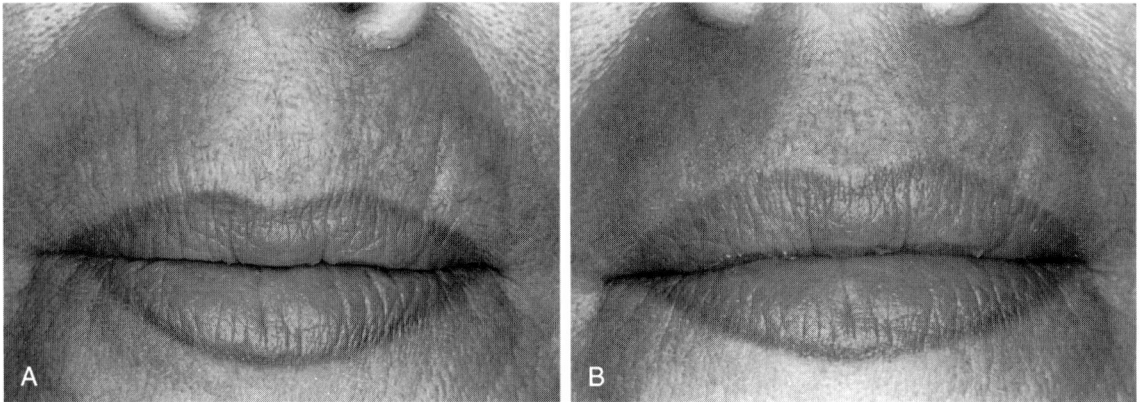

FIGURE 12–30. *A,* Presurgical presentation for perioral rhytidectomy. *B,* Patient presentation 2½ weeks after surgery. (Courtesy of Dr. Larry David.)

have discussed the frontal rhytidectomy procedure, which combines forehead lift with blepharoplasty and skin resurfacing for optimal aesthetic results.

Although the technique differs from conventional surgery in the varying incision portals, different planes and extent of dissection, and different patterns of muscle modification, the advantages to the patient are minimal incisions, which preserve sensation; avoidance of neuromas; a decrease of incisional alopecia; and minimal change in the relationship of hairline to brow. Early results for laser resurfacing are equivalent to or better than results for the chemical peel, with less postoperative edema, scarring, and crusting.

The surgeon is challenged by this new technology, and this protocol appears to be a safe and predictable means of permanently suspending the upper third of the aging face and eliminating periorbital and perioral rhytids. Long-term follow-up is needed to determine adequately the durability and permanency of this suspension technique.

Lasers promise to revolutionize other surgical procedures as applications are investigated: laser-assisted uvulopalatostomy, tonsilectomy, and hair transplantation for micro-grafts and minigrafts are promising areas, although they are not yet perfected. These laser applications have given birth to adjunct surgical accessories and techniques required to optimize the use of the laser surgery. As this work progresses, the surgeon must adopt new paradigms in his or her approach to facial rejuvenation to realize enhanced aesthetic results with less patient trauma.

BIBLIOGRAPHY

Abul-Hassan HS, van Drasek Ascher G, Acland RD: Surgical anatomy and blood supply of the fascial layers of the temporal regions. Plast Reconstr Surg 77:1, 1986.

Baylis HI, Nelson ER, Goldberg RA: Lower eyelid retraction following blepharoplasty. Ophthal Plast Reconstr Surg 8:3, 1992.

Beeson WH, Kabaker S, Keller GS: Carbon dioxide laser blepharoplasty, a comparison to electrosurgery. International Journal of Aesthetic and Restorative Surgery 2:1, 1994.

Beeson WH, McCollough EG: Aesthetic Surgery of the Aging Face. St Louis, CV Mosby Company, 1986.

Bosniak SL: Cosmetic Blepharoplasty. New York, Raven Press, 1990.

Catone G: Selected Readings in Oral and Maxillofacial Surgery, Laser Technology in Oral and Maxillofacial Surgery, Part I: Principles 3:4. The University of Texas Southwestern Medical Center, 1993.

Coleman WP III, Hanke CW, Alt TH, Asken S (eds): Cosmetic Surgery of the Skin, Principles and Techniques. Philadelphia, B.C. Decker Inc., 1991.

Epker BN: Esthetic Maxillofacial Surgery. Philadelphia, Lea and Febiger, 1994.

Flowers RS (guest editor): Clinics in Plastic Surgery, Blepharoplasty and Periorbital Aesthetic Surgery. Philadelphia, W.B. Saunders Company, April, 1993.

Goldman MP, Fitzpatrick RE: Cutaneous Laser Surgery, The Art and Science of Selective Photothermolysis. St Louis, Mosby–Year Book, Inc., 1994.

Green HA, Burd E, Nishioka NS, et al: Middermal wound healing, a comparison between dermatomal excision and pulsed carbon dioxide laser ablation. Arch Dermatol 128:639–645, 1992.

Jelks GW (guest editor): Clinics in Plastic Surgery, Oculoplastic Surgery. Philadelphia, W.B. Saunders Company, April, 1988.

Keller GS: KTP laser rhytidectomy. Fac Plast Surg Clin North Am 1:2, 1993.

Keller GS: Transblepharoplasty brow suspension with the KTP laser. International Journal of Aesthetic and Restorative Surgery 1:2, 1993.

Keller GS: Use of the KTP laser in cosmetic surgery. American Journal of Cosmetic Surgery 9:2, 1992.

Keller GS, Razum NJ, Elliott S, Parks J: Small incision laser lift for forehead creases and glabellar furrows. Arch Otolaryngol Head Neck Surg 119:632–635, 1993.

Kotler R: Clinical Rejuvenation of the Face. St Louis, Mosby–Year Book, Inc., 1992.

Larrabee WF Jr, Makielski KH: Surgical Anatomy of the Face. Raven Press, New York, 1993.

Larrabee WF Jr, Makielski KH, Cupp C: Facelift anatomy. Fac Plast Surg Clin North Am 1:2, 1993.

Lemke BN, Della Rocca RC: Surgery of the Eyelids and Orbit,

an Anatomical Approach. Norwalk, CT, Appleton & Lange, 1990.

Mangat DS (guest editor): Facial Plastic Surgery Clinics of North America, Chemical Peels and Dermabrasion. Philadelphia, W.B. Saunders Company, February, 1994.

McCollough EG, Langsdon PR: Dermabrasion and Chemical Peel, American Academy of Facial Plastic and Reconstructive Surgery. New York, Thieme Medical Publishers, Inc., 1988.

McGrath MH, Turner ML (guest editors): Clinics in Plastic Surgery, Dermatology for Plastic Surgeons. Philadelphia, W.B. Saunders Company, January, 1993.

Menick FJ (guest editor): Clinics in Plastic Surgery, Aesthetic Surgery of the Face. Philadelphia, W.B. Saunders Company, April, 1992.

Meyers AD (ed): Biological Basis of Facial Plastic Surgery,

American Academy of Facial Plastic and Reconstructive Surgery. New York, Thieme Medical Publishers, Inc., 1993.

Putterman AM: Cosmetic Oculoplastic Surgery, 2nd ed. Philadelphia, W.B. Saunders Company, 1993.

Rudolph R, Miller SH (guest editors): Clinics in Plastic Surgery, Wound Healing. Philadelphia, W.B. Saunders Company, July, 1990.

Stegman SJ, Tromovitch TA, Glogau RG: Cosmetic Dermatologic Surgery, 2nd ed. Littleton, MA, Year Book Medical Publishers, Inc., 1990.

Thomas DW, O'Neill ID, Harding KG, Shepherd JP: Cutaneous wound healing: A current perspective. J Oral Maxillofac Surg 53:442–447, 1995.

Tobin HA: The extended subperiosteal coronal lift. The American Journal of Cosmetic Surgery 10:1, 1993.

Tolhurst DE, Carstens MH, Greco RJ, Hurwitz DJ: The surgical anatomy of the scalp. Plast Reconstr Surg 87:4, 1991.

Laser-Assisted Uvulopalatoplasty

ROBERT A. STRAUSS, DDS

Laser-assisted uvulopalatoplasty (LAUP) is a relatively new technique for the management of snoring. The procedure was first reported in France by Kamimi, in 1990, as a simpler and less morbid replacement for the traditional surgical treatment option, uvulopalatopharyngoplasty (UPPP), and is rapidly gaining popularity for treating this all too common problem.[1] Subsequent studies and extensive clinical experience have demonstrated that the procedure has the ability not only to manage snoring effectively but to do so with considerably less morbidity and disability than are associated with UPPP.

The issue of the management of snoring is not trivial. It has been estimated that almost 20% of the population of the United States complain of habitual snoring.[2] In addition, the sound level of some patients' snoring can reach nearly 80 dB, the same level as some jet aircraft and enough actually to cause mild hearing loss in a few patients. This malady can also disrupt the patient's sleep, the bed partner's sleep, and in some cases the sleep of anyone within several hundred feet of the patient. Inadequate quiet sleep can lead to irritability, depression, mood changes, and marital discord. It is not uncommon for snoring patients to have to isolate themselves from their sleep partners, which not only is unfortunate and unpleasant for most patients but also often prevents them from taking trips and vacations that involve a hotel stay with another person. It follows, of course, that patients often are brought for treatment by their spouse or significant other rather than because of their own needs. The LAUP procedure was designed as a simple and rapid method for treating this problem that, in most cases, can be performed on an outpatient basis in

an office setting. It requires approximately 15 minutes of surgical time and generally has been associated with minimal morbidity.

Although the procedure was originally designed to treat snoring, it has also been studied as a possible treatment alternative for patients with obstructive sleep apnea syndrome (OSAS).[3] This was a natural, if somewhat controversial, development, because snoring and sleep apnea are actually just different manifestations of the same physiologic process. Because these processes are so closely related, it is important to examine the pathophysiology of both and how LAUP affects the structures in the airway.

PATHOPHYSIOLOGY

The oronasopharyngeal airway is designed to accomplish two seemingly opposite tasks simultaneously. It must be compliant and flexible enough to allow swallowing and speech vocalization but also stiff enough to prevent collapse during ventilatory efforts. The precise balance of these two processes, which leads to functional airway patency, is effectively accomplished by the velopharyngeal musculature, which must adjust its compliance according to its functional needs at that moment.

In the awake state, the normal neurologic stimulus and subsequent tonus of the pharyngeal musculature is adequate to keep the balance in favor of airway stiffness for patency (except during swallowing, when, of course, compliance is increased). During sleep (especially rapid eye movement [REM] sleep), however, the normal neurologic stimulation and tonus of the velopharyngeal muscu-

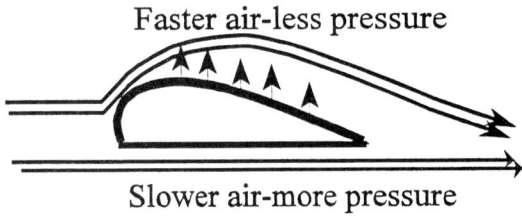

Faster air-less pressure

Slower air-more pressure

FIGURE 13–1. Bernoulli's principle. Air moving over the curved surface of a wing must travel faster than the air moving under the straight surface of the wing to reach the back edge simultaneously. The faster moving air creates less pressure on the wing than the slower moving air and this causes the wing to rise. The same effect can occur in the airway when the quantity of flow is restricted by a partial obstruction somewhere in the nasal or oropharynx, causing a rise in the speed of the flow, pressure differentials, and the subsequent vibration that is heard as snoring.

lature is diminished, and this balance may be upset, which can cause the muscles that maintain the normal airway space to relax, allowing constriction (or even collapse) of the airway during inspiratory efforts.

When the oronasopharyngeal airway is further compromised by anatomic obstruction, redundant or hypertrophic tissue, or excessive compliance, the volume of airflow is decreased and its speed is increased, as a result of the smaller than normal airway. This increased speed of airflow can cause a vibratory effect in the adjacent oral or nasopharyngeal tissues that is manifested as the sounds we associate with snoring. This movement of the tissues is guided by a physical process known as Bernoulli's principle, which states that the faster a gas or liquid moves, the less pressure it exerts on the surrounding structures. It is the same principle that provides the lift for an airplane wing or draws in a shower curtain when the water is turned on full force in the shower (Fig. 13–1). The pressure

differentials that result in the airway from these dynamic airflow changes can lead to rapid elevation and depression of the tissues (i.e., vibration), effects that are manifested clinically as snoring.

The anatomic level of airflow compromise within the airway is very important in the management of this problem. Although it appears that the soft palate and uvula are a common source of snoring, in fact, the level of airway compromise can occur anywhere from the nasal cavity to the larynx (Fig. 13–2). Areas that have been implicated in the literature, beside the soft palate and uvula, include the anterior and posterior nasal cavities, the nasal septum, the lateral walls of the pharynx, tonsils, and adenoids, the base of the tongue, the epiglottis, and the vocal cords themselves. More recent data indicate that in most patients with sleep-related breathing disorders there is often not one but rather multiple levels of obstruction.[4] It has even been postulated that the level of obstruction may change rapidly from place to place within the same patient within short periods of time. This information must always be taken into account when managing either snoring or sleep apnea and must be assessed carefully when deciding on appropriate treatment modalities.

In simple snoring the degree of obstruction is small and the resultant airway effect is physiologic (i.e., it leads to no significant pathologic sequelae). However, when the degree of obstruction at any level is severe enough to cause more extensive reduction of airflow than usually causes simple snoring it is termed *hypopnea* (defined as a greater than 50% decrease in airflow), and when complete obstruction occurs, airflow totally ceases and *apnea* ensues. Obstructive hypopneic and apneic events during sleep are often accompanied by a series of significant and potentially dangerous signs and symptoms that constitute the complications associ-

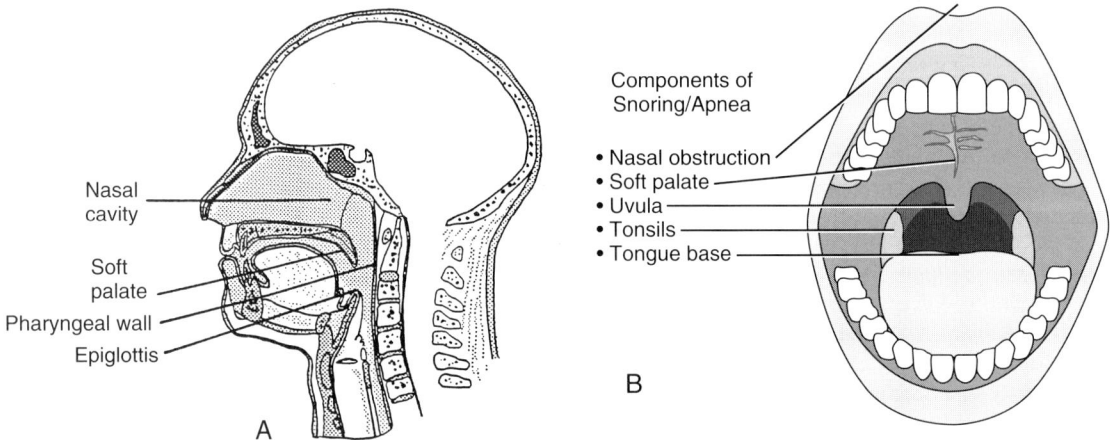

A

Nasal cavity

Soft palate

Pharyngeal wall

Epiglottis

B

Components of Snoring/Apnea

• Nasal obstruction
• Soft palate
• Uvula
• Tonsils
• Tongue base

FIGURE 13–2. Common sites of obstruction in the airway that can lead to snoring or apnea.

TABLE 13–1. Complications of Sleep Apnea Syndrome

Hypoxia
Hypercapnia
Hypertension
Increased incidence of cerebrovascular accident
Impotence
Increased risk of sudden death
Polycythemia
Cor pulmonale
Arrhythmias
Depression

TABLE 13–2. OSAS Work-up Procedures

Detailed history
Complete physical examination
Polysomnography
Flexible nasopharyngoscopy with Mueller's maneuver
Pulmonary function testing
Complete blood count, chemistries, arterial blood gases
Electrocardiography
Chest x-ray study
Computed tomography of head
Cephalometric radiography

ated with OSAS (Table 13–1).[5] Snoring, therefore, may be a benign nuisance that may be left untreated or a *sign* of a syndrome that is associated with great morbidity and, in some cases, even mortality and thus requires immediate attention and intervention. As a result, the practitioner treating snoring must first determine the cause of the snoring, to ensure adequate and correct treatment. This is imperative because the treatment of snoring with the LAUP procedure is usually simple, uncomplicated, and predictable, whereas the treatment of OSAS (by any method, LAUP included) is considerably more complicated and unpredictable. This is also important because a patient treated for snoring with LAUP or any other surgical procedure may or may not demonstrate improvement or be cured of their sleep apnea, if it is present. In theory, much like a patient with hypertension who feels well and therefore does not seek treatment, a patient with OSAS could have the one major symptom (snoring) removed and think—erroneously—that he or she is cured. This could have disastrous consequences in the long run, because the previously mentioned morbidities, many of which are not sensed by the patient, inevitably and inexplicably begin to occur. Even in the short term this could be dangerous if perioperative swelling causes acute respiratory embarrassment after surgery. It is abundantly clear that proper work-up of the snoring patient is essential to correct management, and in light of the ease of the surgical procedure itself, is often the most time-consuming aspect of the treatment.

DIAGNOSIS

The complete diagnosis of snoring and OSAS is rather extensive and the practitioner should certainly avail him- or herself of any one of the many texts and articles that cover this area in greater detail. In general, however, diagnosis has several components (Table 13–2), including a complete history; appropriate physical examination; fiber-optic nasopharyngoscopy; cephalometric radiography;

laboratory testing as needed; and, finally, polysomnography. There are now many reputable sleep laboratories in most major cities that can provide much assistance in the proper work-up of these patients, and it is highly recommended that a working relationship be developed between the surgeon and a sleep disorders specialist.

The history of a snoring patient can be of much value in the diagnostic work-up. Although it is not always conclusive, the history often can help differentiate OSAS from simple snoring. The most common presenting signs and symptoms of OSAS in the history are listed in Table 13–3. Any finding in the history that is consistent with the diagnosis of OSAS should alert the practitioner to seek additional objective data. Obviously, a sleep partner can be invaluable in providing some of the history, and certainly the observation of apneas by the sleep partner should be ascertained. It is important to note, however, that a negative history for signs and symptoms does not necessarily rule out OSAS, because there is a calculable percentage of patients who do not exhibit these manifestations (silent apneics).

Physical examination procedures for evaluating sleep-related disorders can be complex. At the very least, every patient considered for surgery should have a thorough head and neck examination with two purposes in mind: to attempt to ascertain the likely anatomic source or sources of obstruction so that appropriate treatment can be rendered and to rule out any inflammatory, congenital, or neoplastic reasons for the obstruction. This should include a facial proportion examination, speculum examination of the nasal cavity and ears, oral examination, neck examination, and indirect hypopharyngoscopy

TABLE 13–3. OSAS Symptoms

Unusually loud snoring
Excessive daytime sleepiness
Restless, disturbed sleep
Impaired daytime performance
Concomitant sleep disorders
Witnessed apneic episodes

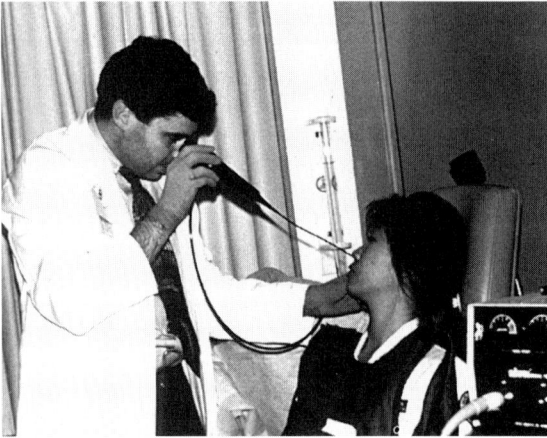

FIGURE 13–3. Nasopharyngoscopy. The procedure is performed using topical anesthesia and allows the practitioner to evaluate possible sources of obstruction as well as examine for any other pathology.

and laryngoscopy. Any areas of swelling, enlargement, hyperplasia, or redundancy should be noted.

Diagnostic nasopharyngoscopy also has an important place in the work-up of these patients. It provides valuable information during the physical examination on anatomic areas not easily visualized clinically, such as the posterior nasal cavity and the nasopharynx. The procedure is performed easily and comfortably with topical anesthesia and requires only a few minutes (Fig. 13–3). Examination should include the anterior and posterior nasal cavities, the choana, the nasopharynx, the soft palate and uvula area, the pharyngeal walls, the tongue base, the hypopharynx, the epiglottis, and the vocal cords.[6]

Aside from ruling out anatomic or pathologic anomalies, the use of the nasopharyngoscope allows the surgeon to perform Mueller's maneuver.[7] This procedure involves placing the patient supine and passing the scope through the nares and into the nasopharynx just above the soft palate and having the patient close the nose and mouth and attempt an inspiration, essentially performing a reverse Valsalva maneuver. The negative pressure created causes the flexible airway to collapse, ideally at the level it would during sleep, mimicking the level and type of obstruction. If the airway collapses at the soft palate this is likely the source of the obstruction, and surgical procedures designed to correct this area (e.g., LAUP and UPPP) should be useful. Conversely, if the collapse is seen to occur at the level of the tongue base rather than the soft palate, these procedures are less likely to work and consideration must be given to procedures that address the base of the tongue, hyoid, or hypopharynx (e.g., mandibular or bimaxillary advancement, hyoid suspension). Although nasopharyngoscopy

does not rule OSAS in or out as a cause of snoring, it does help to characterize the obstruction and is therefore a valuable diagnostic tool.

Cephalometric radiography is a useful adjunct to aid in diagnosis of a possible skeletal-facial deformity that could lead to an airway disturbance.[8] Microgenia, retrognathia, and a posteriorly positioned hyoid have all been implicated in allowing the genial tubercle, and thus, the tongue musculature, to become displaced in a relatively posterior position, allowing for airway compromise. A standard cephalometric film is taken and worked up in the usual fashion with the addition of measurements of (1) the posterior nasal spine (PNS) to the end of the soft palate and uvula, (2) the perpendicular distance from the hyoid to the mandibular plane (MP), and (3) the posterior airway space (PAS). The measurements, and their norms, are depicted in Figure 13–4. A long soft palate and uvula is obviously an indication for LAUP, whereas findings of posteriorly positioned osseous or tongue anatomy may indicate the need for other surgical procedures that more functionally address this region, such as osteotomy.[9]

Because a calculable percentage of patients with OSAS are clinically asymptomatic except for their snoring, polysomnography is the only reliable method of actually assuring the practitioner of the presence or absence of OSAS.[10] Polysomnography is essentially a method of monitoring a patient overnight for a multitude of variables, including electroencephalography, electromyography, electro-

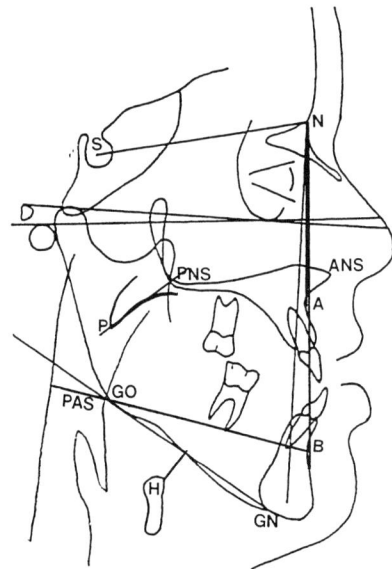

FIGURE 13–4. Cephalometric evaluation. The tracing is performed normally with the addition of the three listed measurements. The normal measure for PAS is 11 mm; for PNS-P 35 mm; and for MP-H 15 mm. Abnormal findings may indicate anatomic abnormalities in the soft palate, mandible, or base of tongue.

oculography, electrocardiography, pulse oximetry, inspiratory effort, airflow, and sleep position. By monitoring for a minimum of 4 hours it is possible to accurately measure three important things: (1) the presence and duration of the stages of sleep experienced by the patient; (2) the presence of any hypopneas and/or apneas during sleep; and (3) any cardiovascular consequences of these respiratory events.

The respiratory disturbance index (RDI) is defined as the total number of apneas and hypopneas per hour experienced by the patient (i.e., a combination of the apnea index and the hypopnea index) and is a good qualitative and quantitative determinant of the presence of OSAS in a snoring patient (assuming, of course, that a conscientious effort is made by the patient and that the apnea is not central in origin). An RDI of less than 5 is considered essentially normal; between 5 and 20 is considered mild to moderate OSAS; greater than 20 is considered severe OSAS and is associated with increased morbidity and mortality levels. The level of maximal oxygen desaturation (anything less than 90% being significant) and the presence of any cardiovascular abnormalities (e.g., arrhythmias) during the respiratory events are also used to determine the level of severity of the OSAS and appropriate courses of treatment.

A finding of OSAS on polysomnography must be carefully weighed when deciding on a treatment plan. Initial therapy for OSAS often begins with nasal continuous positive airway pressure (CPAP) at night, which provides a rapid method for decreasing or eliminating apneic events. A second polysomnogram can be used to perform a trial of the nasal CPAP for the purpose of determining what is the ideal amount of pressure to be supplied by the machine, which the patient can then set up at home for nightly use. Alternatively, the original polysomnogram can be divided into a diagnostic half and a trial CPAP half in a process called a *split night study*. Although this does decrease the cost of the process, a 4-hour polysomnogram is somewhat minimal for obtaining adequate diagnostic information. New home-based machines are now available that can be used to determine if a sleep laboratory test is indicated. This is certainly more convenient for the patient and less expensive, but the reliability and accuracy of these devices has yet to be fully determined and they should be regarded as screening tools only.[11]

Although investigators do not agree on the need for this expensive and labor-intensive diagnostic test on every patient contemplated for LAUP, there is no question that, at the very least, the astute practitioner will have an extremely low threshold for ordering the test if any signs or symptoms of OSAS are present on the history or physical examination. The absolute need for ruling out OSAS before surgical treatment with LAUP has been discussed previously and must be heeded. Consultation and communication with the sleep laboratory will allow each practitioner to develop an acceptable protocol for evaluating patients in an efficient and comprehensive but cost-effective manner.

The primary candidate for the procedure, therefore, is a nonobese patient with uncomplicated snoring that appears on nasopharyngoscopy and cephalometric radiography to be due to an obstruction in the region of the soft palate or uvula. This procedure has received generally excellent reviews for the management of the simple snoring patient with minimal morbidity.

At the time of this writing, it is maintained by some surgeons (albeit highly controversially) that patients with mild to moderate OSAS proved by polysomnography may also be considered for the LAUP procedure if they have minimal or no cardiovascular effects, are not significantly overweight (being overweight dramatically reduces the chance of success),[12] and are receiving concurrent CPAP therapy.[13] This therapy should be continued until the LAUP procedure (including all sessions) is complete and the patient has had a repeat polysomnogram to determine the effect of the surgery. Clinical follow-up—and possibly repeat polysomnography—should be taken on a long-term basis, because some relapse is likely eventually with advancing patient age and may necessitate touch-up surgery. It should be reiterated that this procedure is not universally accepted by all practitioners as a suitable treatment for many OSAS patients, and it is up to the individual clinician to determine the appropriateness of this surgery for their patients. One concern is the difficulty in performing UPPP on a patient with failed LAUP as opposed to the ability to perform LAUP on patients with failed UPPP. Actual success rates in the literature for treating OSAS appear similar for both procedures, although LAUP data are sparse and early. This area will undoubtedly receive more attention and research in the future, and the usefulness of LAUP in OSAS patients will be made more clear.

PRESURGICAL MANAGEMENT

After thorough examination and determination of the cause of the snoring, the patient should be prepared for surgery. A complete discussion of the pathophysiology of snoring should be explained to the patient so that informed consent may be obtained. An explanation of the surgery and the laser itself often helps allay patients' fears. The patient should be told of the need for as many as three to five sessions to obtain maximal benefits, the possibility of procedure failure, and all the pertinent possible complications (described later in this chapter). It is wise to have the patient take nothing by mouth for 2 to 3 hours before the surgery, in the unlikely event that gagging should occur. The patient should also be warned not to use any aspirin or nonsteroidal anti-inflammatory drugs (NSAIDs) for several days before surgery, to limit the possibility of bleeding. Other than nitrous oxide, sedation has not been necessary in this author's experience, so there is usually no need for the patient to be accompanied.

Before the procedure, as with any laser surgery, the patient and office staff must be suitably protected from the laser. This should include wavelength-specific safety glasses with sideshields and avoidance of supplemental oxygenation during the surgery. Presurgical use of oxygen or nitrous oxygen is acceptable, but this should be removed before using the laser. This can be accomplished by providing nitrous for 10 minutes at 30% to 50%, then removing the nasal mask, waiting 1 minute to allow the pharyngeal air to mix with room air, then performing the surgery. If additional nitrous is needed, the process can be repeated as needed.

Although wet gauze or tooth protectors are useful for preventing damage to adjacent teeth and other structures, the nature of the typical backstop-protected LAUP handpiece makes them generally unnecessary in this instance (whereas for standard laser handpieces the use of these safety devices is absolutely indicated).

Finally, because a significant amount of laser plume is generated during this procedure, which is both objectionable to the patient and a pathogen risk to other personnel in the room, adequate smoke evacuation should be available. Ideally, this should be a high-volume independent smoke evacuator with a biologic filter to remove small-caliber particles. A smoke evacuator should be used in addition to small–pore size laser masks for all personnel in the room.

SURGICAL TECHNIQUE

There are two general techniques for performing LAUP. The first—and most common—is the multistage procedure that is completed over a series of three to five appointments, each achieving a small change in the height of the soft palate. Alternatively, some surgeons have elected to perform one-stage LAUP in selected patients to decrease the overall time for the procedure. Although this technique has an obvious time advantage over the long run, it does seem to cause significantly more discomfort and short-term morbidity in some pa-

tients and is recommended, even by its proponents, primarily for young, healthy patients who require a minimal amount of surgical intervention and can better tolerate the increased stress of the one-stage procedure.

It is highly recommended that the surgery be performed with any one of the commercially available LAUP handpieces provided by the manufacturer of the laser being used. This is important, because these handpieces are designed to accomplish the surgery easily with minimal risk to adjacent structures as compared with other techniques for isolating the surgical site with standard carbon dioxide laser handpieces. These special handpieces all have an extended laser delivery handpiece combined with a reflective backstop. In addition, although it would seem reasonable that other wavelengths are potentially usable for this procedure, the only laser that has been documented in the literature at the time of this writing is the carbon dioxide one. Some other wavelengths, such as the Nd:YAG and the argon laser, use contact fiberoptic handpieces that are best used for incisional purposes and provide a relatively small ablational spot size capability but do provide for increased hemostatic penetration, owing to their hemoglobin affinity. Future studies will undoubtedly elucidate which lasers (other than the carbon dioxide) are or are not suitable for this procedure.

The multistage surgery using a hollow-waveguide or articulated-arm carbon dioxide laser with a backstop LAUP handpiece is performed as follows:

1. After preparing the patient as discussed earlier, the patient is placed in the upright sitting position. Topical soft palate and nasal anesthesia is obtained with two sprays of neosynephrine 0.25% administered to each nostril for dilation, followed in 5 minutes by two sprays of 10% lidocaine topical spray in each nostril. This is then followed by two additional sprays of lidocaine intraorally to the soft palate and the base of the tongue. Commercially available combinations of neosynephrine and a local anesthetic are available and may be used if preferred. Using a standard 27-gauge needle, a total of 0.5 to 1.0 ml of lidocaine 2% with 1:100,000 epinephrine is then injected bilaterally into the soft palate, just lateral to the uvula. A small final amount, 0.25 ml or less, is then injected into the base of the uvula (Fig. 13–5). It is important not to inject too much anesthesia, lest it distort the anatomy and interfere with tissue absorption of the carbon dioxide laser wavelength. One milliliter is usually sufficient to perform the procedure in most patients; small amounts are added, if needed during the surgery.

2. The LAUP handpiece backstop is then placed behind the uvula, and the inferior half of the uvula

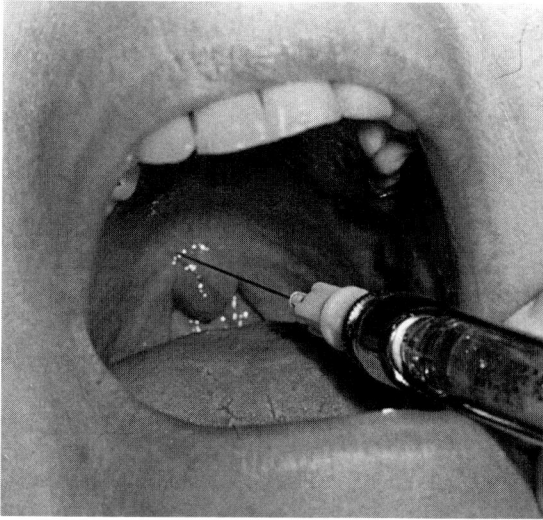

FIGURE 13–5. Injection of the soft palate and uvula following topical anesthesia of the nasal and oral cavities. A total of 1 ml is usually sufficient for the entire procedure.

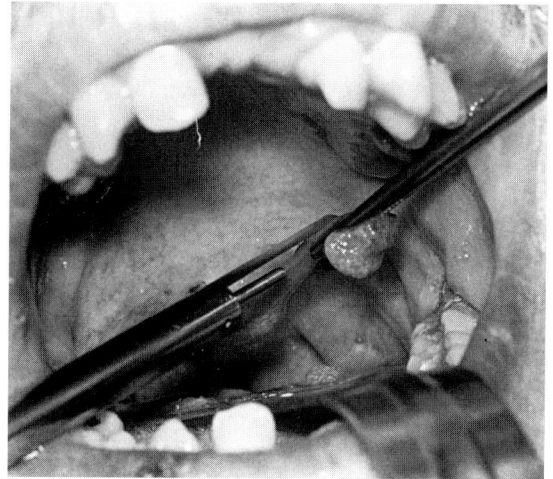

FIGURE 13–7. Excision of the uvula. This is particularly useful for long uvulas or when using a contact fiberoptic-type laser.

is ablated using 12 to 15 W of power in continuous or intermittent fashion (Fig. 13–6). This is accomplished with controlled but swift movements of the handpiece laterally across the bottom of the uvula, ablating one layer of tissue at a time. Depending on the type of laser being used, some carbonization may be seen, and this may be gently removed with a moist cotton swab, if necessary. First-stage surgeries with exceptionally long and thin uvulas may be accomplished by focused laser excision rather than ablation, with subsequent modification or additional removal done by ablation (Fig. 13–7). With normal, shorter and thicker uvulas, or repeat LAUP when the residual uvula is small, ablation may be easier than excision. Uvular papillomas

found during first-stage surgery, which are more common than might be expected, may be excised with the laser simultaneous with the LAUP surgery.

In some cases, the uvula may be too thick to get the backstop easily behind it and perform ablation. This is most likely to occur after several previous LAUP procedures, when the base of the original uvula is being reached or a new uvula has been fashioned from the original soft palate tissue. In this case, the uvula may be grasped gently with forceps and manipulated to aid in the ablation, or it may be placed on a wet tongue blade and further ablation performed carefully using a straight handpiece without the backstop (Fig. 13–8). The wet tongue blade provides adequate protection as long as the patient does not swallow during the lasing

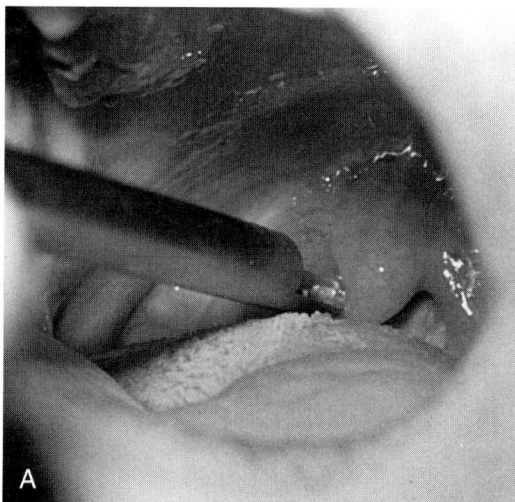

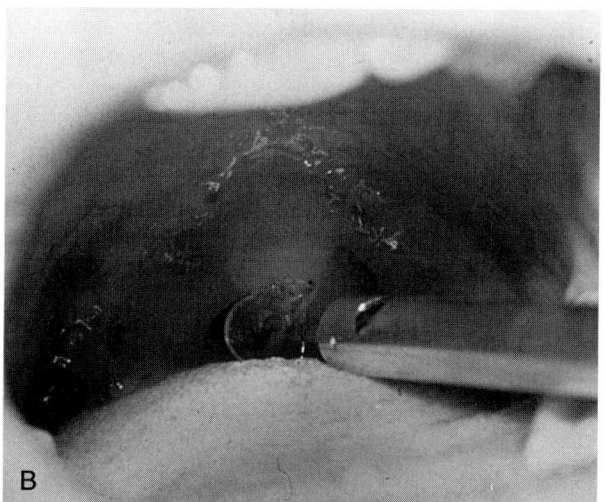

FIGURE 13–6. *A*, Ablation of the uvula (lateral approach). *B*, Ablation of the uvula—posterior pharyngeal wall protection.

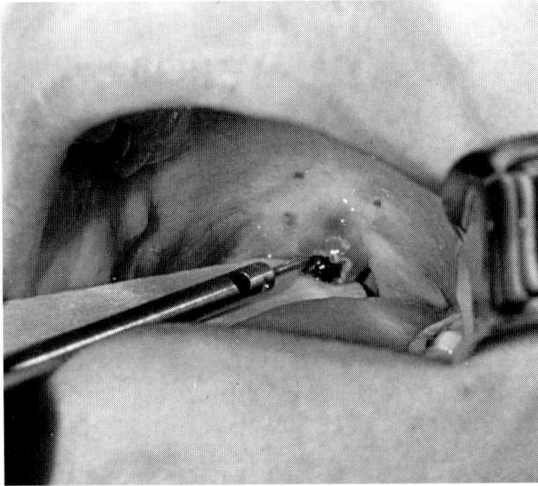

FIGURE 13–8. In cases in which the backstop cannot be used, the uvula may be placed on a wet tongue blade and ablated without the backstop.

FIGURE 13–10. Tonsillar pillar ablation. This method is useful in widening the airway considerably but increases postoperative discomfort.

process. If the palate is suddenly elevated, a pharyngeal wound could be created. Although this has occurred, the wound is usually minor as long as the laser is stopped immediately, and no morbidity has resulted.

3. The handpiece is then placed just lateral to the uvula, and a 5- to 10-mm vertical cut is made in focused mode through the soft palate using the same 12- to 15-W power settings. These lateral trenches should be full thickness, allowing visualization of the posterior pharyngeal wall through the soft palate. This maneuver should enlarge the airway space and re-establish the original contour of the soft palate (Fig. 13–9). When access or mobility necessitates, the uvula ablation and the vertical cuts may be performed in reverse order. This is espe-

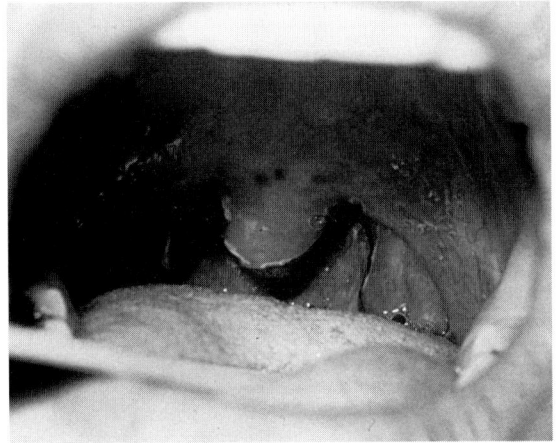

cially useful when a thick uvula does not easily allow maneuvering to vaporize its posterior aspect. Performing the vertical trenches in effect lengthens the uvula and allows significantly increased mobility and easier ablation or excision of the uvula.

4. When necessitated by anatomic features (e.g., webbing) the tonsillar pillars may be ablated superficially by turning the handpiece laterally and carefully lasing the medial aspect of the pillar. This further enlarges the airway space and is very useful in patients with this type of anatomy, but it does increase the postoperative discomfort in many patients (Fig. 13–10). Although ablation of the tonsils themselves has been reported in the literature with some success, it can be associated with significant bleeding and probably is best avoided in these cases. In extreme cases in which the tonsils are believed to be a major factor in the snoring, the

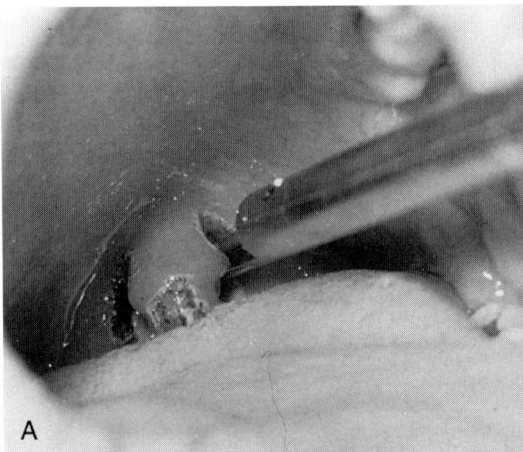

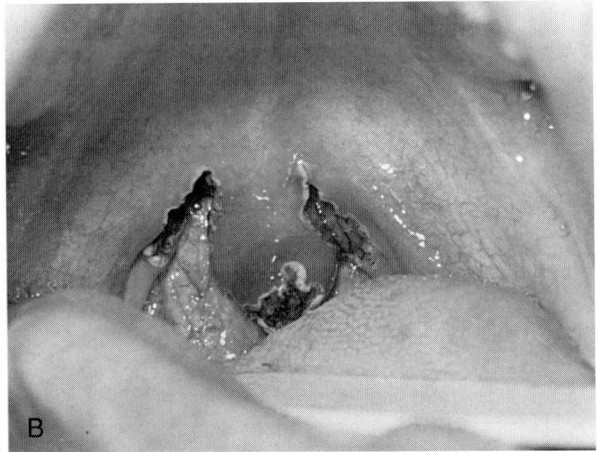

FIGURE 13–9. *A*, Creating the vertical incisions in the soft palate. These are carried through the entire thickness of the palate. The height of the cut should not extend beyond the levator muscle, regardless of whether the procedure is done one stage at a time or in multiple stages. *B*, Posterior pharyngeal wall seen through vertical laser incisions.

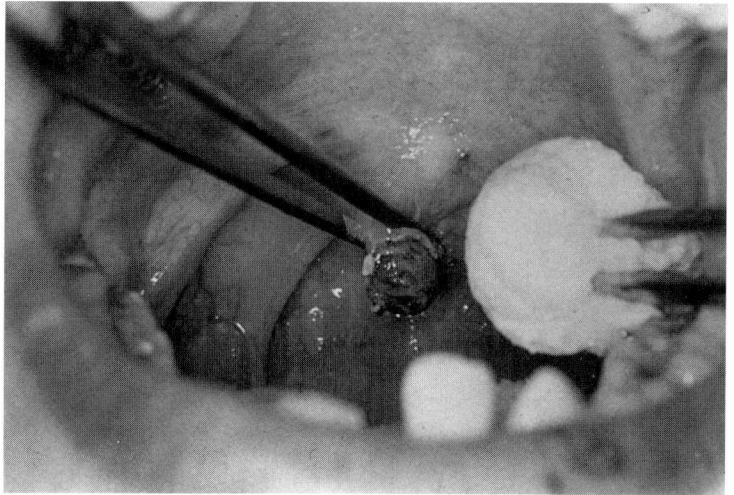

FIGURE 13–11. Char layer removal. If a char layer should form, it can be removed by gently wiping with a moist cotton swab.

patient may require tonsillectomy before, or after, the LAUP. It is not uncommon for the tonsils to rotate medially after LAUP as a result of the muscular changes associated with tonsillar pillar ablation, and this may affect the need for postoperative tonsillar surgery. Unless the tonsils are hyperplastic initially, it is reasonable, in adults, to attempt LAUP first and to seek secondary tonsil removal, if needed.

5. If desired, a moist cotton swab may be used to remove any char that has formed on the uvula or in the vertical trenches. The uvula is easily stabilized with forceps to assist in this process if necessary (Fig. 13–11).

6. After postoperative instructions are provided, the patient may be discharged. No special wound care is required at this point, and all physiologic functions, such as speech and swallowing, remain intact.

The one-stage procedure is performed with the following modifications:

1. The vertical trenches are performed first and are carried just short of the insertion of the levator palatini muscle, which is identified presurgically and may be marked with methylene blue or by needle puncture. Infringement on the muscle proper may cause functional disturbances and must be avoided.

2. The uvula now appears long because the original uvula is added to the additional apparent uvula created artificially by the vertical trench cuts. The laser is then used in focused mode to excise this tissue in an amount adequate to create a new uvula that appears normal in size and shape.

3. Otherwise, the patient is managed identically to those who undergo the multistage procedure.

POSTOPERATIVE INSTRUCTIONS

Before discharge the patient should be thoroughly informed of the expected and unexpected postoperative sequelae associated with this procedure, along with their management or prevention, or both. The usual postoperative instructions are listed in Table 13–4.

Although the efficacy of perioperative and postoperative steroids has yet to be determined for this procedure, they are used by many practitioners to limit the inevitable swelling seen after the surgery. Unlike most other laser surgical procedures, significant edema is seen with the LAUP. The uvula enlarges to the point where it is often felt and described by the patient as "something hanging in the back of my throat." This sensation is initially disconcerting to the patient but diminishes quickly (Fig. 13–12A to C). Hydrocortisone or dexamethasone given parenterally at the time of surgery, or a tapering Medrol dosepak or equivalent given orally for postoperative use has worked well in this author's hands and does seem to diminish postoperative edema and discomfort.

Because an impressive sore throat invariably follows this procedure, appropriate analgesics should be prescribed. Acetaminophen with codeine, in tablet or elixir form, is generally adequate for most

TABLE 13–4. Patient Instructions After Surgery

Analgesic prescription (generally acetaminophen with codeine tablets or elixir, or an equivalent).
Steroids (generally a Medrol dosepak or equivalent).
Soft, room-temperature diet for 7–10 days.
Hydrogen peroxide gargles b.i.d.
Elevate head of bed 45 degrees for sleeping for first 48 to 72 hours.
Must sleep in same room as another responsible adult for 48 hours.
Avoid acid or citrus products for 7 to 10 days.
Avoid acetylsalicylic acid or NSAIDs for 5 to 7 days, if possible.
CPAP therapy should be continued beginning first postoperative night.

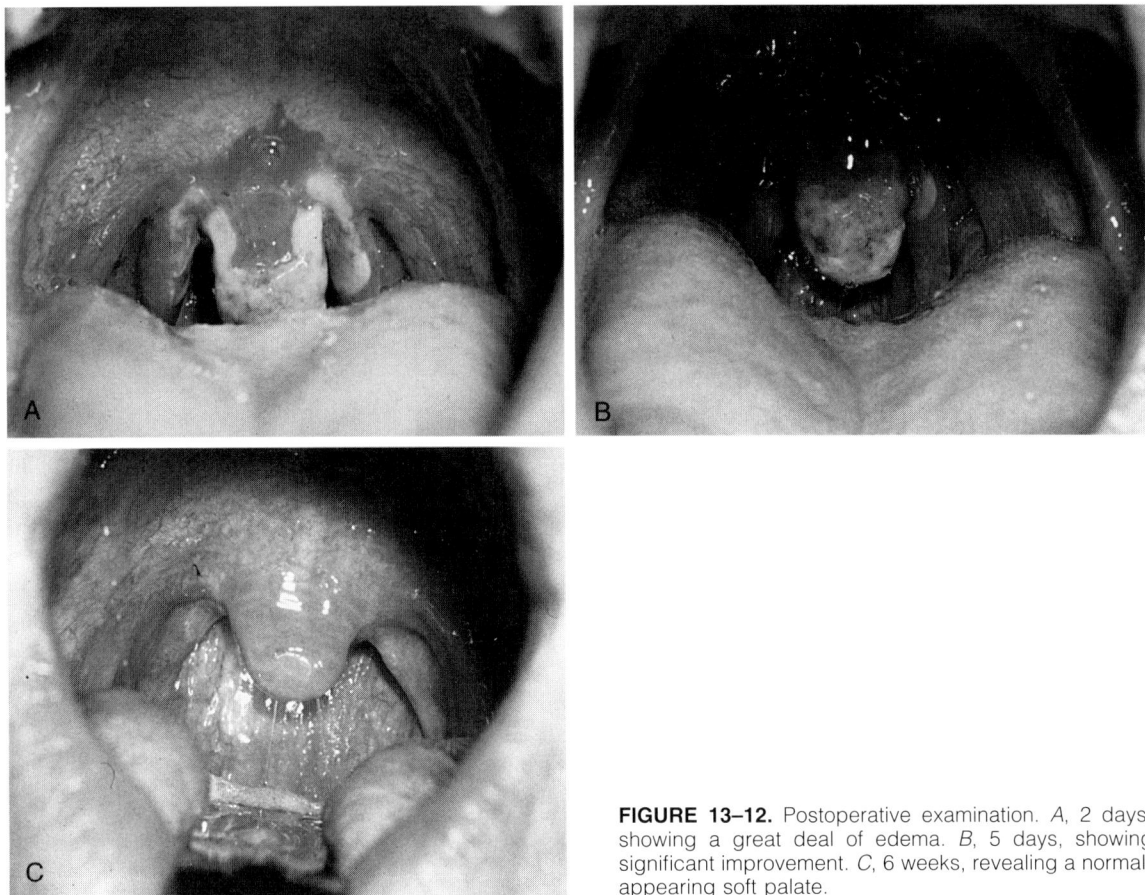

FIGURE 13–12. Postoperative examination. *A*, 2 days, showing a great deal of edema. *B*, 5 days, showing significant improvement. *C*, 6 weeks, revealing a normal-appearing soft palate.

patients and is taken every 3 to 4 hours, as needed. Additional analgesia may be obtained by the use of topical agents in lozenge or spray form (e.g., Chloraseptic spray or Cēpastat lozenges). When used frequently as needed between narcotic doses, these can be of great benefit in allowing the patient to function normally in the postoperative period, and they should not be overlooked. The sore throat lasts 10 to 12 days, waxing and waning in intensity (mostly related to diet).

Antibiotics such as amoxicillin have been prescribed by some practitioners, but as with any intraoral surgery, their prophylactic benefit is suspect and their use is probably unnecessary. Infections of the surgical site are rare and often fungal, undoubtedly secondary to the use of the antibiotics rather than the surgery.

For obvious reasons a soft diet is recommended after surgery. This diet should be maintained for 5 to 7 days at a minimum, and patients should be cautioned against attempting to eat normal foods too early, because it prolongs discomfort. Aside from mechanical consistency, excessive thermal extremes (hot or cold), spiciness, and the acid content of foods affect their acceptability. Dairy products

(but not ice cream) are soothing but lead to increased viscosity of secretions and phlegm production, making swallowing more difficult. Their use, therefore, should be decided on by each patient after experimentation.

Oral hygiene following surgery is important and consists of normal brushing and flossing as well as hydrogen peroxide gargles twice a day (1 tablespoon in a glass of water). This procedure aids healing and manages any minor bleeding that may occur. Smoking should, of course, be discouraged. The use of chlorhexidine is probably unnecessary and, aside from leading to increased total procedure costs, may cause additional discomfort.

Although postoperative respiratory embarrassment is unlikely, patients should be instructed to sleep in the same room with another responsible adult for the first one to two nights, as a routine precaution. Sleeping in the semiupright position can be of some benefit in maintaining the airway and may help with the postoperative edema. In addition, patients on CPAP therapy must use the device beginning the night of surgery and continuing until they are told otherwise, as dictated by repeat polysomnography.

Following surgery, patients may be allowed to return to their normal daily routine. They should be instructed that driving and operating machinery should be avoided if narcotics are used for analgesia but that they will tolerate the postoperative course best if they are performing whatever functions they normally do every day. They should also be reminded that, despite the sore throat, they are not infectious to anyone.

COMPLICATIONS

In general, the LAUP procedure is a relatively benign surgery, but it does have the potential for a few serious, or even catastrophic, complications. The primary complication is the inevitable sore throat that accompanies the surgery. Although it may be moderate in some patients, the majority of patients describe the discomfort as moderately severe or worse. Unlike most other laser procedures, which usually do not manifest discomfort for 3 or 4 days, the LAUP is associated with pain the first night after surgery. The problem is usually worst in the mornings and often is associated with swallowing. The pain may increase for the next 24 to 48 hours then level off until it usually begins to subside at 7 to 9 days. Eating inappropriate foods, smoking, and failure to use the prescribed topical and systemic analgesics both exacerbate and prolong the discomfort. It is important when obtaining informed consent for this elective procedure to verify that the patient understands the expected level of discomfort and that the surgeon does not underestimate this normal sequela.

Bleeding following LAUP is rare and usually minor. Most commonly, bleeding during or after surgery comes from the height of the vertical trenches and is easily controlled with hydrogen peroxide gargles, or if persistent, by chemical or electrical cauterization. Even less commonly, bleeding may come from a small artery within the uvula, which may require suture ligation if electrical cauterization is unsuccessful. It is recommended that the patient avoid the use of aspirin or other NSAIDs, because the prolonged bleeding time may increase the risk of hemorrhage.

Although it has not been well documented in the literature, the potential for serious postoperative airway embarrassment does exist, especially in patients with unrecognized or untreated OSAS. The airway in most normal patients appears to have adequate reserve to accommodate the postoperative swelling from the LAUP procedure. In OSAS patients, this reserve is already limited, and the additional burden of the surgery could prove to be overwhelming, leading to dangerous or potentially fatal airway obstruction in the perioperative period.

Steroids (for all patients) and CPAP therapy (for OSAS patients) may be useful in limiting this effect.

Although working in the pharyngeal area always carries the risk of adversely affecting the velopharyngeal mechanism, this does not seem to be a serious long-term risk with the LAUP procedure. Velopharyngeal insufficiency, as evidenced by hypernasal speech or nasal reflux, is not seen to any significant extent. Speech and vocalization are also generally unaffected, but patients who speak ethnic dialects that rely on certain palatally induced sounds (e.g., trill sounds) should be warned of the possibility that they may not be able to produce these sounds reliably. In some instances, this may constitute a relative contraindication to the procedure.

DISCUSSION

Throughout its history of more than 5 years' use in clinical practice, the LAUP procedure has been associated with considerable controversy. Although its use for the management of uncomplicated snoring is fairly well accepted by most clinicians, its application to treatment of documented OSAS has met with more skepticism and caution (as it should, given the seriousness of the disease). In addition, despite its widespread clinical use, there are remarkably few objective data on the procedure, its effectiveness, or its safety.

Kamimi first reported the procedure in 1990.[7] In this unselected pool of 37 patients, Kamimi observed total cessation of snoring in 77.4% of patients and dramatic improvement in the remaining 22.6%. Interestingly, the patients noted improvement in their other symptoms and their perceived ease of nighttime breathing before the improvement in their snoring. Carenfelt, comparing the LAUP and UPPP procedures for non-OSAS snorers, found essentially no difference in the effectiveness of the two procedures (range of success 85% to 90%).[13]

It should be noted that both of these studies relied on subjective patient and family information rather than any objective testing methods as the determinant of success. Given these data, it would appear that both of these surgical procedures are suitable, effective, and appropriate for the management of uncomplicated snoring. The LAUP procedure, however, has the distinct advantage of reduced morbidity, as described earlier.

For OSAS patients, as compared with uncomplicated snorers, LAUP is associated with a statistically higher incidence of morbidity. Not only is the risk of the procedure itself higher, as a result of the limited respiratory reserve in OSAS patients, but the possibility exists of unknowingly removing the symptom of snoring without affecting the underlying OSAS, giving the patient a false sense of being cured. In addition, some clinicians have noted that performing UPPP in a patient in whom LAUP fails is more difficult, or in some cases impossible; this makes UPPP the first surgery of choice in some surgeons' eyes, despite the increased morbidity and expense.

Conversely, LAUP has been used successfully on occasion to correct failed UPPP or the complications sometimes seen with it (such as velopharyngeal insufficiency), by incising through contracted scar tissue and improving mobility of the tissues. It is important that studies looking at OSAS patients use objective polysomnographic techniques to determine the postoperative effect of the procedure—not only on the snoring but on the apnea as well. Naturally, any OSAS patient treated with either of these procedures should have postoperative polysomnography for the same reason, and this should be performed every 1 to 2 years to ensure long-term success.

In a 1994 study Kamimi used preoperative and postoperative polysomnography to evaluate 53 OSAS patients undergoing the LAUP procedure. His findings indicated that 47 of them had a 50% or better decrease in their RDI as well as significant improvement in their clinical symptoms.[3] As expected, patient weight played an important part in the success of the procedure, and it is clear that weight reduction should be stressed to these patients. Although this was a preliminary article and the clinical efficacy of this surgery is still in question, it is of little doubt that the LAUP will have some role to play in the treatment of this disease. Riley and coworkers and other authors in a series of articles on the surgical management of OSAS, have described a staged protocol that utilizes a combination of nasal surgery, UPPP, genioplasty, and orthognathic surgery quite effectively to control the manifestations of the OSAS.[9, 14] For the LAUP to be beneficial, it must have not only less morbidity but also documented results showing at least as good a success rate as UPPP, which is very effective for snoring but only approximately 50% effective for OSAS.[15, 16] Perhaps LAUP, given more time to study its precise indications and usefulness, will

find a place in such a protocol, providing surgeons one more tool with which to combat this serious disease. Without question, however, it is already proving an excellent aid in the treatment of uncomplicated snoring.

REFERENCES

1. Kamimi YV: Laser CO_2 for snoring—preliminary results. Acta Otorhinolaryngol Belg 44:451–456, 1990.
2. Young T, Palta M, Pemsey J: The occurrence of sleep-disordered breathing among middle-aged adults. N Engl J Med 328:1230–1235, 1993.
3. Kamimi YV: Ambulatory treatment of sleep apnea syndrome with CO_2 laser—a review of 53 cases. J Fr Otorhinolaryngol 43(3):183–188, 1994.
4. Crumley RI, Stein S, Gamsu G: Determination of obstructive sites in obstructive sleep apnea. Laryngoscope 97:301–308, 1987.
5. Klitzman DA, Miller A: Obstructive sleep apnea syndrome. Mt Sinai J Med 61(2):113–122, 1994.
6. Hausfeld JN: Fiberoptic manipulation of the upper airway and the preoperative assessment for uvulopalatopharyngoplasty. Laryngoscope 95(6):738, 1985.
7. Sher AE, Thorpy MJ, Shrintzel RJ: Predictive value of Muller maneuver in selection of patients for uvulopalatopharyngoplasty. Laryngoscope 95:1483–1486, 1985.
8. Fujita S: Obstructive sleep apnea syndrome: Pathophysiology, upper airway evaluation and surgical treatment. ENT J 72(1):67–76, 1993.
9. Riley RW, Powell NB, Guilleminault C: Obstructive sleep apnea syndrome: A review of 306 consecutively treated surgical patients. Otolaryngol Head Neck Surg 108:117–125, 1993.
10. Rundell OH, Jones RK: Polysomnographic methods and interpretations. Otolaryngol Clin North Am 23(4):583–592, 1990.
11. Emsellem HA, Corson WA, Rappaport BA: Verification of sleep apnea using a portable sleep apnea screening device. South Med J 83:749–752, 1990.
12. Smith PL, Gold AR, Meyers DA: Weight loss in mildly to moderately obese patients with obstructive sleep apnea. Ann Intern Med 103:850–855, 1985.
13. Carenfelt C: Laser uvulopalatoplasty in treatment of habitual snoring. Ann Otol Rhinol Laryngol 100:451–454, 1991.
14. Koopman CF, Moran WB: Surgical management of obstructive sleep apnea. Otolaryngol Clin North Am 23(4):787–808, 1990.
15. Fujita S, Conway WA, Zorick FJ: Evaluation of the effectiveness of uvulopalatopharyngoplasty. Laryngoscope 95:70–74, 1985.
16. Davis JA, Fine ED, Maniglia AJ: Uvulopalatopharyngoplasty for obstructive sleep apnea in adults: Clinical correlation with polysomnographic results. ENT J 72(1):63–66, 1993.

Complications and Side Effects of Laser Surgery

CHARLES C. ALLING III, DDS, MS

When safety procedures and sound surgical principles are followed, the possibility of a complication or an undesired side effect from the surgical use of laser equipment is negligible. The surgeon who has both an appreciation of the physics of laser energy and an in-depth understanding of the biologic effects of the laser on soft and, in some instances, hard tissues will protect the patient and the surgical team from side effects and complications. As laser equipment improves and the techniques progress, the accuracy, versatility, and precision of laser energy will complement and, in many situations, supplant the scalpel.

Although the tactile and proprioceptive sensations associated with the scalpel and dissecting instruments are absent during surgery with lasers, complications associated with surgical technique are negligible. The laser, as Carlson observed, allows an accomplished surgeon to perform finer procedures.[1]

The usual undesired side effects and complications associated with laser surgery are related to the extremely high levels of thermal energy used. Burns are hazards to patients, the surgical team, and others in the range of the beam. This chapter intentionally overlaps with other chapters to reinforce the need for laser safety to prevent complications and undesired side effects of thermal energy and burns. Keon wrote, "Unless properly handled, lasers can harm the patient or the operating room personnel. The high-intensity beam can damage the eye, burn the skin, or ignite flammable materials (e.g., the endotracheal tube, breathing circuit, ointments, prepara-

tion solutions, or surgical drapes). The laser device is high-voltage equipment, and it can cause electrical burns, including electrocution, if it malfunctions or is mishandled. Injury can also occur by inhalation of noxious fumes produced by laser beam combustion of tissue. The laser beam is reflected by shiny flat or concave surfaces and when so deflected, it may go in unintended directions, potentially causing injury."[2]

THERMAL INJURIES

Undesired side effects and complications of laser surgery have a common denominator of thermal injury. Any laser produces heat in the target tissues with an ideal of instantaneous vaporization without effect on contiguous tissues. Some of the heat is dissipated as steam in the plume, and the remainder is absorbed by the surrounding tissues. Ideally, again, the tissue immediately adjacent to the site of the laser energy must both absorb the heat without an undue inflammatory response and conduct the heat away from the site by radiation and by the vascular system. As Chinn wrote, "This process has been termed *thermal* or *zonal necrosis* and is related directly to the amount of radiant energy the tissue receives."[3] Correctly controlled and applied laser energy produces a relatively narrow width of vaporized tissue and permits early repair, comparable to that produced by scalpel incision and better than that produced by electrocoagulation.[4, 5]

The superpulsed carbon dioxide lasers use the

highest irradiance level with the least exposure time, and thus, the thermal effect is minimal and the heat is diffused by the adjacent tissues. Surrounding the surgical site with gauzes soaked in a sterile solution and constant sponging of the surgical site helps dissipate the heat.

For the sake of completeness, it should be noted that the use of the contact lasers (neodymium: yttrium-aluminum-garnet [Nd:YAG] and holmium: yttrium-aluminum-garnet [Ho:YAG]) for temporomandibular joint arthroscopic surgery appears to control side effects and complications resulting from the generation of heat. For example, Bradrick and colleagues, using dogs as subjects during temporomandibular joint (TMJ) surgery with a Nd:YAG laser, noted: "Laser damage to the condylar marrow under an articular disk wound was unexpectedly found." They discussed a thermal blooming due to refraction of the energy at the saline and target interfaces; however, when the Nd:YAG laser was used in the contact technique within the TM joint, backscatter side effects and complications were controlled. They suggested that the addition of "... sapphire contact probes to the Nd:YAG fiber may eliminate deep-tissue effects and improve the safety of TMJ laser arthroscopy."[6]

In a definitive article, Hendler and colleagues reviewed the physical properties and biologic responses of the Ho:YAG laser in TMJ arthroscopy; they noted the minimal side effects, ease of handling the equipment, and the precision of operation that was possible using this type of laser.[7] As Koslin and Martin wrote, "Although not technically a 'cold laser,' the holmium laser produced almost no heat in the temporomandibular joint. The average intraarticular increase in temperature recorded was 10 degrees F (range 1.2 degrees F to 22.6 degrees F)."[8]

Overlasing the Surgical Target

Delivering laser energy at too high a level for the lesion being treated or for the planned reaction of tissues in the target area obviously will produce a burn. A char is produced during lasing that must be wiped away to prevent it being relased. If a char is exposed to continuing laser energy, temperatures measuring in the range of 4000°C are generated, which will conduct damaging thermal injuries to the contiguous normal tissues. The results include undesired side effects of delayed repair, pain, and edema.

Reflected Laser Energy

Sliney wrote, "The principal hazard to personnel in the vicinity of an operating laser results from specular (mirror-like) reflections."[9] Highly polished metallic surfaces and convex curvatures on instruments and equipment have no place in a laser surgery operating room. Reflections of laser beams from the polished surfaces and concentration of beams by convex curvatures produce uncontrolled and damaging laser energy.

Instruments used in laser surgery and in laser-assisted surgery should have surfaces that are ebonized or brushed in texture. When possible, the instruments should have convex curves to avoid the refocusing of laser beams that may occur by reflection off convex curves.

The Surgical Team

As summarized by Carlson, "If the surgeon and staff members interrupt the laser beam path, they may suffer burns as a result. These accidental encounters with the laser are commonplace, especially when the surgeon is working with a new or inexperienced assistant. The individuals in the procedure room must be familiar with the potential for harm and take appropriate evasive action."[1]

Explosive Potentials

Materials with an explosive potential when exposed to an igniting heat, such as inhalation anesthetic agents and topical anesthetic skin-freeze spray preparations, absolutely should not be used in conjunction with laser surgery and should not be stocked in cabinets that may be exposed to a laser beam.

Rectal gases have an explosive potential and should be controlled with preoperative preparation of the patient or, if necessary, by closing the rectum with moistened gauzes.

OCULAR INJURIES

Ocular injuries are a preeminent concern associated with laser surgery. The photoablative and thermal characteristics of the laser can produce, depending on the wavelength in use, corneal or retinal burns. The injury either to the lens or to the retina may be acute or incurred over time on a chronic basis.

The carbon dioxide laser, which has a longer wavelength, is absorbed by water, and this factor puts all surface areas at risk, but, especially, the cornea of the eye. Carbon dioxide laser energy produces corneal burns, ulcerations, and opacification.

Eye damage from impact of the Nd:YAG and

other lasers with shorter wavelengths typically may occur in the pigmented tissues of the retina, because frequencies less than 2.5 nm pass through the cornea and be absorbed by the dark pigment of the retina.

As emphasized throughout the writings and teachings associated with laser surgery, the use of protective eyewear specific to the laser wavelength in use is mandatory; the eyewear is equipped with side protectors to prevent damage from reflected laser energy. The eyewear must be used by the surgical team and others in the area. The patient's eyes are protected with either saline-soaked sponges placed over taped eyelids or appropriate protective eyewear.

Chronic injury to the retina may follow exposure of the eyes to ultraviolet light that is produced by carbon arcing. The carbon arcing, associated with extremely high temperatures when a char is lased, can produce cumulative damage to the retina, as may occur with welders; therefore, the eyewear should include a protective shield against ultraviolet light.

To decrease the probability of ocular damage from lasers, in addition to the usual protection of the patient and the laser surgical team, the laser system should be in a controlled access area. Warning signs should be placed at the entrance to the operating room, and protective wavelength-specific eyewear should be available at the entrance.

GENERAL ANESTHETIC AIRWAY

A major concern for general anesthesia in the presence of laser energy has been the possible ignition of the tube in the presence of flammable gases, which may produce a devastating blowtorch effect. The use of laser-resistant endotracheal tubes and the use of nitrogen or helium instead of nitrous oxide as the carrier gas have decreased the risk. [10–13]

Garry summarized the general anesthetic airway risks as follows, "Laser surgery on the airway is associated with a greater risk of fire and explosion than with its use elsewhere in the body with the possible exception of an unprepared large bowel. The patient is ventilated with an oxygen-rich atmosphere through conduits that are at least minimal flammable in the presence of a high ignition source. There have been many reports of fires in the airway with grave consequences caused by ignition of endotracheal tubes." [14]

Keon observed, "A devastating complication of laser surgery is ignition and burning of an endotracheal tube. Such laser-generated fire causes thermal and chemical injury. Direct thermal injury results from exposure to the flame, heating of the endotracheal tube, and the blowtorch effect that occurs due to the high concentration of oxygen. Chemical injury occurs with the inhalation of smoke, hydrogen chloride (polyvinylchloride combustion), and carbon monoxide (rubber combustion). The tube may be ignited indirectly by burning pieces of tissue that lie next to the tip or near an unprotected portion of the tube." [2]

If a tracheal fire should occur, the immediate removal of the burning endotracheal tube or catheter followed by mask ventilation and reintubation are performed on an emergency basis. The earliest objectives are to protect the trachea and lung from thermal injury, smoke, noxious fumes, and debris. [15]

INHALATION OF THE PLUME

The impact of laser beams on tissues produces a plume of superheated water vapor that contains particulate cellular matter. Protection from the plume, an irritant to the pulmonary tree and a carrier of particles of tissue and of microorganisms, is controlled by evacuation systems. Mancuso reported that, "It is possible to eliminate 98.6% of the laser plume using a laser plume evacuation device at a distance of 1.0 cm. This substantially decreases to 50% by lengthening the distance to a mere 2.0 cm." [16]

The usual surgical masks do not filter all of the particles, tissues, and microorganisms contained in the laser plume. Specially constructed laser surgical filtration masks that filter down to 0.1 μ provide protection to the surgical team.

The precautions of using specially designed masks are necessary to protect the pulmonary system from irritants and to decrease the possibility of an infection by microorganisms; for example, papillomavirus may survive a low-power laser beam used while eradicating a papilloma. In an outstanding review of three decades of dermatologic laser surgery, Alster and Kohn commented on the plume as follows: "Perhaps the most worrisome disadvantage of laser use is the unknown risk of inhalation of laser smoke." [17] When laser energy is used for dermabrasion, Wentzell and colleagues noted that particles with diameters between 0.1 and 1.0 μ could be found in the laser plume and may penetrate into distal lung branches; they referred to the particles as lung-damaging dust. [18] In addition to the irritants, intact human papillomavirus DNA and human immunodeficiency virus (HIV) have been isolated in the plume. [19–21]

SURGICAL SITE

Surgery is surgery, no matter how elegantly performed and no matter the cutting instrument used.

With laser surgery, there is a possibility of augmentation of undesired side effects of tissue responses and postoperative pain, comparable to that associated with surgery with a scalpel, especially if the application of the laser energy is not exact.

Hypertrophic Cutaneous Fibrosis

Following laser surgery through cutaneous tissues, hypertrophic scarring is the most frequent undesirable dermatologic side effect.[17] The thermal energy of the laser alters the contiguous tissues and sets the stage for hypertrophic scarring; the greater the depth of necrosis by the laser, the greater the alterations in the contiguous tissues. The total reparative cellular response produces irregular and often exuberant growth, resulting in the formation of excessive fibrosis. However, a carbon dioxide laser in the superpulsed mode produces the least amount of thermal damage because of its high radiance level and low exposure time. Reduction of thermal effects at the cellular level is aided by the use of saline-soaked gauze, which speeds intracellular cooling. If laser penetration is limited to the superficial fascia, scar tissue and fibrosis are negligible.

Postoperative Discomfort

Not surprisingly, postoperative pain is related to the thermal effects of lasers on the contiguous tissues. The greater the penetration of the laser energy, the greater the inflammatory response and the more intense the hyperesthesia. Penetration through the superficial fascia may permit herniation of adipose tissue, increased pain due to neuritic damage, and delayed healing due to thermal effects.

Infection

The usual preoperative and postoperative care of the surgical site, as for any type of surgery, should be performed. It is possible that the decreased vitality of the contiguous tissues, owing to the thermal damage, may provide a regional site for opportunist microorganisms to flourish if there has been contamination. Mancuso observed, "Because the laser itself is able to act as a sterilization medium, most soft tissue infections that do occur are caused by a break in asepsis postoperatively from an external source."[16]

A systemic infection secondary to laser surgery may be thwarted by the sealing of blood and lymphatic vessels during the vaporization of tissue. Kaminer and associates found the bacteremia in hamsters following incisions using carbon dioxide laser was not statistically different from the control (nonsurgery) group; however, significant bacteremia occurred following scalpel and electrosurgery.[22]

UNFOUNDED CONCERNS

The aura of new technology may produce unfounded apprehensions and claims of complications in relation to laser surgery.[9]

There is no scientific basis for believing lasers could be a hazard to a fetus. The misunderstanding probably is an outgrowth of confusion between laser radiation and ionizing radiation.

A visitor to a surgical area using laser surgery may believe that a malady arising months or years later was due to the hazards in the atmosphere resulting from laser beams. This unfounded association has occurred many times in industrial laser facilities.

REFERENCES

1. Carlson BA: Complications associated with laser surgery. Clin Podiatr Med Surg 4:823–828, 1987.
2. Keon TP: Anesthetic management during laser surgery. Int Anesthesiol Clin 30:99–107, 1992.
3. Chinn SD: Complications of surgery; safety, risks, and the plume. Clin Podiatr Med Surg 3:763–779, 1992.
4. Pogrel MA, Yen C-K, Hansen LS: A comparison of carbon dioxide laser, liquid nitrogen cryosurgery, and scalpel wounds in healing. Oral Surg Oral Med Oral Pathol 69:269–273, 1990.
5. Pogrel MA, McCracken KJ, Daniels TE: Histologic evaluation of the width of soft tissue necrosis adjacent to carbon dioxide laser incisions. Oral Surg Oral Med Oral Pathol 70:564–568, 1990.
6. Bradrick JP, Eckhauser ML, Indresano AT: Early response of canine temporomandibular joint tissues to arthroscopically guided neodymium:YAG laser wounds. J Oral Maxillofac Surg 50:835–842, 1992.
7. Hendler BH, Gateno J, Mooar P, Sherk HH: YAG laser arthroscopy of the temporomandibular joint. J Oral Maxillofac Surg 50:931–934, 1992.
8. Koslin MG, Martin JC: The use of holmium laser for temporomandibular joint arthroscopic surgery. J Oral Maxillofac Surg 51:122–123, 1993.
9. Sliney DH: Laser safety in general surgery. In Joffe SN (ed): Lasers in surgery. Baltimore, Williams & Wilkins, 1989, pp 16–23.
10. Burgess GE, LeJeune FE: Endotracheal tube ignition during laser surgery of the larynx. Arch Otolaryngol 106:561–562, 1979.
11. Hirshman CA, Smith J: Indirect ignition of the endotracheal tube during carbon dioxide laser surgery. Arch Otolaryngol 106:639–641, 1979.
12. Snow JC, Norton ML, Saluia TS, Estanislao AF: Fire hazard during CO_2 laser microsurgery on the larynx and trachea. Anesth Analg 55:146–147, 1976.
13. Cozine K, Rosenbaum LM, Askanazi J, Rosenbaum SH: Laser-induced endotracheal tube fire. Anesthesiology 55:683–685, 1981.
14. Garry BP: Anesthetic technique for safe laser use in surgery. Semin Surg Oncol 6:184–188, 1990.
15. Spiess BD, Ivankovich AD: Anesthetic management of laser airway surgery. Semin Surg Oncol 6:189–193, 1993.

16. Mancuso JE: Laser surgery. Clin Podiatr Med Surg 8:399–408, 1991.
17. Alster TS, Kohn SR: Dermatologic lasers: Three decades of progress. Int J Dermatol 31:601–610, 1992.
18. Wentzell JM, Robinson JK, Wentzell JR, et al: Physical properties of aerosols produced by dermabrasion. Arch Dermatol 125:1637–1643, 1989.
19. Gardon JM, O'Banion MK, Shelnitz LS, et al: Papillomavirus in the vapor of carbon dioxide–laser–treated verrucae. JAMA 259:1199–1202, 1988.
20. Sawchuck WS, Weber PJ, Lawy DR, et al: Infectious papillomavirus in the vapor of warts treated with carbon dioxide laser or electrocoagulation: Detection and protection. J Am Dermatol 20:41–49, 1989.
21. Baggish MS, Polesz BJ, Joret D, et al: Presence of human immunodeficiency virus DNA in laser smoke. Lasers Surg Med 11:197–203, 1991.
22. Kaminer R, Liebow C, Margarone JE, Zambon JJ: Bacteremia following laser and conventional surgery in hamsters. J Oral Maxillofac Surg 48:45–48, 1990.

BIBLIOGRAPHY

Catone, GA: Lasers in dentoalveolar surgery. Oral Surg Clin North Am 5:45–61, 1993.
Editor: Laser energy and its dangers to eyes. Health Devices 22:159–204, 1993.
Holmes JA: A summary of safety considerations for the medical and surgical practitioner. *In* Apfelberg DB (ed): Evaluation and installation of surgical laser systems. New York, Springer-Verlag, 1987, pp 69–95.
Nirankari VS, Richards RD: Complications associated with the use of neodymium:YAG laser. Ophthalmology 92:1371–1375, 1985.
Ossoff RH: Laser safety in otolaryngology—head and neck surgery: Anesthetic and educational considerations for laryngeal surgery. Laryngoscope 99:1–25, 1989.
Prendiville PL, McDonnell PJ: Complications in laser surgery. Int Ophthalmol Clin 32:179–204, 1992.
Schroder TM, Puolakkainen, Hahl J, Ramo OJ: Fatal air embolism as a complication of laser induced hyperthermia. Lasers Surg Med 2:183–185, 1989.

CHAPTER 15

Cutaneous Facial Laser Resurfacing

EDWARD HALUSIC JR, DMD

GUY A. CATONE, DMD

For hundreds of years humanity has made efforts to retard the aging process. They have ranged from the ancient Egyptians' use of oils, salt, and alabaster to improve the skin to Ponce de Leon's search for the Fountain of Youth.[1, 2] This search continues as the population continues to live longer. Current reports indicate that the over-65 age group is projected to increase to more than 20% of the population within the next 50 years. The life span has increased significantly. In 1965 the average life span was 65 years; in 1990 it was 78 years.[3] As a greater percentage of our population ages, there will be a greater demand for rejuvenation procedures as patients desire to look as good as they feel.

Chemical peeling and dermabrasion have been the workhorses of surgeons for treating rhytids, scars, and sun-damaged skin.[4] Rejuvenation of facial skin has been revolutionized with a new-generation laser that is an effective alternative to chemical peel and dermabrasion.[5, 6] In this chapter, we will discuss the rationale behind this new technology, its advantages and disadvantages, and its clinical applications.

LASER RESURFACING

Rationale

Laser surgery can be defined as tissue denaturation through the direct thermal effects of intense electromagnetic radiation.[7] The electromagnetic radiation of the carbon dioxide laser has a wavelength of 10,600 nm, its target tissue (chromophore) being water. Water, which constitutes 85% of soft tissues, absorbs the energy of the laser beam, causing the water to boil explosively and resulting in ablation of the tissue.[8] This concept has led to the use of the carbon dioxide laser for cutaneous disorders and intraoral lesions.[9, 10] However, many surgeons have realized that carbon dioxide lasers produce a significant amount of undesirable thermal trauma leading to scarring.[9, 11, 12] The scarring is caused by injury to the lower reticular dermis, which houses the adnexal structures capable of regenerating the epidermis.[13, 14] Injury to the lower reticular dermis is caused by conduction of heat from surrounding tissues causing coagulative necrosis. The key to laser resurfacing is to minimize thermal damage by ablating tissue faster than heat is conducted to surrounding tissues.[8] This ensures that coagulation is limited to the absorption length of the laser and is not undesirably extended to underlying tissues. The process by which heat is conducted to underlying tissues is called *thermal relaxation*.[8] Therefore, if one decreases or avoids thermal relaxation and delivers adequate pulse energy, tissue can be ablated in discrete layers down to the midreticular dermis, preserving the adnexal structures, thus permitting re-epithelialization with restoration of normal vertical polarity of the epidermis and elimination of pigmentary variations and keratoses.[4] Clinical improvement is also related to healing of the dermis. The appearance of new elastic fibers within the upper dermis, as well as the realignment of collagen fibers into the more parallel patterns of youthful skin, correlates with the clinical smoothing of skin.[4, 14]

Tissue has an inherent resistance to lateral heat conduction. It takes approximately 695 microseconds for heat at the site of impact to overcome tissue resistance and result in significant conduction to underlying tissues (thermal relaxation).[8, 15, 16] It has been shown in animal studies that pulse widths of 200 microseconds and 600 microseconds limit heat diffusion.[15, 17] It is thought that a pulse width less than 950 μ sec is short enough to prevent significant thermal trauma.[16] At this pulse width, the energy can be contained within the target tissue specific to the wavelength of the laser beam, thus increasing photovaporization. Conversely, if energy is delivered in a manner that significantly exceeds the thermal relaxation time, the energy is absorbed by the target tissue specific to the carbon dioxide wavelength *and* conducted into the underlying tissue, thus increasing photocoagulation and producing unwanted thermal necrosis.[7] This thermal diffusion can result in a band of thermal necrosis measuring 1 to 5 mm, as opposed to a narrow zone of thermal damage of 50 to 100 microns.[16] Although use of low-dose energies (fluences) has been advocated by some authors to treat thin epidermal lesions,[18–22] this low energy results in a nonspecific laser injury that is similar to tissue damage caused by a hot water bath or heated copper template.[23–25] The use of the carbon dioxide laser in such a nonablative manner results in a situation in which conduction is the only heat transfer process, thus causing desiccation of tissues, charring, and burning.[4, 16] Tissue ablation that is clean, bloodless, and char free requires that a single laser impact have enough fluence (250 millijoules minimum at a 3.0-mm spot size[26]) to vaporize tissue so that remnants can be removed before heat is conducted into adjacent nontarget tissue. To put it another way, the ablation front travels faster than the thermal conduction front. Effective pulsing also requires a frequency of less than 1000 pulses per second and a pulse length of less than one third of the time between pulses,[26] which gives the tissue appropriate cooling time between pulses, thus decreasing thermal conduction.

It has been shown that high power densities (irradiance) result in less tissue injury than attempting to ablate tissue at lower power densities.[8, 27, 28] Thus, combining the requirements of a pulse duration shorter than the thermal relaxation time to minimize thermal trauma and high peak powers to maximize tissue vaporization led to the development of superpulsed lasers. Most superpulsed lasers, however, have inadequate energy per pulse to ablate tissue. Therefore, to accumulate enough heat for vaporization to occur, the pulses must be spaced relatively close together so that tissue cannot cool between pulses.[16] The disadvantage of this type of vaporization is conduction of heat deep or lateral to the intended target, creating thermal necrosis (Fig. 15–1). To solve the problem of undesirable thermal damage, the idea of superpulsing was further modified with the introduction of the UltraPulse laser by Coherent Medical Lasers. This carbon dioxide laser

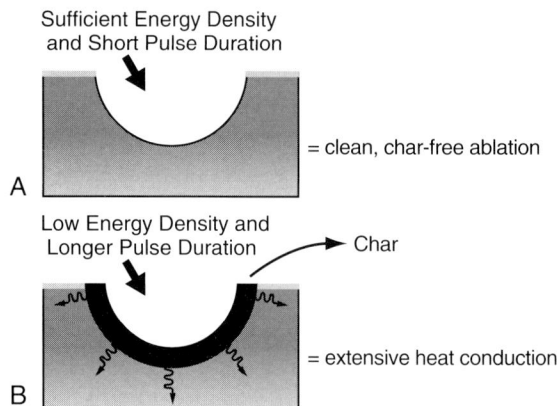

FIGURE 15–1. The degree of thermal damage is depicted with different types of lasers. *A,* The pulse duration is less than the thermal relaxation time of tissue, and the energy density is sufficient to cause clean, char-free ablation of tissue at the intended target without significant thermal damage extending to adjacent tissues. *B,* With lower energy density, and a longer pulse duration as provided by superpulse or continuous-wave technology, the intended target is ablated but not without extending thermal damage to adjacent tissues. (Adapted with permission from Reid R: Physical and surgical principles governing carbon dioxide laser surgery on the skin. Dermatol Clin 9:297, 1991.)

enables the practitioner to ablate the target tissue while minimizing thermal damage to surrounding tissues.[8] The UltraPulse laser fulfills the requirement of high power densities with energies five to seven times greater than those of conventional superpulsed lasers. It also fulfills the requirement of a short pulse duration by keeping it under 1 millisecond.

Advantages of Carbon Dioxide Laser for Resurfacing

The UltraPulse laser has several advantages over conventional resurfacing procedures such as dermabrasion and chemical peeling.[6, 7, 9] There is extreme precision of depth[13, 29, 30] that can be monitored in a bloodless field owing to photocoagulation of blood vessels 0.5 mm in diameter or smaller.[4, 9, 28, 31–34] Visualization of the endpoint is good although dependent on operator experience. Unlike dermabrasion or chemical peel, laser resurfacing affords immediate visual assessment of the result so large or very small areas can be further modified as needed. Also unlike dermabrasion, there is no blood spatter; thus, the risk of viral transmission through blood-borne contaminants is decreased.[26, 35] It appears to be much safer than dermabrasion in the periocular and perioral areas as the risk of damaging the delicate lids or lips with rotary instruments is avoided. Additionally, variables are applicable to dermabrasion, such as doing it with or without freezing the skin. The depth of freeze and the number of times the area is frozen introduce different degrees of tissue injury. Instrumentation can vary from a wire brush to a diamond fraise, which can interfere with the standardization of treatment.[14] There are reports that there is much less risk of hypopigmentation as compared with dermabrasion.[35, 36] Also, it is reported that the incidence of hyperpigmentation is rare.[35] When it does occur, it is reported to resolve spontaneously, or with the help of melanocyte-suppressing compounds such as hydroquinone.[5, 6, 26]

With respect to chemical peeling, systemic risks such as renal, cardiac, or possible allergic reactions are avoided. Standardization of treatment with chemical peel is limited by multiple factors, including the type and concentration of chemicals used, the skin preparation performed before peeling, the method of application of the chemicals, and the skin contact time of the chemicals.[26] Additionally, when the laser-resurfacing procedure is completed there is no chemical damage that can continue to occur in the remaining tissue. Other advantages include a very low incidence of hypertrophic scarring.[35] It has also been reported that there is less pain[4] and less swelling with laser resurfacing, owing to the laser's ability to seal small nerve endings and lymphatics.[4, 35, 37, 38] Patients are reported to recover more rapidly[26] because of decreased swelling, decreased pain, and fairly rapid re-epithelialization of 7 to 10 days.[6, 26, 36]

Disadvantages include the cost of the equipment, but this factor can be balanced by the increase in patient procedures. In the authors' experience, patients seem to accept laser resurfacing much more readily than chemical peel or dermabrasion. Additionally, although we do not consider this a disadvantage, the learning curve must be addressed in a very deliberate manner, whether or not an operator has experience with other resurfacing procedures or with other laser procedures. For older technologies such as continuous-wave and superpulse lasers there is a much steeper learning curve. It is difficult to teach, and visualization of the endpoint can be a real challenge. With the newer UltraPulse laser technology, no less judgment or knowledge is required but the method is easier to learn and to perform.[39]

Indications

The UltraPulse laser has many indications, including treatment of facial rhytids, facial scarring, and aging or sun-damaged skin.[5, 9, 16, 26, 27] Perioral wrinkles, vertical lip furrows, forehead wrinkles, crow's feet, and infraorbital rhytids have all been treated successfully with the UltraPulse laser (Fig. 15–2).[26, 35] Rhytids related to muscle activity, such

as glabellar lines, forehead wrinkles, and nasolabial folds, will not respond as favorably over the long term as lines caused by sun or nonmuscular activity; however, improvement can be significant and can last up to several years.[26, 40] Also, patients who have had other types of resurfacing procedures such as chemical peel or dermabrasion may have different degrees of tissue fibrosis and the result with laser resurfacing on these patients may be less impressive.[26] Laser resurfacing is not contraindicated for these patients provided they have healed without scarring from previous procedures.

Transconjunctival lower lid blepharoplasty in conjunction with infraorbital resurfacing has replaced the external skin muscle incision blepharoplasty in many instances.[35] The transconjunctival approach avoids violating the orbital septum and avoids skin and muscle excision, all of which can lead to unfavorable scleral show and ectropion.[35, 41–43] The combination of lower transconjunctival blepharoplasty with simultaneous cutaneous resurfacing provides excellent results with minimal complications.[35]

Other indications for laser resurfacing include treatment of actinic cheilitis (Fig. 15–3),[9, 26, 44–50, 51] rhinophyma,[9, 26, 52–65] removal of eyeliner tattoo,[9, 66] epidermal nevi,[9, 67, 68] xanthelasma (Fig. 15–4),[9, 16, 26] syringomas, and sebaceous hyperplasia.[26] Resurfacing of scars from acne, trauma, and surgery using the UltraPulse carbon dioxide laser has been reported to have results superior to those of other forms of treatment. Resurfacing following initial wound repair or secondary scar revision should be scheduled within 6 to 8 weeks to maximize collagen reorganization during normal wound repair to reduce the amount of visible scar tissue.[26]

The carbon dioxide laser resurfacing procedure is not indicated for telangiectasia[9, 69, 70] or port-wine stain.[9, 71–74] These vascular lesions are better treated with the flashlamp-pumped pulsed-dye laser.[75] Hypertrophic or erythematous or pigmented scars can be treated with the flashlamp-pumped pulsed-dye laser.[75] Thin, flat epidermal pigmented lesions such as café-au-lait macules, or lentigines respond better to the Q-switched Nd:YAG laser.[9, 76, 77] Black and blue pigmented tattoos can be successfully removed using the Q-switched alexandrite laser,[78] whereas red tattoo pigment seems to be best removed with the flashlamp-pumped pulsed-dye laser.[79]

Patient Selection

A thorough history and an examination are critical, because prevention is the best treatment for hypertrophic scarring. Any history of illness or treatment that could affect the function of the adnexal structures is a red flag. Patients taking isotreti-

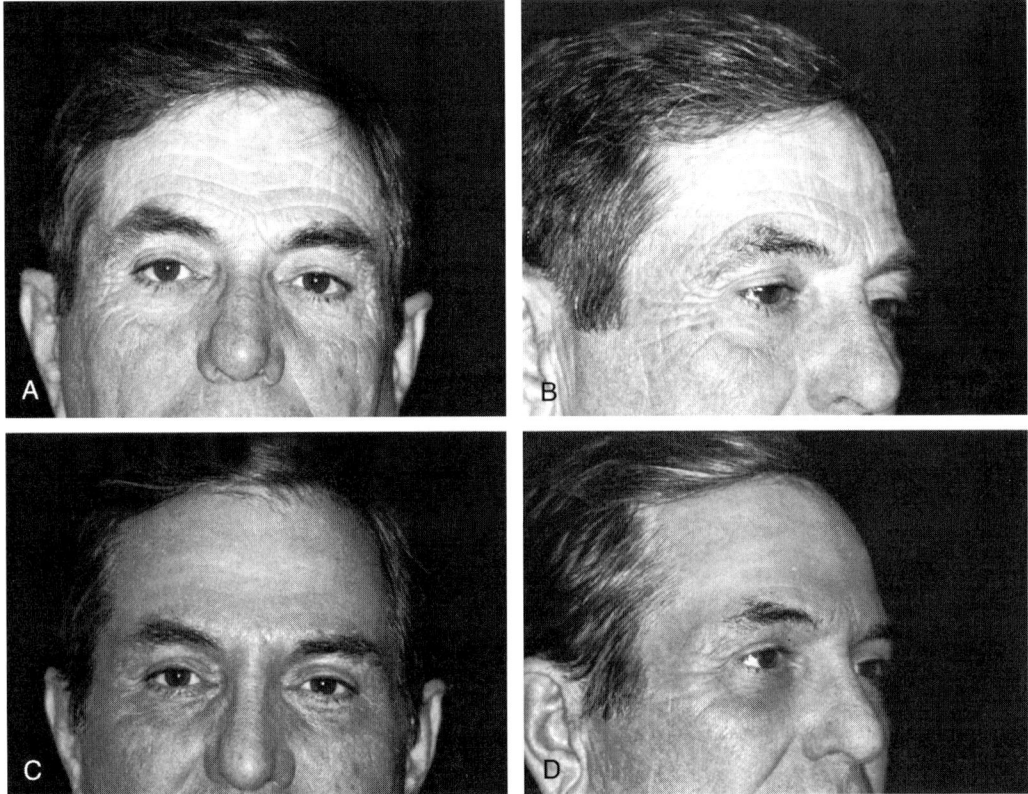

FIGURE 15–2. This patient has undergone laser resurfacing of the forehead and infraorbital areas in conjunction with a bilateral cervicofacial rhytidectomy. Note the significant effacement of forehead and periorbital rhytids when comparing the preoperative photos (*A* and *B*) with the postoperative photos (*C* and *D*). (Courtesy of Dr. Tom Faerber, Midwest Facial Surgery, Kansas City, Kansas.)

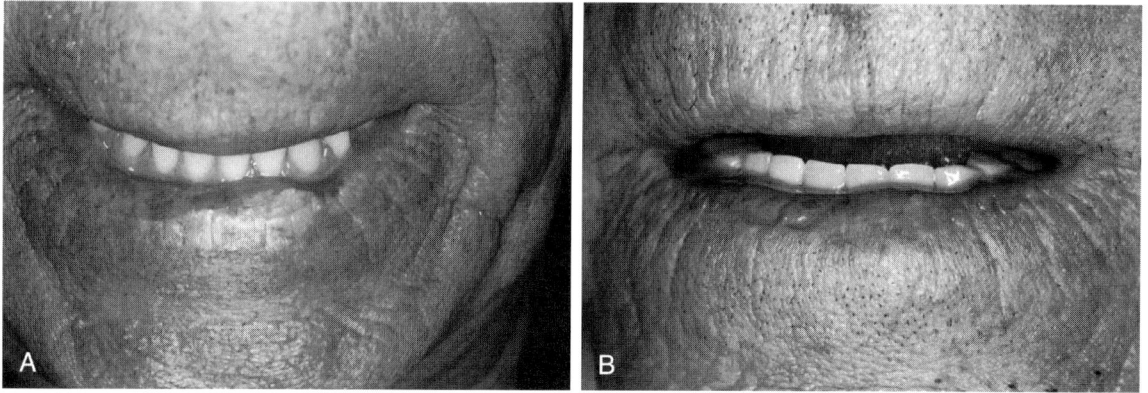

FIGURE 15–3. This patient had a diagnosis of actinic cheilitis. He was treated with UltraPulse laser therapy with two passes at 200 millijoules and a density of 7 with the computer pattern generator set at pattern 3, size 4 (34 in Fig. 15–10*B*), and a third pass with 150 millijoules with a density of 4 using the same pattern. *A,* Preoperative appearance. *B,* Postoperative appearance.

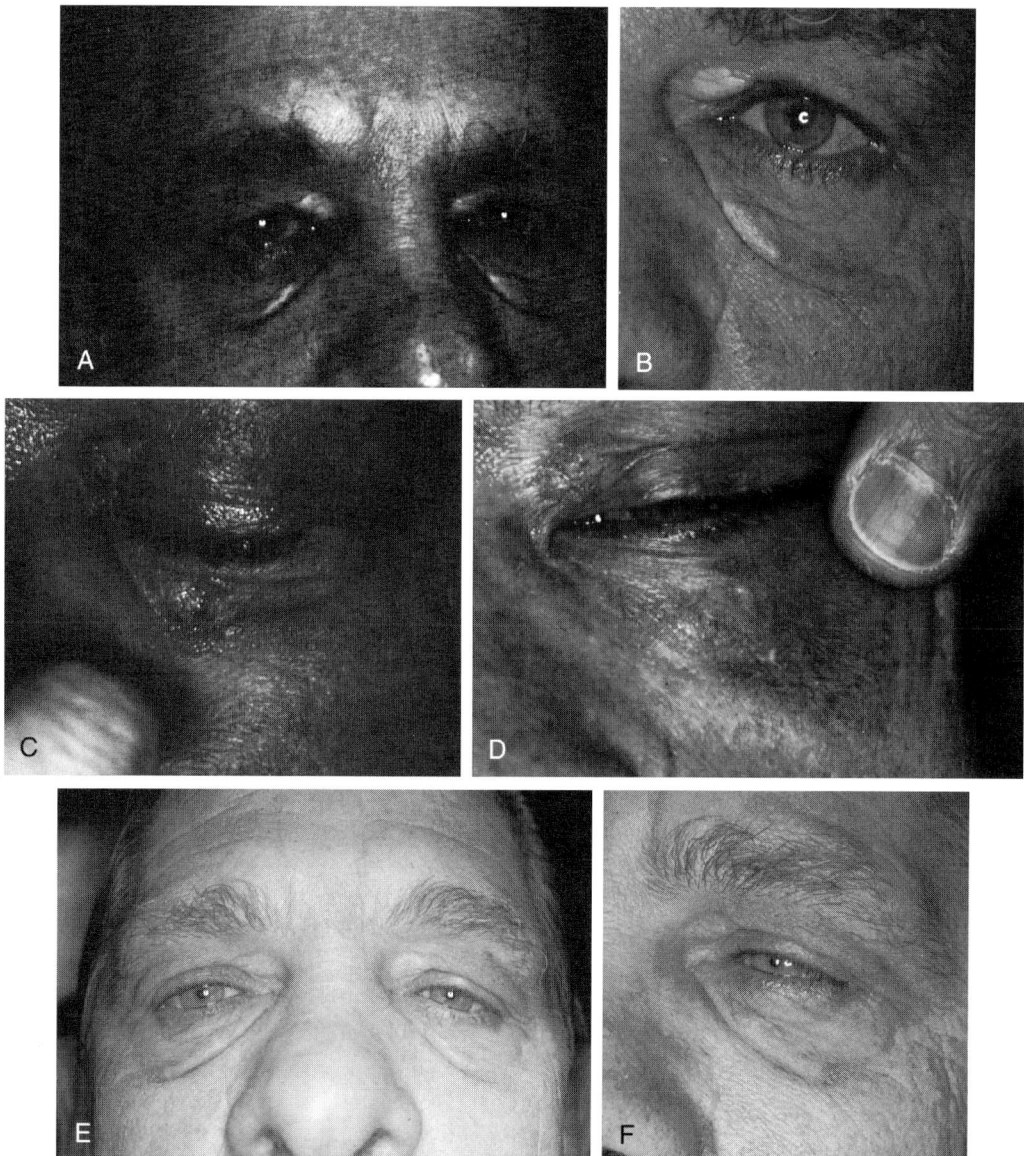

FIGURE 15–4. This patient was treated for xanthelasma using the UltraPulse laser. Four passes with the 3.0-mm handpiece at 4 W (16 pulses/sec) were used. *A* and *B,* Preoperative appearance. *C,* Immediate postoperative appearance. *D,* Ten days postoperative appearance. *E* and *F,* Three weeks postoperative appearance.

noin (Accutane) should not be considered candidates for this procedure within a minimum of 2 years from treatment.[26] Because it is impossible to predict the recovery of adnexal structures when the patient previously used isotretinoin, it is imperative that a test spot be done before any laser resurfacing. Because the risk of hypertrophic scarring is considerably increased, it may be appropriate to eliminate isotretinoin patients as candidates for facial resurfacing. This dictum also holds true for patients who have had electrolysis of certain facial areas, usually the upper lip. Patients with a history of scleroderma also have questionable adnexal function and should be excluded as candidates, as should those who have scarring secondary to a burn. Anyone with a history of hypertrophic scarring or keloid formation should be approached with extreme caution. Patients who have had radiation therapy to facial areas, including those with a history of superficial x-ray treatment for acne, need to be assessed carefully by evaluating the presence of vellus hairs or by punch biopsy. Additionally, the neck should be avoided in resurfacing, owing to the potential for increased scarring secondary to the decreased concentration of adnexal structures.[14]

As with chemical peel and dermabrasion the ideal patients for laser resurfacing are fair skinned.[14, 26] Darker skin types can also be treated with satisfactory results, but the tendency to develop transient postinflammatory hyperpigmentation is greater.[26, 80] These pigmentation changes usually resolve spontaneously, but hydroquinone can be used immediately (10 to 14 days) after re-epithelialization to resolve it faster.[5, 26, 36, 80] There is no reported experience with type 4 skin (Table 15–1), and caution must be exercised here. Until there are more case reports of blacks, the senior author believes that the risk of hypopigmentation is too great to warrant the procedure.

Preoperative Consultation

One of the major goals of the preoperative consultation is to find out what the patient's expectations are and to assess how realistic they are. Computer imaging is very helpful as a communication

tool in this regard; however, caution must be exercised when using the computer, because it is easy with a wisk of the stylus to overcorrect the patient far beyond realistic expectations. The surgeon needs to be conservative when generating the postoperative prediction images. The patient will always be happy if the actual improvements are better than the prediction shown in the computer image. On the other hand, they will generally be dissatisfied if the actual results are not as good as the predicted ones. Along these lines, specific informed consent for the computer imaging should be used before reviewing predicted computerized results with the patient. The informed consent should indicate that the images are predictions only and that no guarantees can be made about the final result.

After the patient's goals have been discussed and the patient appears to have accepted reasonable expectations, informed consent should be discussed. This should include a slide or photo presentation to the patient indicating what he or she will look like for the first 7 days, and additional slides or photos to show healing at 2, 4, 8, and 12 weeks. This visual presentation is critical for enabling the patient to understand that the skin will be red for at least several weeks, and indeed, the redness, which most likely is secondary to capillary ingrowth, may last 3 to 6 months.

It should also be emphasized to the patient that a conservative treatment is one that reduces the risk of scarring and that additional therapy may be necessary several months afterward if the patient desires further improvement. There is evidence to support waiting at least 6 months before repeating the procedure, because significant dermal vascularity was observed when it was repeated at 3 months.[6] Additionally, there is evidence that in some patients, improvement from baseline is greater at 3 and 6 months than at 1 month after laser resurfacing.[6]

All potential complications should be discussed, including mild hypopigmentation, hyperpigmentation (usually transient and self-limiting), scarring, redness that will last several weeks or months, induration that may need to be treated with steroid injections, and increased scleral show or ectropion for infraorbital procedures.[5, 6, 26, 35, 36, 80] Scleral show and ectropion are usually transient but may be more pronounced if infraorbital laser resurfacing is performed before correcting any lid margin laxity.[35] Additionally, lag ophthalmus will sometimes occur with blunting of the lateral canthus when resurfacing the infraorbital areas. This usually resolves in 2 to 4 weeks.

It is critical to emphasize to the patient the importance of postoperative care, both in the office and at home, and the need for frequent follow-up visits

TABLE 15–1. Fitzpatrick Skin Types

Type	Hair Color	Skin Color	Eye Color
1	Red	Light	Blue/green
2	Blonde	Light	Blue
3	Brown	Medium	Brown
4	Brown/black	Medium/dark	Brown/black
5	Black	Dark	Dark
6	Black	Black	Black

within the first week. The specifics of this care will be discussed later in this chapter.

Visual Endpoints and Depths of Wounding

The goal of laser resurfacing is to ablate tissue to a level no deeper than the midreticular dermis. Injury to the lower reticular dermis damages adnexal structures and causes scarring. To avoid this unfortunate sequela, endpoint visual guidelines have been published. Although these guidelines are helpful, they are not absolutely definitive, because some discrepancies exist, as discussed later.

Using a pulse duration of 600 to 900 milliseconds at an energy level of 500 millijoules with a 3-mm spot size, the laser usually ablates the epidermis with entrance into the papillary dermis (Figs. 15–5 and 15–6). The color attributed to the papillary dermis by some authors is pink[7, 36]; others describe a gray tinge.[4] The lower papillary dermis has been described as yellow.[36] A chamois cloth appearance has been attributed to the deeper papillary dermis,[7] midpapillary dermis,[36] and the reticular dermis.[4] A waterlogged cotton thread appearance has also been used to describe the midreticular dermis.[7] Our experience indicates a pink color for papillary dermis.

Once into the papillary dermis, further laser bursts enable the surgeon to visualize actual contraction of the collagen. Once the surgeon can no longer visualize contraction of the tissue (collagen shortening), a yellow endpoint should be visible. This yellow endpoint must be used with caution in areas of the face with thinner dermis, as one may actually be in the lower reticular dermis (Fig. 15–7) when it is seen. This level of penetration is best avoided, as one is getting precariously close to adnexal structures. Ablation to this level is extremely deep and can lead to significant postoperative scarring.

The foregoing discussion of visual endpoints in relation to depth of wounding should not be relied on in cookbook fashion. It must be emphasized that the dermis varies in thickness in various parts of the face. With each pass of the laser the endpoints must be visualized and interpreted by the operator to determine the histologic effect that has been achieved. For example, on some areas of the face it is possible to perform six or seven passes using the same laser parameters for each pass and still be within the upper reticular dermis, whereas in other areas the level of ablation would be into fat. Obviously, surgeons can get more aggressive with treatment as their caseload increases, giving them the experience to be confident in interpreting the various levels. It is always better to be cautious and err

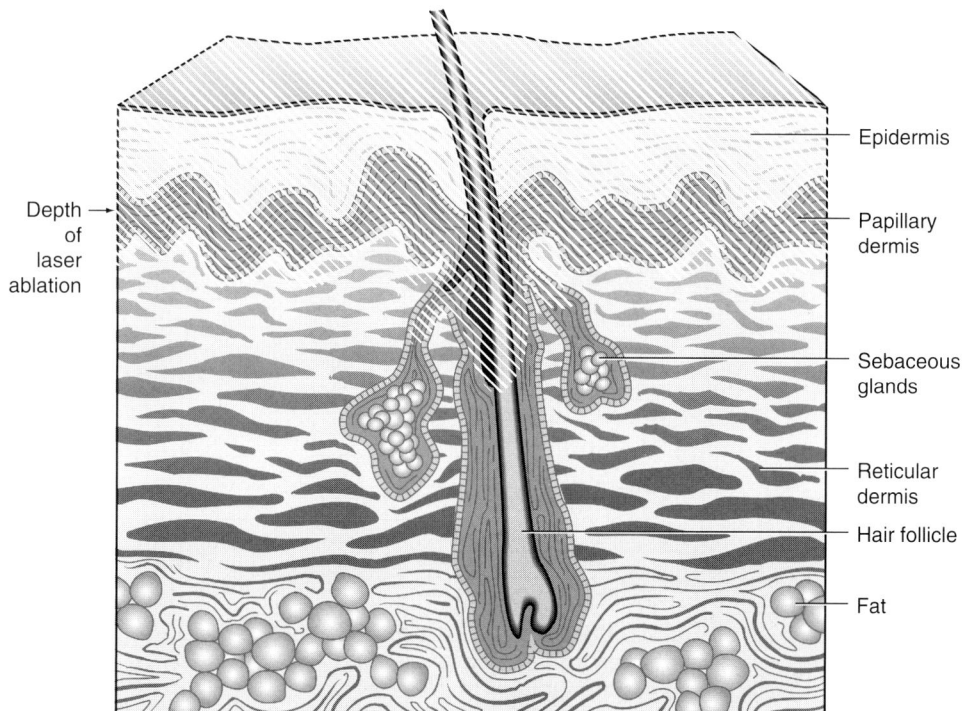

FIGURE 15–5. This drawing depicts ablating the epidermis with entrance into the papillary dermis. Hatch marks indicate area of laser ablation. (Adapted with permission from Reid R: Physical and surgical principles governing carbon dioxide laser surgery on the skin. Dermatol Clin 9:297, 1991.)

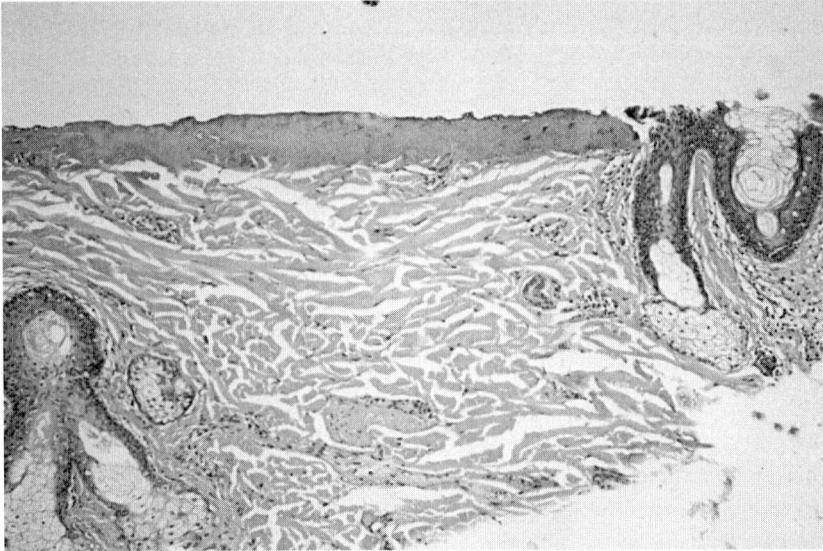

FIGURE 15–6. This photomicrograph of laser-treated skin from the forehead shows ablation of the epidermis with entrance into the papillary dermis. The reticular layer is not entered into, and this level of ablation is well above the adnexal structures. The depth of this injury is 0.06 mm. (The skin was treated with two passes using a Coherent UltraPulse Laser 5000c with a density of 9, and millijoules of 300 on the first pass, and 250 on the second pass.) (Histology courtesy of Dr. Jerry E. Bouquot, Director, Head and Neck Diagnostics of America, Morgantown, West Virginia. Laser courtesy of Dr. Marion M. Vujevich, Pittsburgh, Pennsylvania.)

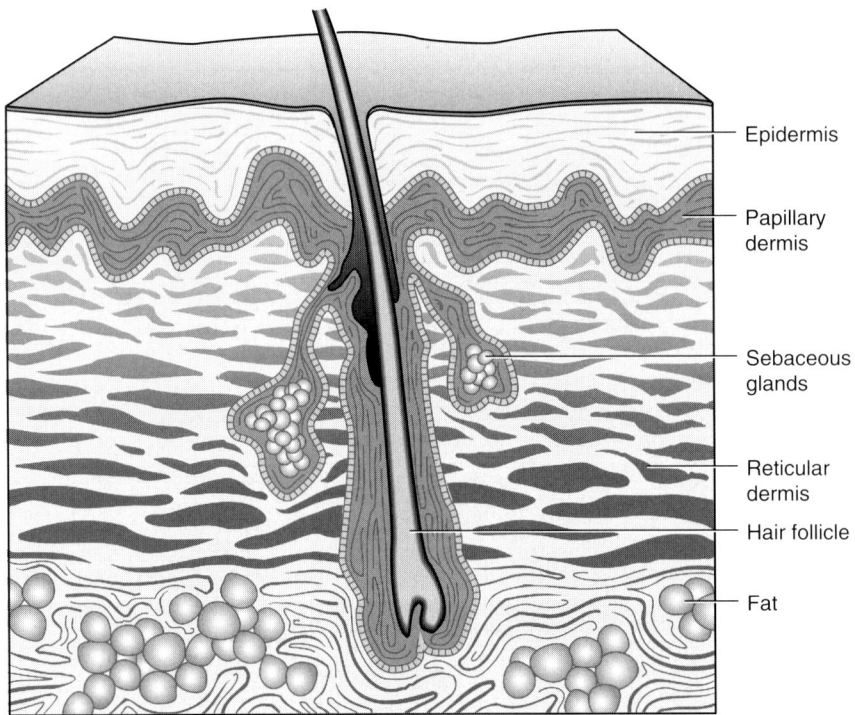

FIGURE 15–7. This drawing depicts thermal damage caused by heat conduction down to the deep reticular dermis. Injury at this depth is dangerous because increased scarring will result from damage to the adnexal structures. Without the keratinocytes housed within the adnexal structures, re-epithelialization will not occur. Exposing these skin appendages is equivalent to the creation of a third-degree burn. (From Reid R: Physical and surgical principles governing carbon dioxide laser surgery on the skin. Dermatol Clin 9:297, 1991.)

on the conservative side. Repeated laser resurfacing procedures in an attempt to improve the result are always accepted better by the patient than a scar.

Procedure

The procedural protocol must take into account laser safety. Every office using lasers should have a designated laser safety officer, and routine safety measures need to be followed. A written policy is essential and should be prepared and discussed with all staff members before the first in-office laser procedure. Fire and ocular injury are two significant risks that must be treated with great respect. The fire prevention standards dictated by the American National Standards Institute[81] require that the patient be draped with wet towels. Some practitioners prefer draping with aluminum foil, because of the possible discomfort to the patient as the wet towels saturate through the drapes. This has been solved by placing an inexpensive plastic waterproof drape over the patient before draping with wet towels. Wet towels are preferred because it has been observed that the aluminum foil does not always stay in place and could expose the patient's underlying hair or surgical bonnet. Inadvertent or misguided firing of the laser could ignite the patient's hair or bonnet. If aluminum foil is used, the dull side should be placed facing outward to decrease the chance of beam reflection (Fig. 15–8).

Other fire safety precautions need to be taken, including having available a fire extinguisher and a bowl of water in the operating room. Of course, the best way to fight a fire is to prevent it. Prevention should include avoiding surgical scrub or prepara-tion solutions that are flammable, such as acetone, Hibiclens, or any alcohol-based solution. Additionally, oxygen should be used with care because it supports combustion. If intravenous sedation is used, the nasal or oral cannula can be used to deliver supplemental oxygen before lasing begins. If the Po_2 decreases to a level at which supplemental oxygen is necessary, lasing can cease until the patient is properly oxygenated. If a patient cannot be treated without supplemental oxygen the nasal or oral cannula will have to be covered with either aluminum foil or wet drapes. Extreme care must be taken while lasing so that the laser beam does not encroach on or cross the oxygen supply, lest serious consequences occur. For patients undergoing general endotracheal anesthesia, special laser-safe anode tubes are preferred.[28]

Ocular injury—to both patient and operator—is certainly avoidable. Plastic glasses with side shields for the operating personnel are mandatory. Proper signage on the operating room door with an extra pair of safety glasses hanging by the sign is an essential reminder to anyone entering the operating suite that eye protection is needed. Glass prescription lenses can be shattered by a high power density beam and should be avoided.

Eye protection for the patient should include "sunnies" (see Fig. 15–8) if the laser will not be used in the periorbital areas. For periorbital resurfacing procedures, corneal metal eye shields need to be used (Fig. 15–9). Plastic corneal protectors should never be used, as the energy produced by the laser may melt them, resulting in thermal or mechanical damage to the eye.

Anesthesia can consist of only local analgesia, although this is generally reserved for smaller cos-

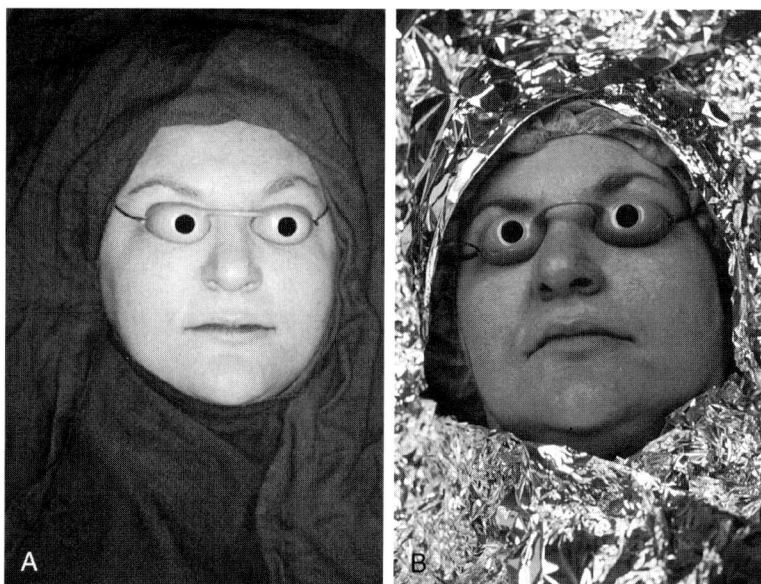

FIGURE 15–8. Proper draping of the patient is shown in *A*. Note how the wet towels fit snugly around the patient. In *B*, the aluminum foil has a tendency to migrate because of its stiffness. This exposes the patient's surgical bonnet or hair thus increasing the danger of an aberrant laser beam causing a fire. The aluminum foil also has its shiny side out. This is improper. If aluminum foil is used, the dull side should be facing outward. Also note the patient's safety lenses.

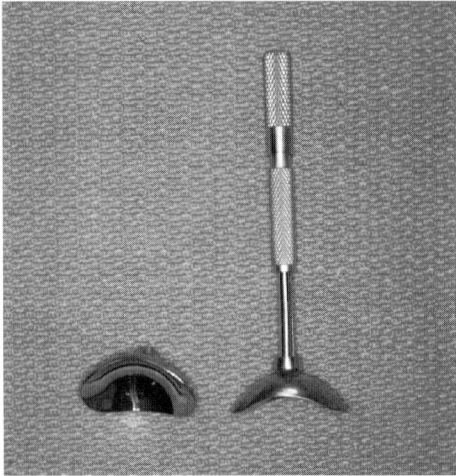

FIGURE 15–9. Eye protection is an absolute necessity when performing laser surgery. These stainless steel scleral shields are useful when performing periorbital laser resurfacing. They have a polished inside surface where they contact the cornea, and a nonreflective, matte finish on the outside.

metic units such as perioral or periocular areas. As the cosmetic resurfacing procedure begins to involve multiple cosmetic units, intravenous sedation is preferred. Because most oral and maxillofacial surgeons are well versed in anesthesia, details of regional blocks and intravenous anesthesia are not discussed in this chapter.

Although there is some disagreement over routine pretreatment of the skin with topical tretinoin, glycolic acid,[26] and hydroquinone, there appears to be good rationale for the use of these agents.[5, 36, 80, 81, 82] Studies show that topical tretinoin in 0.1% cream applied for 2 weeks before a 35% trichloroacetic acid peel or dermabrasion reduces healing time.[83–85] This may be due to widened vascular lumina or true angiogenesis secondary to the topical tretinoin, which most likely increases the response of inflammatory mediators that function as chemoattractants for neutrophils, macrophages, and lymphocytes.[82] Additionally, it has been shown by electron microscopy that topical tretinoin increases collagen formation with increased fibroblasts.[82] Glycolic acid treatment is also thought to increase angiogenesis, collagen formation, and epidermal cohesion.[86] Based on this information, pretreatment with topical tretinoin and glycolic acid most likely increases the rate of healing, and, therefore, should reduce the rate of complications.

Hydroquinone interferes with the melanocyte system, resulting in decreased production of melanin. Because melanin is distributed mainly in the basal and suprabasal keratinocytes that are removed with the epidermis during resurfacing, one may question the value of preoperatively depressing pro-

duction of melanin. Melanin, however, is also found in the lower levels of the dermis,[14] so it may be useful to decrease melanin production preoperatively. It is a definite advantage to use hydroquinone postoperatively after re-epithelialization is complete (in 7 to 14 days), to decrease the risk of hyperpigmentation.

The patient is also premedicated with acyclovir (Zovirax) beginning the day before surgery using 200 mg five times per day and continuing for 7 to 10 days until re-epithelialization is complete. It is started 24 hours before surgery to establish steady-state plasma levels by the day of surgery.[87] Premedicating with acyclovir is necessary because an outbreak of herpes can create significant complications that result in delayed healing, significant pain, and scarring. If herpes does occur postoperatively, the dosage of acyclovir should be increased to 400 mg five times per day.

Immediately before the procedure, the patient is also premedicated with an antibiotic, usually a cephalosporin. This is usually continued for 7 to 10 days until re-epithelialization is nearly complete. Steroids are also given preoperatively to help decrease postoperative edema in a dose of 0.5 mg/kg up to 20 mg intravenously for Decadron. Decadron can also be prescribed postoperatively in a dose of 8 mg b.i.d. for 5 days.

After appropriate evaluation, informed consent, premedication, and anesthesia, laser resurfacing can begin. The skin is prepped with an alcohol-free solution such as Betadine or pHisoHex. In addition to avoiding alcohol-based preps such as Hibiclens, any other preparation (e.g., acetone) that is flammable or will support combustion should be avoided.

The resurfacing procedure should be performed in discrete cosmetic units. It is acceptable to do small areas in Fitzpatrick type 1 and type 2 skin (see Table 15–1), but the patient needs to be informed that some hyperpigmentation may occur and may be noticeable. There is a much better chance of concealing color change such as hyperpigmentation if the entire cosmetic unit is done. Hyperpigmentation is self-limiting and will resolve with time. It can resolve sooner—or even be avoided—if 4% hydroquinone is started approximately 10 to 15 days after resurfacing, at which time re-epithelialization should be complete. In addition to the hydroquinone, patients are again given topical retinoids and glycolic acid following re-epithelialization.

The actual laser resurfacing can be performed with either a 3-mm handpiece, which lays down single bursts of laser energy, or a computer pattern generator (CPG), which lays down multiple bursts of laser energy using a 2.25-mm spot that is preset to a specific pattern and density (Fig. 15–10). The CPG is much more efficient, and is associated with

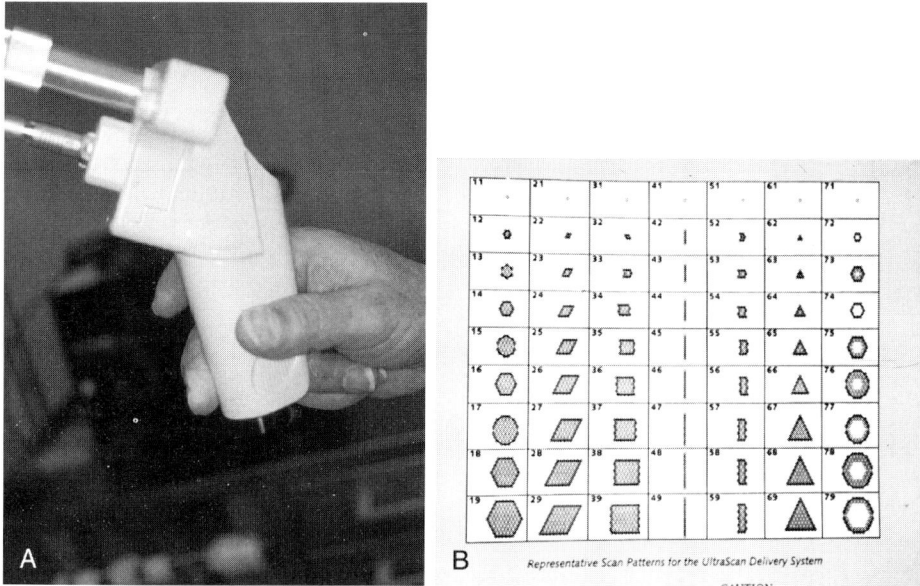

FIGURE 15–10. The computer pattern generator (CPG) *(A)* lays down multiple bursts of laser energy according to the preselected size, pattern, and density. The patterns available are seen in *B.*

greater safety of depth because it affords more control over density. This results in more uniform distribution of energy, which correlates with greater uniformity of tissue wounding.[39] Also, the CPG helps make the procedure less operator dependent because the density and speed of the laser bursts are preset and do not depend on the operator's hand movement (Figs. 15–11 and 15–12).

Finally, the CPG markedly reduces the time it takes to complete a procedure.[39] This results in less anesthesia time for the patient and less operating time for patient, physician, and staff. The parame-

ters that the surgeon controls during the resurfacing are millijoules per pulse and wattage. In addition, pattern shape, size, and density need to be selected for the CPG (Fig. 15–13).

Millijoules per pulse is the fluence, or the amount of energy that is going to strike the target. The range of millijoules used is 250 to 500 millijoules when using the 3.0-mm single-burst handpiece. When the CPG is used one must take into account a smaller focal spot of 2.25 mm. Because the energy per pulse of the laser will now be concentrated within a smaller diameter spot, it will be necessary

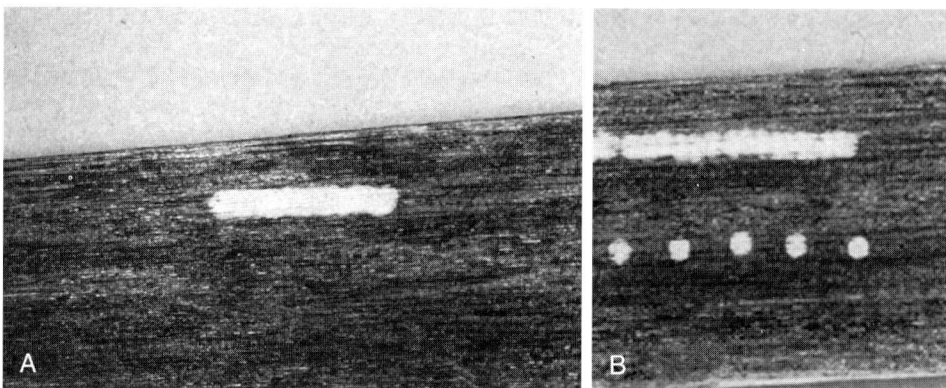

FIGURE 15–11. These three linear patterns were created using the single-spot handpiece. The millijoules (400 millijoules) and wattage (4 W) were the same. The only difference is the rate of hand movement. Note that the dots get closer together as the speed of the hand decreases. In *A*, hand speed was very slow in creating a solid groove in the wood without any evidence of individual spots. In *B*, the top pattern indicates a faster hand speed, and some dots are recognizable. The bottom pattern indicates an even faster hand speed, resulting in individual dots. Both the density and the amount of char are related to speed of hand movement. If one significantly overlaps the spots, charring will occur, resulting in a deeper wound through conduction. This means that the depth of the wounding is related not only to the millijoules but also to the speed of hand movement, making the procedure more operator dependent.

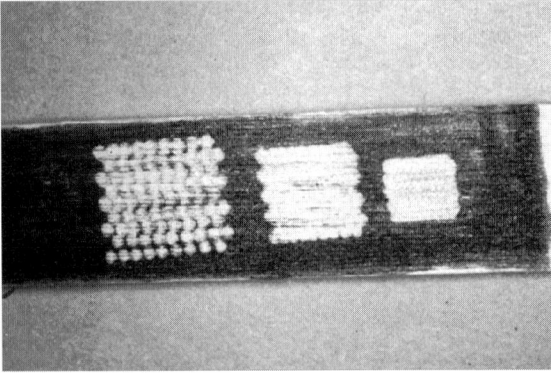

FIGURE 15–12. The CPG created these tongue blade patterns. This is very rapid fire because the wattage determines the rate of fire, and this wattage setting was 100 W. The rate is over 300 pulses per second. Millijoules determine the strength of the laser burst and can be correlated with the depth of wounding. Even though the wattage creates a rapid fire situation, the CPG creates a higher margin of safety because the density is preset and the hand does not move in order to create the above pattern. Unlike the single-spot handpiece, density is not a function of hand movement with the CPG. These are all pattern 3, size 9, with densities of 5, 7, and 9 from left to right. Note that as the density increases, the size gets smaller.

mediate to experienced surgeons. Some very skilled surgeons increase the wattage to produce a repetition rate of 12 pulses per second or faster. With the CPG, the wattage can be set high (100 W) because the pattern is generated without hand movement. The CPG can produce patterns of various sizes, shapes, and density at rates of more than 300 pulses per second. Obviously, the human hand is not capable of this precision speed and reproducibility using single pulses. One can see from this discussion that the CPG saves time, increases safety, and reduces operator fatigue.

The density of the CPG is usually set at 4, 5, or 6. As the density number increases, there is increasing overlap. For example, a grid pattern of density 6 has 35% overlap whereas a pattern of density 9 has 60% overlap. Figure 15–14 shows the same pattern and shape at different densities.

Regardless of which handpiece is used, some general principles must be followed. Magnification of 2 × to 2.5 × is extremely helpful in evaluating the results of each pass. The handpiece should be held at right angles to the skin. The entire cosmetic unit can be treated with the first pass, or some surgeons focus initially on the rhytids and shoulders

to decrease the energy (millijoules per pulse) by 40%. Therefore, the range for the CPG is 150 to 300 millijoules.

Wattage is related to the rate of pulse delivery. With the 3.0-mm handpiece set at 500 millijoules per pulse, 4 W delivers eight pulses per second (energy [millijoules per pulse] × rate [pulse/second] = power [watts]). If the wattage is reduced to 2 W, four pulses per second is delivered. Therefore, depending on the surgeon's skill level and speed of movement, one can select a rate of pulse delivery. Usually, four pulses per second is appropriate for the beginner and eight pulses per second for inter-

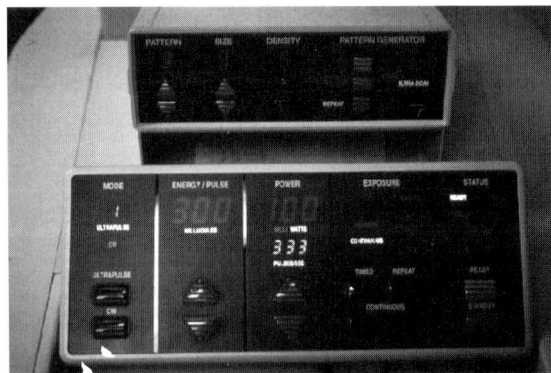

FIGURE 15–13. The parameters selected by the surgeon are millijoules, wattage, pattern, size, and density. Wattage correlates directly with the pulses per second. Note that these settings are for the CPG. Thus, the wattage is 100 with a very fast delivery rate of 333 pulses per second.

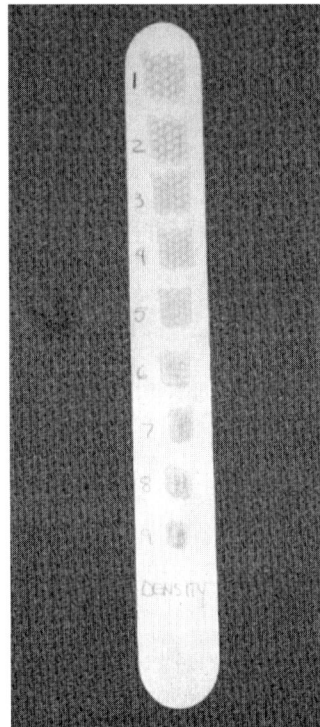

FIGURE 15–14. This photograph shows the same pattern and shape at different densities. Note as the density increases, the percentage of overlap increases, and the actual size of the pattern decreases. Overlap is as follows with the density in parentheses: (1), −10%; (2), 0%; (3), +10%; (4), +20%; (5), +30%; (6), +35%; (7), +40%; (8), +50%; (9), +60%.

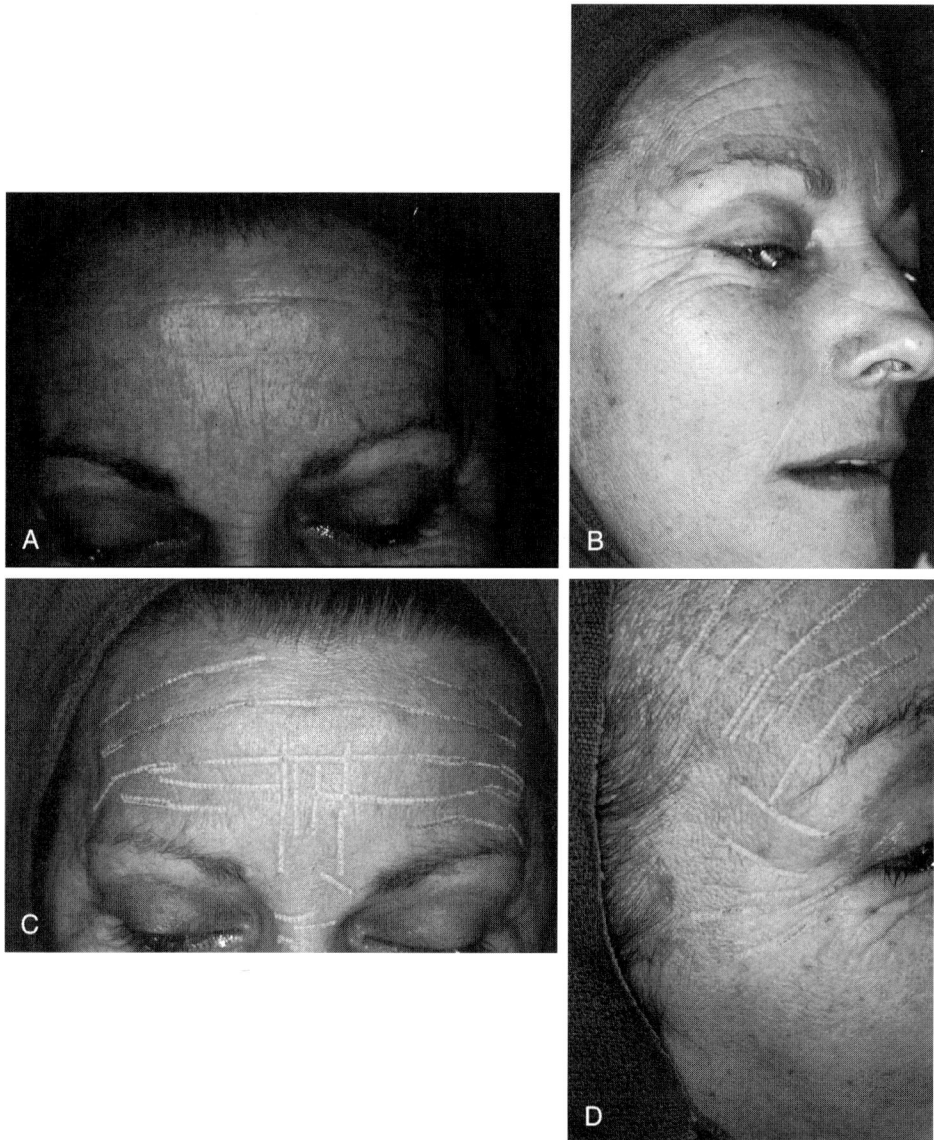

FIGURE 15–15. Laser resurfacing of the forehead and periorbital areas. *A* and *B*, Preoperative photographs. *C* and *D*, Rhytids are lased with linear pattern at 300 millijoules, pattern 4, size 9, and a density of 5.

Illustration continued on following page

of the rhytids. It is also a good idea to change the orientation of the handpiece after each pass. With each additional pass of the laser one must keep in mind the area of the face that is being treated and must err on the conservative side. At times, one may be tempted to do "just one more pass" in an effort to obliterate a rhytid. Very deep rhytids are at the level of the mid- to deep reticular dermis, and attempts to treat at this level increase the risk of scarring. One must also remember that new collagen formation will be taking place in the rhytid area for several months postoperatively. This new collagen formation also helps efface the rhytid and is an effect that is not seen immediately. In one study, patients improved markedly at 2, 4, and 6 months as compared with their results at 1 month.[6]

Another extremely important principle is to keep the amount of char to a minimum. The residue of vaporized epidermis must be wiped off with moist gauze or a cotton-tipped applicator after each pass. Failing to perform this simple maneuver results in a conduction burn with the risk of extending this wound deeper than one desires. Conduction burns can also occur by overlapping patterns or spots; therefore, care should be taken to align the CPG patterns up against each other and avoid overlap.

In order to assist in blending the treated and nontreated areas, feathering can be performed by

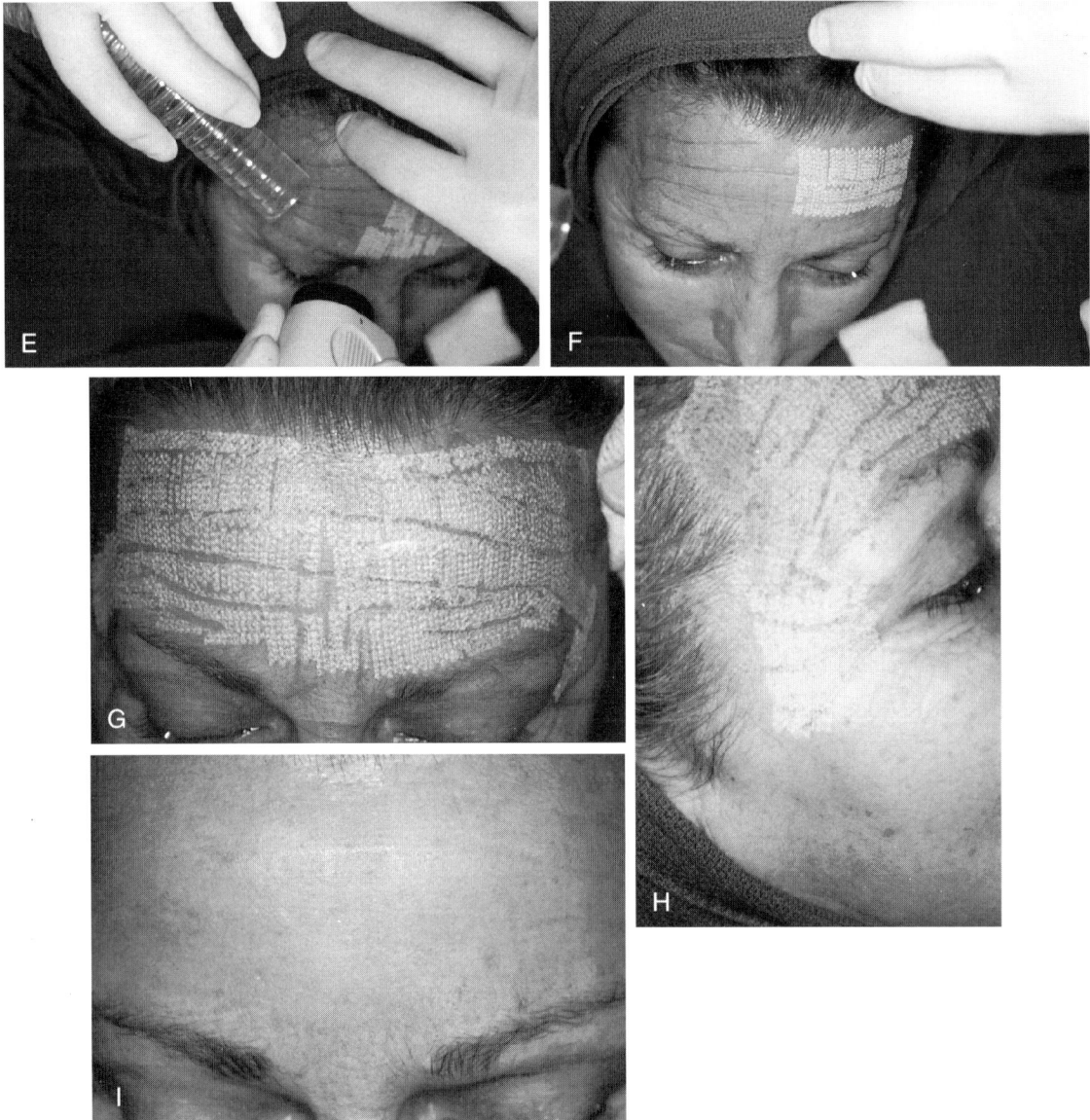

FIGURE 15–15 *Continued E* to *I,* First pass at 300 millijoules, pattern 3, size 9, density 5. An additional pass with the same parameters was also performed, resulting in entry into the mid- to upper reticular dermis. Clinically, this is seen as a yellow endpoint.

decreasing the energy per pulse or decreasing the pattern density.

The periorbital area (Fig. 15–15; see also Color Plate 7) is usually treated inferiorly and laterally. The globe should be protected with scleral shields like those shown in Figure 15–10. Because the resurfacing procedure could damage the eyelashes, they need to be protected with a wet handle of a cotton-tipped applicator. Using the 3.0-mm handpiece, one to two passes can be made in the infraorbital area at 3 to 7 W and 250 to 500 millijoules, while laterally it may take an additional one or two passes, owing to the generally thicker skin—and possibly deeper rhytids. The CPG can also be used

by selecting the appropriate patterns and reducing the millijoules to 300.

In the lower lid, ectropion can occur, which is usually transient. However, if patients have lower lid laxity, it is advisable to do a lateral canthal suspension before the resurfacing procedure.

With perioral resurfacing, it is acceptable to cross the vermilion border. A final pass along the vermilion border with a single spot can be used in an attempt to better define it. Millijoules used with the 3-mm handpiece are 400 to 500, and the wattage is 3 to 7. The CPG can also be used, and it is preferred by most surgeons owing to the increased speed of resurfacing. The millijoules setting for the CPG

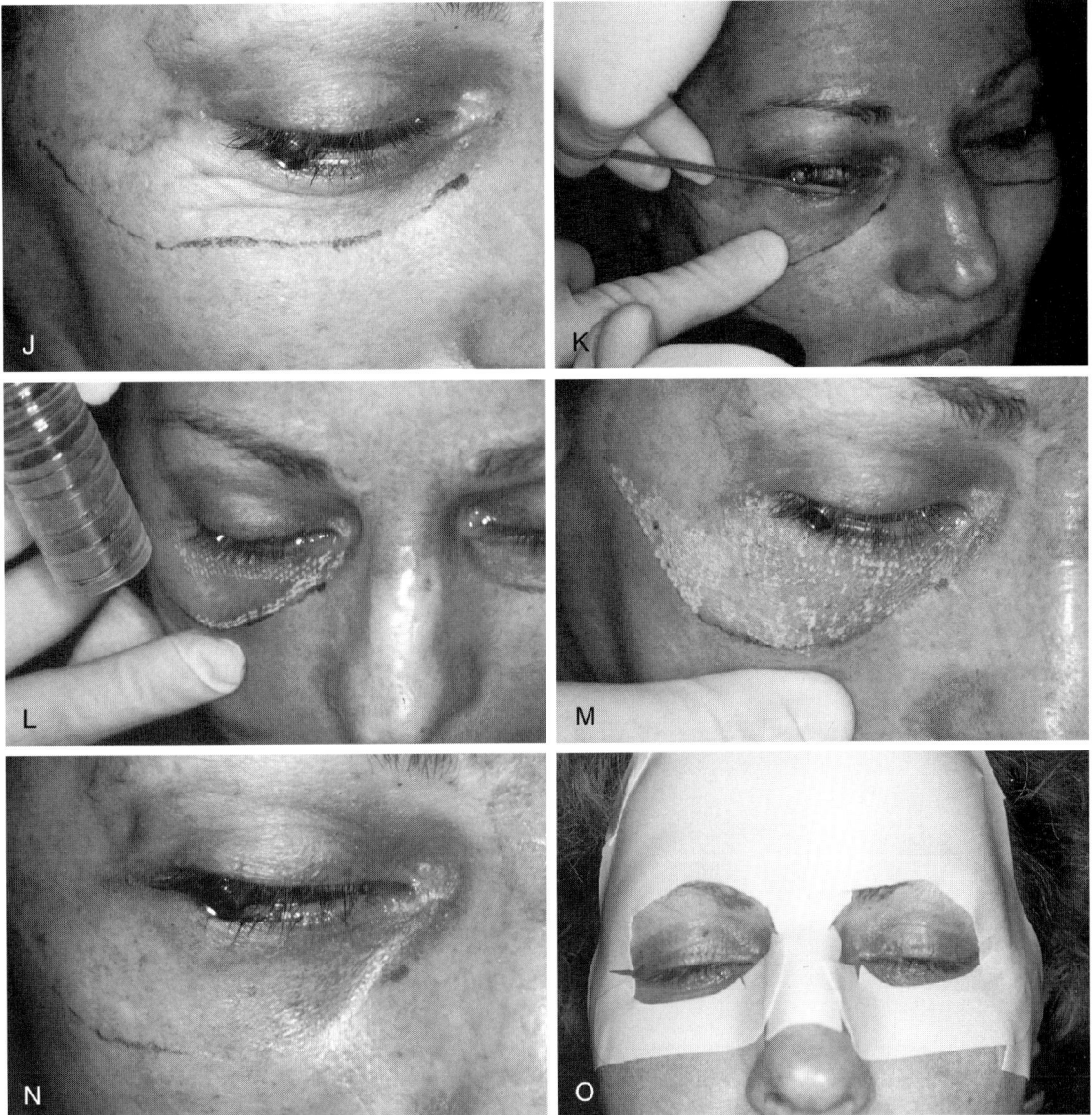

FIGURE 15–15 *Continued J* to *N,* Infraorbital area resurfaced as an individual cosmetic unit. Note how the wet handle of cotton-tipped applicator is being used to protect the lashes. A scleral shield is in place. Lasing is performed at 125 millijoules, pattern 3, size 3, density 5. Part of resurfacing was performed with pattern 3, size 5, density 5. Two passes were made at these settings. *O,* Flexzan dressing is applied. This dressing is changed daily until it adheres firmly, then it is permitted to remain in place for 7 days.

Illustration continued on following page

would be 250 to 300, and two to five passes are made, as required. Pattern sizes can be selected and altered as necessary. With all of the shapes and sizes available, one rarely needs to resort to the 3.0-mm handpiece. The one exception may be nasal resurfacing, when significant curved surfaces need to be treated. Use of the pattern generator in this area would most likely find a portion of the pattern that is not perpendicular to the skin, which could result in uncertainty with respect to both the actual energy striking the target, the density of the pattern, and the geometric configuration of the pattern.

The entire forehead (see Fig. 15–15) can be resurfaced using 450 to 500 millijoules at 3 to 10 W. Usually, two to five passes are necessary. Alternatively, the CPG can be used at 300 millijoules with a pattern of the operator's choice. A large pattern is very suitable for this area. Depending on the brow position and severity of rhytids, a forehead lift with frontalis, corrugator, and procerus resection may be the preferred procedure.

Actinic cheilitis can be treated with one pass of 500 millijoules for the 3.0-mm handpiece, and 300 millijoules for the CPG. After the initial pass, it

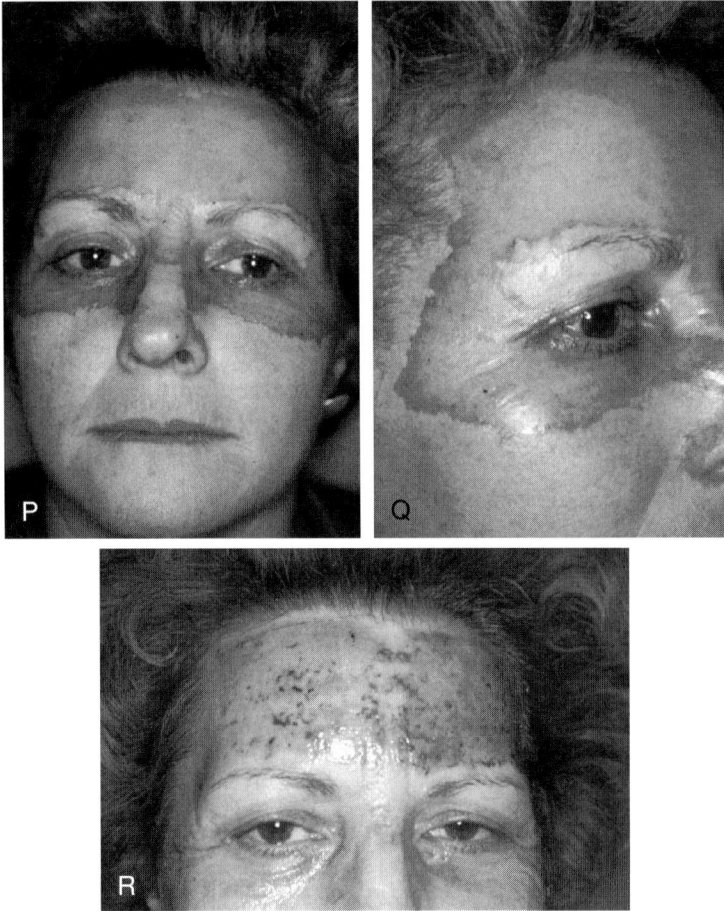

FIGURE 15–15 *Continued P* and *Q,* One day after laser resurfacing. *R,* One week after laser resurfacing.

may be necessary to make additional passes over areas that appear to be abnormal. Usually, one additional pass is significant (see Fig. 15–4).

Treating the cheeks is similar to other areas and can be done with one to four passes and 450 to 500 millijoules, with wattage of 3 to 7. The CPG can again be used by decreasing the energy delivered per pulse to 270 to 300 millijoules. Acne scars can be treated by initially lasing with a donut pattern around the scar to lower the shoulders, and then continue to ablate the entire area with a second pass (Fig. 15–16). Passes are continued until the scars are relatively effaced or the visual endpoint is reached.

As with any resurfacing procedure, additional touch-up procedures may be necessary or desirable. As discussed earlier, this is best performed 6 months after the initial resurfacing procedure. For deeply pitted scars, punch grafting following excision may be required. It has been advocated to resurface the skin after excision of the scar and

before placement of the graft.[40] This supposedly causes a nice blend of grafted and original skin.

Postoperative Care

The key to good wound healing is moisture. It is well known that the water content of a wound is an extremely important factor that influences the migration speed of epithelial cells. Studies show that occluded wounds undergo re-epithelialization faster than open wounds.[88] One reason this occurs is because the epidermis does not need to grow deep into the dermis as for an open, desiccated wound. If eschar is allowed to form, the epidermal cells must migrate beneath this crust to reach a plane of hydration. This epidermal dive can be responsible for delayed wound healing and, possibly, for geometric depression of the healed epidermis, resulting in an unfavorable cosmetic result.

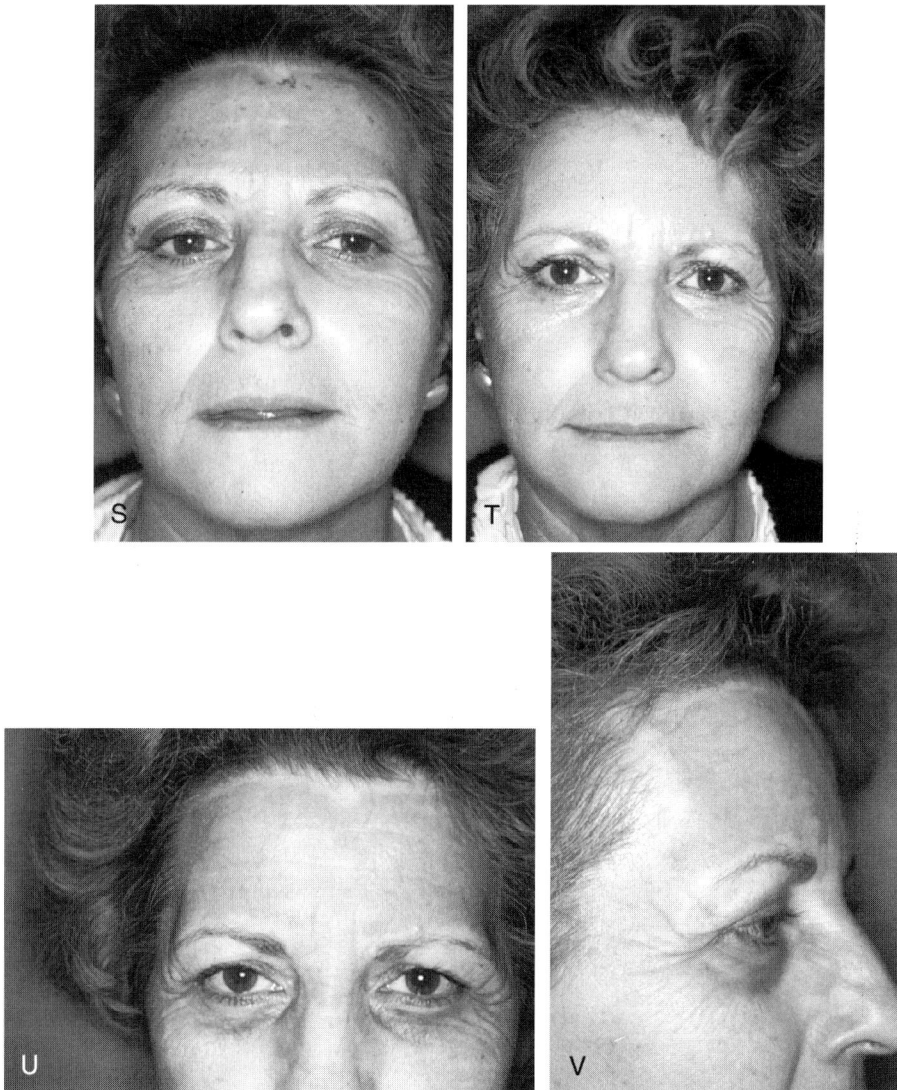

FIGURE 15–15 *Continued S,* Ten days after laser resurfacing. *T,* Ten days after laser resurfacing with makeup. *U* and *V,* Twenty-four days after laser resurfacing. (See also Color Plate 7.)

Several methods have been employed to keep wounds moist after resurfacing. These include Vaseline, Preparation H, Crisco, topical antibiotics, and facial dressings such as Vigilon and Flexzan. Flexzan, a polyurethane foam adhesive, is our first choice because it seems to adhere better than other dressings we have tried. The first step of application is blow drying the skin with a hair dryer on a cool setting. The Flexzan is then cut and applied over the resurfaced areas (see Fig. 15–16). It is changed on the first postoperative day, and, again, the hair dryer is used on a cool setting to dry the skin before reapplication of Flexzan. After the first or second dressing change the Flexzan usually adheres firmly to the wound, and it is permitted to remain in place for 7 days; then it can be peeled off. At this point, re-epithelialization is well on its way to completion

and ointments are now used to keep the skin moist. One may find that the perioral area requires more frequent dressing changes, owing to the possible accumulation of food on the dressings. Therefore, these patients may need daily evaluation of their perioral dressing.

Patient compliance is very important for successful postoperative management. Compliant patients clean their wounds and apply ointments frequently, thus promoting healing. Even the most responsible patients, however, have difficulty keeping the wounds moist during sleep, and the result is significant nocturnal pain, described as a burning sensation. Semiocclusive dressings such as Vigilon or Flexzan are superior to ointments for keeping wounds moist. Also, it is much easier for patients to comply with postoperative care when it is taken

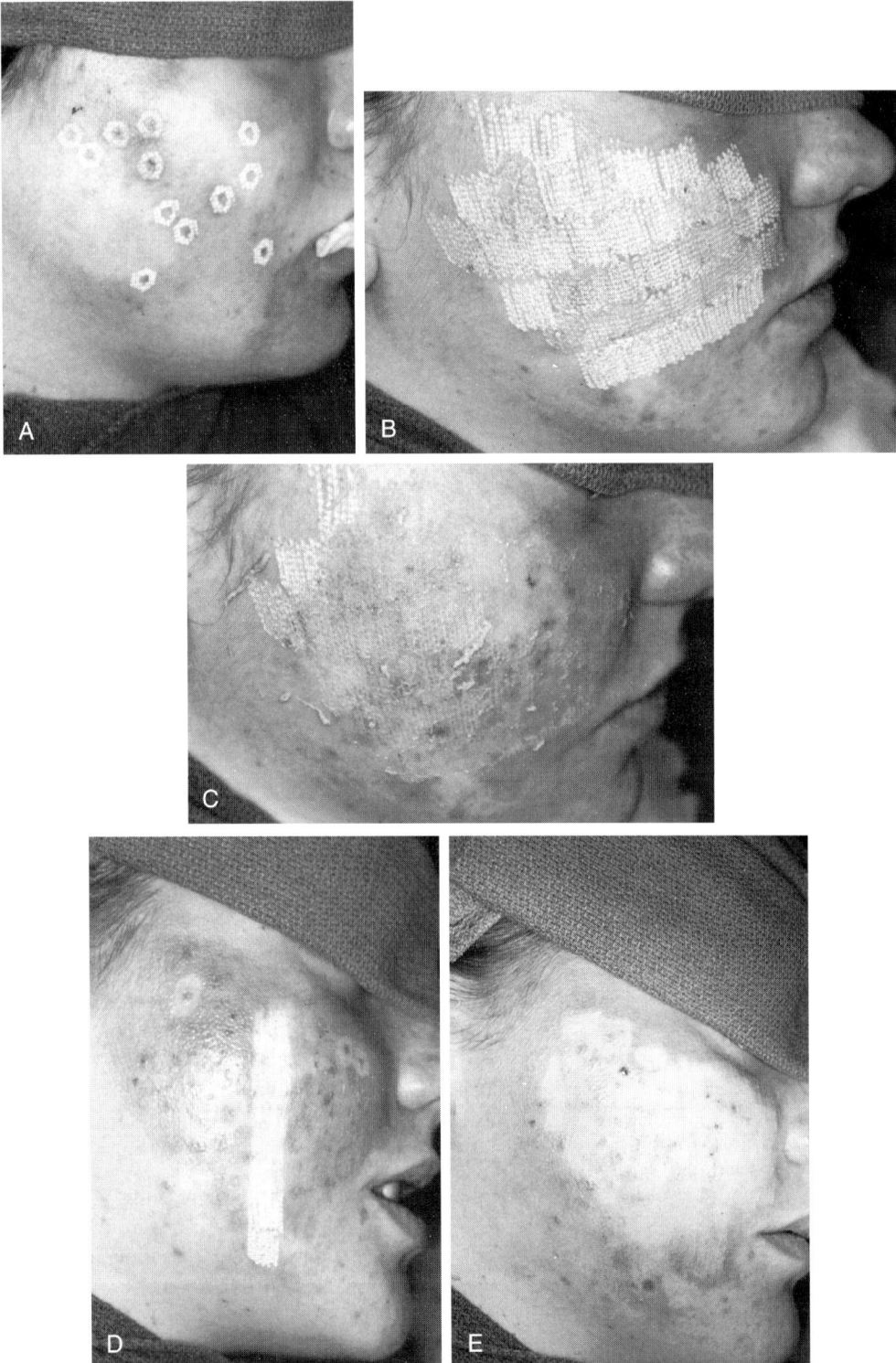

FIGURE 15–16. Laser resurfacing of skin with acne scarring. *A,* Donut pattern at 200 millijoules, pattern 7, size 5, density 7. *B,* Square pattern at 200 millijoules, pattern 3, size 9, density 7. Two passes were made at these settings. *C,* Note the wiping of the lased epidermal remnants. This wiping is necessary to avoid thermal conduction burn of the underlying tissue. *D,* One strip of the final pass. At this stage, one can actually see the tissue contract as the laser energy strikes the tissue. *E,* Second pass is complete.

out of their hands. With semiocclusive dressings patients do not have to be concerned about managing their wounds, but it is imperative that they diligently keep their postoperative appointments—daily for the first 3 to 5 days, then weekly for 2 weeks, then at 3 months or until redness resolves. It is wise to follow them closely to spot any possible complications early. If the patient begins to have significant pain, herpes should be suspected. Other complications have been discussed previously in this chapter. It is also advantageous to recall patients annually to re-evaluate the laser-resurfacing results. These annual follow-up evaluations also afford an opportunity to discuss additional facial changes secondary to aging and may result in inquiries about other cosmetic surgical procedures.

Following laser resurfacing, antibiotics, steroids, and acyclovir are continued, as explained previously. Topical tretinoin, hydroquinone, and glycolic acids are started approximately 12 to 15 days after the resurfacing procedure if re-epithelialization is complete. Makeup can also be worn after re-epithelialization is complete. The risk of hyperpigmentation is reduced by the daily use of sun block (SPF 15), which will protect the skin from UV light, thus avoiding melanocyte stimulation and reducing the risk of hyperpigmentation.

SUMMARY

Laser resurfacing can be used effectively to rejuvenate facial skin. It appears to be replacing chemical peel and dermabrasion as the state-of-the-art technique for resurfacing. Some of the advantages include greater precision of resurfacing with virtually no hypopigmentation and a very low rate of scarring. The learning curve is reasonable, and with appropriate training, this procedure can be added to any competent oral and maxillofacial surgeon's armamentarium.

REFERENCES

1. Bryan CP: Ancient Egyptian Medicine; The Papyrus Ebers [translation]. Chicago, Ares Publishers, 1974, pp 158–161.
2. Marmelzat WL: A historical review of chemical rejuvenation of the face. *In* Kistler R (ed): Chemical Rejuvenation of the Face. St. Louis, Mosby–Year Book, 1992.
3. Misch CE: Contemporary Implant Dentistry. St. Louis, Mosby–Year Book, 1993.
4. Chernoff WG: Cutaneous laser resurfacing. Int J Aesthet Restor Surg 3:57–68, 1995.
5. Lowe NJ: Laser skin resurfacing. Dermatol Surg Dec: 1017–1019, 1995.
6. Lowe NJ: Skin resurfacing with ultrapulse CO_2 laser—observation in 100 patients. Dermatol Surg Dec: 1025–1028, 1995.
7. Reid R: Physical and surgical principles governing carbon dioxide laser surgery on the skin. Clin Dermatol 9:297–314, 1991.
8. Trost D, Zacherl A, Smith M: Surgical laser properties and their tissue interaction, St. Louis, Mosby–Year Book, 1992.
9. Fitzpatrick R, Goldman M: Advances in carbon dioxide laser surgery. Dermatol Surg 13:35–47, 1995.
10. Catone G: Laser technology in oral and maxillofacial surgery; Part II. *In* Sinn D (ed): Selected Readings in Oral and Maxillofacial Surgery. Dallas, Texas, University of Texas Southwestern Science Center, 1993.
11. Friedman M, Kebid G: Scars as a result of CO_2 laser for molluscum contagiosum. Obstet Gynecol 70:394–396, 1987.
12. Shipshay S, Rebeiz E, Bohigian R, et al: Benign lesions of the larynx: Should the laser be used? Laryngoscope 100:953–957, 1990.
13. Green HA, Burd H, Bruggemann N, et al: Middermal wound healing. A comparison between dermatomal excision and pulsed carbon dioxide laser ablation. Arch Dermatol 128:639–645, 1992.
14. McCollough EG, Langsdon PR: Dermabrasion and chemical peel. New York, Thieme, 1988.
15. Walsh J, Flotte T, Anderson R, et al: Pulsed CO_2 laser tissue ablation: Effect of tissue type and pulse duration on thermal damage. Laser Surg Med 8:108, 1988.
16. Fitzpatrick R, Goldman M: CO_2 laser surgery. *In* Goldman MP, Fitzpatrick RE (eds) Cutaneous Laser Surgery. St. Louis, CV Mosby, 1994, pp 199–258.
17. Green H, Domankevitz Y, Nishioka N: Pulsed carbon dioxide laser ablation of burned skin: In vitro and in vivo analysis. Laser Surg Med 10:476, 1990.
18. Hallock GG, Rice DC: In utero fetal surgery using a milliwatt carbon dioxide laser. Lasers Surg Med 9: 482, 1989.
19. Dover JS, Smoller BR, Stern RS, et al: Low-fluence CO_2 laser irradiation: Selective epidermal damage to human skin. J Invest Dermatol 93:75, 1989.
20. Kamatt BR, Tang SV, Arndt KA, et al: Low-fluence CO_2 laser irradiation: Selective epidermal damage to human skin. J Invest Dermatol 85:274, 1985.
21. Benedict LM, Cohen B: Treatment of Peutz-Jeghers lentigines with the carbon dioxide laser. J Dermatol Surg Oncol 17:954, 1991.
22. Herbich G: Epidermal changes limited to the epidermis of guinea pig skin by low-power carbon dioxide laser irradiation. Arch Dermatol 122:132, 1986.
23. Moritz AR, Henriques FC: Studies of thermal injury. II. The relative importance of time and surface temperatures in the causation of cutaneous burns. Am J Pathol 23:695, 1947.
24. Henriques FC, Moritz AR: Studies of thermal injury. I. The conduction of heat to and through the skin and the temperatures attained therein. A theoretical and experimental investigation. Am J Pathol 23:531, 1947.
25. Zweig AD, Weber HP: Mechanical and thermal parameters in pulsed laser cutting of tissue. IEEE J Quantum Electronics 10:1787, 1987.
26. Alster T, Apfelberg D: Cosmetic Laser Surgery. New York, Wiley-Liss, 1996.
27. McKenzie A: How far does thermal damage extend beneath the surface of CO_2 laser incision? Phys Med Biol 28:905–912, 1983.
28. Catone G: Laser technology in oral and maxillofacial surgery; Part I. *In* Sinn D (ed): Selected Readings in Oral and Maxillofacial Surgery. Dallas, Texas, University of Texas Southwestern Medical Center, 1993.
29. Walsh JT, Flotte TJ, Anderson RR, et al: Pulsed CO_2 laser ablation: Effects of tissue type and pulse duration on thermal damage. Lasers Surg Med 8:108–118, 1988.
30. Green HA, Domankevitz Y, Nishioka NS: Pulsed carbon dioxide laser ablation of burned skin: In vitro and in vivo analysis. Lasers Surg Med 10:476–484, 1990.
31. Hall RR: Haemostatic incisions of the liver. CO_2 laser compared with surgical diathermy. Br J Surg 58:538–540, 1971.
32. Fidler JP, Hoefer RW, Polanri TG, et al: Laser surgery in exsanguinating liver injury. Surg Forum 23:350–352, 1972.

33. Kirschner RA: Cutaneous plastic surgery with the CO_2 laser. Surg Clin North Am 64(5):871–883, 1984.
34. Slutzki S, Shafir R, Bornstein LA: Use of the carbon dioxide laser for large excisions with minimal blood loss. Plast Reconstr Surg 60:250–255, 1977.
35. Weinstein C: Ultrapulse carbon dioxide laser removal for periocular wrinkles in association with laser blepharoplasty. J Clin Laser Med Surg 12:205–209, 1994.
36. Lowe NJ: Laser skin resurfacing with the silk touch scanner for facial rhytids. Dermatol Surg Dec: 1021, 1995.
37. Aschler P, Ingolitsch E, Walter G, et al: Ultrastructural findings in CNS tissue with CO_2 laser. In Kaplan I (ed): Laser Surgery II. Jerusalem, Academic Press, 1976.
38. Ben-Bassat M, Ben-Bassat J, Kaplan I: An ultrastructural study of the cut edges of skin and mucous membrane specimens excised by carbon dioxide laser. In Kaplan I (ed): Laser Surgery II. Jerusalem, Academic Press, 1976.
39. David LM, Sarne AJ, Unger WE: Rapid laser scanning. Dermatol Surg Dec: 1031, 1995.
40. Weinstein C: CO_2 laser resurfacing workshop. Washington, DC, Center for Laser Surgery, 1995.
41. Shorr N, Goldber RA: Lower lid retraction following blepharoplasty. Am J Cosmetic Surg 6:72–82, 1989.
42. Shorr N, Enzer Y: Considerations in aesthetic eyelid surgery. J Dermatol Surg Oncol 18:1081–1095, 1992.
43. Asken S: The preseptal and retroseptal approaches in transconjunctival blepharoplasty. J Dermatol Surg Oncol 18:1110–1116, 1992.
44. Schmitt CK, Folsom TC: Histologic evaluation of degenerative changes of the lower lip. J Oral Surg 26:51–56, 1968.
45. Defresne RG, Garrett AB, Bailin PL, et al: Carbon dioxide laser treatment of chronic actinic cheilitis. J Am Acad Dermatol 19:876–878, 1988.
46. Goldman L, Shumrick DA, Rockwell J, et al: The laser in maxillofacial surgery—Preliminary investigative surgery. Arch Surg 96:397–400, 1968.
47. David LM: Laser vermilion ablation for actinic cheilitis. J Dermatol Surg Oncol 11:605–608, 1985.
48. Whitaker DC: Microscopically proven cure of actinic cheilitis by CO_2 laser. Lasers Surg Med 7:520–523, 1987.
49. Stanley RJ, Roenigk RK: Actinic cheilitis: Treatment with the carbon dioxide laser. Mayo Clin Proc 63:230–235, 1988.
50. Zelvekson BD, Roenigk RK: Actinic cheilitis. Treatment with the carbon dioxide laser. Cancer 65:1307–1311, 1990.
51. Johnson TM, Sebastien TS, Lowe L, et al: Carbon dioxide laser treatment of actinic cheilitis: Clinicohistopathologic correlation to determine the optimal depth of destruction. J Am Acad Dermatol 27:737–740, 1992.
52. Greenbaum SS, Krull EA, Watnick K: Comparison of CO_2 laser and electrosurgery in the treatment of rhinophyma. J Am Acad Dermatol 18:363–368, 1988.
53. Eisen RF, Katz AE, Bohigian RK, et al: Surgical treatment of rhinophyma with the Shaw scalpel. Arch Dermatol 122:307–309, 1986.
54. Ali KM, Callari RH, Mobley DL: Resection of rhinophyma with CO_2 laser. Laryngoscope 99:453–455, 1989.
55. Bohigian RK, Shapshay SM, Hybels RL: Management of rhinophyma with carbon dioxide laser: Lahey Clinic experience. Lasers Surg Med 8:397–401, 1988.
56. Roenigk RK: CO_2 laser vaporization for treatment of rhinophyma. Mayo Clin Proc 62:676–680, 1987.
57. Wheeland RG, Bailin PL, Ratz JL: Combined carbon dioxide laser excision and vaporization in the treatment of rhinophyma. J Dermatol Surg Oncol 13:172–177, 1987.
58. Shapshay SM, Strong MS, Anastasi GW, et al: Removal of rhinophyma with the carbon dioxide laser. Arch Otolaryngol 106:257–259, 1980.
59. Goldman L, Perry E, Stefanovsky D: A flexible sealed tube transverse radio frequency–excited carbon dioxide laser for dermatologic surgery. Lasers Surg Med 2:317–322, 1983.
60. Amedee RG, Routman MH: Methods and complications of rhinophyma excision. Laryngoscope 97:1316–1318, 1987.
61. Hassard AD: Carbon dioxide laser treatment of acne rosacea and rhinophyma: How I do it. J Otolaryngol 17:336–337, 1988.
62. Hallock GG: Laser treatment of rhinophyma. Aesthetic Plast Surg 12:171–174, 1988.
63. Haas A, Wheeland RG: Treatment of massive rhinophyma with the carbon dioxide laser. J Dermatol Surg Oncol 16:645–649, 1990.
64. Greenbaum SS, Krull EA, Watnick K: Comparison of CO_2 laser and electrosurgery in the treatment of rhinophyma. J Am Acad Dermatol 18:363–368, 1988.
65. El-Ashary R, Roenigk RK, Wang TD: Spectrum of results after treatment of rhinophyma with the carbon dioxide laser. Mayo Clin Proc 66:899–905, 1991.
66. Fitzpatrick RE, Goldman MP, Dierickx C: Laser ablation of facial cosmetic tattoos. Aesth Plast Surg 18:91–98, 1994.
67. Ratz JL, Bailin PL, Lakeland RF: Carbon dioxide laser treatment of epidermal nevi. J Dermatol Surg Oncol 12:567–570, 1986.
68. Garden JM, Geronemus RG: Dermatologic laser surgery. J Dermatol Surg Oncol 16:156–168, 1990.
69. Labandter H, Kaplan I: Experience with a "continuous" laser in the treatment of suitable cutaneous conditions: Preliminary report. J Dermatol Surg Oncol 3:527–530, 1977.
70. Kaplan I, Peled I: The CO_2 laser in the treatment of superficial telangiectases. Br J Plast Surg 28:214–215, 1975.
71. Ratz JL, Bailin PL, Levine HL: CO_2 laser treatment of portwine stains: A preliminary report. J Dermatol Surg Oncol 8:1039–1044, 1982.
72. Lanigan SW, Cotterill JA: The treatment of port wine stains with the carbon dioxide laser. Br J Dermatol 123:229–235, 1990.
73. Fitzpatrick R, Goldman M: Advances in cutaneous laser surgery. Western J Med Oct:509–510, 1995.
74. Fitzpatrick R, Lowe N, Goldman M, et al: Flashlamp-pumped pulsed dye laser treatment of port-wine stains. Dermatol Surg 20:743–748, 1994.
75. Dierickx C, Goldman M, Fitzpatrick R: Laser treatment of erythematous/hypertrophic and pigmented scars in 26 patients. Plastic Reconstr Surg Jan:84–90, 1995.
76. Dover JS, Smoller BR, Stern RS, et al: Low-fluence carbon dioxide laser irradiation of lentigines. Arch Dermatol 124:1219–1224, 1988.
77. Kamat BR, Tang SV, Arndt KA, et al: Low-fluence CO_2 laser irradiation: Selective epidermal damage to human skin. J Invest Dermatol 85:274–278, 1985.
78. Fitzpatrick R, Goldman M: Tattoo removal using the alexandrite laser. Arch Dermatol 130:1508–1514, 1994.
79. Fitzpatrick R, Goldman M, Dierickx C: Laser ablation of facial cosmetic tattoos. Aesth Plast Surg 18:91–98, 1994.
80. Ho C: Laser resurfacing in pigmented skin. Dermatol Surg Dec:1035, 1995.
81. American National Standards Institute: American National Standards for the Safe Use of Lasers. Standard; 1993:Z136.1. New York, AVSI Publications, 1993.
82. Brody H: Chemical Peeling. St. Louis, Mosby–Year Book, 1992, pp 7–31.
83. Mandy S: Tretinoin in the preoperative and postoperative management of dermabrasion. J Am Acad Dermatol 15(suppl):878–879, 1986.
84. Hevia O, Nemeth AJ, Taylor JR: Tretinoin accelerates healing after trichloroacetic acid chemical peel. Arch Dermatol 127:678–682, 1991.
85. Hung VC, Lee JY, Zitelli JA, et al: Topical tretinoin and epithelial wound healing. Arch Dermatol 125:65–69, 1989.
86. Ellis DA, Trimas S, Ellis C: The use of glycolic acid as a micro-peel. Facial Plast Surg Clin North Am 2:15–20, 1994.
87. Physicians Desk Reference, 49th ed. Montvale, New Jersey, Medical Economics Data Production Company, 1995.
88. Maibach HF, Rovee DT: Epidermal Wound Healing. St. Louis, Mosby–Year Book, 1972.

CHAPTER 16

Medical-Legal Considerations in Laser Surgery

FRANK L. NELSON, DDS, JD

Before any specific discussion of liability issues in the use of lasers in dental and oral surgical procedures, a simplified overview of the malpractice maze is in order. It is not the purpose of this chapter to make the practitioner an expert in medical malpractice, but rather to inform the practitioner to the extent that reasonableness and understanding are used in the treatment planning for patients, in light of the litigious nature of the public today. There is a national malpractice hysteria, inflamed by occasional bad verdicts against practitioners, incomplete and sensationalistic reporting by media and insurance companies, and of course, a large number of cases filed by attorneys that have no merit. The phenomenon is ongoing.

An example of the confusion produced by the media can be seen in the following case. There was a reported award of over a million dollars to a psychic who claimed she had lost her psychic powers due to a simple radiologic examination. The facts reported were so bizarre that this author researched the case and found the true result of the matter. In fact, there was a claim that the psychic powers were lost, but that claim was summarily dismissed by the court. The true, underlying matters for which this award was made dealt with the fact that the patient was allergic to iodine and reported this to her physician. The radiologic examination was an intravenous pyelogram in which an iodine-based dye was used despite the allergy warning label on her hospital chart. The resulting injury was a cardiac arrest, resuscitation, and permanent neurologic and other physical damages, which led

to long-term rehabilitative treatment in a hospital setting and a lifetime of medical needs. The individual was also unable to secure gainful employment. Certainly, this paints a significantly different picture of the cause, damages, and resultant award.

Keeping in mind that providers of any product or service must see a profit, as costs of defending lawsuits increase with increased public awareness and demands for favorable results in medicine coupled with the apparent present day refusal to accept one's own responsibility for actions and inactions, there is no solution other than increased costs to the consumer. These increases in cost result from increased professional liability costs, increased use of minimally necessary laboratory and radiographic tests, and other defensive practices by the providers. These costs are passed on to the consumer and cause health insurance premiums to soar. As this occurs, there are those once insured either individually or as a group who can no longer afford the insurance. An increase in the proportion of the population who are uninsured results in lost income to the provider, either through bankrupting of claims or diminished payments from Medicare or Medicaid. This loss must be borne by the consumer, and the spiral continues.

As with all professions, the medical, dental, and legal professions are composed of people the vast majority of whom are sincere individuals pursuing their profession. There is a small number of individuals who are either inept, infirm, insincere, or otherwise unable to reach the level of professionalism or performance that is required of them. Our different organizations have attempted to develop rules of professional conduct, standards of care and performance, and guidelines as to what is acceptable and unacceptable in pursuit of our professions. The more the professions police themselves and weed out that small number of problematic individuals mentioned earlier, the closer we will be to arriving at a solution to the malpractice crisis in the professions. If the individuals of the professions allow colleagues to perform improper procedures, continue to practice in the face of chemical dependency, or otherwise not reach the standard of care of the profession without intervening, then it is no wonder that the profession is subject to outside attack. The primary concern must be what is best for the patient, not how to avoid a lawsuit.

PROOF OF MALPRACTICE CLAIMS

The result of a negligent act of a practitioner in the treatment or diagnosis of his or her patient, which directly or indirectly causes damage or injury to the patient, may result in a claim of malpractice against the practitioner by the patient. Malpractice claims are based, in most states, on specific legislation that interweaves contract law with the principles of common law in torts (civil wrongs). Every state has its own particular minutia requirements for proving a malpractice claim. The general principles and requirements are fairly similar nationwide. Because this author is both an oral and maxillofacial surgeon and an attorney at law in the State of Alabama, the specific references to the law will be based on the Alabama standards.

A malpractice claim requires proof of four separate events or relationships. These events or relationships are proof (1) of a duty of care or otherwise a provider-patient relationship; (2) that the standard of care was breached by the provider or simply that there was negligence in the treatment or diagnosis; (3) that as a result of the negligence, an injury occurred; and (4) that the patient suffered damages as a result of the injury. Each of the elements of proof of a malpractice claim are more fully explained in the following paragraphs.

There must be a duty of care from the provider to the patient. Not only is there a duty of care resulting from the normal patient-provider fee-for-service relationship, it may also arise from an offhand answer given at a social gathering, if the layperson reasonably believes the response to be sincere and relies on the response. The contract is formed because the layperson has sought advice from one who is seen as a professional and who has both the education and training as well as a duty to provide medical treatment to those in need. This, in contract law, would be termed detrimental reliance by the layperson. Obviously, the usual sequence of events includes the giving of something of value (consultation or treatment fees) wherein the contract is initiated and the duty to the layperson is established. This scenario occurs when the patient consults the provider at the provider's office or when the provider visits the patient in the hospital in response to a consultation request.

The negligently delivered service to the patient or negligent omission of a service would include negligent misdiagnosis, and failure to protect the patient from injury before, during, and after the treatment, such as failure to provide antibiotic coverage when necessary, failure to warn of the need of preanesthetic fasting, and failure to give adequate postoperative instructions and care, to mention only a few. Negligence is determined today in most states by a national standard. The standard is determined by the practitioner's access to information. Thus, the national standard is a result of the ability to receive instantaneous transmission of information worldwide and hence, information is available to any practitioner regardless of location. Added to this determination of negligence and the national standard, any generalist who undertakes a procedure that is within the realm of a recognized specialty nationwide must perform that procedure to the standard of care developed and espoused by that specialty. That is to say that a general dentist who surgically removes third molars must conform to the standards of treatment and procedure that are recognized by oral and maxillofacial surgeons. One of the requirements for maintaining the standard of care is to apprise the patient of the risks and alternatives of treatment so that he or she may give informed consent to the treatment.

The Doctrine of Informed Consent has been developed nationally; however, each state has its own particular requirements. Again, using the State of Alabama as an example, the courts went through a multiphased metamorphosis to reach the current standard for determining proximate cause for the doctrine of informed consent.

In the United States, the right of a patient to determine what treatment is to be administered was established firmly in the landmark decision of *Schloendorff v. Society of New York Hospital* by the late Justice Benjamin Nathan Cardozo (1870–1938). In that case, a woman claimed she had not given permission for an operation performed during an examination. The court concluded that an operation performed without the consent of the patient constituted an actionable offense. Justice Cardozo stated, "Every human being of adult years and sound mind has a right to determine what shall be done with his own body; and a surgeon who performs an operation without his patient's consent commits an assault. . . ." With this legal principle in mind, the courts rule that a patient's consent to a proposed course of treatment is not valid unless the patient is informed by the practitioner as to what is to be done, the risks involved, and the alternatives available.

A violation of the doctrine of informed consent consists of three basic elements to be proved: (1) the practitioner's failure to inform the patient, (2) an injurious result, and (3) causation of the injury by the treatment rendered.

The practitioner has a duty to inform the patient. Under this duty, a lawsuit may be brought if the practitioner failed to properly diagnose the condition and inform the patient that other practitioners may reach a different diagnosis. Included in this, accountability may be found if the practitioner fails to advise the patient to see a specialist or one with more specialized skill. Failure to recognize and recommend tests or radiographs may also be found to be a liability on the practitioner's part. The practitioner may be held accountable for failing to disclose the risks of refusing the treatment. If the practitioner learns of newly discovered dangers relating to the treatment previously provided, there is a duty to inform the patient. Even if the practitioner complies with all of these duties, the practitioner may still be held liable for the negligence of the specialist to whom the patient is referred under the legal theory of negligent referral.

Two separate standards were used to establish the level of the duty to inform the patient. The first of these was the medical standard. This simply requires the practitioner to inform the patient of risks that any reasonable practitioner would disclose to the patient. Expert testimony is required to establish this standard, and hence, it was based on the expert's personal interpretation and integrity. The materiality standard, based on the patient's need to know, uses a lay standard of reasonableness to determine the depth and scope of disclosure. The practitioner is not required to make disclosures when the risks are common knowledge, when disclosure would threaten the patient's health, or when an emergency situation renders the patient incapable of making a decision. Decisions not to inform based on the above-mentioned reasons remain the practitioner's burden to defend in court.

To add to the problem of determination of what constitutes proper disclosure by the practitioner, the courts remained uncommitted as to whether this should be determined subjectively based on a patient's hindsight, colored by the results of the procedure, or by the practitioner's objective determination. Both the medical and the materiality standards allowed self-serving expert defense testimony, because those who would be judged were allowed to set the standards by which they were judged. The Alabama Courts adopted a hybrid standard, which requires consideration by the factfinder (the

jury) of what a reasonable person with all of the characteristics of the plaintiff, including his or her idiosyncrasies and religious beliefs, would have done under the same circumstances.

Finally, there must be an injury to the patient, which is the result of the negligent breach of the standard of care by the provider. Logically, treatment by chemotherapy or radiation will cause some injury to the patient. Surgery, including laser surgery, requires that some tissues be violated and injured. As long as that injury is an integral part of the procedure or treatment, there is no injury for which a lawsuit may be filed. If the injury is one that can be explained to be a consequence to the treatment but is in fact a result of negligence in the treatment and care in the particular case, the injury is one for which there is an actionable claim if the other requirements for litigation are met. An actionable injury must be a direct or indirect result of the negligent act of the practitioner.

This author, owing to the uniqueness of his professional combination of oral and maxillofacial surgeon and attorney, has been called to evaluate potential malpractice cases and render opinions as to the presence or absence of actionable negligence and resulting injury. Many of the referred cases revealed egregious errors and omissions and lack of documentation of the procedures. Although the lack of records would have little or nothing to do with the actual injury or damage to the patient, their nonexistence allowed conjecture and innuendo to be used by the plaintiff. Concise and accurate documentation is usually the only recorded historical account of the alleged treatment in a malpractice case. For example, the failure to obtain a preoperative radiograph before extraction of a tooth is below the standard of care nationally; however, it would be very unlikely to have anything to do with a patient suffering a cardiac arrest during the extraction. If that same practitioner had not obtained an adequate medical history and vital signs before performing the extraction, then there would possibly be a nexus or connection of causation of the cardiac arrest if the patient had a history of cardiac problems, and it could be proved that the taking of vital signs and a medical history might have revealed a contraindication to surgery at that time.

The question of negligence, substandard treatment, and the above-mentioned causation requires testimony of an expert in the field of health care that is being scrutinized. The Alabama courts require that the expert who is to give testimony be licensed to practice and, in fact, did practice in the field for which testimony is to be given during the same time period in which the complained action by the provider occurred.

One can easily see from the previous discussion that there are innumerable medical and legal pitfalls for practitioners. It is imperative for all practitioners to continue to remain as up to date as possible on the available treatments, newfound risks and problems associated with treatments and procedures, and most of all, what is considered to be the standard of care in each and every diagnosis, treatment, or procedure with which their patient may be involved. Vivid memories remain with this author of the exciting news of the original Sargenti technique and paste for root canal therapy. It was believed that the need to fit silver points or gutta percha points in the aperture of the root tip was gone. Just as vivid are the memories of the subsequent realization that there were significant injurious results reported in the literature. When the time came for lawsuits concerning the harmful effects, those practitioners who had ceased using the technique within a reasonable time after publication of these results were usually not found negligent. However, those practitioners who did not heed the warnings or did not cease using the materials after they were removed from the market were found to have fallen below the standard of care based on the requirement that they remain current in their treatment modalities. Sargenti paste has been reformulated and is an effective alternative filling material in endodontic treatment.

The general principles of proper care in surgical settings dealing with preoperative histories, examinations, tests, and imagery; intraoperative sterile technique and the procedure itself; and the postoperative care and treatment follow-up should be as instinctive as dressing oneself in the morning. These principles are not, as was said in this writer's presence during a trial, to please the lawyers; rather, they are necessary to provide the patient with the best possible outcome with the least possible risk. Accurate, timely, and complete, detailed records should be kept for the sake of all concerned. For the practitioner, it is a written record of the sequence of diagnosis, treatment, and recovery, which allows the practitioner to record the responses to the treatment and technique, and thus, is the provision of raw data for possible improvements in patient care. Incidentally, the information can be used to provide answers and proof in a court of law years after the event; for legal use, the collected data should not have been altered.

GENERAL LIABILITY CONSIDERATIONS IN LASER SURGERY

Safety is vital to all surgical techniques. This usually refers to the safety of the patient. In the case of lasers, it refers to the safety of all, including the operating team and the support staff. All lasers have several risk factors in common, and each type of laser has unique risk factors. A commonsense approach to potential hazards should be implemented to avoid negligence liability claims. A review of cases shows that as of this writing, there are few reported cases that deal with what this writer would term laser malpractice.

The following examples and discussion are the opinion of the writer, and are the product of the research of articles, opinions, industry recommendations, and common sense. They do not represent any one set of standards of care, rather, a conglomerate of many, including the American National Standards Institute (ANSI): Safe Use of Lasers in the Health Care Environment. Liability and responsibility for injuries are with the laser manufacturer, the owner, the operator, and any combination of these agents. Manufacturers would be liable if there was a design or production flaw in the laser. This product liability would also depend on proof that the laser had not been altered, or abused, and was maintained according to the manufacturer's specifications and used as it was intended. There are guidelines and regulations as to the production of lasers that are promulgated by the Food and Drug Administration's Center for Devices and Radiological Health (CDRH). ANSI and the FDA's CDRH have almost the same classification standards for lasers according to their potential hazards. The lasers used in the surgical setting are either level III or IV, which is on the high end of the scale.

Owner liability would occur if the individual responsible for the maintenance and repair and overseeing the use of the laser negligently failed to do so. In other words, if the laser is owned by a medical or surgical center, there will be someone on the staff designated as the person responsible for the maintenance and care of the laser. Negligence by that person in performance of that responsibility will carry back to the owner. If it is not spelled out in written policy form, then the responsibility would fall on the operating room director. The Joint Commission on Accreditation of Hospitals (JCAHO) standards require that hospitals that own lasers must have a written policy providing a preventive maintenance program for them. The written policy should address the legally responsible party for the care and maintenance of the laser, the use of the laser, and training of the staff involved. The policy should further specify what maintenance should be performed, by whom, and at what intervals so as to comply with the manufacturer's suggestions on each laser. As with all other aspects of health care, records must be maintained both to record what maintenance and care have been performed to predict possible future equipment problems and for the purpose of proof of adherence to the written policy should a negligence claim arise. There should be a checklist that requires the actual physical examination of the laser, which should be completed before each and every use of the laser. Liability could reach the operator who does not check to determine the laser was properly maintained and cared for. A visual examination for frayed wires, worn connections, and improperly maintained tips should be a minimal routine for any operator. Although the operator is generally not responsible for the actual care and maintenance of the equipment, the operator should check to ensure that the care and maintenance has been performed according to policy. Pilots must go through a preflight checklist before taking off in their aircraft. Firefighters wash or clean the fire engine and each piece of equipment it carries every day as they change shifts. These routines are not to make sure the equipment is clean, rather they are done to ensure that it has been inspected and tested before it is needed or before its possible failure may mean disaster.

The owner could be liable for injuries to the patient or staff on the principle of negligent entrustment if the owner has not established a reasonable set of standards of training and continuing education requirements for both the staff and the operator of the laser. This liability would be the same as if an adult entrusted his or her automobile to a child who did not have a driver's license. Lasers are dangerous instruments that must be used appropriately and only by those who are properly trained. At this point, this writer is unaware of any universally accepted standard of training. It, then, once again, falls on the individual surgical center to establish its own criteria using common sense with the basic intent being to protect patients, staff, and operators from injuries due to lack of knowledge or experience.

Owners and operators who are familiar with lasers and their continuing improvement should be aware that modification of the laser unit by the individual, without the specific knowledge and advice of the manufacturer, would most probably not only void the warranty of the manufacturer, but also would shift the burden of liability for product failure away from the manufacturer. Manufacturer upgrades generally would cost the owner significantly more than to have his or her own bioengineering staff perform the same upgrade. However, in the long run, failure of the manufacturer's upgrade remains a product liability problem for the manufacturer, whereas the bioengineering upgrade, in all probability, shifts that liability to the owner.

Operator liability would primarily arise in the face of improper surgical technique. The surgical laser has no set direction for incision or ablation of the tissues. In this case, the laser is much like a bur in a handpiece. The surgical sites are very small and demand a steady and accurate surgical approach by the operator. Care should be taken to assist the patient to remain motionless. Failure to do so would likely cause a claim of negligence to be brought against the operator should there be any untoward tissue destruction. Liability can be reduced or even done away with if there is thorough patient education and responsibility for remaining motionless is reasonably allocated to the patient. Should the procedure being performed be one that requires only local anesthesia, cooperation between the operator and patient is a must. The operator should assist the patient in any way possible to remain motionless and should provide communication intraoperatively as to when the patient can move and when to remain motionless. As with any other procedure, if the patient's actions cause the injury in the face of all of the above-mentioned precautions taken by the operator, more likely than not the patient would be found liable for his or her own injuries on the basis of contributory negligence or even comparative negligence.

SPECIFIC LIABILITY CONSIDERATIONS IN LASER SURGERY

There is no way to address each and every liability issue, variant of responsibility for safety, potential danger, and subsequent liability for injuries arising from a laser mishap. With the privilege of using state-of-the-art surgical lasers comes the responsibility of each member of the team, whether manufacturer, owner, staff, operator, and, even to some extent, the patient, to respect the fact that there are significant inherent dangers in using lasers. The laser has been proved to be a very effective and efficient surgical instrument. As a result of its effectiveness as a surgical instrument, there is minimal or no room for operator error during its use. Complete education and hands-on training are a must before the operator attempts to use the laser. The use of the laser without a full understanding of its surgical capability coupled with a demanding commonsense approach in its use is to assume the liability for mishap without any defense. The following discussions are examples of the commonsense approach to laser use. They are neither all inclusive as to hazards, nor can they be viewed as the only solution to the specific problems discussed.

Notice to all individuals who are present or potentially present during the use of lasers is a must. This includes staff, operator, and observers. Warning signs should be posted to warn everyone entering the area that lasers are in use. Access to the area should be restricted to a minimal number of individuals. This includes observers being present only on an as-needed basis, not just out of curiosity. A combination of a permanently affixed sign indicating the use of the particular area for lasers and a warning light that is activated when the laser is being used in a case would be a minimal requirement. Safety eyewear, appropriate for the wavelength of laser being used, should be available for individuals who are entering the laser area to put on before they enter. Because several types of lasers are currently being used, the particular type in use should be indicated and written precautionary instructions should be posted at each ingress and egress point of the operating area. Any individual who intends to enter the area should either be intimately familiar with those precautions or should be required to read them before entering the area.

With the understanding that the laser beam is like a scalpel of indeterminate length, care must be taken to prevent inadvertent exposure of those outside the area of operation through windows or doors. Curtains or shields should cover all windows. All avenues of ingress to and egress from the area where laser surgery is taking place should be controlled either by the use of a short laser lock hallway, a laser safe curtain, or some other partitioning device to prevent accidental escape of the laser beam from the operating area into the common area of the facility.

Much discussion has concerned whether there should be a door interlock connected to the laser. This would act as a kill switch to deactivate the laser when the door opened. Although this would protect the hallways and individuals who entered the room from accidental laser exposure, there is a great risk that the door would be opened at a time when deactivation of the laser would create a hazard for the patient.

The presence of water leakage or spills on the floor at or near the laser or its connection to the electrical circuitry should be avoided. Wires should be inspected each time the unit is used. The failure to check these items would be considered negligence if an accident occurred that was caused by electrocution or explosion due to electric arcing.

There must be a smoke evacuator because live viruses have been found in the plume resulting from use of the laser on tissues. The evacuator system should be checked for proper function prior to the implementation of the laser. The evacuation system already in place in the operating room may be adequate for this usage. The plume is composed of vaporized tissue and smoke, and tends to leave residue in the evacuation tubes. This residue may cause a clogging and ineffectiveness of the regular surgical evacuation system, necessitating the use of a free-standing smoke evacuator.

The evacuator tips as well as other instruments used at or near the procedure site should conform to suggested measures for minimizing reflection of the beam. These measures include anodizing, matte finish, and the use of plastics when feasible. The use

of reflective or minimally reflective instrumentation would most assuredly be considered negligence and perhaps even gross negligence in the face of all of the standards and research information presently available.

The laser itself should be checked for proper function prior to each and every use in surgery. A systems checklist should be developed, wherein tips are checked, the internal power meter is checked, and the output beams are checked for power and alignment. The laser is a sensitive piece of equipment and hence should not be transported frequently and should be stored in a safe environment, out of the way of heavy traffic areas. A checklist should be developed wherein routine maintenance is performed in a timely fashion by qualified individuals. Records of these checklists should be maintained for medicolegal information. Also, these records may be used to recognize and correct system degeneration rather than incurring a breakdown in the midst of a critical stage of an operation using the laser.

The laser should have only one operating switch, which is usually a foot switch. During the time that the laser is not in use, it should be placed in the standby mode so that it could not be activated inadvertently. The operating switch should be one that is a continuous pressure–activated switch; hence, removal of the pressure deactivates the beam. There should also be a panic or kill switch so that if there is a malfunction of the operating switch or other problem, the kill switch could be activated and the laser could be shut down. Without these measures, the laser could be activated by accidental application of pressure to an operating switch or it could remain activated and uncontrolled. Both of these situations, if they caused injuries, would create liability for those injuries.

Proper draping of the surgical site and protection of the patient's eyes is determined by the type of laser used. The patient should have, as a minimum, the same eyewear protection as the operator and staff. Preferably, the eyewear should be affixed so that accidental dislodging is a minimal risk. The use of moistened sponges covering the patient's eyes in addition to the eyewear would add protection for the patient. This would also further limit liability in situations in which negligence is alleged in reference to application of surgical safeguards for the patient.

The use of general anesthesia brings with it its own special problems. Because the laser generates heat, flammable gases should not be allowed to accumulate to a critical concentration. In all cases of general anesthesia in oral and maxillofacial surgical procedures, careful protection of the endotracheal tube is a must. The smoke evacuator mentioned earlier should be adequate to remove the high concentrations of oxygen at the same time as it removes the plume. Care should be taken not to direct the beam on objects at or near the tip of the evacuator.

The laser should be stored out of the way of normal traffic to protect it from bumping or damage, which could cause misalignment of the mechanism. It should also have a locked cover on the main console so that curiosity would not allow those not trained in its use or aware of its dangers to turn it on and potentially injure themselves or others or to otherwise damage the laser itself. Key control should be with either the operating room director or that individual designated to be responsible for the care and maintenance of the laser.

The operator must be thoroughly familiar with all aspects of the specific laser that is being used, including energy absorption by soft tissues, the depth of penetration of the laser beam into the soft tissue, the type of eyewear needed for proper protection, and all of its other unique qualities. The use of lasers requires that the operator know which laser is best suited for the surgery at hand.

Informed consent by the patient requires that all practical surgical alternatives be discussed with the patient. The practitioner surely can give an opinion as to what is preferable; however, the final decision rests with the patient. With the advent of laser surgery, not only the pros and cons of laser versus conventional treatment must be discussed with the patient but also the choice among types of lasers, when there is a choice. Failure to completely inform the patient leaves the practitioner open to a negligence claim based on the lack of informed consent.

HYPOTHETICAL CASE HISTORIES

Case Profile 1. Dr. A sees a pigmented lesion inside the mouth of patient B. Dr. A explains the niceties of laser surgery, with its reduced postoperative pain and relatively bloodless intraoperative procedure. Dr. A has only the carbon dioxide laser available to him and fails to mention that if the argon laser available to Dr. Z were used, there would possibly be no intraoral lesion because the argon laser could attack only the pigment and leave the epithelium intact. Later, Dr. A is confronted by an irate patient B, whose sister had the very same type of lesion removed with minimal postoperative pain compared with the week of postoperative pain patient B suffered. Dr. A was not wrong for using the carbon dioxide laser; it was appropriate because it attacks any tissue containing water. He was wrong and could have a malpractice claim filed against him because he knew of a technology that could be

preferable to the patient and did not inform the patient of its availability.

Case Profile 2. However, consider if Dr. A explained the argon laser to the patient, who then desired a referral to Dr. Z. In the ensuing treatment, Dr. Z, in his usual fashion, which was known to Dr. A, failed to adequately protect the patient's eyes and blinded patient B. Who is liable? Patient B can file suit against Dr. Z without a doubt in most any jurisdiction in the United States. Patient B can also file a negligent referral action against Dr. A in some jurisdictions also.

Case Profile 3. Dr. A was demonstrating the new carbon dioxide laser to certain members of the operating room staff. The staff all had on protective eyewear, the warning signs and light on the entrance to the operating suite were properly affixed, and eyewear was available at the entrance. The curtains were drawn to cover the windows. In an effort to show the dramatic effects of bouncing the laser off a highly reflective surface, Dr. A had just activated the beam, directing it at the mirror in an attempt to divert it to a piece of raw meat across the room. At that same instant one of the staff sneezed loudly causing Dr. A to flinch and misdirect the beam. The laser beam was diverted and hit nurse C's hand causing tissue damage. Nurse C screamed and jumped back away from the beam. In doing so, she bumped into two or three other individuals who fell like dominoes. One of those individuals fell across a stool and hit her head on the floor, causing permanent brain damage. The nurse who sneezed is not liable to anyone for anything. Nurse C is not liable to the head-injured individual. Dr. A and the hospital would have to fight against a claim that involved negligence in the use and demonstration of the laser, which was the proximate cause of Nurse C's injuries and the brain damage to the other individual. Why? The laser was intended for surgical use, not to demonstrate the result of not following protocol. When Dr. A decided to intentionally misuse the laser, even in an effort to demonstrate the dangers as part of the education process, Dr. A assumed the liability for the consequences. The hospital, through its responsible agent (the operating room director), either did not oversee the demonstration and not allow the misuse or knew of the intentions of Dr. A and condoned them, thus assuming the same liability as Dr. A.

Case Profile 4. Dr. A was performing ablative surgery on hyperplastic tissue on the crest of the anterior mandibular ridge. He had intended to perform a frenectomy using the laser also. During the surgery, prior to the ablation of adequate hyperplastic tissue, the laser malfunctioned. All of the preoperative checks had been performed, and all of the routine care and maintenance to the laser were up to date. Dr. A abandoned the use of the laser and completed the removal of the hyperplastic tissue using conventional surgical methods. He had informed the patient that conventional surgery in his case would not yield as favorable results as would laser ablation. At that point, Dr. A, who was very concerned about the patient's reaction, completed the removal of the hyperplastic tissue and performed the frenectomy. Several months later, in a discussion with the attorney representing the doctor, much to Dr. A's surprise, the attorney recommended a settlement in the case. Dr. A was furious and explained that all of the precautions had been taken, and that there was no fault in the laser's failure. The attorney agreed and explained that the settlement was not for the laser's failure and subsequent conventional approach used to complete the removal of the hyperplastic tissue. He explained that even though the patient had signed an operative permission specifically stating that the laser would be used, the doctor had been correct in completing the surgery using conventional methods because there was no other choice. The problem was that the frenectomy had not been initiated before the laser malfunctioned and that Dr. A was not justified in using conventional surgery for that procedure.

SUMMARY

The above-mentioned hypothetical cases are stretching the limit of reasonableness. In today's society, that limit is frequently stretched. There was no reason to present the obvious problems with failure to conform to standards and protocols. To do this would be to insult the reader's intelligence. It is the writer's intent to show the reader that it is impossible to treat patients with actions designed strictly to limit liability claims. If you are of the mindset to practice defensive surgery, STOP! There is no possible way to perform any activity, especially surgery, without calling on one's judgment to decide the course of action to take. Once judgment is used, then disagreement with the decision can be elicited from someone. Treat the patient, not the law or the courts. If one follows the course of action and treatment, which is reasonable in judgment and decision making, which puts the safety and well-being of the patient first and foremost, which is based on sound principles and knowledge of the subject, then even if a cause of action is brought, in all likelihood, it will not prevail. Cutting corners, allowing expediency to compromise patient care, and using cold professionalism that does not communicate rather than the warm, concerned approach of a caring practitioner will create the atmosphere of nonpersonal provision of services. This is the prime environment that triggers the filing of a lawsuit.

Awesome instrumentation is both of the present and of the future. It is the affirmative responsibility of practitioners to educate themselves as to its advantages and drawbacks. The laser offers an exciting new approach to surgical techniques. It is this writer's belief that in the near future, the failure of the surgeon to offer the choice between surgery using the laser and conventional surgery as we know it today will in itself be a negligent act in cases in which laser surgery is appropriate. This could very well lead to an increase in negligence claims filed based on the lack of informed consent.

APPENDIX

Glossary of Laser Terms

Ablative surgery. Gross removal of tissue, as in tumor removal, debulking, or vaporization.

Absorption coefficient. The measure of the capability of a laser wavelength to be absorbed in water. The point at which maximum energy is absorbed.

Absorption. Energy transfer caused by the action of a photon impacting on another photon usually causing an energy transition that drives an electron to a higher energy state. A transformation of radiant energy to a different form of energy by the interaction of matter.

Active medium. The pumped medium that supplies the energy to a lasant or laser medium.

Angstrom (Å). A unit of length, 1 Å equals 10^{-4} microns equals 10^{-10} meters (0.1 nm).

Argon laser. A visible light laser producing radiant energy of a 488- or 514-nm wavelength in which argon gas is the active medium after ionization either by an electric charge (electron beam) or by energy from a diode laser.

Attenuation. The observed decline in energy as a beam passes through an absorbing or scattering medium.

Beam diameter. A measure of the distance between diametrically opposed points in the cross section of a beam where the power density is 1/e times that of the peak power per unit area.

Beam. Any collection of radiant electromagnetic rays that may be divergent, convergent, or parallel.

Beam divergence. The observed gradual increase in beam diameter with distance from the exit aperture of the laser. (See *Divergence*.)

Beam spot size (spot size). The radius or diameter of the laser beam or area of the beam cross section. Usually referenced as the diameter.

Carbon dioxide laser. A laser of the molecular lasers class that produces laser radiant energy by distortions of the carbon dioxide molecule. The laser beam is emitted in the far infrared portion of the electromagnetic spectrum with a wavelength of 10.6 microns, or 10,600 nm. The radiant energy is 99% absorbed by tissue to a depth of about 90 microns.

Chromophore. A light-absorbing compound or molecule normally occurring in tissues and critical in certain effects produced by lasers of specific wavelengths (e.g., hemoglobin, melanin).

Coagulation (photocoagulation). An observed irreversible denaturation of tissue proteins heated to between 50° and 100°C.

Coherence. A state in which all light waves are temporally and spatially in phase.

Collimation. The state in which all rays are parallel with virtually negligible beam divergence of less than one milliradian at 1 km.

Collision pumping. An external power source that receives its energy by collision of particles or species.

Complicated mode. A beam intensity pattern or profile characterized by multiple spots.

Continuous mode. A manner of applying laser energy in which beam power density remains constant with time. It is used in laser surgery when broad areas of tissue surfaces are to be lased.

CW laser. A laser that emits a continuous laser beam without pulses.

Diffraction. The bending of a light ray as the light passes through a small hole in a barrier or passes by the edge of a barrier.

Divergence. An observed degree of spread of the laser beam as it increases its distance from the emission aperture of the laser. Laser radiation has a low degree of divergence.

Dye laser. A laser in which an organic dye is dissolved in a solvent and is the active medium. These lasers are tunable by adjusting the dye medium and the excitation radiation.

Electromagnetic radiation. Flow of energy consisting of orthogonally vibrating electric and magnetic fields lying transverse to the direction of radiation wave propagation.

Electromagnetic spectrum. The accepted spectrum of radiation emitted in frequencies and wavelengths originating from atomic systems.

Energy (energy density). Expressed as joules; that is, watts $\times$ time. (See *Irradiance, Fluence*.)

Energy. The energy in laser systems is determined by factoring time as a variable and consisting of watts per square centimeter multiplied by time (sec). Energy is expressed as joules.

Excited state. An atom or molecule with an electron or molecular configuration in a high-energy state.

External power source. An energy system outside the laser chamber or resonator cavity that provides the energy to cause hyperexcitation of the laser within the cavity.

Extinction length. The thickness of a substance in which 98% of the incident energy is absorbed, measured in cm^{-1}.

Fluence. The energy per unit area measured in joules per square centimeter. (See *Irradiance*.)

Focal length. The distance between the focusing lens and the focal point usually measured in millimeters. This refers to the laser handpiece as well as the laser-incorporated microscope.

Focus (focal point). The precise locus where laser radiant energy is at peak power.

Frequency. The number of waves or cycles of light waves that pass a given point in a unit of time (usually per second), or cycles per second also referred to as *hertz* (Hz).

Gas lasers. The class of lasers that have a noble or rare gas as the lasant.

Gaussian curve. The cross section of the radiant power density at a transverse electromagnetic mode of the lowest order, TEM_{oo}.

Handpiece. An instrument attached to the distal portion of a laser delivery system that contains the focusing lens system. It may also refer to the distal instrument of a contact laser system (Nd:YAG) on which is mounted the sapphire contact probe where there are no focusing devices per se (i.e., lenses).

Helium-neon laser. A laser operating in the visible portion of the electromagnetic spectrum in which a mixture of helium and neon gases is the lasant. It is usually used as a coaxial red aiming beam for many lasers, especially infrared lasers. It is also used for some medical purposes.

Hertz (Hz). The unit in which frequency is measured. One hertz is one complete cycle or one complete oscillation per second.

HpD. The initials for hematoporphyrin derivation, a tissue-sensitizing agent that is usually used with the tuneable dye laser. (See *Photosensitizers*.)

Ideal mode. A square wave of equal cross-sectional intensity.

Intensity. The total amount of power applied to a given area, also known as irradiance, energy density, and power density. However, power density does not include the variable of time and therefore cannot express total power.

Interference. The phenomenon that results when two or more waves of the same type pass simultaneously through the same point(s) and form a combined wave.

Irradiance. Total power per unit area, measured in watts per square centimeter. Power density, also termed internal irradiance, determines the rate of tissue thermal effect.

Joule. A unit in physics to represent energy; 1 joule equals 1 watt-second.

Lasant. A material with the ability to be the source of radiant energy. A lasant may be an ion, atom, molecule, or rare gas *(species)* that is capable of a population inversion upon the application of external energy (e.g., flash lamp, electricity, radio waves) or other laser source, such as diode lasers and x-rays.

Laser. L(ight) A(mplification by) S(timulated) E(mission of) R(adiation). A device that emits an intense coherent directional beam of radiant energy by stimulated electronic or molecular transitions to a lower energy level.

Laser beam (laser light). Radiant energy emitted from the laser cavity.

Laser cavity (chamber-resonator cavity). A resonator space with many variations of design, which may consist of two reflecting mirrors mounted parallel at each end. The radiant energy produced by excitation within the cavity to and fro (theoretically, infinitely) causing the energized photons to increase in number by multiple impacts of stimulated photons on the lasant, eventually to be released from the cavity as the formal laser beam.

Laser medium. Any substance capable of giving rise to a laser radiation source. (See *Lasant*.)

Laser pumping. The application of external or internal energy that results in activation or excitation of the lasant.

Meter. A unit of length, by definition the fixed number of wavelengths in vacuum of the orange-red line of the spectrum of krypton 86. The meter (m) is subdivided: 1 centimeter (cm) = 10^{-2} m, and nanometer (nm) = 10^{-9} m.

Micromanipulator (Joystick). A device that controls the direction of the laser beam by finger manipulation when attached to a microscope on which the laser is mounted coaxial with the optics of the microscope.

Mode. Normally, the geometric patterns of coherent radiation, as in transverse electromagnetic mode, which indicates the pattern of the focal spot produced by the laser beam. It may also refer to the manner in which the laser is pulsed (e.g., continuous [wave], pattern mode, and superpulse mode).

Mode-locked. A state in which the laser is adjusted so that the phase or amplitude of the laser wave output is locked in order to exit the laser chamber in a controlled train of ultrashort-duration pulses.

Monochromatic. Having identical visible light wavelengths, or color.

Monochromaticity. The state of having only one wavelength, or color.

Multimode. Laser emission at several closely spaced frequencies.

Neodymium:yttrium aluminum garnet (Nd:YAG) laser. The laser is composed of a medium consisting of a YAG crystal "doped" with a rare earth element, neodymium. This laser is capable of stimulated emission when excited by external energy (e.g., xenon flash lamp) and can emit radiant energy at 1.06 microns, which is absorbed within 30 mm of tissue with moderate lateral scattering. Nd:YAG is known as a doped-insulator laser, the YAG acting as the insulator and the Nd as the dope.

Optical cavity. Laser chamber, laser cavity, or resonator chamber or cavity.

Optical pumping. A method of imparting additional energy to the lasant in the laser cavity.

Photocoagulation. The use of a laser beam to heat tissue below the temperature of vaporization (50° to 100°C) causing irreversible tissue denaturation and, in some instances, affecting hemostasis.

Photon. From quantum physics, light energy composed of discrete packets of energy emitted by excited atoms, ions, molecules, or gases.

Photosensitizers. Agents that increase the sensitivity of a material (in photobiology, tissue) to the effects of electromagnetic radiation.

Plume (fume). The smoke observed when a laser beam

vaporizes tissue. It is composed of particulate matter, cellular debris, carbonaceous material, and potentially biohazardous active viruses (e.g., human papillomavirus, which causes condylomata).

Polarization plane. Refers to a particular class of waves for which the oscillation occurs in one particular direction (e.g., the vertical direction for a wave that is travelling along the horizontal).

Population inversion. A state within the laser cavity in which the quantity of excited species in a lasant exceeds that of unexcited species and renders the lasant capable of emitting a beam of radiant energy.

Power density. Power in watts multiplied by the area of the focal spot (πr^2) of the beam, multiplied by 100 as the numerator over the size of the lased area in square centimeters.

Pulsed beam. A beam of radiant energy modified to be produced in short bursts of radiant energy.

Pulse duration. The time lapses for one laser pulse.

Pumped medium. The state in which the laser medium or lasant has been subjected to external energy and has reached a critical energy state or population inversion and is ready for beam emission.

Pumping. Refers to the process of applying energy usually externally to the laser medium.

Q-Switched. A laser system which employs a "Q" switch, or very fast shutter, which allows the build-up of photon energy within the laser cavity, thus preventing its release until a desired time, at which a "giant pulse" of extremely high energy is produced. In the usual Q-switched pulse maneuver, the pulse is approximately 30 nanoseconds (30×10^{-9} m).

Radiant energy. Energy transferred by radiation, especially by an electromagnetic wave.

Reflectance reflectivity. The ratio of the total reflected radiant power to the total incidence power.

Refraction. Refers to the bending of a light ray as the light passes from one material into another.

Resonant cavity. Laser cavity, chamber; optical cavity, chamber.

Selective photothermolysis. In this laser maneuver, precise thermal tissue damage can be achieved in tissue targets that absorb well-focused emitted wavelengths when the pulse duration (exposure time) is shorter than the cooling or recovery time or thermal coagulation time of the target tissue.

Semiconductor laser. A laser in which the lasant is a layer of semiconductor materials.

Single mode. A laser emission at a single TEM mode, usually the smallest focused spot available.

Sine. One of several mathematic functions utilized in trigonometry. In a right triangle the sine of an angle is defined as the ratio of the length of the side opposite the right angle to the length of the hypotenuse.

Speed of light. In a vacuum light travels at the rate of 2.988×10^8 m/sec.

Spontaneous emission. The release of a photon of absorbed energy from an excited species.

Stimulated emission. The emission of electromagnetic radiation (photons) from a higher-energy state to a lower-energy state in an excited laser medium as postulated by Einstein.

Superpulse. A pulsed laser emission option in which extremely high peak powers per pulse are generated for very short pulse widths with variable repetition.

TEM. T(transverse) E(lectromagnetic) M(ode): the pattern produced by the laser beam or spot on its target.

TEM$_{oo}$. The lowest-order mode available, a bell-shaped (gaussian) distribution of radiant energy intensity across the laser beam cross section. The irradiance is highest in the center of the spot and gradually decreases toward the periphery.

Thermal effect. Usually refers to the observation that radiant energy emitted via a carbon dioxide laser is absorbed in water and minimizes the heat conductivity through the tissues, the ultimate effect of most lasers in producing heating of target and contiguous tissues/cells.

Transmission. The passage of electromagnetic radiation through any medium.

Transmittance. The ratio of the total transmitted radiant power to the total incident radiant power.

Tunable laser. A laser system (usually a dye laser but others have the capability) that can be tuned to emit radiant energy over a continuous range of wavelengths or frequencies.

Ultraviolet radiation. Electromagnetic radiation with wavelengths smaller than those of the visible spectrum (0.1–0.38 microns).

Vaporization. The physical process of converting a solid or liquid into a vapor. This is observed in laser photobiology when thermal impact exceeds 50° to 100°C.

Visible radiation (light). Electromagnetic radiation that can be detected by the human eye. Wavelengths between 0.38 and 0.7 microns.

Watt. The unit of power or radiant flux.

Wave. A disturbance or oscillation propagated from point to point in a medium or in space and described by mathematic specification of its amplitude, velocity, frequency, and phase.

Wavelength. The distance from crest to crest in any electromagnetic wave or the distance between two points in a periodic wave that have the same phase.

YAG. Active solid-state laser material in the form of a garnet crystal which is composed of ^{3}Y, ^{5}Al, ^{12}O (Y, yttrium; Al, aluminum; O, oxygen). In the Nd:YAG laser, 0.6% to 1.2% of the Al atoms are substituted for by neodymium Nd^{+3}, a rare earth element with output in the red portion of the visible spectrum. The energized neodymium atoms are the site of laser action.

Index

Note: Page numbers in *italics* refer to illustrations; page numbers followed by t refer to tables.

ISBN 0-7216-5020-1

90038

9 780721 650203